AF679423

Neurotrauma and Critical Care of the Brain

Neurotrauma and Critical Care of the Brain

Editor: Franklin McDonough

AMERICAN
MEDICAL PUBLISHERS
www.americanmedicalpublishers.com

AMERICAN
MEDICAL PUBLISHERS
www.americanmedicalpublishers.com

Cataloging-in-Publication Data

Neurotrauma and critical care of the brain / edited by Franklin McDonough.
p. cm.
Includes bibliographical references and index.
ISBN 978-1-63927-320-1
1. Nervous system--Wounds and injuries. 2. Neurological intensive care. 3. Brain damage. 4. Neurology.
5. Critical care medicine. I. McDonough, Franklin.
RD593 .N48 2022
617.48--dc23

© American Medical Publishers, 2022

American Medical Publishers,
41 Flatbush Avenue,
1st Floor, New York,
NY 11217, USA

ISBN 978-1-63927-320-1 (Hardback)

This book contains information obtained from authentic and highly regarded sources. Copyright for all individual chapters remain with the respective authors as indicated. All chapters are published with permission under the Creative Commons Attribution License or equivalent. A wide variety of references are listed. Permission and sources are indicated; for detailed attributions, please refer to the permissions page and list of contributors. Reasonable efforts have been made to publish reliable data and information, but the authors, editors and publisher cannot assume any responsibility for the validity of all materials or the consequences of their use.

Trademark Notice: Registered trademark of products or corporate names are used only for explanation and identification without intent to infringe.

Contents

Preface

The main aim of this book is to educate learners and enhance their research focus by presenting diverse topics covering this vast field. This is an advanced book which compiles significant studies by distinguished experts in the area of analysis. This book addresses successive solutions to the challenges arising in the area of application, along with it; the book provides scope for future developments.

Neurotrauma refers to an injury to the brain or the spinal cord. It includes the degeneration or destruction of brain cells that often leads to serious medical conditions such as paralysis, brain damage and death. The symptoms of neurotrauma vary, based on the severity of the brain injury. Mild brain injury often causes headaches, confusion, fatigue and tinnitus. Moderate and severe brain injuries include symptoms such as slurred speech, coma, nausea, convulsions and abnormal dilation of the eyes. The medical field which provides critical care in life threatening conditions related to the nervous system is known as neurocritical care or neurointensive care. Some of the procedures which are used in neurocritical care are hypothermia, intracranial pressure management and basic life support monitoring. This book presents researches and studies performed by experts across the globe. It provides comprehensive insights into neurotrauma and critical care of the brain. This book will serve as a valuable source of reference for graduate and post graduate students.

It was a great honour to edit this book, though there were challenges, as it involved a lot of communication and networking between me and the editorial team. However, the end result was this all-inclusive book covering diverse themes in the field.

Finally, it is important to acknowledge the efforts of the contributors for their excellent chapters, through which a wide variety of issues have been addressed. I would also like to thank my colleagues for their valuable feedback during the making of this book.

Editor

1

Inflammatory cytokine and chemokine profiles are associated with patient outcome and the hyperadrenergic state following acute brain injury

Alex P. Di Battista[1,2*], Shawn G. Rhind[1,3], Michael G. Hutchison[3,4], Syed Hassan[1,2], Maria Y. Shiu[1,3], Kenji Inaba[5,6], Jane Topolovec-Vranic[4], Antonio Capone Neto[10], Sandro B. Rizoli[4,7,8,9] and Andrew J. Baker[2,4,7,8,9]

Abstract

Background: Traumatic brain injury (TBI) elicits intense sympathetic nervous system (SNS) activation with profuse catecholamine secretion. The resultant hyperadrenergic state is linked to immunomodulation both within the brain and systemically. Dysregulated inflammation post-TBI exacerbates secondary brain injury and contributes to unfavorable patient outcomes including death. The aim of this study was to characterize the early dynamic profile of circulating inflammatory cytokines/chemokines in patients admitted for moderate-to-severe TBI, to examine interrelationships between these mediators and catecholamines, as well as clinical indices of injury severity and neurological outcome.

Methods: Blood was sampled from 166 isolated TBI patients (aged 45 ± 20.3 years; 74.7 % male) on admission, 6-, 12-, and 24-h post-injury and from healthy controls ($N = 21$). Plasma cytokine [interleukin (IL)-1β, -2, -4, -5, -10, -12p70, -13, tumor necrosis factor (TNF)-α, interferon (IFN)-γ] and chemokine [IL-8, eotaxin, eotaxin-3, IFN-γ-induced protein (IP)-10, monocyte chemoattractant protein (MCP)-1, -4, macrophage-derived chemokine (MDC), macrophage inflammatory protein (MIP)-1β, thymus activation regulated chemokine (TARC)] concentrations were analyzed using high-sensitivity electrochemiluminescence multiplex immunoassays. Plasma catecholamines [epinephrine (Epi), norepinephrine (NE)] were measured by immunoassay. Neurological outcome at 6 months was assessed using the extended Glasgow outcome scale (GOSE) dichotomized as good (>4) or poor (≤4) outcomes.

Results: Patients showed altered levels of IL-10 and all chemokines assayed relative to controls. Significant differences in a number of markers were evident between moderate and severe TBI cohorts. Elevated IL-8, IL-10, and TNF-α, as well as alterations in 8 of 9 chemokines, were associated with poor outcome at 6 months. Notably, a positive association was found between Epi and IL-1β, IL-10, Eotaxin, IL-8, and MCP-1. NE was positively associated with IL-1β, IL-10, TNF-α, eotaxin, IL-8, IP-10, and MCP-1.

Conclusions: Our results provide further evidence that exaggerated SNS activation acutely after isolated TBI in humans may contribute to harmful peripheral inflammatory cytokine/chemokine dysregulation. These findings are consistent with a potentially beneficial role for therapies aimed at modulating the inflammatory response and hyperadrenergic state acutely post-injury.

Keywords: Catecholamines, Traumatic brain injury, Systemic inflammation, Sympathetic nervous system activation, Epinephrine, Norepinephrine, IL-10, IL-1β

* Correspondence: dibattista.alex@gmail.com
[1]Defence Research & Development Canada, Toronto Research Centre, Toronto, ON, Canada
[2]Institute of Medical Science, University of Toronto, Toronto, ON, Canada
Full list of author information is available at the end of the article

Background

Growing experimental and clinical evidence indicates that inflammation is an integral component to the pathogenesis of secondary injury after traumatic brain injury (TBI) [1, 2]. Its effects are not limited to the brain parenchyma, as systemic inflammation is a noted consequence of TBI, and can impact patient outcome by exacerbating cerebral tissue injury and contributing to systemic complications such as nosocomial infection and multiple organ failure [2–4]. While potentially harmful, bi-directional neuroimmune communication between the central nervous system (CNS) and the periphery is essential for neuronal repair and regeneration [5]. The duality of this process is highlighted by a number of failed clinical trials aimed broadly at reducing or inhibiting inflammation [6]. Hence, a better understanding of the underlying mechanisms governing the inflammatory response to isolated TBI in humans can help guide future therapeutic strategies and improve patient outcome.

In an effort to restore vital homeostasis in the face of TBI, activation of the sympathetic nervous system (SNS) results in a massive secretion of catecholamines [epinephrine (Epi), norepinephrine (NE)] into the periphery as part of the generalized host stress response to trauma [7–13]. Moreover, we have recently demonstrated in a large group of moderate-to-severe TBI patients, that both NE and Epi are elevated in a dose-dependent fashion according to injury severity, and that prolonged elevation of NE and Epi throughout the first 24 h after hospital admission is highly correlated with adverse patient outcomes [14].

It has been hypothesized that early SNS activation after TBI may influence the inflammatory response both locally and systemically. This occurs prototypically as a response to elevations in cerebral IL-1β concentrations and subsequent initiation of both the local and systemic acute phase response [4, 15–18]. In addition, trauma-induced activation of NE terminals in peripheral organs such as the liver and spleen may lead to the systemic release of inflammatory mediators into the circulation [4, 19, 20]. It is also possible that elevated concentrations of peripheral catecholamines can differentially alter cytokine/chemokine production in circulating lymphocytes [21]. NE and Epi interact with α- and β-adrenergic receptors expressed on leukocytes and other tissues, influencing the production of inflammatory mediators from these cells [22–25]. Furthermore, β-blocker therapy in human TBI has been associated with improved outcome [26, 27], and a number of animal studies using pharmacological blockade of β-adrenergic receptors have shown concomitant attenuation of the inflammatory response and improved outcome after treatment [28–30]. However, no previous clinical studies have evaluated the relationship between the SNS and systemic inflammation in isolated TBI patients.

Elevations in a number of cytokines, including interleukin (IL)-1β, -6, -10, and TNF-α, have been identified in the circulation of TBI patients within hours of injury [31–36]. However, their relationship to patient survival and outcome is less clear, likely owing to the heterogeneous nature of both primary brain injury (i.e., focal vs. blunt trauma and extracranial complications) and the complexity of secondary injury processes. Additionally, correlations have been found between early elevations in peripheral cytokines and poor patient outcome [37–40], although others have found no association [34, 41] or have even identified inverse relationships between cytokines and risk of infection after injury [42]. Moreover, chemokines appear to play an important role in TBI pathophysiology [43], though human studies to date have focused predominantly on IL-8 and MCP-1 [39, 44, 45] and require further characterization.

Therefore, the purpose of this study was to (1) identify the temporal profile of a panel of circulating cytokines and chemokines acutely after injury in both moderate and severe isolated blunt TBI patients; (2) identify possible interrelationships between circulating catecholamines and cytokines/chemokines post-injury; (3) to evaluate these markers in patients stratified according to 6-month neurological outcome and mortality.

Methods

Ethics statement

The study protocol complied with the ethical guidelines of the Declaration of Helsinki of 1975 and was approved by the Research Ethics Boards and Institutional Review Boards of the participating hospitals. All patients' families received a comprehensive description of the study and gave written informed consent for their relatives' participation. In the absence of a substitute decision-maker, consent was delayed in accordance with the Tri-Council Policy Agreement for Research in Emergency Health Situations (Article 2.8); delayed written consent for participation in the study was subsequently obtained from next-of-kin or, where possible, directly from the patient once they had recovered sufficiently. Informed consent for a single blood sample was also obtained from healthy (control) volunteers.

Patients and controls

Potential study participants were admitted to Sunnybrook Health Sciences Centre (Toronto, ON, Canada), St. Michael's Hospital (Toronto, ON, Canada), and Los Angeles County + University of Southern California (USC) Medical Center (Los Angeles, CA). Upon admission, patients with an isolated TBI, defined by a Glasgow coma scale (GCS) score of <13 and a non-head abbreviated injury score (AIS) of ≤ 2, were considered for inclusion. Patients with an elapsed time between trauma and hospital admission of >3 h, with a penetrating brain injury, <16 years of age, pregnant, taking β-blockers, lacking vital signs prior to admission, or clinically brain dead on admission were excluded. A healthy control group with no history of brain injury was included for a single blood donation for analysis of the selected panel of soluble inflammatory markers.

Study design and procedures

Upon hospital admission, clinical and demographic data were obtained from eligible patients: *demographics*—age and sex ; *clinical information*—mechanism of injury, elapsed time from the trauma to the emergency room, injury severity score (ISS), and AIS head; *neurological status*—level of consciousness categorized by the GCS, pupil size and reactivity, seizures, and alcohol level; *clinical status*—blood pressure, tracheal intubation, spontaneous vs. mechanical ventilation, oxygen saturation, and temperature; and *medical history*—past medical history, present medications including β-blockers and anticoagulants. Routine laboratory exams and imaging were also completed upon admission, including chest radiography and computerized tomography (CT) scans. All significant clinical events during the first 24 h were recorded, including, but not limited to, sepsis/infection, organ failure, any medical treatments administered, surgical procedures, and any other significant changes in clinical parameters. Organ failure was defined by the following criteria: (1) arterial hypoxemia—$PaO_2/FiO_2 < 300$; (2) acute oliguria—urine output <0.5 mL/kg/h for at least 2 h despite adequate fluid resuscitation; (3) creatine increase—>0.5 mg/dL or 44.2 μmol/L; (4) coagulation abnormalities—INR > 1.5 or aPTT > 60 s; (5) ileus—absent bowel sounds; (6) thrombocytopenia—platelet count <100,000 μ/L; and (7) hyperbilirubinemia—plasma total bilirubin >4 mg/dL or 70 μmol/L.

For patients who died, the cause of death was recorded and classified as TBI-related or non-TBI related. Upon hospital discharge, at 28 days and at 6-months, patient outcome was assessed using the extended Glasgow outcome scale (GOSE) .

Blood sample collection

Venous blood samples were drawn as soon as possible after admission to the trauma room or emergency department, and again at 6-, 12-, and 24-h post-injury. Samples were drawn into either 10 mL K_2EDTA [with 4 mM sodium metabisulfite ($Na_2S_2O_5$)] or 10-mL sodium heparin vacutainers (Vacutainer, Becton Dickinson, Rutherford, NJ). Specimens were immediately centrifuged at 1600×*g* for 15 min at 4 °C; the plasma supernatant was then separated into six (1–2 mL) aliquots and frozen at −70 °C until subsequent analysis.

Multiplex cytokine and chemokine measurements

Immunoreactive plasma levels of selected cytokines and chemokines were analyzed with Meso Scale Discovery (MSD) 96-Well MULTI-SPOT® Ultra-Sensitive Human Immunoassay Kits, using electrochemiluminescence detection on an MSD Sector Imager™ 6000 with Discovery Workbench software (version 3.0.18) (MSD®, Gaitherburg, MD, USA). Cytokines were measured using the TH1/TH2 10-plex kit, which included nine markers (excluding IL-8): IFN-γ, IL-1 β, -2, -4, -5, -10, -12p70, -13, and TNF-α. Chemokines were measured using the Chemokine 9-plex, which also included nine markers: eotaxin, eotaxin-3, MIP-1β, thymus activation regulated chemokine (TARC), IP-10, IL-8, MCP-1, MDC, and MCP-4 (Additional file 1: Table S1). All assays were performed according to manufacturer's instructions, in duplicates, and without alterations to the recommended standard curve dilutions. Briefly, samples were thawed on ice and added to a 96-well MULTI-SPOT® plate coated with capture antibodies in a spatially distinct fashion. SULFO-TAG® labeled detection antibodies were then added to each of the wells to complete the sandwich format, and a read buffer was added to alter the chemical environment for electrochemiluminescence. The subsequent reaction resulted in the emission of light from the labeled analytes, which was then quantified to approximate the concentration (pg/mL) of each protein present in the sample.

Catecholamine measurements

Plasma Epi and NE levels were determined from duplicate samples using a competitive enzyme immunoassay method according to the manufacturer's instructions (Bi-CAT EIA, ALPCO Diagnostics, Salem, NH). Briefly, plasma Epi and NE were extracted using a cis-diol-specific affinity gel, acylated and then derivatized enzymatically into *N*-acylmetanephrine and *N*-acylnormetanephrine, respectively. Antibody bound to the solid-phase catecholamines were detected by an anti-rabbit IgG-peroxidase conjugate using tetramethylbenzidine as a substrate. Quantification of unknown samples was achieved by comparing their absorbance with a reference curve prepared with known standard concentrations included in the kit.

Statistical analysis

Demographic and clinical parameters are expressed as the mean ± standard deviation (SD) unless otherwise stated, while blood marker concentrations are graphically displayed as the median and interquartile range. Comparison of inflammatory marker levels between TBI patients at each sampled time point and healthy control subjects was performed using a Kruskal-Wallis analysis of variance, with Dunn's multiple comparisons post hoc test. To assess 6-month neurological outcome, patients were dichotomized into favorable (GOSE 5–8) and unfavorable (GOSE

1–4) outcomes. Mortality was assessed by stratifying patients into two groups, "survivors" and "non-survivors." Death was further stratified as either "neurologic" or "non-neurologic." Differences in cytokine and chemokine concentrations between moderate and severe TBI patients, unfavorable and favorable outcome, survivors and non-survivors, and neurologic and non-neurologic death were assessed by Mann-Whitney *U*. To identify possible correlations between catecholamines and inflammatory marker concentrations, pooled data over all time points was evaluated by Spearman's ρ. To generate an aggregate inflammation score (IS), peak quartile rank scores from each marker associated with both unfavorable outcome and survival were summed [36, 46]. For each marker, values >75th percentile were given a score of 4, values between the 50th and 75th percentile were given a score of 3, values between the 25th and 50th percentile were given a score of 2, and values <25th percentile were given a score of 1. When lower concentrations of a marker were associated with unfavorable patient outcome, the scoring system was reversed, hence values <25th percentile were given a score of 4, while values >75th percentile were given a score of 1. Quartile scores of each marker were added, resulting in an aggregate score; six markers were included, allowing for a score ranging from 6 to 24. Patients were then dichotomized into high- vs. low-inflammation categories based on the median aggregate IS [47]. In addition, to assess the ability of cytokines and chemokines to predict poor patient outcome and death while controlling for injury severity, a multivariate binomial logistic regression analysis was employed. All markers were quartiled in order to standardize unit increases for statistical comparison. Each individual marker was added independently to a model containing GCS and AIS head scores. The binary dependent outcome variables were 6-month GOSE or survival. Biomarker data was not statistically analyzed or graphically displayed unless at least 50 % of the samples analyzed were within the detection range of the assay, or contained replicate values with a coefficient of variation (CV) <25 %. Statistical significance in all analyses was indicated by a *p* value of ≤0.05. All data were analyzed using GraphPad Prism Version 6.0d (GraphPad Inc, CA, USA) and Stata Version 13.1 (StataCorp, TX, USA).

Results

Demographics and clinical characteristics

Table 1 summarizes the demographic, clinical, and outcome data for the 166 (33 moderate, 133 severe) patients analyzed in the study. Subjects were predominantly male ($n = 124$, 74.7 %), with an average age of 45.8 ± 20.3 years . The majority of patients had an unfavorable outcome at 6 months, classified as a GOSE score of 1–4 ($n = 102$, 61.4 %). Eighteen patients (10.8 %) developed organ failure, and there were 45 (27.1 %) deaths. Among the 21 healthy control subjects, 71.4 % were males ($n = 15$), and the mean age was 32.7 ± 7.8 years (data not shown).

Table 1 Demographic and clinical characteristics for TBI patients

Characteristics	All TBI patients ($n = 166$)	Moderate TBI ($n = 33$)	Severe TBI ($n = 133$)
Demographics			
Age (years)	45.8 ± 20.3	49.5 ± 19.7	44.9 ± 20.4
Male —*n* (%)	124 (74.7)	23 (69.7)	101 (75.9)
Clinical characteristics			
Time to ED (min)	77.6 ± 63.5	74.7 ± 64.8	78.3 ± 63.4
ISS score	24.4 ± 11.8	18.8 ± 11.5	25.9 ± 11.5
AIS head	4.1 ± 1.1	3.5 ± 1.2	4.3 ± 1.0
GCS	5.9 ± 3.0	10.5 ± 1.3	4.7 ± 1.9
Marshall score—*n* (%)			
I	28 (16.9)	11 (33.3)	17 (12.8)
II	76 (45.8)	16 (48.5)	60 (45.1)
III	13 (7.8)	1 (3.0)	12 (9.0)
IV	27 (16.3)	3 (9.1)	24 (18.0)
Evacuated mass lesion	21 (12.6)	2 (6.1)	19 (14.3)
Non-evacuated mass lesion	1 (0.6)	0 (0.0)	1 (0.7)
Pre-injury comorbidities—*n* (%)	45 (27.1)	14 (42.4)	31 (23.3)
Outcomes			
Mortality—*n* (%)	45 (27.1)	1 (3.0)	44 (33.0)
Neurosurgery performed—*n* (%)	47 (28.3)	5 (15.1)	42 (31.6)
Sepsis/infection—*n* (%)	42 (25.3)	7 (21.2)	35 (26.3)
Organ failure—*n* (%)	18 (10.8)	0 (0.0)	18 (13.5)
6-month GOSE	4.0 ± 2.5	5.7 ± 2.1	3.6 ± 2.5

Unless otherwise stated, results are expressed as mean ± standard deviation (SD)
Abbreviations: *TBI* traumatic brain injury, *ED* emergency department, *ISS* injury severity score, *AIS* abbreviated injury scale, *GCS* Glasgow coma scale, *GOSE* extended Glasgow outcome scale

Plasma concentrations of inflammatory markers in moderate and severe TBI patients

Plasma concentrations of cytokines and chemokines stratified according to moderate (GCS 9–12) and severe (GCS 3–8) TBI are shown in Fig. 1. IL-10 was the only cytokine altered in patients compared with healthy controls—median admission IL-10 levels were 5 - and 9 - fold higher, respectively, in moderate and severe TBI patients, and were significantly elevated at all time points (Fig. 1a). Furthermore, at 6, 12, and 24 h after hospital admission, mean IL-10 levels in severe TBI patients were significantly elevated (~2-fold at admission, 6, and 24 h) compared to moderate TBI patients (Fig. 1a).

Significant alterations in all nine chemokines were detected in TBI patients dichotomized by injury severity vs. healthy controls (Fig. 1c–k). The most dramatic increase

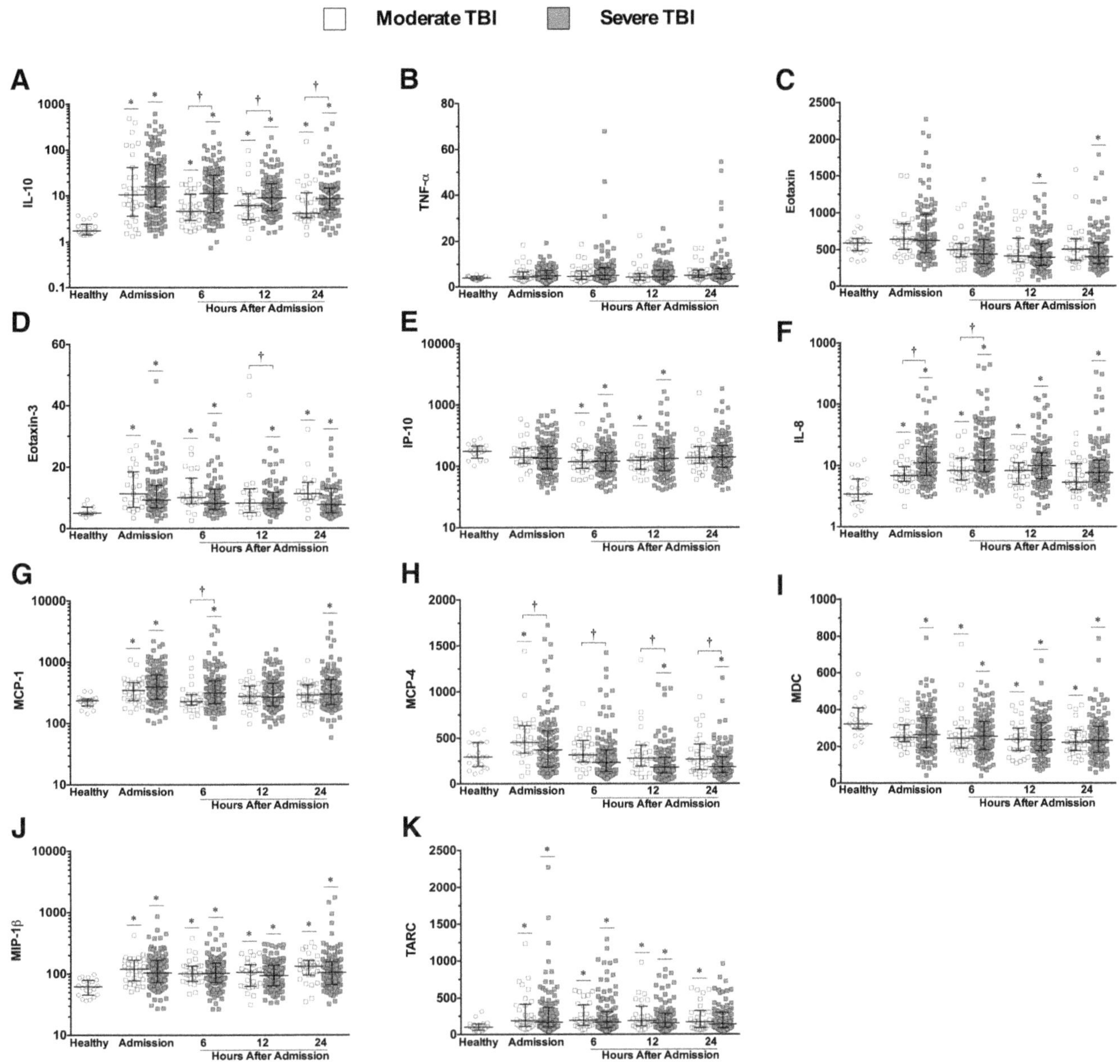

Fig. 1 Plasma cytokine and chemokine concentrations in moderate and severe TBI patients sampled over 24 h. Cytokines interleukin (*IL*)-10 (**a**), tumor necrosis factor (*TNF*)-α (**b**). Chemokines eotaxin, eotaxin-3, interferon-gamma induced protein (*IP*)-10, IL-8, monocyte chemoattractant protein (*MCP*)-1, -4, macrophage-derived chemokine (*MDC*), macrophage inflammatory protein (*MIP*)-1β, and thymus and activation regulated chemokine (*TARC*) (**c**–**k**) in moderate (GCS 9–12, $n = 33$, *open squares*) and severe (GCS 3–8, $n = 133$, *closed squares*) TBI patients within the first 24 h of hospital admission vs. healthy control subjects (no TBI, $n = 21$, *open circles*). *Lines* represent the median and interquartile range. *$p < 0.05$ vs. healthy controls by Kruskal-Wallis. †$p < 0.05$ vs. moderate TBI by Mann-Whitney *U* test

was seen in IL-8: patient concentrations peaked at 6 h after hospital admission and were nearly 3.5-fold higher in those with severe TBI vs. healthy control subjects (median concentrations, 12.2 vs. 3.5 pg/mL, respectively) (Fig. 1f). In addition, at admission and 6 h, mean IL-8 levels were higher in patients with severe TBI compared to those with moderate TBI (Fig. 1f). Significant increases in MCP-1 concentrations in severe vs. moderate TBI patients were also identified (6 h) (Fig. 1g). Conversely, IP-10 and MDC concentrations were decreased in both moderate and severe TBI patients compared with controls (Fig. 1e, i, respectively), while eotaxin was decreased in severe TBI patients only (Fig. 1c). MCP-4 levels were elevated on admission in moderate TBI patients compared with healthy subjects, but were lower in severe TBI patients compared with healthy subjects at 12 and 24 h (Fig. 1h). Furthermore, MCP-4 levels were lower in severe TBI patients at all sampled time points compared to moderate TBI patients (Fig. 1h). Eotaxin levels were elevated in severe TBI patients at admission, but similar to MCP-4, were decreased at 12 and 24 h (Fig. 1c).

Correlation between SNS and inflammatory markers

Pooled concentrations of NE and Epi were associated with a number of inflammatory markers acutely after TBI (Table 2). IL-1β and IL-10 were positively correlated to Epi, with IL-10 displaying the strongest correlation ($r = 0.44$, $P < 0.01$) (Table 3). NE concentrations were positively related to IL-1β, IL-10, and TNF-α (Table 2). Similar to Epi, NE was most strongly correlated to IL-10 ($r = 0.45$, $P < 0.01$). In addition, IL-1β displayed a stronger positive association with NE ($r = 0.28$, $P < 0.01$) than with Epi ($r = 0.11$, $P < 0.03$) (Table 2).

E otaxin, IL-8, and MCP-1 were positively related to both NE and Epi, while IP-10 was associated with NE only (Table 2). The strongest relationship between catecholamines and chemokines was found between IL-8 and NE ($r = 0.39$, $P < 0.01$); IL-8 also displayed the highest correlation of any chemokine with Epi ($r = 0.35$, $P < 0.01$) (Table 2).

Six-month neurological outcome

Within 24 h of hospital admission, significant differences in plasma levels of three cytokines and three chemokines were observed between patients with favorable and unfavorable 6-month neurological outcome (Fig. 2a–f respectively). IL-10 displayed the most profound difference of all cytokines assessed: concentrations at 6 h were near 3-fold higher in patients with unfavorable vs. favorable 6-month outcome (median concentrations, 13.3 vs. 4.5 pg/mL, respectively) and were significantly elevated at all sampled time points (Fig. 2b). In addition, both IL-1β and TNF-α concentrations were elevated at 6 and 12 h in patients with unfavorable vs. favorable outcome (Fig. 2a, c, respectively). IL-8 levels were significantly elevated at all sampled time points, with a peak difference at 6 h (13.6 vs. 8.7 pg/mL in unfavorable vs. favorable outcome, respectively), while MCP-1 concentrations were significantly elevated at admission and 24 h in patients with unfavorable vs. favorable outcome (Fig. 2d, e, respectively).

Mortality

Alterations in inflammatory marker concentrations were observed in patients who lived vs. those who died; differences were noted in three cytokines and eight chemokines (Fig. 3a–k, respectively). IL-10 levels were elevated at 6, 12, and 24 h after admission in patients who died compared to those who lived. In non-survivors, IL-1β concentrations were 2- fold higher at 12 h (median concentrations, 0.9 vs. 0.4 pg/mL, respectively), and IL-10 concentrations were 4- fold higher at 6 h (median concentrations, 28.1 vs. 6.5 pg/mL, respectively) (Fig. 3a, b, respectively). Similar to the 6-month neurological outcome, IL-8 levels displayed the greatest elevation of all chemokines assessed in patients who died vs. those who lived (Fig. 3d). IL-8 concentrations were significantly elevated at all sampled time points, with the greatest disparity at 6 h, where patients who died had concentrations >2-fold higher than those who lived (median concentrations, 23.9 vs. 9.3 pg/mL, respectively) (Fig. 3d). Conversely, MCP-4, MDC, and TARC concentrations at 24 h after hospital admission were significantly lower in TBI patients who died compared to survivors (Fig. 3g, h, j, respectively).

Secondary complications controlled for injury severity

Six-month GOSE

When controlled for admission GCS and AIS head scores, and standardized according to ranked quartiles, IL-1β (peak, 6 h; OR (odds ratio) 1.84; 95 % confidence interval (CI) 0.90–2.25), IL-10 (peak, 6 h; OR 1.76; 95 % CI 1.25–2.70), and TNF-α (peak, 6 h; OR 1.61; 95 % CI

Table 2 Catecholamine and inflammatory marker correlations

Marker	Catecholamines			
	Epinephrine		Norepinephrine	
	r	*P* value	*r*	*P* value
Cytokines (pg/mL)				
IL-1β	0.11	0.04*	0.28	<0.01*
IL-5	−0.07	0.19	0.01	0.90
IL-10	0.44	<0.01*	0.45	<0.01*
TNF-α	0.00	0.93	0.14	<0.01*
Chemokines (pg/mL)				
Eotaxin	0.16	<0.01*	0.16	0.01*
Eotaxin-3	0.08	0.15	0.05	0.31
IL-8	0.35	<0.01*	0.39	<0.01*
IP-10	−0.00	0.88	0.10	0.02*
MCP-1	0.23	<0.01*	0.33	<0.01*
MCP-4	0.06	0.17	0.05	0.24
MDC	−0.00	0.98	−0.09	0.04*
MIP-1β	−0.00	0.97	0.16	<0.01
TARC	−0.05	0.24	0.03	0.43

Abbreviations: *IL* interleukin, *TNF-α* tumor necrosis factor-alpha, *IP-10* interferon-gamma induced protein-10, *MCP* monocyte chemoattractant protein, *MDC* macrophage-derived chemokine, *MIP-1β* macrophage inflammatory protein-1β, *TARC* thymus and activation regulated chemokine
*$p < 0.05$ via Spearman's ρ

Table 3 Binomial logistic regression models assessing the ability of inflammatory markers to predict poor patient outcome, controlling for injury severity

Marker	Admission		Hours after admission					
			6		12		24	
	OR	*P* value	OR	*P* value	OR	*P* value	OR	*P* value
Unfavorable 6-month GOSE								
IL-1β	0.84	0.489	1.84*	0.002	1.65*	0.009	0.91	0.673
IL-10	1.18	0.376	1.76*	0.005	1.57*	0.019	1.48*	0.034
TNF-α	1.49*	0.024	1.61*	0.008	1.50*	0.021	1.30	0.138
IL-8	1.66*	0.007	1.48*	0.030	1.44*	0.036	1.33	0.104
MCP-1	1.42	0.052	1.09	0.603	1.24	0.213	1.39	0.067
MDC	1.10	0.586	0.90	0.515	1.45	0.037*	0.85	0.363
Mortality								
IL-1β	1.02	0.935	1.06	0.825	1.85*	0.038	1.15	0.598
IL-10	1.19	0.417	2.82*	<0.001	2.09*	0.003	2.20*	0.003*
TNF-α	1.58*	0.027	1.77*	0.007	1.58*	0.033	1.19	0.395
IL-8	1.31	0.168	1.89*	0.005	1.84	0.010*	1.37	0.176
IP-10	3.11*	<0.001	2.06*	0.002	1.59*	0.030	1.19	0.400
MCP-1	1.26	0.230	1.46	0.069	1.57*	0.035	0.91	0.674
MCP-4	1.43	0.090	1.49	0.065	0.99	0.964	0.57*	0.023
MDC	1.03	0.864	0.91	0.620	1.14	0.529	0.71	0.114
MIP-1β	1.13	0.544	1.27	0.243	1.29	0.221	0.89	0.592
TARC	0.95	0.801	1.00	0.991	0.77	0.231	0.56*	0.015
Eotaxin	1.90*	0.005	1.90*	0.007	1.33	0.208	0.79	0.304

Models were controlled for admission GCS and AIS head scores
All blood biomarker concentrations were standardized by quartiles. A one-unit increase is equivalent to a 25 % increase in biomarker concentration
Abbreviations: *OR* odds ratio, *GOSE* extended Glasgow outcome scale, *IL* interleukin, *TNF-α* tumor necrosis factor-alpha, *MCP* monocyte chemoattractant protein, *MDC* macrophage-derived chemokine, *IP-10* interferon-gamma induced protein-10, *MIP-1β* macrophage inflammatory protein-1β, *TARC* thymus and activation regulated chemokine
*$p < 0.05$

1.13–2.29) were significant independent predictors of unfavorable 6-month outcome (GOSE 1–4) (Table 3). In addition, IL-8 (peak, admission; OR 1.66; 95 % CI 1.15–2.39) and MDC (peak, 12 h; OR 1.45; 95 % CI 1.02–2.05) were independent predictors of unfavorable outcome (Table 3).

Mortality

Controlled for admission GCS and AIS head scores, patient death was independently associated with three cytokines and four chemokines (Table 3). IL-10 was the greatest predictor of death of all cytokines analyzed (peak, 6 h; OR 2.82; 95 % CI 1.63–4.87). However, the strongest predictor of death among chemokines as well as all evaluated inflammatory markers was IP-10 (peak, admission; OR 3.11; 95 % CI 1.83–5.27) (Table 3).

Neurologic vs non-neurologic death

Differences in specific inflammatory biomarkers were observed between patients who lived vs. those who died by neurologic or non-neurologic organ failure. IL-1β was significantly elevated in patients who died by neurologic death vs. those who survived at 6, 12, and 24 h; no difference was found between those who died by organ failure and those who survived (Fig. 4a). IL-10 levels were elevated in patients succumbing to both neurologic and non-neurologic death compared to those who survived at all time points except admission (Fig. 4b). Similarly, IL-8 concentrations were elevated in neurologic and non-neurologic death compared to patients who died at 6 h, but were elevated only in patients succumbing to neurologic death at all other sampled time points (Fig. 4c). MCP-1 concentrations were elevated in neurologic death vs. survival at admission, 6, and 12 h, but were lower at 24 h in patients who died by non-neurologic organ failure vs. neurologic death (Fig. 4f). In addition, MIP-1β concentrations were significantly lower in patients who died by non-neurologic organ failure vs. neurologic death at 6 and 24 h (Fig. 4g).

Combined inflammatory score and patient characteristics

A combined IS was created in a subset of 76 patients using three cytokines (IL-1β, -10, and TNF-α) and three chemokines (IL-8, MCP-1, MDC) that were associated with both unfavorable patient outcome at 6 months and mortality. Compared to patients with low a IS (<15), patients with a high IS (≥15) had significantly greater mean NE levels over 24 h from hospital admission, while Epi levels did not statistically differ (Table 4). Greater injury severity, as assessed by admission GCS, AIS head, and ISS scores, was associated with a high IS. In addition, patients with poor outcomes (unfavorable 6-month GOSE and death) had high IS scores (Table 4).

Discussion

In this study we demonstrated that following isolated TBI, acute alterations in systemic cytokine and chemokine levels were associated with unfavorable patient outcome and death. Our sample size of 166 patients is, to our knowledge, the largest study to date to characterize the systemic inflammatory response in isolated TBI. A compelling finding of this work was the identification of a relationship between SNS activity and systemic inflammation acutely post-injury. In addition, our findings addressed the heterogeneous and complex nature of TBI which has confounded our understanding of the pathophysiology and clinical relevance of post-traumatic systemic inflammation [1]. Specifically, our study population consisted of isolated TBI patients with non-penetrating injuries, stratified according to injury severity, and sampled acutely at four

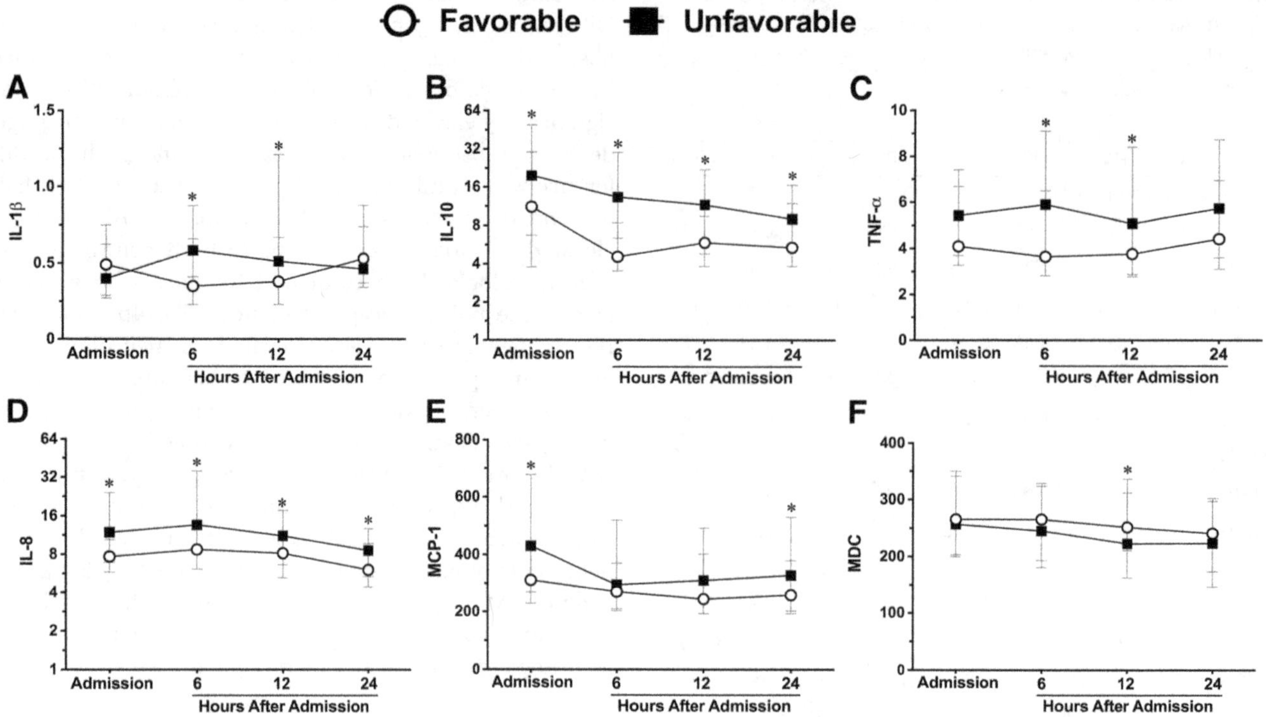

Fig. 2 Plasma cytokine and chemokine concentrations in TBI patients stratified according to the 6-month GOSE. I nterleukin (*IL*)-1β, -10, tumor necrosis factor (*TNF*)-α (**a**–**c**). IL-8, monocyte chemoattractant protein (*MCP*)-1, macrophage-derived chemokine (*MDC*) (**d**–**f**) in TBI patients with unfavorable (GOSE 1–4, $n = 102$) vs. favorable (GOSE 5–8, $n = 61$) 6-month neurological outcome. *Lines* represent the median and interquartile range. $^{*}p < 0.05$ *vs*. favorable outcome by Mann-Whitney *U* test

time points over the first 24 h from hospital admission (Additional file 2: Table S2).

We found IL-10 was the most prominently altered of all cytokines acutely after injury, and was positively correlated with injury severity. While this is in general agreement with previous findings [21, 37, 48, 49], few studies have assessed IL-10 in isolated TBI patients [21, 49]. Furthermore, we are aware of only one previous report that evaluated IL-10 in isolated TBI patients dichotomized by injury severity, albeit in a population of 26 patients that assessed injury severity at 7 days post-injury [50]. Also, in agreement with previous research, unfavorable patient outcome and mortality were associated with elevated peripheral concentrations of IL-1β, IL-10, and TNF-α [32, 37, 46, 48]. Importantly, the relationships between cytokines and patient outcome were significant even after controlling for injury severity, suggesting a possible independent role of these mediators in secondary injury pathogenesis. Moreover, our results provide evidence that certain cytokines may be associated with specific outcomes. For example, IL-1β and TNF-α were elevated only in patients who died from neurologic death, while IL-10 was higher in patients who died as a result of both neurologic and non-neurologic organ failure. Taken together, these findings not only reinforce the globally detrimental role of IL-10 acutely after TBI, but also suggest that peripheral blood may be a viable source for biomarkers related to brain injury-specific outcomes.

Systemic concentrations of all nine chemokines analyzed were significantly different in TBI patients compared to healthy subjects, and alterations in eight of the nine chemokines were associated with poor patient outcome. In addition, we found eotaxin-3, IL-8, MCP-1, and MCP -4 were associated with injury severity. Similar to our cytokine analysis, when controlled for injury severity, seven of the nine chemokines were still related to poor patient outcome, with increases in admission IP-10 levels displaying the strongest relationship to death of all inflammatory markers analyzed. Notably, while higher IP-10 levels in patients were independently associated with mortality, on average, levels were lower in patients vs. healthy controls. The reasons for this are unclear, but it is possible that our total patient values were skewed by lower IP-10 concentrations in survivors vs. those who died. Furthermore, that a number of chemokines were lower in patients compared to controls, or lower in patients with unfavorable vs. favorable outcomes, may speak to the complex and divergent roles of chemokines in mediating secondary

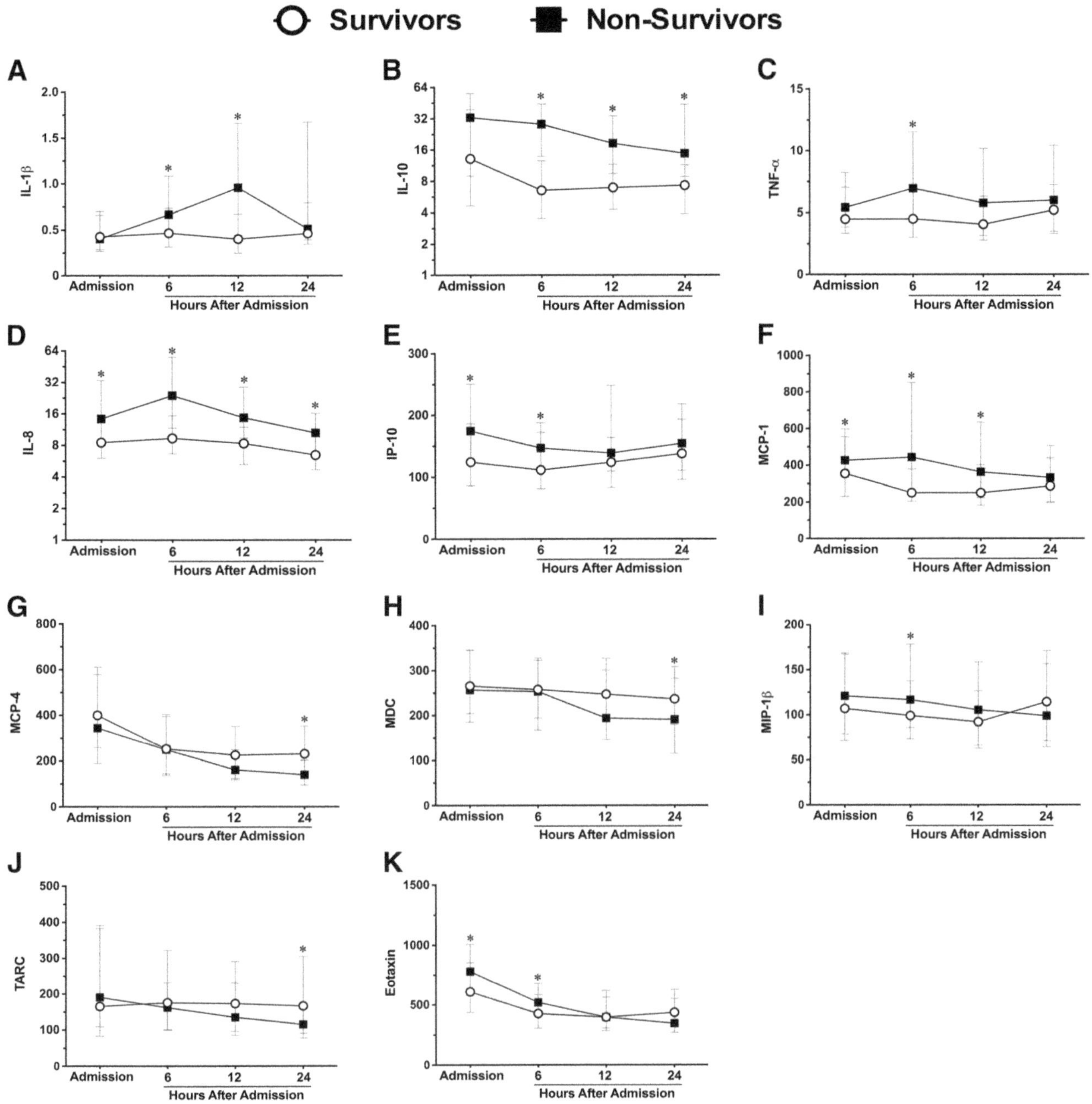

Fig. 3 Plasma cytokine and chemokine concentrations in TBI patients stratified by mortality. Cytokines interleukin (*IL*)-1β, -10, tumor necrosis factor (*TNF*)-α (**a**–**c**). Chemokines IL-8, interferon-gamma producing protein (*IP*)-10, monocyte chemoattractant protein (*MCP*)-1, -4, macrophage-derived chemokine (*MDC*), macrophage inflammatory protein (*MIP*)-1β, thymus and activation regulated chemokine (*TARC*), and eotaxin (**d**–**k**) in TBI patients who died ($n = 45$) vs. those who lived ($n = 119$). *Lines* represent the median and interquartile range. $^{*}p < 0.05$ vs. lived by Mann-Whitney *U* test

injury. Our findings are in general agreement with others who have identified elevations in systemic IL-8 and MCP-1 after TBI [31, 39, 44, 51, 52] and identified the relationship between this and poor patient outcome [38, 40, 45]. However, to our knowledge, no previous studies have characterized this diverse array of chemokines in the peripheral blood after human TBI. Interestingly, Helmy et al. [53] evaluated a number of cytokines and chemokines in the brain extracellular fluid in 12 TBI patients post-injury. These authors concluded that among other inflammatory mediators evaluated, IL-8, MCP-1, IP-10, and MIP-1β were elevated in the brain extracellular fluid relative to plasma, and may be centrally produced after TBI. However, this study did not evaluate plasma levels of these

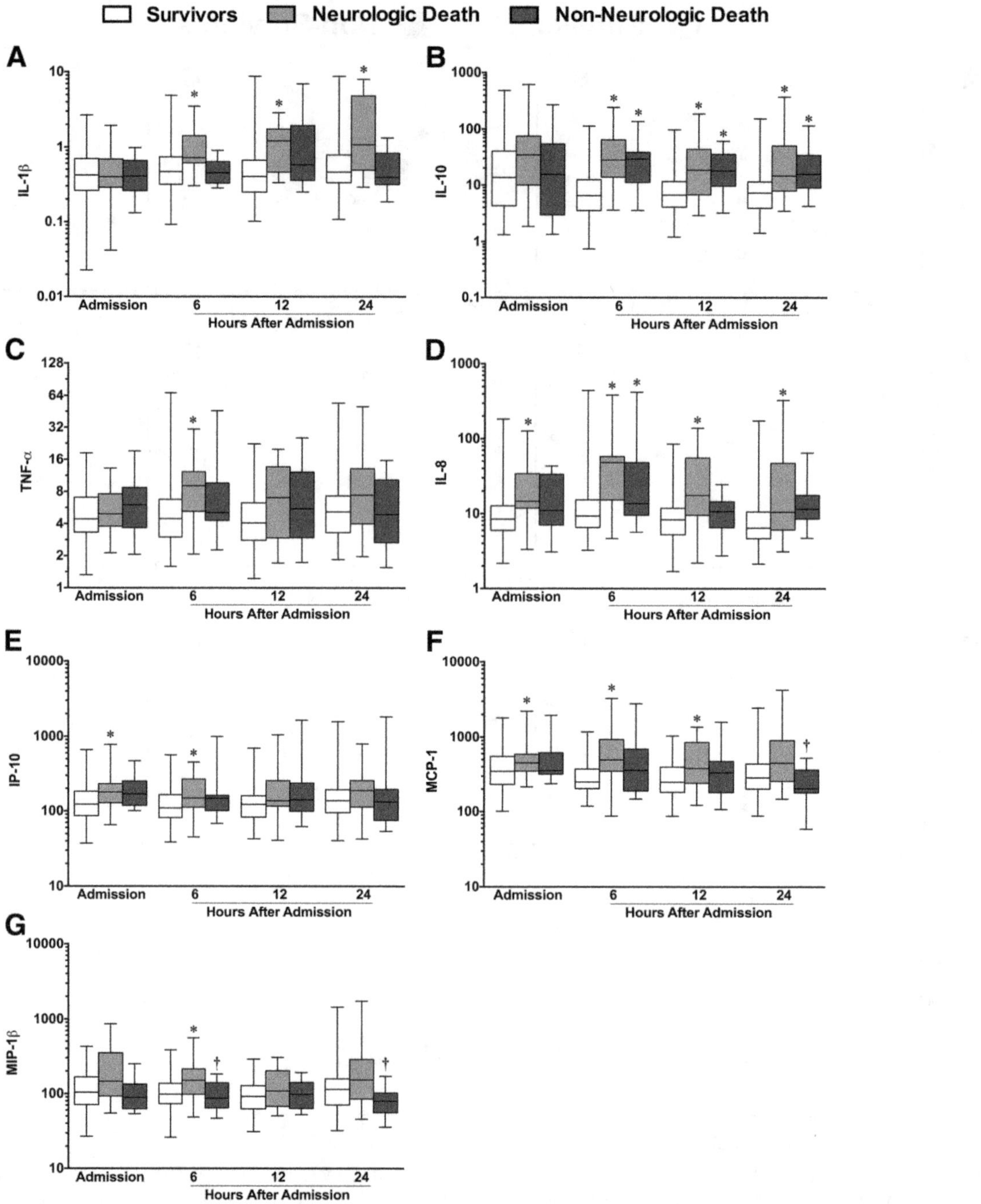

Fig. 4 Plasma cytokine and chemokine concentrations in TBI patients according to the cause of death. I nterleukin (*IL*)-1β, -10, tumor necrosis factor (*TNF*)-α (**a**–**c**). IL-8, interferon-gamma producing protein (*IP*)-10, monocyte chemoattractant protein (*MCP*)-1, and macrophage inflammatory protein (*MIP*)-1β (**d**–**g**) in TBI patients who survived ($n = 119$) vs. those who died by neurologic death ($n = 28$) or by non-neurologic organ failure ($n = 17$). *Boxes* represent the median and interquartile ranges, and *whisker plot lines* represent the range. *$p < 0.05$ vs. patients who survived; $^{\dagger}p <$ 0.05 vs. patients who succumbed to neurologic death, by Kruskal-Wallis

markers in comparison to healthy controls and subsequently, the relative systemic changes were not determined. Furthermore, Chen et al. [54] recently found serum levels of CXCL12 were significantly related to injury severity and patient death after isolated human TBI. Collectively, these recent findings and those of the current study support the deleterious involvement of chemokines beyond IL-8 and MCP-1 in secondary injury pathophysiology, and warrants further investigation.

We identified a number of specific correlations between systemic catecholamines and inflammatory mediators that are consistent with previous experimental

Table 4 Clinical characteristics according to dichotomized inflammatory scores

Characteristics	Inflammation—low (IS < 15, *n* = 33)	Inflammation—high (IS ≥ 15, *n* = 43)	*P* value
Catecholamine levels[a] (pmol/L)			
Epi	1131.5 (656.0–1901.9)	1655.0 (733.2–4307.4)	0.110
NE	6064.3 (3081.0–18373.4)	12,110.0* (7653.1–37,939.8)	0.013
Injury severity			
GCS	7.0 (4.0–9.0)	3.0* (3.0–7.0)	0.002
AIS head	4.0 (3.0–5.0)	5.0* (4.0–5.0)	0.006
ISS	20.5 (16.5–29.5)	29.5* (20.0–35.0)	0.014
Outcome (*n*)			
Sepsis/infection	13	9	0.079
Unfavorable 6-month GOSE	14	33*	0.002
Overall mortality	4	16*	0.014
Neurologic death	2	13*	0.009

Values described as the median and interquartile range unless otherwise stated. IS variables consist of peak differences between unfavorable and favorable outcome over 24 h in IL-1β (6 h), IL-10 (6 h), TNF-α (6 h), IL-8 (6 h), MCP-1 (admission), and MDC (12 h)

Abbreviations: *IS* inflammation score, *Epi* epinephrine, *NE* norepinephrine, *GCS* Glasgow coma scale, *AIS* abbreviated injury scale, *ISS* injury severity score, *GOSE* extended Glasgow outcome scale

*$p < 0.05$ vs. low inflammatory score by Mann-Whitney *U* or chi-square, where appropriate

[a]Average catecholamine concentrations over 24 h

findings. For example, Woisciechowsky et al. [24] found that SNS activation after brain trauma results in the systemic release of IL-10. The authors showed that NE and Epi signaling through peripheral blood monocyte β_2-adrenergic receptors caused an increase in circulating IL-10 concentrations, deactivation of circulating monocytes, and subsequent immunosuppression and infection [24]. That we found a strong association between both NE, Epi, and IL-10 is consistent with the experimental findings of Woiciechowsky et al. and suggests a mechanistic role for catecholamines in mediating IL-10 production in the acute period after isolated TBI. Additionally, it has been hypothesized that IL-1β may induce SNS activation after brain trauma [55–57]. Experimental studies have shown that both CNS and peripherally injected IL-1β have the ability to stimulate the SNS [55, 58], which may then mediate leukocyte mobilization and initiate the hepatic acute phase response [15–18, 55]. This is consistent with the associations we found between IL-1β and both NE/Epi . Furthermore, we identified a positive correlation between NE, Epi, and IL-8 and MCP-1. It has been suggested that the production and release of chemokines from the liver, particularly IL-8 and MCP-1, is an important component of the systemic acute phase response after TBI [4, 16–18], particularly in mediating the mobilization and recruitment of leukocytes to the brain [17, 18, 59, 60]. In a review by Catania and colleagues [4], it was hypothesized that systemic chemokine production and release from the liver post-injury may be mediated by SNS activation and, specifically, the activation of sympathetic nerve terminals and subsequent interaction between tissue macrophages and synaptic NE [18]. In addition, NE has been found to interact with β-adrenergic receptors on cultured peripheral blood mononuclear cells to produce MCP-1 [61], and Epi has been shown in multiple studies to potentiate LPS-induced IL-8 production in monocytes [22, 62]. While the specific mechanism(s) has/have yet to be determined, the results of the current study are supportive of catecholamine- mediated chemokine production after isolated TBI.

While the pathogenesis of systemic inflammation after TBI remains uncertain, our results provide evidence consistent with a detrimental role for the innate immune system in the acute period after injury and further supports the concept that SNS hyperactivity mediates this process. Indeed, the application of an inflammation-based prognostic score showed that the net inflammatory effect seen acutely after TBI is associated with poor patient outcomes, injury severity, and significant elevations in NE. Furthermore, our findings are generally consistent with the revised interpretation of the systemic inflammatory response syndrome (SIRS) and compensatory anti-inflammatory response syndrome (CARS) noted after trauma and sepsis, which suggests that pro- and anti-inflammatory processes occur concurrently, not in a phase delayed manner as was previously hypothesized [63, 64]. We and others have consistently observed that the anti-inflammatory molecule IL-10 is among the earliest detectable mediators after trauma [48, 50, 65] and is elevated concurrently with pro-inflammatory IL-1β, IL-8, TNF-α, and numerous other chemokines in patients with poor outcomes.

Notably, we did not find any association between acute inflammation and the onset of sepsis/infections. However, this study did not directly characterize cellular immune function, and previous studies have reported that immunosuppression and subsequent infection after brain trauma may be related to impaired cellular immunity, including monocyte deactivation [24, 65] and/or suppression of T cell function [66, 67].

The results of this study should be interpreted in the context of its limitations. Despite a well-controlled clinical design and moderately sized cohort of 166 TBI patients, a larger sample size would have allowed for further stratification of our patient population, particularly regarding variables such as sex, age and isolated sepsis. Also, we were only able to assess the level of inflammatory markers in patients' blood samples for the first 24 h post-injury, and a longer sampling period may have been advantageous to assess the potential for hyperadrenergic mediated immunosuppression. In spite of these limitations, this investigation is one of the most comprehensive inflammatory studies in isolated human TBI to date. The results demonstrated a pronounced systemic cytokine/chemokine response acutely after isolated head injury and suggest that this response is associated with the degree of SNS activation.

Conclusions

A number of peripheral cytokines and chemokines are altered in the acute period after moderate and severe isolated TBI. These alterations are associated with unfavorable patient outcomes. Moreover, the systemic inflammatory response after TBI appears to be mediated, at least in part, by a profound trauma-induced hyperadrenergic state. In the present study, we found marked increases in circulating IL-10 and alterations in all chemokines assessed within 24 h of hospital admission. Poor patient outcome was associated with alterations in IL-1β, IL-10, TNF-α, and all chemokines with the exception of eotaxin-3. Furthermore, circulating NE and Epi levels were positively correlated with IL-1β, IL-10, IL-8, eotaxin, and MCP-1. Future controlled clinical studies should continue to emphasize potential therapeutic interventions that modulate excessive SNS activation and inflammation, including treatment with selective adrenergic blocking agents.

Competing interests

The authors declare that they have no competing interests.

Authors' contributions

SGR, AJB, KI, AC, JTV, and SBR were involved in the conception and design of the study. AD, SH, and MS acquired the data for the study. AD, MH, MS, and SH analyzed and interpreted the data. All authors were involved in drafting, revising, and providing intellectual contribution for the manuscript. All authors read and approved the final manuscript.

Acknowledgements

The authors gratefully acknowledge the assistance of Sandy Trpcic, Yangmei Li, Marlene Santos, Ingrid Smith, and Martin Chapman. This research was funded by the Physicians' Services Incorporated Foundation and Defence Research and Development Canada Technology Investment Fund Programme. This study was approved by the Canadian Armed Forces (CAF) Surgeon General's Health Research Program. In accordance with the Department of National Defence (DND) policy, the paper was reviewed and approved for submission without modification by the DRDC Publications Office.

Author details

[1]Defence Research & Development Canada, Toronto Research Centre, Toronto, ON, Canada. [2]Institute of Medical Science, University of Toronto, Toronto, ON, Canada. [3]Faculty of Kinesiology & Physical Education, University of Toronto, Toronto, ON, Canada. [4]Keenan Research Centre, Li Ka Shing Knowledge Institute, St. Michael's Hopsital, Toronto, ON, Canada. [5]Division of Trauma & Critical Care, University of Southern California, Los Angeles, CA, USA. [6]LA County+ USC Medical Center, Los Angeles, CA, USA. [7]Department of Critical Care, St. Michael's Hospital, University of Toronto, Toronto, ON, Canada. [8]Department of Anesthesia, St. Michael's Hospital, University of Toronto, Toronto, ON, Canada. [9]Department of Surgery, St. Michael's Hospital, University of Toronto, Toronto, ON, Canada. [10]Institute for Healthcare Improvement (IHI) Fellow, Cambridge, MA, USA.

References

1. Hinson HE, Rowell S, Schreiber M. Clinical evidence of inflammation driving secondary brain injury: a systematic review. J Trauma Acute Care Surg. 2015;78:184–91.
2. Lu J, Goh SJ, Tng PYL, Deng YY, Ling E-A, Moochhala S. Systemic inflammatory response following acute traumatic brain injury. Front Biosci. 2009;14:3795–813.
3. Anthony DC, Couch Y. The systemic response to CNS injury. Exp Neurol. 2014;258:105–11.
4. Catania A, Lonati C, Sordi A, Gatti S. Detrimental consequences of brain injury on peripheral cells. Brain Behav Immun. 2009;23:877–84.
5. Morganti-Kossmann MC, Rancan M, Stahel PF, Kossmann T. Inflammatory response in acute traumatic brain injury: a double-edged sword. Curr Opin Crit Care. 2002;8:101–5.
6. Bergold PJ. Treatment of traumatic brain injury with anti-inflammatory drugs. Exp Neurol. 2016;275 Pt 3:367–80.
7. Desborough JP. The stress response to trauma and surgery. Br J Anaesth. 2000;85:109–17.
8. Hörtnagl DDH, Hammerle AF, Hackl JM, Brücke T, Rumpl E, Hörtnagl H. The activity of the sympathetic nervous system following severe head injury. Intensive Care Med. 1980;6:169–77.
9. Clifton GL, Robertson CS, Kyper K, Taylor AA, Dhekne RD, Grossman RG. Cardiovascular response to severe head injury. J Neurosurg. 1983;59:447–54.
10. Clifton GL, Ziegler MG, Grossman RG. Circulating catecholamines and sympathetic activity after head injury. Neurosurgery. 1981;8:10–4.
11. Hamill RW, Woolf PD, McDonald JV, Lee LA, Kelly M. Catecholamines predict outcome in traumatic brain injury. Ann Neurol. 1987;21:438–43.
12. Woolf PDP, Hamill RWR, Lee LAL, McDonald JVJ. Free and total catecholamines in critical illness. Am J Physiol. 1988;254:E287–91.
13. Woolf PD, Hamill RW, Lee LA, Cox C, McDonald JV. The predictive value of catecholamines in assessing outcome in traumatic brain injury. J Neurosurg. 1987;66:875–82.
14. Da Luz LT, Capone Neto A, DaCosta LD, Inaba K, Rhind SG, Nascimento B, et al. Catecholamines as outcome markers in traumatic brain injury. Can J Surg. 2015;18:S7–8.
15. Wilcockson DC, Campbell SJ, Anthony DC, Perry VH. The systemic and local acute phase response following acute brain injury. J Cereb Blood Flow Metab. 2002;22:318–26.

16. Campbell SJ, Perry VH, Pitossi FJ, Butchart AG, Chertoff M, Waters S, et al. Central nervous system injury triggers hepatic CC and CXC chemokine expression that is associated with leukocyte mobilization and recruitment to both the central nervous system and the liver. Am J Pathol. 2005;166:1487–97.
17. Campbell SJ, Wilcockson DC, Butchart AG, Perry VH, Anthony DC. Altered chemokine expression in the spinal cord and brain contributes to differential interleukin-1beta-induced neutrophil recruitment. J Neurochem. 2002;83:432–41.
18. Campbell SJ, Hughes PM, Iredale JP, Wilcockson DC, Waters S, Docagne F, et al. CINC-1 is an acute-phase protein induced by focal brain injury causing leukocyte mobilization and liver injury. FASEB J. 2003;17:1168–70.
19. Li M, Li F, Luo C, Shan Y, Zhang L, Qian Z, et al. Immediate splenectomy decreases mortality and improves cognitive function of rats after severe traumatic brain injury. J Trauma. 2011;71:141–7.
20. Chu W, Li M, Li F, Hu R, Chen Z, Lin J, et al. Immediate splenectomy down-regulates the MAPK-NF-κB signaling pathway in rat brain after severe traumatic brain injury. J Trauma Acute Care Surg. 2013;74:1446–53.
21. Shimonkevitz R, Bar-Or D, Harris L, Dole K, McLaughlin L, Yukl R. Transient monocyte release of interleukin-10 in response to traumatic brain injury. Shock. 1999;12:10–6.
22. van der Poll T, Lowry SF. Lipopolysaccharide-induced interleukin 8 production by human whole blood is enhanced by epinephrine and inhibited by hydrocortisone. Infect Immun. 1997;65:2378–81.
23. van der Poll T, Coyle SM, Barbosa K, Braxton CC, Lowry SF. Epinephrine inhibits tumor necrosis factor-alpha and potentiates interleukin 10 production during human endotoxemia. J Clin Invest. 1996;97:713–9.
24. Woiciechowsky C, Asadullah K, Nestler D, Eberhardt B, Platzer C, Schöning B, et al. Sympathetic activation triggers systemic interleukin-10 release in immunodepression induced by brain injury. Nat Med. 1998;4:808–13.
25. Bierhaus A, Wolf J, Andrassy M, Rohleder N, Humpert PM, Petrov D, et al. A mechanism converting psychosocial stress into mononuclear cell activation. Proc Natl Acad Sci U S A. 2003;100:1920–5.
26. Schroeppel TJ, Fischer PE, Zarzaur BL, Magnotti LJ, Clement LP, Fabian TC, et al. Beta-adrenergic blockade and traumatic brain injury: protective? J Trauma Acute Care Surg. 2010;69:776–82.
27. Schroeppel TJ, Sharpe JP, Magnotti LJ, Weinberg JA, Clement LP, Croce MA, et al. Traumatic brain injury and β-blockers: not all drugs are created equal. J Trauma Acute Care Surg. 2014;76:504–9. discussion 509.
28. Xu L, Yu W-K, Lin Z-L, Tan S-J, Bai X-W, Ding K, et al. Impact of β-adrenoceptor blockade on systemic inflammation and coagulation disturbances in rats with acute traumatic coagulopathy. Med Sci Monit. 2015;21:468–76.
29. Rough J, Engdahl R, Opperman K, Yerrum S, Monroy MA, Daly JM. β2 adrenoreceptor blockade attenuates the hyperinflammatory response induced by traumatic injury. Surgery. 2009;145:235–42.
30. Ley EJ, Clond MA, Bukur M, Park R, Chervonski M, Dagliyan G, et al. β-Adrenergic receptor inhibition affects cerebral glucose metabolism, motor performance, and inflammatory response after traumatic brain injury. J Trauma Acute Care Surg. 2012;73:33–40.
31. Maier B, Schwerdtfeger K, Mautes A, Holanda M, Müller M, Steudel WI, et al. Differential release of interleukines 6, 8, and 10 in cerebrospinal fluid and plasma after traumatic brain injury. Shock. 2001;15:421–6.
32. Taşçi A, Okay O, Gezici AR, Ergün R, Ergüngör F. Prognostic value of interleukin-1 beta levels after acute brain injury. Neurol Res. 2003;25:871–4.
33. Chiaretti A, Genovese O, Aloe L, Antonelli A, Piastra M, Polidori G, et al. Interleukin 1β and interleukin 6 relationship with paediatric head trauma severity and outcome. Childs Nerv Syst. 2005;21:185–93.
34. Venetsanou K, Vlachos K, Moles A, Fragakis G, Fildissis G, Baltopoulos G. Hypolipoproteinemia and hyperinflammatory cytokines in serum of severe and moderate traumatic brain injury (TBI) patients. Eur Cytokine Netw. 2007;18:206–9.
35. Goodman JC, Robertson CS, Grossman RG, Narayan RK. Elevation of tumor necrosis factor in head injury. J Neuroimmunol. 1990;30:213–7.
36. Santarsieri M, Kumar RG, Kochanek PM, Berga S, Wagner AK. Variable neuroendocrine-immune dysfunction in individuals with unfavorable outcome after severe traumatic brain injury. Brain Behav Immun. 2015;45:15–27.
37. Schneider Soares FM, Menezes de Souza N, Libório Schwarzbold M, Paim Diaz A, Costa Nunes J, Hohl A, et al. Interleukin-10 is an independent biomarker of severe traumatic brain injury prognosis. Neuroimmunomodulation. 2012;19:377–85.
38. Gopcevic A, Mazul-Sunko B, Marout J, Sekulic A, Antoljak N, Siranovic M, et al. Plasma interleukin-8 as a potential predictor of mortality in adult patients with severe traumatic brain injury. Tohoku J Exp Med. 2007;211:387–93.
39. Rhodes J, Sharkey J, Andrews P. Serum IL-8 and MCP-1 concentration do not identify patients with enlarging contusions after traumatic brain injury. J Trauma. 2009;66:1591–8.
40. Kushi H, Saito T, Makino K, Hayashi N. IL-8 is a key mediator of neuroinflammation in severe traumatic brain injuries. Acta Neurochir Suppl. 2003;86:347–50.
41. Stein DM, Lindell A, Murdock KR, Kufera JA, Menaker J, Keledjian K, et al. Relationship of serum and cerebrospinal fluid biomarkers with intracranial hypertension and cerebral hypoperfusion after severe traumatic brain injury. J Trauma. 2011;70:1096–103.
42. Dziurdzik P, Krawczyk L, Jalowiecki P, Kondera-Anasz Z, Menon L. Serum interleukin-10 in ICU patients with severe acute central nervous system injuries. Inflamm Res. 2004;53:338–43.
43. Jaerve A, Müller HW. Chemokines in CNS injury and repair. Cell Tissue Res. 2012;349:229–48.
44. Buonora JE, Yarnell AM, Lazarus RC, Mousseau M, Latour LL, Rizoli SB, et al. Multivariate analysis of traumatic brain injury: development of an assessment score. Front Neurol. 2015;6:68.
45. Di Battista AP, Buonora JE, Rhind SG, Hutchison MG, Baker AJ, Rizoli SB, et al. Blood biomarkers in moderate-to-severe traumatic brain injury: potential utility of a multi-marker approach in characterizing outcome. Front Neurol. 2015;6:110.
46. Kumar RG, Boles JA, Wagner AK. Chronic inflammation after severe traumatic brain injury: characterization and associations with outcome at 6 and 12 months postinjury. J Head Trauma Rehabil. 2015;30:369–81.
47. Grund B, Sabin C. Analysis of biomarker data: logs, odds ratios, and receiver operating characteristic curves. Curr Opin HIV AIDS. 2010;5:473–9.
48. Ferreira LCB, Regner A, Miotto KDL, de Moura S, Ikuta N, Vargas AE, et al. Increased levels of interleukin-6, -8 and -10 are associated with fatal outcome following severe traumatic brain injury. Brain Inj. 2014;28:1311–6.
49. Hensler T, Sauerland S, Riess P, Hess S, Helling HJ, Andermahr J, et al. The effect of additional brain injury on systemic interleukin (IL)-10 and IL-13 levels in trauma patients. Inflamm Res. 2000;49:524–8.
50. Woiciechowsky C, Schöning B, Cobanov J, Lanksch WR, Volk H-D, Döcke W-D. Early IL-6 plasma concentrations correlate with severity of brain injury and pneumonia in brain-injured patients. J Trauma. 2002;52:339–45.
51. Mussack T, Biberthaler P, Kanz K-G, Wiedemann E, Gippner-Steppert C, Mutschler W, et al. Serum S-100B and interleukin-8 as predictive markers for comparative neurologic outcome analysis of patients after cardiac arrest and severe traumatic brain injury. Crit Care Med. 2002;30:2669–74.
52. Sohrevardi SM, Ahmadinejad M, Said K, Sarafzadeh F, Zadeh SS, Yousefi M, et al. Evaluation of TGF β1, IL-8 and nitric oxide in the serum of diffuse axonal injury patients and its association with clinical status and outcome. Turk Neurosurg. 2013;23:151–4.
53. Helmy A, De Simoni M-G, Guilfoyle MR, Carpenter KLH, Hutchinson PJ. Cytokines and innate inflammation in the pathogenesis of human traumatic brain injury. Prog Neurobiol. 2011;95:352–72.
54. Chen T-J, Wu W-Q, Ying G-R, Fu Q-Y, Xiong K. Serum CXCL12 concentration in patients with severe traumatic brain injury are associated with mortality. Clin Chim Acta. 2015;454:6–9.
55. Kenney MJ, Blecha F, Wang Y, McMurphy R, Fels RJ. Sympathoexcitation to intravenous interleukin-1β is dependent on forebrain neural circuits. Am J Physiol Heart Circ Physiol. 2002;283:H501–5.
56. Saindon CS, Blecha F, Musch TI, Morgan DA, Fels RJ, Kenney MJ. Effect of cervical vagotomy on sympathetic nerve responses to peripheral interleukin-1beta. Auton Neurosci. 2001;87:243–8.
57. Woiciechowsky C, Volk HD. Increased intracranial pressure induces a rapid systemic interleukin-10 release through activation of the sympathetic nervous system. Acta Neurochir Suppl. 2005;95:373–6.
58. Woiciechowsky C, Schöning B, Daberkow N, Asche K, Lanksch WR, Döcke WD, et al. Brain IL-1beta increases neutrophil and decreases lymphocyte counts through stimulation of neuroimmune pathways. Neurobiol Dis. 1999;6:200–8.
59. Campbell SJ, Jiang Y, Davis AEM, Farrands R, Holbrook J, Leppert D, et al. Immunomodulatory effects of etanercept in a model of brain injury act through attenuation of the acute-phase response. J Neurochem. 2007;103:2245–55.
60. Giles JA, Greenhalgh AD, Davies CL, Denes A, Shaw T, Coutts G, et al. Requirement for interleukin-1 to drive brain inflammation reveals tissue-specific mechanisms of innate immunity. Eur J Immunol. 2015;45:525–30.

61. Takahashi H, Tsuda Y, Kobayashi M, Herndon DN, Suzuki F. Increased norepinephrine production associated with burn injuries results in CCL2 production and type 2 T cell generation. Burns. 2004;30:317–21.
62. Kavelaars A, van de Pol M, Zijlstra J, Heijnen CJ. Beta 2-adrenergic activation enhances interleukin-8 production by human monocytes. J Neuroimmunol. 1997;77:211–6.
63. Gentile LF, Cuenca AG, Efron PA, Ang D, Bihorac A, McKinley BA, et al. Persistent inflammation and immunosuppression: a common syndrome and new horizon for surgical intensive care. J Trauma Acute Care Surg. 2012;72: 1491–501.
64. Osuchowski MF, Welch K, Siddiqui J, Remick DG. Circulating cytokine/ inhibitor profiles reshape the understanding of the SIRS/CARS continuum in sepsis and predict mortality. J Immunol. 2006;177:1967–74.
65. Rizoli SB, Rhind SG, Shek PN, Inaba K, Filips D, Tien H, et al. The immunomodulatory effects of hypertonic saline resuscitation in patients sustaining traumatic hemorrhagic shock. Ann Surg. 2006;243:47–57.
66. Quattrocchi KB, Frank EH, Miller CH, MacDermott JP, Hein L, Frey L, et al. Suppression of cellular immune activity following severe head injury. J Neurotrauma. 1990;7:77–87.
67. Wolach B, Sazbon L, Gavrieli R, Broda A, Schlesinger M. Early immunological defects in comatose patients after acute brain injury. J Neurosurg. 2001;94:706–11.

2

Netrin-1 attenuates brain injury after middle cerebral artery occlusion via downregulation of astrocyte activation in mice

Xiaosong He[1,2†], Yanqun Liu[3†], Xiaohong Lin[1,2†], Falei Yuan[4], Dahong Long[1,2], Zhijun Zhang[5], Yongting Wang[5], Aiguo Xuan[1,2,7*] and Guo-Yuan Yang[5,6,8*]

Abstract

Background: Netrin-1 functions largely via combined receptors and downstream effectors. Evidence has shown that astrocytes express netrin-1 receptors, including DCC and UNC5H2. However, whether netrin-1 influences the function of astrocytes was previously unknown.

Methods: Lipopolysaccharide was used to stimulate the primary cultured astrocytes; interleukin release was used to track astrocyte activation. In vivo, shRNA and netrin-1 protein were injected in the mouse brain. Infarct volume, astrocyte activation, and interleukin release were used to observe the function of netrin-1 in neuroinflammation and brain injury after middle cerebral artery occlusion.

Results: Our results demonstrated that netrin-1 reduced lipopolysaccharide-induced interleukin-1β and interleukin-12β release in cultured astrocytes, and blockade of the UNC5H2 receptor with an antibody reversed this effect. Additionally, netrin-1 increased p-AKT and PPAR-γ expression in primary cultured astrocytes. In vivo studies showed that knockdown of netrin-1 increased astrocyte activation in the mouse brain after middle cerebral artery occlusion ($p < 0.05$). Moreover, injection of netrin-1 attenuated GFAP expression (netrin-1 0.27 ± 0.06 vs. BSA 0.62 ± 0.04, $p < 0.001$) and the release of interleukins and reduced infarct volume after brain ischemia (netrin-1 0.27 ± 0.06 vs. BSA 0.62 ± 0.04 mm^3, $p < 0.05$).

Conclusion: Our results indicate that netrin-1 is an important molecule in regulating astrocyte activation and neuroinflammation in cerebral ischemia and provides a potential target for ischemic stroke therapy.

Keywords: Astrocyte, Brain, Ischemia, Inflammation, Netrin-1, UNC5H2

Background

Stroke is a leading cause of death and disability worldwide. Currently, no effective drugs have shown benefit for patients in the acute phase of ischemic stroke except for tissue-type plasminogen activator (tPA). However, the short time window and the side effects limit the effective application of tPA. It is estimated that only 5% of ischemic stroke patients could benefit from tPA treatment [1]. Although numerous studies have shown that neuroprotection reduces brain injury after ischemic stroke in laboratory research, most neuroprotective attempts have failed when translated into the clinic. The lack of effective treatments for ischemic stroke has turned the efforts of researchers and physicians to the neuroprotective effects of not only neurons but also other cell types including astrocytes [2].

Astrocytes are the most abundant cells in the mammalian brain and display diverse functions including blood flow regulation, neurotransmitter metabolism, and endogenous neural stem cell development [3]. Under the

* Correspondence: xag2005@sohu.com; gyyang0626@163.com
†Xiaosong He, Yanqun Liu and Xiaohong Lin contributed equally to this work.
[1]Key Laboratory of Neuroscience, the Second Affiliated Hospital Guangzhou Medical University, Guangzhou, China
[5]Neuroscience and Neuroengineering Research Center, Med-X Research Institute and School of Biomedical Engineering, Shanghai Jiao Tong University, Shanghai, China
Full list of author information is available at the end of the article

cerebral ischemia condition, astrocytes are activated, which is characterized by an increase in glial fibrillary acidic protein (GFAP) expression and elongation of neural processes, as well as secretion of interleukins (ILs) [4]. Astrocytes play multiple roles in ischemic stroke pathology and can be a therapeutic target in promoting functional recovery after cerebral ischemia [5, 6]. Astrocytes respond differently to ischemic injury based on the distance from the lesion, on the severity, and on the phase course of ischemic stroke. In the acute phase, astrocytes produce inflammatory mediators such as ILs and chemokines, which initiate focal inflammatory and immune responses and aggravate brain injury after ischemia/reperfusion [7]. Meanwhile, the astrocytes adjacent to the lesion are activated and form a glial scar. In the first few days, the glial scar restricts the damage to remote areas [6]. However, glial scars have also been shown to inhibit the axon sprouting in the recovery phase of injury. In the chronic phase, studies demonstrated that activated astrocytes could secrete growth factors to aid the recovery [8]. Recently, it was demonstrated that activated astrocytes could form a glial scar, which may promote axon regeneration following severe spinal cord injury [9]. Despite the controversial role of astrocytes, it was widely accepted that astrocytes regulate neuroinflammation. Alleviating ischemia-induced astrocyte activation could promote recovery [10]. Hence, to explore the molecular mechanisms of astrocyte activation could assist the recovery post stroke.

The initiation function of netrin-1 (NT-1) in the brain is axon guidance and regulation of vascular development [11]. Recent studies have shown that NT-1 also exhibited an anti-inflammatory effect. For instance, NT-1 inhibited leukocytes migrating from the endothelium to the parenchyma in vitro and in vivo [12]. Exogenous NT-1 administration attenuated pulmonary inflammation during acute lung injury [13]. After brain ischemia, NT-1 improved recovery through enhanced remodeling ability and brain protection [14, 15]. However, whether NT-1 influences the neuroinflammation in the ischemic brain is unclear. The function of NT-1 mainly depends on the combined receptors such as Deleted in Colorectal Cancer (DCC) and UNC5H2. These receptors are expressed on astrocytes [16, 17]. However, the effect of NT-1 on astrocyte activation including the detailed molecular mechanism was previously unknown. Here, we explore the role of NT-1 in astrocyte activation and the neuroinflammation status after middle cerebral artery occlusion (MCAO) in mice.

Methods

Experimental design

Animal experiment procedure was approved by the Institutional Animal Care and Use Committee (IACUC), Guangzhou Medical University, China. Adult male CD-1 mice weighing 25 to 30 g were divided into five groups: (1) NT-1 injection group, mice underwent 2 μl NT-1 protein solution (100 ng/μl, dissolved in PBS containing 0.1% BSA) injection 1 day before MCAO; (2) BSA group, mice underwent BSA injection 1 day before MCAO; (3) NT-1 shRNA group, mice underwent lentivirus-carried NT-1shRNA injection 2 weeks before MCAO (shRNA sequence: GGGTGCCCTTCCAGTTCTA [18]); (4) GFP group, as control mice for the NT-1 shRNA group, these mice underwent GFP gene transfer through lentiviral vector injection; and (5) sham group, the mice underwent vessel occlusion without suture injection.

Astrocyte culture

Primary astrocytes were prepared from C57BL/6 mice at the stage of P0 as previously described [8]. Astrocytes were cultured in six-well plates and were allowed to reach 90% confluence. Ten micrograms per milliliter of lipopolysaccharide was added in each well for 24 h to induce the interleukin release. NT-1 protein (500 ng/ml) and antibodies (UNC5H2, 5 μg/μl) were added into the medium 12 h before LPS intervention.

Viral vector or NT-1 treatment

Adult CD-1 mice, weighted 25–28 g, were intraperitoneally anesthetized with pentobarbital (10 mg/kg body weight). The mouse skull was fixed on a stereotaxic plate (RWD, Shenzhen, China). A 0.5-mm bone hole was drilled by a hand drill (Fine Science Tool, Foster City, CA). Lentiviral vector (2.5 μl, 4×10^8 IU/ml) or NT-1 was slowly injected into the left striatum (AP = − 0.02 mm, ML = − 2.5 mm, DV = 3 mm relative to the bregma) at the speed of 0.1 μl/min. After 20 min of injection, the needle was maintained in the brain for an additional 5 min. The bone hole was then sealed by bone wax and the skin was sutured. Animals were returned to their cages after being awaken. Two hundred nanograms of NT-1 protein (R&D system) was injected into the brain. NT-1 and BSA injection was performed 1 day before MCAO, lentiviral vectors carried NT-1 shRNA, or GFP gene was injected 2 weeks before MCAO.

Mouse model of MCAO

The mouse model of MCAO was performed as previously reported [19]. Briefly, adult mice were anesthetized intraperitoneally with pentobarbital (10 mg/kg). Then, a 6-0 suture (Covidien, Mansfield, MA) with a round and silicone-coated tip was inserted from the left external carotid artery (ECA) into the internal carotid artery (ICA) to occlude the origin of middle cerebral artery (MCA). The animal body temperature was regularly maintained at 37 °C by a heating pad. After the surgery, animals were placed at room temperature and returned to the cage until awake. The CBF was measured at the MCA territory on the skull before surgery, after the occlusion and reperfusion respectively used a laser Doppler flowmetry (Moor instrument, Devon, UK). The CBF down to less than 10–15% after occlusion and return to more than 70% of baseline after reperfusion was recognized as the success of MCAO as shown in Table 1; no significance was observed among groups. In the sham group, mice underwent the same procedure as MCAO mice except suture injection. Three days after MCAO, mice were sacrificed and brain tissues were collected for further analysis.

Immunohistochemistry

After animals were sacrificed, mice were perfused with saline and sequenced 4% paraformaldehyde fixation solution through the left ventricle and then quickly frozen in precooled isopentane. The brain was coronal sectioned to a 20-μm-thick slice. For immunofluorescence staining, sections were rinsed three times by PBS for 5 min, blocked by 5% normal donkey serum for 60 min, incubated with GFAP (1:300 dilution, Millipore Inc., Billerica, MA) and NT-1 (1:200 dilutions, Abcam, CA) antibodies at 4 °C overnight. After rinsing, sections were incubated with IgG for 60 min. For double immunofluorescence staining, sections were pretreated as described above; antibodies for DCC (1:100 dilutions, Santa Cruz, CA) and GFAP, A2B (1:200 dilutions, Santa Cruz) and GFAP, and UNC5H2 (1:100 dilutions, Abcam, Shanghai, China) and GFAP were incubated together; and corresponded secondary antibodies were incubated individually. The pictures were taken under confocal or fluorescent microscopes.

Behavioral tests in mice

Modified neurologic severity scores (mNSS) of the animals were graded on a scale of 0 to 14, which is a composite of motor, reflex, and balance tests. The higher score reflected more severe injury. The elevated body swing test was performed as previously reported [20]. In this test, mice were held by the tail and raised 10 cm above the surface. The initial direction of swing was recorded in 20 trials in each mouse. The number of turns in each (left or right) direction was recorded for each mouse.

Real-time PCR determination

Total RNA from astrocytes was isolated using TRIzol Reagent (Invitrogen). The RNA concentration was determined by a spectrophotometer (NanoDrop1000, Thermo, Wilmington, DE), followed by a reverse transcription process using PrimeScript RT reagent kit (TaKaRa, Dalian, China). RT-PCR amplification reactions were performed using SYBR Premix Ex Tag Kit according to the manufacturer by two steps under the following conditions: 95 °C for 30 s followed by 40 cycles of 95 °C for 5 s and 60 °C for 30 s. The primers used are listed in Table 2. The ΔCT method was used to detect the NT-1 receptors as described previously [21]. To quantify the mRNA levels of chemokines, the ΔΔCT method was used.

Table 1 CBF measurement (Pu)

Groups	Before surgery	After occlusion	After reperfusion
NT-1 shRNA	277 ± 40	21 ± 6	270 ± 35
Scramble	266 ± 43	21 ± 6	233 ± 40
NT-1	265 ± 39	23 ± 4	230 ± 34
BSA	276 ± 34	25 ± 4	261 ± 35

Western blot and ELISA analysis

After MCAO, mice were anesthetized by pentobarbital intraperitoneally as described above. Brains were quickly removed from a cooled brain mold and then cut into four coronal sections with 2 mm apart; the second section including ischemic core was collected. The section was divided into the cortex and striatum. For protein extraction, tissues were first homogenized by ultrasonic on ice and then centrifuged. Equal amount of total protein (40 μg) was loaded on 10% (*W*/*V*) SDS-PAGE and transferred to nitrocellulose membrane (Whatman, Piscataway, NJ). The membrane was blocked with 5% non-fat milk for 60 min at room temperature and subsequently with anti-NT-1 or anti-GFAP antibody (1:1000 dilutions, Abcam) and anti-β-actin antibody (1:1000 dilution, Santa Cruz) at 4 °C overnight. The membrane was washed in Tris-buffered saline Tween-20 (TBST) and incubated with appropriate horseradish peroxidase-conjugated anti-rabbit or anti-goat IgG for 120 min at room temperature and then reacted with an enhanced ECL substrate (Pierce, Rockford, IL). The result of chemiluminescence was recorded and semi-quantified by Quantity One imaging software (Bio-Rad, Hercules, CA).

The ELISA analysis was used to test the protein level of IL-1β and IL-12β in animals using ELISA kits (Neobioscience, China). Absorbance at 450 nm was recorded and the concentration of the target protein was quantified according to the standard curve. Result was expressed as picogram per milligram protein.

Infarct volume measurement

For measuring brain infarct volume, a series of 20-μm-thick coronal sections with a 300-μm interval were cut. The sections were stained with 1% cresyl violet (Sigma) for 30 min at room temperature. Infarct volume was calculated by NIH Image J software. Infarct size equaled to the total contralateral hemisphere size minus total ipsilateral hemisphere size. Infarct volume between two adjacent sections was calculated by the formula: $V = \sum_1^n [(S_n + \sqrt{S_n \times S_{n+1}} + S_{n+1}) \times \frac{h}{3}]$, in which h was the distance between two adjacent sections and S_n and S_{n+1} were the infarction areas of

Table 2 Primers used for quantitative analysis of gene expression

Gene symbol	Forward primer 5′–3′	Reverse primer 5′–3′
DCC	CTCTTCACAGGATTGGAGAAAGGC	GAGGAGGTGTCCAACTCATGATG
UNC5H2	TGGATCTTTCAGCTCAAGACCCAG	AAGATGGCCAGCTGGAGCCG
A2B	TTGGCATTGGATTGACTC	TATGAGCAGTGGAGGAAG
IL-1β	GCAACTGTTCCTGAACTCAACT	ATCTTTTGGGGTCCGTCAACT
IL-12β	TGGTTTGCCATCGTTTTGCTG	ACAGGTGAGGTTCACTGTTTCT
GAPDH	AGGTCGGTGTGAACGGATTTG	TGTAGACCATGTAGTTGAGGTCA

two adjacent sections. Total infarct volume was the sum of each adjacent section.

Statistical analysis

Quantitative or semi-quantitative data are expressed as mean ± SD. ANOVA with Tukey multiple comparisons post-test was used for the analysis of multi groups. Comparisons between two groups were made by Student's t test. A $p < 0.05$ was considered significantly different. Statistical analysis was carried out with Prism GraphPad 6 (GraphPad Software, Inc., La Jolla, CA).

Results

NT-1 attenuated the release of IL-1β and IL-12β in cultured astrocytes

Primary astrocytes were obtained from the cortex of P0 mice. Through counting the GFAP-positive cells, we determined that the purity of the cultured astrocytes was higher than 95% (Fig. 1a). No ionized calcium-binding adaptor molecule 1 (IBA1)-positive microglia were observed in the cultured cells (Additional file 1: Figure S1). To reveal the effects of NT-1 on astrocyte activation, primary astrocytes were stimulated by lipopolysaccharide (LPS). Although there are differences in gene expression and cellular mechanisms between LPS- and MCAO-induced astrocyte activation [22], LPS is widely used to stimulate astrocyte activation in ischemia condition [10]. In the present study, the release of IL-1β and IL-12β was used to track astrocyte activation. We found that LPS induced the release of IL-1β and IL-12β from cultured astrocytes, and NT-1 treatment before LPS intervention significantly attenuated IL-1β (118 ± 10.6 vs. 64 ± 28.3, $p < 0.05$) and IL-12β (118 ± 14.8 vs. 60 ± 20.1, $p < 0.05$) release, suggesting that NT-1 could be an important target in regulating astrocyte activation during neuroinflammation (Fig. 1b).

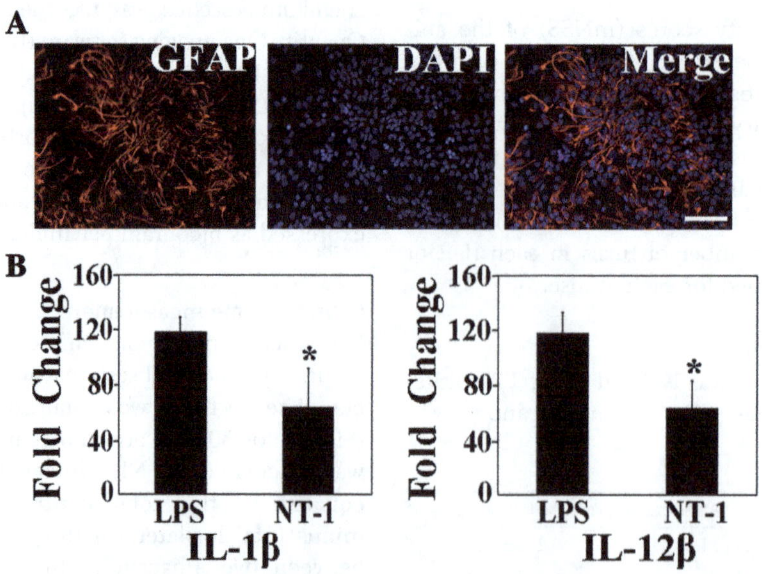

Fig. 1 NT-1 inhibited interleukin release in primary cultured astrocytes. **a** The primary cultured astrocytes; the red indicates GFAP-positive cells, the blue represents the nucleus, and the merge shows the cultured GFAP-positive astrocytes; bar = 100 μm. **b** mRNA expression of the interleukin IL-1β and IL-12β in primary cultured astrocytes induced by LPS and NT-1 treatment; *$p < 0.05$ compared with the LPS group

UNC5H2 was the NT-1 receptor responsible for sustaining astrocyte activation

The effect of NT-1 depends on combined receptors [23]. Therefore, we tested NT-1 receptor expression. We found that the NT-1 receptors DCC, A2B, and UNC5H2 were expressed in the cultured astrocytes at the mRNA level (Fig. 2a, c, e). The immunostaining results demonstrated that DCC, A2B, and UNC5H2 were also present on astrocytes in the MCAO mouse brain tissue (Fig. 2b, d, f).

To define the receptors that are responsible for mediating the effect of NT-1 on astrocyte activation, we applied antibodies or an inhibitor in the cultured astrocytes to respectively neutralize or block the receptors before NT-1 intervention and LPS stimulation. The results showed that NT-1 pretreatment significantly attenuated IL-1β and IL-12β release, and administration of the UNC5H2 antibody in the culture medium reversed the inhibitory function of NT-1 (NT-1 + anti-UNC5H2 170 ± 46.6 vs. NT-1 51 ± 7.72, $p < 0.05$, Fig. 2g, h). In contrast, blocking NT-1 receptors by the DCC antibody or A2B receptor inhibitor did not alter IL-1β or IL-12β release compared to the control conditions. These results indicated that UNC5H2 was the key receptor in regulating astrocyte activation.

NT-1 phosphorylated AKT and increased PPAR-γ expression

To identify the signaling pathways and the downstream molecular effectors involved in astrocyte activation, we performed Western blot to quantify phosphorylated extracellular signal-related kinase (p-ERK) and phosphorylated protein kinase B (p-AKT) expression in cultured astrocytes. Compared to the LPS-treated group, the group pretreated with NT-1 showed an increased p-AKT level in the primary astrocytes ($p < 0.05$, Fig. 3a, b) but not in p-ERK expression (Fig. 3c, d). In addition, Western blot results also showed that the expression of nuclear transcription factor peroxisome proliferator-activated receptor gamma (PPAR-γ) displayed a similar trend as p-AKT

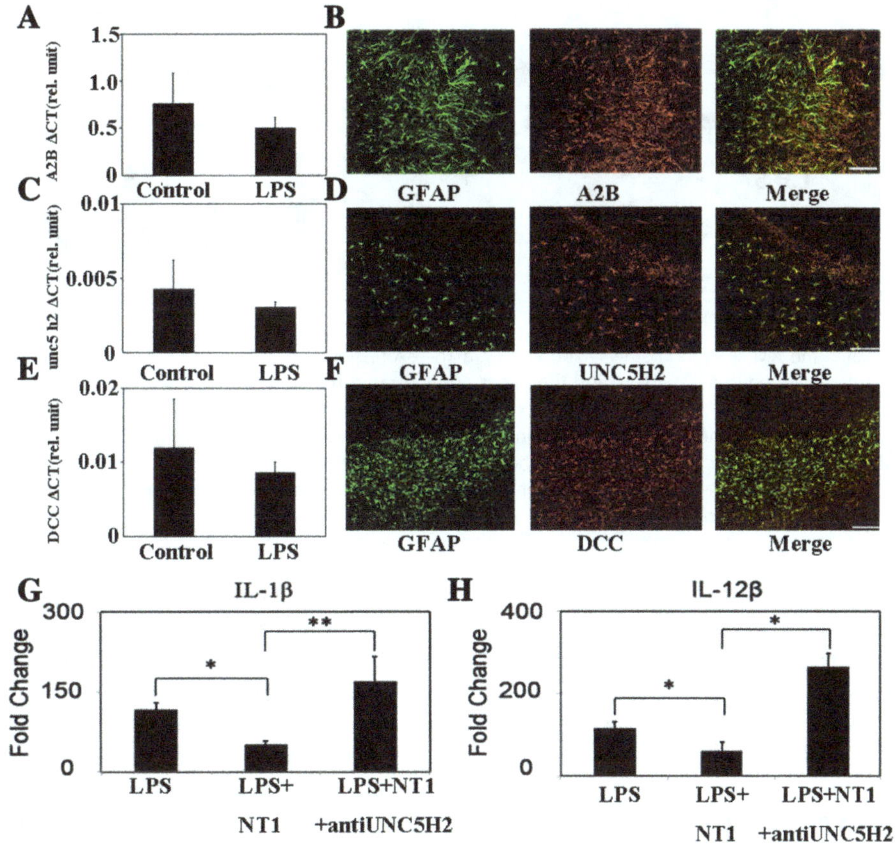

Fig. 2 NT-1-induced inhibition of interleukin release in primary cultured astrocytes was dependent upon UNC5H2 receptors. **a** Bar graph exhibits the mRNA expression of A2B in the cultured astrocytes in different conditions. **b** The immunofluorescence results show A2B expression in the brain sections after ischemia; bar = 100 μm. **c** Bar graph exhibits the mRNA expression of UNC5H2 in the cultured astrocytes in different conditions. **d** The immunofluorescence results show UNC5H2 expression in the brain sections after ischemia; bar = 50 μm. **e** Bar graph exhibits the RNA expression of DCC in the cultured astrocytes in different conditions. **f** The immunofluorescence results show DCC expression in the brain sections after ischemia; bar = 100 μm. **g** IL-1β release in the astrocytes under different interventions; *$p < 0.05$, **$p < 0.01$. **h** IL-12β release in the astrocytes under different interventions; *$p < 0.05$, **$p < 0.01$

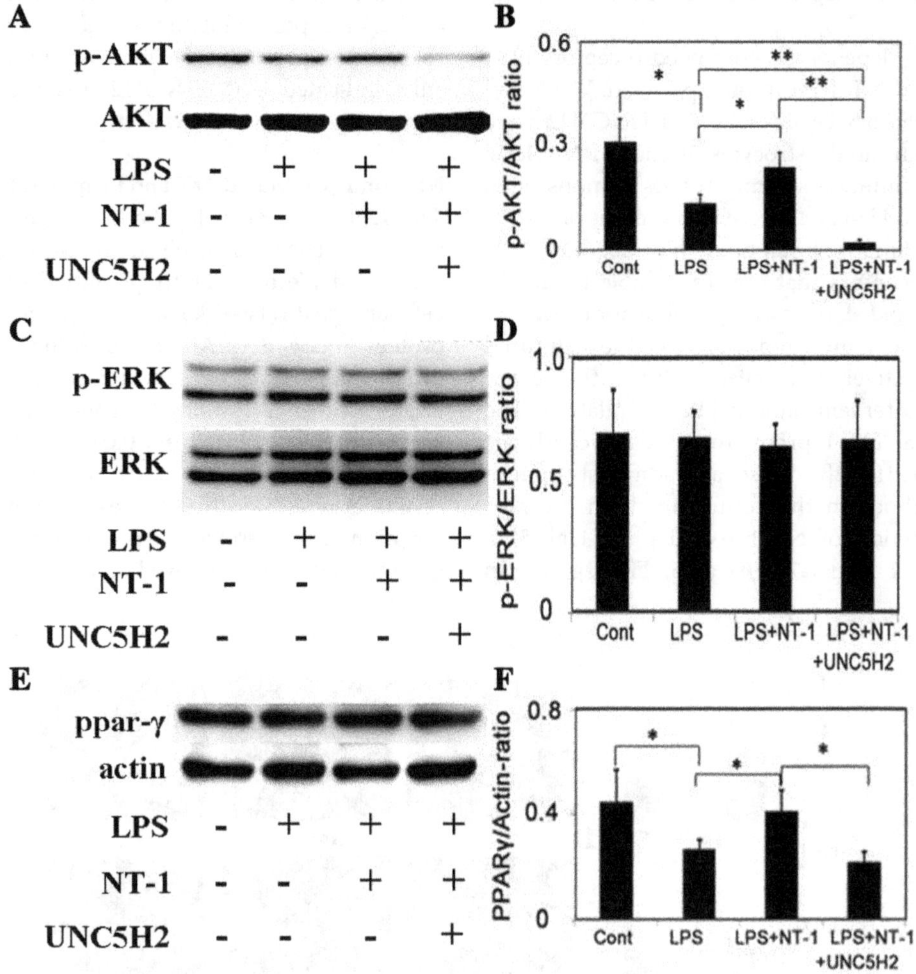

Fig. 3 NT-1/UNC5H2 activated the AKT signaling pathway and PPAR-γ. **a** The expression of p-AKT and AKT analyzed by Western blot; the plus sign represents the material was added to the medium and the minus sign indicates the material was absent from the culture medium. **b** Bar graph represents the statistical results of p-AKT and AKT expression. **c** The expression of P-ERK and ERK examined by Western blot; the plus sign represents the material was added to the medium; the minus sign indicates the material was absent from the culture medium. **d** Bar graph represents the statistical results of p-AKT and AKT expression. **e** The expression of PPAR-γ and actin analyzed by Western blot; the plus sign represents the material was added to the medium; the minus sign indicates the material was absent from the culture medium. **f** Bar graph represents the statistical results of p-AKT and AKT expression; *$p < 0.05$, **$p < 0.01$

expression ($p < 0.05$, Fig. 3e, f). Furthermore, the UNC5H2 antibody attenuated p-AKT and PPAR-γ expression. These results suggest that the phosphoinositide 3-kinase (PI3K)/AKT signaling pathway is an important factor in mediating the function of NT-1 in astrocytes, and PPAR-γ is involved in this progress.

NT-1 regulated astrocyte activation in an ischemic stroke animal model

Astrocyte activation is an important process that influences post-stroke recovery. To investigate whether NT-1 influences astrocyte activation after ischemic stroke, a lentivirus carrying NT-1 shRNA was injected into the mouse striatum to knock down NT-1 expression before the MCAO surgery and observe GFAP expression. To confirm the viral vector transduction in the brain, the viral vector-carried shRNA or GFP was injected into the peri-focal region (striatum). Consistent with our previous results [19], the GFP was majorly expressed in the striatum region 14 days after viral vector transduction (Additional file 2: Figure S2), where the peri-focal region is in our suture MCAO model.

Next, Western Blot was performed to detect NT-1 and GFAP protein expression. The results showed that the NT-1 protein level was significantly reduced in the mouse striatum 2 weeks after the NT-1 shRNA injection ($p < 0.01$, Fig. 4a, b, c). Furthermore, the NT-1 shRNA injection enhanced astrocyte activation, as indicated by GFAP expression ($p < 0.01$, Fig. 4d, e, f). These results suggest that NT-1 is an important regulator for astrocyte activation.

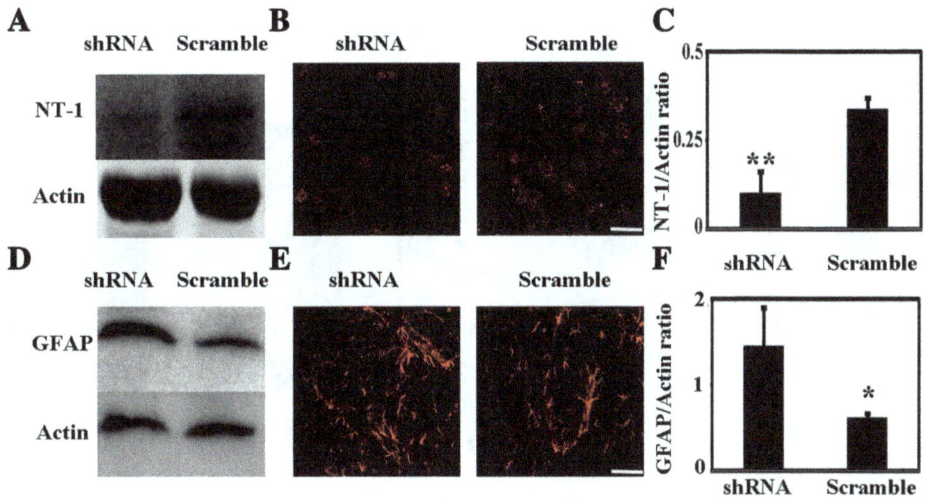

Fig. 4 NT-1 knockdown promoted astrocyte activation in an animal model of MCAO. **a** NT-1 expression in the NT-1 shRNA-injected mice and the control group. **b** The immunofluorescence staining of NT-1 in the shRNA and control groups; bar = 30 μm. **c** The statistical results of NT-1 expression analyzed by Western blot; $^{**}p < 0.01$. **d** GFAP expression in the NT-1 shRNA-injected mice and the control group after ischemic stroke. **e** The immunofluorescence results of GFAP expression in the shRNA and control groups; bar = 30 μm. **f** The statistical results of NT-1 expression examined by Western blot analysis; $^{*}p < 0.05$, $n = 3–5$ in each group

NT-1 attenuated neuroinflammation and brain injury after MCAO

Inhibiting astrocyte activation could attenuate neuroinflammation and alleviate brain injury [24]. Given the role of NT-1 in astrocyte activation, we tested whether an NT-1 injection could alleviate neuroinflammation and reduce brain injury in an ischemic stroke animal model. NT-1 was injected in the mouse striatal area 1 day before MCAO surgery, and the neurological score and body swing test were used to assess behavioral performance 3 days after MCAO. To test the penetration of injected protein, Western blot analysis was performed to quantify NT-1 protein. The protein was extracted from the tissue surrounding the peri-focal region. Two hundred nanograms of recombinant mouse NT-1 was used as a positive control in Western blot tests. As shown in Additional file 3: Figure S3, NT-1 was increased in the brain 1 h after the NT-1 injection compared to the BSA-treated group, indicating the successful injection of protein.

As shown in Fig. 5a, the infarct volume was significantly reduced in the NT-1 pretreatment group (NT-1 22.9 ± 7.5 vs. bovine serum albumin [BSA] 37.9 ± 7.8 mm^3, $p < 0.01$), indicating that NT-1 alleviated brain injury 3 days after MCAO, and this was further shown by the neurological score ($p < 0.05$) and the number of times the animals turned to the right in the body swing test ($p < 0.05$, Fig. 5c, d). The Western blot results showed that the NT-1 injection attenuated GFAP expression ($p < 0.05$, Fig. 6a, b, c). The ELISA results indicated that injecting NT-1 attenuated chemokine IL-1β and IL-12β release (Fig. 6d). In addition, NT-1 has no influence on astrocyte activation or interleukin release in mice that did not undergo the MCAO surgery (Additional file 4: Figure S4). These results imply that NT-1 can attenuate neuroinflammation induced by ischemic stroke.

Discussion

The effect of NT-1 in the brain depends on the combined receptors, the downstream signaling pathway, and the molecular effectors. Previous studies have demonstrated that DCC and UNC5H2 are expressed on astrocytes. However, the effect of NT-1 on astrocytes was not previously explored. In the present study, we demonstrated that pretreatment with NT-1 alleviated LPS-induced IL-1 and IL-12 release in cultured astrocytes. UNC5H2 was the receptor responsible for regulating the effect of NT-1 on astrocyte activation. Furthermore, NT-1 and UNC5H2 relied on the AKT pathway and PPAR-γ in regulating astrocyte activation. In the animal model, NT-1 knockdown via RNA silencing augmented the stroke-induced astrocyte activation, and NT-1 protein injection attenuated the ischemia-induced injury and subsequent neuroinflammation. In summary, we demonstrated a novel role of NT-1 in the prevention of ischemic stroke.

Recently, NT-1 was discovered to possess anti-inflam mation potential in various disease models including acute lung injury and intestinal inflammation [25, 26]. Evidence also demonstrated that NT-1 was an important regulator in sustaining the integrity of the blood-brain barrier (BBB) during experimental autoimmune encephalomyelitis, traumatic brain injury, and ischemic

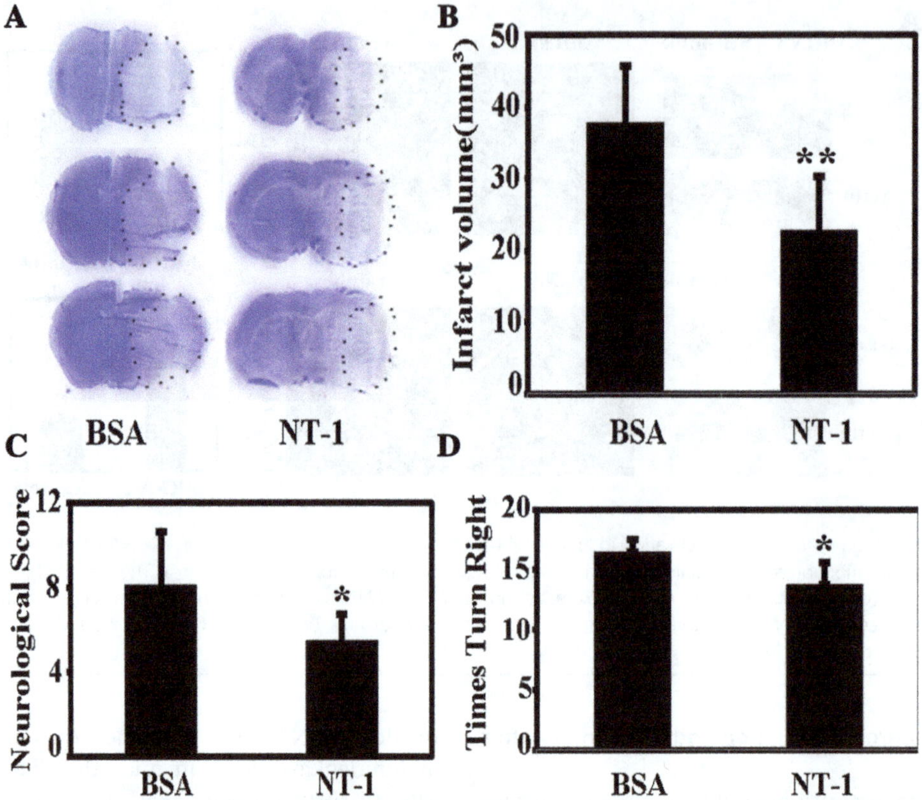

Fig. 5 NT-1 alleviated brain injury and promoted recovery after MCAO in mice. **a** Crystal violet staining in the NT-1 protein- and BSA-injected groups 3 days after MCAO surgery. **b** The statistical results of infarct volume; $^{**}p < 0.01$, $n = 3$ in each group. **c** The neurological scores of the two groups 3 days after MCAO surgery; $^{*}p < 0.05$, $n = 7$ in each group. **d** The number of times the animals turned right in the body swing test; $^{*}p < 0.05$, $n = 7$ in each group

stroke [21]. In the BBB, NT-1 was secreted by endothelial cells and provided anti-inflammation effects through decreasing chemokine secretion and protecting against cytokine-induced barrier disruption. Notably, NT-1 expression on endothelial cells was regulated by astrocyte-derived sonic hedgehog, which led us to hypothesize the effects of NT-1 on astrocytes. In this study, NT-1 protein was added to primary cultured astrocytes before LPS intervention, and we found that IL release was significantly reduced, indicating that NT-1 is an important factor in regulating the function of astrocytes. Furthermore, the in vivo results showed that NT-1 knockdown significantly increased GFAP expression, indicating that NT-1 is a key regulator in the process of astrocyte activation.

Receptors are the first factors that influence the function of NT-1. NT-1 has an array of receptors that are known to support the effect of NT-1, including DCC, UNC5H2, and A2B. In the present study, we found that three receptors could be detected in cultured astrocytes using real-time PCR and immunostaining in brain sections. Using an antibody or inhibitor blockade in vitro, we found that UNC5H2 was the receptor responsible for mediating the effect of NT-1 on astrocyte activation. UNC5H2 was also the prominent receptor while inducing the repelling function in guiding axon outgrowth and sustaining endothelial cell proliferation [27]. UNC5H2 was also required to inhibit leukocyte migration during inflammation and chemokine secretion and to induce the proliferation of Schwann cells [12, 28, 29]. Our results showed that the UNC5H2 antibody blockade significantly reversed the effects of NT-1 by inhibiting chemokine release from the cultured astrocytes. Interestingly, the concentration of the chemokines IL-1β and IL-12β released from astrocytes were even higher than that in the LPS group. Since antibody neutralizing was executed before NT-1 and LPS incubation, we believe that (1) UNC5H2 was the receptor responsible for NT-1-attenuated astrocyte activation and (2) NT-1 was not the only ligand of UNC5H2 in regulating astrocyte activation. In support of our postulation, using a knockout animal model, Yung et al. demonstrated that UNC5H2 was not the dominant receptor in mediating the action of NT-1 [30]. Of note, our data suggested that UNC5H2 was the receptor of NT-1 involved in regulating astrocyte activation.

NT-1 activates various signaling pathways and downstream effectors. For example, NT-1 interacted with DCC

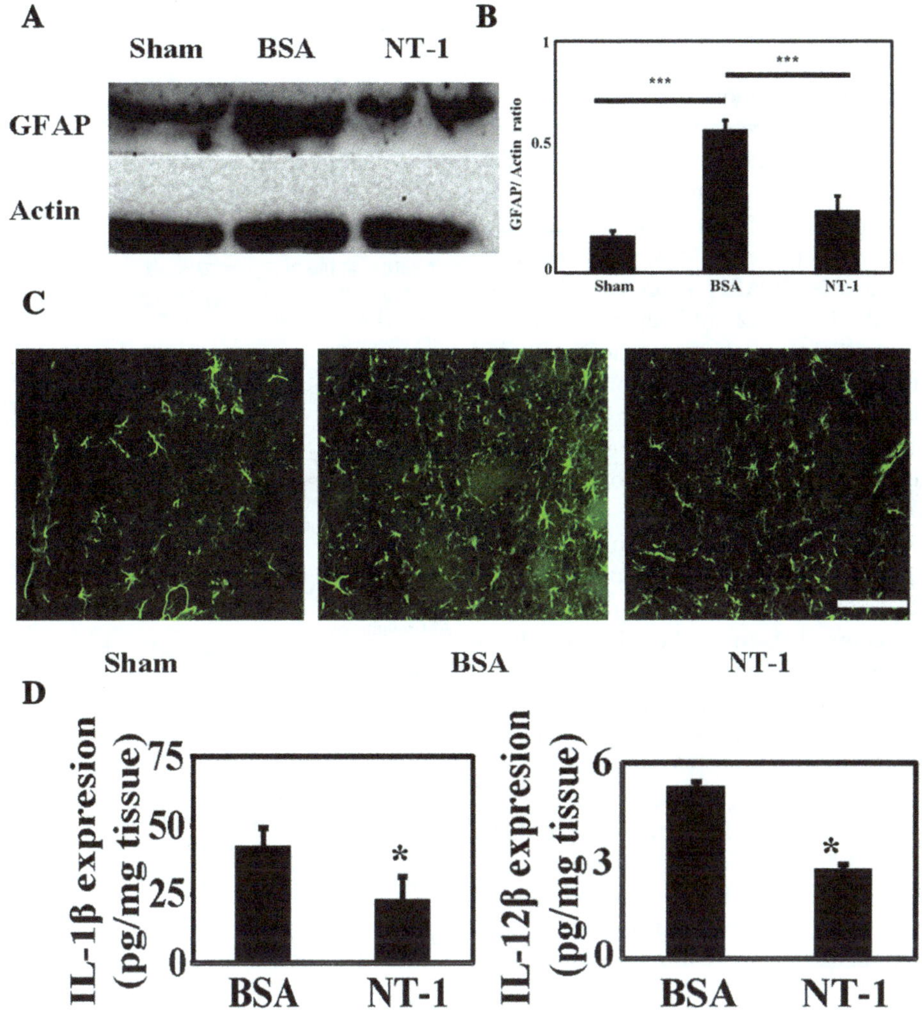

Fig. 6 NT-1 reduced astrocyte activation and interleukin release after brain ischemia. **a** GFAP expression in the sham mice, NT-1 protein-injected mice, and the BSA-injected mice 3 days after MCAO. **b** The statistical results of GFAP expression in the NT-1 and control groups; $^{***}p < 0.001$. **c** The immunofluorescence results of GFAP staining in the peri-infarct area in the NT-1 and control groups; bar = 50 μm, $n = 3$ in each group. **d** ELISA results of the expression of chemokines IL-1β and IL-12β in the NT-1-injected mice and the control mice after ischemic stroke. The left graph indicates the IL-1β expression; the right graph indicates the IL-12β expression; $^{*}p < 0.05$, $n = 3$–5 in each group

and activated the ERK pathway to promote the proliferation of endothelial cells and angiogenesis [31]. NT-1 combined with DCC to reduce the DNA damage and apoptosis in cultured primary neurons [32]. UNC5H2 was the receptor responsible for protecting BBB breakdown [33]. NT-1 also inhibited the notch signaling pathway after ischemic stroke [34]. In the process of angiogenesis and vascular remodeling, an NT-1/focal adhesion kinase (FAK)/Src signaling axis was also reported to be an important pathway [35]. In addition, NT-1 phosphorylated AMP-activated protein kinase (AMPK) and reduced the phosphorylation of mammalian target of rapamycin (mTOR) and P70S6K in a spinal cord injury model [36]. NT-1 also activated APPL1-AKT signing pathway via combining with DCC receptor to reduce apoptosis after subarachnoid hemorrhage in rats [37]. When introducing to astrocytes, AKT signing pathway was reported to protect astrocytes from activation [38]. In our study, we found a significant increase of *p*-AKT expression, while no change could be observed of ERK phosphorylation, when treated with NT-1 in astrocytes, indicating that NT-1 influenced the AKT pathway instead of the ERK pathways in inhibiting astrocyte activation.

Molecular effectors are crucial in regulating the effect of NT-1. When introduced to proliferating endothelial cells, NT-1 was reported to increase the expression of inducible nitric oxide synthase (iNOS) and cluster of differentiation (CD) 151 [31, 35]. NT-1 was also shown to be a regulator of nuclear factor kappa B (NF-κB) when inhibiting prostaglandin E2 (PGE-2) production [39]. NT-1 was also reported to be a key upstream regulator of PPAR-γ in reducing ischemia-induced inflammation

[40]. PPAR-γ belongs to the nuclear hormone receptor family and was demonstrated to be an important target in the treatment of ischemic stroke. For example, PPAR-γ agonists were widely reported to attenuate ischemic brain injury through attenuating apoptosis and neuroinflammation [41]. PPAR-γ was also highly expressed on astrocytes and activation of PPAR-γ could protect astrocytes from apoptosis induced by ischemia [42]. Partly consistent with reported studies, we found that NT-1 significantly increased PPAR-γ expression in cultured astrocytes, and the UNC5H2 antibody blockade reversed the expression of PPAR-γ, indicating that PPAR-γ is an important effector in supporting the function of NT-1.

Numerous studies have demonstrated that NT-1 is an important factor influencing the recovery after ischemic stroke through various mechanisms [43]. For example, in the acute phase of brain ischemia, NT-1 attenuated apoptosis and promoted neural stem cell migration to alleviate brain injury [15]. It was also reported that NT-1 was able to enhance the local field potential (LFP) and reduce memory loss in a whole-brain ischemic model [44]. Recently, NT-1 was shown to attenuate injury through inhibiting autophagy [36]. In the chronic course of ischemic stroke, our previous results demonstrated that NT-1 was able to improve the remodeling process through enhanced angiogenesis, neurogenesis, and oligodendrogenesis [45–47]. Here, we report that NT-1 attenuates brain injury and reduces neuroinflammation via inhibiting astrocyte activation. Astrocyte activation has dual roles in post-stroke recovery depending on the upregulated genes. As reported, activated astrocytes can divide into the A1 and A2 types, where the A1 type loses much astrocyte-benefiting function and gains neurotoxic function, and the A2 type upregulates many neurotrophic factors [48]. Under ischemic conditions, astrocytes undergo apoptosis, which may increase the permeation of the BBB. However, the balance between apoptosis and proliferation sustains the astrocyte numbers [49]. In addition, it remains unknown which type of astrocytes could help to preserve the function of the BBB after ischemic stroke. Our results showed that NT-1 can inhibit GFAP expression, reduce chemokine release, and promote recovery, partly through reducing astrocytes activation, which expands the role of NT-1 in stroke pathology.

Conclusion

In conclusion, our study demonstrated that NT-1 was a crucial factor in regulating astrocyte activation. The interaction of NT-1 with UNC5H2 was an important process in regulating astrocyte activation. NT-1 attenuated ischemia-induced inflammation through inhibiting astrocyte activation. Identification of this novel function of NT-1 has implications for research into the mechanisms of astrocyte activation and for the treatment of ischemic stroke.

Additional files

Additional file 1: Figure S1. IBA1 staining in primary cultured cells. The red indicates IBA1-positive cells; the blue represents the nuclei; the merge shows the cultured IBA1-positive microglia.

Additional file 2: Figure S2. Virus expression in the brain. Lentivirus carried ShRNA, and GFP was majorly expressed in the striatum area 14 days after virus injection; green indicated GFP expression and blue represented Dapi. Bar = 500 μm.

Additional file 3: Figure S3. Protein penetration in the brain. NT-1 expression 1 h after injection; 200 ng recombinant mouse NT-1 was used as positive control. Actin was absent in the positive-control groups.

Additional file 4: Figure S4. NT-1 did not induce astrocyte activation in the intact mouse brain. a) GFAP expression in NT-1- and saline-treated mice that did not undergo MCAO. b) Cytokine IL-1β and IL-12β release in mice that did not undergo MCAO.

Abbreviations

DCC: Deleted in Colorectal Cancer; GFAP: Glial fibrillary acidic protein; MCAO: Middle cerebral artery occlusion; NeuN: Neuronal nuclei; NT-1: Netrin-1; tPA: Tissue-type plasminogen activator; VEGF: Vascular endothelial growth factor

Acknowledgements

The authors thank Jianwei Dai, Xiang Gu, and Jin Xu for their technical assistance and collaborative support.

Funding

This study is supported by the NSFC Projects #81501014 (HXS), 81501029 (LYQ), and #81371305 (YW) and Guangdong Natural Science Foundation #Q17056016 (HXS), Science and Technology Planning Project of Guangdong Province #2017A020211009 (DJW).

Authors' contributions

XS designed the experiment, collected and analyzed data, and drafted the manuscript. YQ carried out the astrocyte culture and subsequent tests in the astrocytes. XH participated in animal surgery and data collection. FL revised the manuscript. DH, ZJ, and YT provided study material and revised the manuscript. AG provided materials and revised the manuscript. GY designed the study, provided study material, and revised the manuscript. All authors have read and approved the final submitted manuscript.

Consent for publication

Not applicable.

Competing interests

The authors declare that they have no competing interests.

Author details

[1]Key Laboratory of Neuroscience, the Second Affiliated Hospital Guangzhou Medical University, Guangzhou, China. [2]Department of Anatomy, School of Basic Medical Science, Guangzhou Medical University, Guangzhou, China.

[3]Department of Neurology, Changhai Hospital, Naval Military Medical University, Shanghai, China. [4]Hailisheng Biomarine Research Institute, Zhoushan, China. [5]Neuroscience and Neuroengineering Research Center, Med-X Research Institute and School of Biomedical Engineering, Shanghai Jiao Tong University, Shanghai, China. [6]Department of Neurology, Ruijin Hospital, School of Medicine, Shanghai Jiao Tong University, Shanghai, China. [7]Department of Anatomy, Guangzhou Medical college, Guangzhou 511546, China. [8]Med-X Research Institute and School of Biomedical Engineering, 1954 Hua-shan Road, Shanghai 200030, China.

References

1. Campbell BC, Meretoja A, Donnan GA, Davis SM. Twenty-year history of the evolution of stroke thrombolysis with intravenous alteplase to reduce long-term disability. Stroke. 2015;46:2341–6.
2. Barreto G, White RE, Ouyang Y, Xu L, Giffard RG. Astrocytes: targets for neuroprotection in stroke. Cent Nerv Syst Agents Med Chem. 2011;11:164–73.
3. Haydon P, Carmignoto G. Astrocyte control of synaptic transmission and neurovascular coupling. Physiol Rev. 2006;86:1009.
4. Gleichman AJ, Carmichael ST. Astrocytic therapies for neuronal repair in stroke. Neurosci Lett. 2013;565:47–52.
5. Sims NR, Yew WP. Reactive astrogliosis in stroke: contributions of astrocytes to recovery of neurological function. Neurochem Int. 2017;107:88–103.
6. Liu Z, Chopp M. Astrocytes, therapeutic targets for neuroprotection and neurorestoration in ischemic stroke. Prog Neurobiol. 2015;144:103–20.
7. Li M, Li Z, Yao Y, Jin WN, Wood K, Liu Q, Shi FD, Hao J. Astrocyte-derived interleukin-15 exacerbates ischemic brain injury via propagation of cellular immunity. Proc Natl Acad Sci U S A. 2016;114:E396–405.
8. Tang G, Liu Y, Zhang Z, Lu Y, Wang Y, Huang J, Li Y, Chen X, Gu X, Yang GY. Mesenchymal stem cells maintain blood-brain barrier integrity by inhibiting aquaporin-4 upregulation after cerebral ischemia. Stem Cells. 2014;32:3150–62.
9. Anderson MA, Burda JE, Ren Y, Ao Y, O'Shea TM, Kawaguchi R, Coppola G, Khakh BS, Deming TJ, Sofroniew MV. Astrocyte scar formation aids central nervous system axon regeneration. Nature. 2016;532:195–200.
10. Liu T, Zhang T, Yu H, Shen H, Xia W. Adjudin protects against cerebral ischemia reperfusion injury by inhibition of neuroinflammation and blood-brain barrier disruption. J Neuroinflammation. 2014;11:107.
11. Bradford D, Cole SJ, Cooper HM. Netrin-1: diversity in development. Int J Biochem Cell Biol. 2009;41:487–93.
12. Ly NP, Komatsuzaki K, Fraser IP, Tseng AA, Prodhan P, Moore KJ, Kinane TB. Netrin-1 inhibits leukocyte migration in vitro and in vivo. Proc Natl Acad Sci U S A. 2005;102:14729–34.
13. Mutz C, Mirakaj V, Vagts DA, Westermann P, Waibler K, Konig K, Iber T, Noldge-Schomburg G, Rosenberger P. The neuronal guidance protein netrin-1 reduces alveolar inflammation in a porcine model of acute lung injury. Crit Care. 2010;14:R189.
14. Sun H, Le T, Chang TTJ, Habib A, Wu S, Shen F, Young WL, Su H, Liu J. AAV-mediated netrin-1 overexpression increases peri-infarct blood vessel density and improves motor function recovery after experimental stroke. Neurobiol Dis. 2011;1:73–83.
15. Wu TW, Li WW, Li H. Netrin-1 attenuates ischemic stroke-induced apoptosis. Neuroscience. 2008;156:475–82.
16. Wang X, Xu J, Gong J, Shen H. Expression of netrin-1 and its receptors, deleted in colorectal cancer and uncoordinated locomotion-5 homolog B, in rat brain following focal cerebral ischemia reperfusion injury. Neural Regen Res. 2013;8:64–9.
17. Liu N, Huang H, Lin F, Chen A, Zhang Y, Chen R, Du H. Effects of treadmill exercise on the expression of netrin-1 and its receptors in rat brain after cerebral ischemia. Neuroscience. 2011;194:349–58.
18. Xu H, Liu J, Xiong S, Le YZ, Xia X. Suppression of retinal neovascularization by lentivirus-mediated netrin-1 small hairpin RNA. Ophthalmic Res. 2012;47:163–9.
19. He X, Lu Y, Lin X, Jiang L, Tang Y, Tang G, Chen X, Zhang Z, Wang Y, Yang GY. Optical inhibition of striatal neurons promotes focal neurogenesis and neurobehavioral recovery in mice after middle cerebral artery occlusion. J Cereb Blood Flow Metab. 2017;37:837–47.
20. Li J, Tang Y, Wang Y, Tang R, Jiang W, Yang GY, Gao WQ. Neurovascular recovery via co-transplanted neural and vascular progenitors leads to improved functional restoration after ischemic stroke in rats. Stem Cell Reports. 2014;3:101–14.
21. Podjaski C, Alvarez JI, Bourbonniere L, Larouche S, Terouz S, Bin JM, Lecuyer MA, Saint-Laurent O, Larochelle C, Darlington PJ, et al. Netrin 1 regulates blood-brain barrier function and neuroinflammation. Brain. 2015;138:1598–612.
22. Zamanian JL, Xu L, Foo LC, Nouri N, Zhou L, Giffard RG, Barres BA. Genomic analysis of reactive astrogliosis. J Neurosci. 2012;32:6391–410.
23. Xu K, Wu Z, Renier N, Antipenko A, Tzvetkova-Robev D, Xu Y, Minchenko M, Nardi-Dei V, Rajashankar KR, Himanen J, et al. Neural migration. Structures of netrin-1 bound to two receptors provide insight into its axon guidance mechanism. Science. 2014;344:1275–9.
24. Shao W, Zhang SZ, Tang M, Zhang XH, Zhou Z, Yin YQ, Zhou QB, Huang YY, Liu YJ, Wawrousek E, et al. Suppression of neuroinflammation by astrocytic dopamine D2 receptors via alphaB-crystallin. Nature. 2012;494:90–4.
25. He J, Zhao Y, Deng W, Wang DX. Netrin-1 promotes epithelial sodium channel-mediated alveolar fluid clearance via activation of the adenosine 2B receptor in lipopolysaccharide-induced acute lung injury. Respiration. 2014; 87:394–407.
26. Aherne CM, Collins CB, Eltzschig HK. Netrin-1 guides inflammatory cell migration to control mucosal immune responses during intestinal inflammation. Tissue Barriers. 2014;1:e24957.
27. Larrivee B, Freitas C, Trombe M, Lv X, Delafarge B, Yuan L, Bouvree K, Breant C, Del Toro R, Brechot N, et al. Activation of the UNC5B receptor by Netrin-1 inhibits sprouting angiogenesis. Genes Dev. 2007;21:2433–47.
28. Tadagavadi RK, Wang W, Ramesh G. Netrin-1 regulates Th1/Th2/Th17 cytokine production and inflammation through UNC5B receptor and protects kidney against ischemia–reperfusion injury. J Immunol. 2010;185:3750–8.
29. Lee HK, Seo I, Seo E, Seo SY, Lee HJ, Park HT. Netrin-1 induces proliferation of Schwann cells through Unc5b receptor. Biochem Biophys Res Commun. 2007;362:1057–62.
30. Yung AR, Nishitani AM, Goodrich LV. Phenotypic analysis of mice completely lacking netrin 1. Development. 2015;142:3686–91.
31. Nguyen A, Cai H. Netrin-1 induces angiogenesis via a DCC-dependent ERK1/2-eNOS feed-forward mechanism. Proc Natl Acad Sci. 2006;103:6530–5.
32. Chen J, Du H, Zhang Y, Chen H, Zheng M, Lin P, Lan Q, Yuan Q, Lai Y, Pan X, et al. Netrin-1 prevents rat primary cortical neurons from apoptosis via the DCC/ERK pathway. Front Cell Neurosci. 2017;11:387.
33. Yu J, Li C, Ding Q, Que J, Liu K, Wang H, Liao S. Netrin-1 ameliorates blood-brain barrier impairment secondary to ischemic stroke via the activation of PI3K pathway. Front Neurosci. 2017;11:700.
34. Yang X, Li S, Li B, Wang X, Sun C, Qin H, Sun H. Netrin-1 overexpression improves neurobehavioral outcomes and reduces infarct size via inhibition of the notch1 pathway following experimental stroke. J Neurosci Res. 2017;95:1850–7.
35. Yang X, Li S, Zhong J, Zhang W, Hua X, Li B, Sun H. CD151 mediates netrin-1-induced angiogenesis through the Src-FAK-Paxillin pathway. J Cell Mol Med. 2016;21:72–80.
36. Bai L, Mei X, Shen Z, Bi Y, Yuan Y, Guo Z, Wang H, Zhao H, Zhou Z, Wang C, et al. Netrin-1 improves functional recovery through autophagy regulation by activating the AMPK/mTOR signaling pathway in rats with spinal cord injury. Sci Rep. 2017;7:42288.
37. Xie Z, Huang L, Enkhjargal B, Reis C, Wan W, Tang J, Cheng Y, Zhang JH. Intranasal administration of recombinant Netrin-1 attenuates neuronal apoptosis by activating DCC/APPL-1/AKT signaling pathway after subarachnoid hemorrhage in rats. Neuropharmacology. 2017;119:123–33.
38. Sankar SB, Donegan RK, Shah KJ, Reddi AR, Wood LB. Heme and hemoglobin suppress amyloid β-mediated inflammatory activation of mouse astrocytes. J Biol Chem. 2018; https://doi.org/10.1074/jbc.RA117.001050.
39. Ranganathan PV, Jayakumar C, Mohamed R, Dong Z, Ramesh G. Netrin-1 regulates the inflammatory response of neutrophils and macrophages, and suppresses ischemic acute kidney injury by inhibiting COX-2-mediated PGE2 production. Kidney Int. 2013;83:1087–98.
40. Ranganathan PV, Jayakumar C, Ramesh G. Netrin-1-treated macrophages protect the kidney against ischemia-reperfusion injury and suppress inflammation by inducing M2 polarization. Am J Physiol Renal Physiol. 2013; 304:F948–57.
41. Cuartero MI, Ballesteros I, Moraga A, Nombela F, Vivancos J, Hamilton JA, Corbí ÁL, Lizasoain I, Moro MA. N2 neutrophils, novel players in brain inflammation after stroke: modulation by the PPARγ agonist rosiglitazone. Stroke. 2013;44:3498–508.
42. Xia P, Pan Y, Zhang F, Wang N, Wang E, Guo Q, Ye Z. Pioglitazone confers neuroprotection against ischemia-induced pyroptosis due to its inhibitory effects on HMGB-1/RAGE and Rac1/ROS pathway by activating PPAR. Cell Physiol Biochem. 2018;45:2351–68.

43. Tsuchiya A, Hayashi T, Deguchi K, Sehara Y, Yamashita T, Zhang H, Lukic V, Nagai M, Kamiya T, Abe K. Expression of netrin-1 and its receptors DCC and neogenin in rat brain after ischemia. Brain Res. 2007;1159:1–7.
44. Bayat M, Baluchnejadmojarad T, Roghani M, Goshadrou F, Ronaghi A, Mehdizadeh M. Netrin-1 improves spatial memory and synaptic plasticity impairment following global ischemia in the rat. Brain Res. 2012;1452:185–94.
45. Lu H, Wang Y, He X, Yuan F, Lin X, Xie B, Tang G, Huang J, Tang Y, Jin K, et al. Netrin-1 hyperexpression in mouse brain promotes angiogenesis and long-term neurological recovery after transient focal ischemia. Stroke. 2012; 43:838–43.
46. Lu H, Song X, Wang F, Wang G, Wu Y, Wang Q, Wang Y, Yang GY, Zhang Z. Hyperexpressed netrin-1 promoted neural stem cells migration in mice after focal cerebral ischemia. Front Cell Neurosci. 2016;10:223.
47. He X, Li Y, Lu H, Zhang Z, Wang Y, Yang GY. Netrin-1 overexpression promotes white matter repairing and remodeling after focal cerebral ischemia in mice. J Cereb Blood Flow Metab. 2013;33:1921–7.
48. Liddelow SA, Guttenplan KA, Clarke LE, Bennett FC, Bohlen CJ, Schirmer L, Bennett ML, Munch AE, Chung WS, Peterson TC, et al. Neurotoxic reactive astrocytes are induced by activated microglia. Nature. 2017;541:481–7.
49. Barreto GE, Sun X, Xu L, Giffard RG. Astrocyte proliferation following stroke in the mouse depends on distance from the infarct. PLoS One. 2011;6:e27881.

3

Macrophages in trigeminal ganglion contribute to ectopic mechanical hypersensitivity following inferior alveolar nerve injury in rats

Dulguun Batbold[1], Masamichi Shinoda[2*], Kuniya Honda[2], Akihiko Furukawa[3], Momoko Koizumi[4], Ryuta Akasaka[3], Satoshi Yamaguchi[1] and Koichi Iwata[2]

Abstract

Background: Accidental mandibular nerve injury may occur during tooth extraction or implant procedures, causing ectopic orofacial pain. The exact mechanisms underlying ectopic orofacial pain following mandibular nerve injury is still unknown. Here, we investigated the role of macrophages and tumor necrosis factor alpha (TNFα) in the trigeminal ganglion (TG) in ectopic orofacial pain following inferior alveolar nerve transection (IANX).

Methods: IANX was performed and the mechanical head-withdrawal threshold (MHWT) in the whisker pad skin ipsilateral to IANX was measured for 15 days. Expression of Iba1 in the TG was examined on day 3 after IANX, and the MHWT in the whisker pad skin ipsilateral to IANX was measured following successive intra-ganglion administration of the macrophage depletion agent liposomal clodronate Clophosome-A (LCCA). TNFα expression in the TG and the MHWT in the whisker pad skin ipsilateral to IANX following successive intra-ganglion administration of the TNFα blocker etanercept were measured on day 3 after IANX, and tumor necrosis factor receptor-1 (TNFR1) immunoreactive (IR) cells in the TG were analyzed immunohistochemically on day 3.

Results: The MHWT in the whisker pad skin was significantly decreased for 15 days, and the number of Iba1-IR cells was significantly increased in the TG on day 3 after IANX. Successive intra-ganglion administration of the macrophage depletion agent LCCA significantly reduced the increased number of Iba1-IR cells in the TG and reversed the IANX-induced decrease in MHWT in the whisker pad skin. TNFα expression was increased in the TG on day 3 after IANX and was reduced following successive intra-ganglion administration of the TNFα inhibitor etanercept. The decreased MHWT was also recovered by etanercept administration, and TNFR1-IR cells in the TG were increased on day 3 following IANX.

Conclusions: These findings suggest that signaling cascades resulting from the production of TNFα by infiltrated macrophages in the TG contributes to the development of ectopic mechanical allodynia in whisker pad skin following IANX.

Keywords: Trigeminal ganglion, Tumor necrosis factor alpha, Macrophage, Ectopic orofacial pain, Inferior alveolar nerve transection, Mechanical allodynia

* Correspondence: shinoda.masamichi@nihon-u.ac.jp
[2]Department of Physiology, School of Dentistry, Nihon University, 1-8-13 Kandasurugadai, Chiyoda-ku, Tokyo 101-8310, Japan
Full list of author information is available at the end of the article

Background

There are several causes of orofacial neuropathic pain, including accidental nerve injury or compression of the trigeminal nerve during dental treatments such as dental implant surgery and tooth extractions or facial trauma [1–3]. The orofacial pain may occasionally spread to intact orofacial regions, and clinicians struggle to alleviate the symptoms of ectopic orofacial pain. However, the detailed mechanisms of ectopic neuropathic pain are not fully understood.

Previous studies have indicated that pathological changes in the intra-trigeminal ganglion (TG) signaling mechanisms following trigeminal nerve injury are involved in the development of ectopic orofacial neuropathic pain. For example, nitric oxide released from the injured TG neurons and satellite glial activation via connexin 43 signaling modulates the excitability of intact TG neurons following inferior alveolar nerve injury (IANX) [4, 5]. Recently, immune cells that are infiltrated following peripheral nerve injury have been shown to play an important and diverse role in pathological neuronal changes. Sciatic nerve transection induces macrophage proliferation around axotomized dorsal root ganglion neurons and contributes to the regeneration of transected afferent nerve fibers [6–8]. Furthermore, sciatic nerve injury-induced macrophage invasion into the injured site and injury-induced mechanical and thermal hypersensitivity was abolished by macrophage depletion [9, 10]. The infiltration of activated macrophages into the dorsal root ganglion results in the development of behavioral hypersensitivity in rats which induced chemotherapy-induced peripheral neuropathy [11].

Tumor necrosis factor alpha (TNFα) is well known as a proinflammatory cytokine involved in the development and maintenance of neuropathic pain. Increased TNFα was observed in the injured region in a model of sciatic nerve injury-induced mechanical and thermal hyperalgesia, and inhibition of TNFα synthesis abolished the hyperalgesia [12]. Activated macrophages are known to produce and release TNFα [13]. These results suggest that TNFα production by infiltrating macrophages may be involved in pain hypersensitivity following peripheral nerve injury.

Therefore, we hypothesized that the proliferation of activated macrophages in the TG contributes to the development of orofacial ectopic neuropathic pain following inferior alveolar nerve transection (IANX). In this study, we examined the relation between mechanical allodynia following IANX with the infiltration of macrophages into the TG and elucidated their functional roles in the development of ectopic orofacial neuropathic pain.

Methods

Animals

We used male Sprague-Dawley rats ($n = 101$, Japan SLC, Shizuoka, Japan) weighing 170–260 g. All rats were housed individually in transparent polycarbonate cages (length 48 cm; width 26.5 cm; height 21 cm) with paper shavings as bedding. The room temperature was controlled (23 °C) with a 12 h light/dark cycle (lights on at 7:00, off at 19:00), and animals were allowed ad libitum access to food and water. All experiments were performed according to the National Institutes of Health Guide for the Care and Use of Laboratory Animals and the guidelines of the International Association for the Study of Pain [14]. This study was approved by the Animal Experimentation Committee at Nihon University (AP16D010).

Inferior alveolar nerve transection

IANX was performed as described previously under deep anesthesia with intraperitoneal (i.p.) butorphanol (2.5 mg/kg, Meiji Seika Pharma, Tokyo, Japan), medetomidine (0.375 mg/kg, Zenoaq, Fukushima, Japan), and midazolam (2.0 mg/kg, Sandoz, Tokyo, Japan) [15]. Briefly, a small incision was made in the skin of the left cheek, and the masseter muscle was dissected to expose the mandibular bone surface. The surface of the mandible was scraped using a low-speed dental drill bur to expose the inferior alveolar nerve. The exposed inferior alveolar nerve was gently pulled, transected, and replaced into the mandibular canal. In the control group, the skin incision, muscle dissection, and bone scraping without IANX were performed (sham operation). The dissected muscle and skin incision were sutured with 6-0 silk.

Measuring mechanical sensitivity of the whisker pad skin

Rats were trained daily for 5 to 7 days to protrude their snout from a cage that had a small fenestration and to withdraw their snout freely following application of mechanical stimuli to the whisker pad skin by von Frey filaments (Touch-Test Sensory Evaluator, North Coast Medical, Morgan Hill, CA) as described previously [4]. After stabilizing the mechanical head-withdrawal threshold (MHWT), IANX or sham operation was performed and followed by behavioral testing under the same conditions every other day for 15 days. The MHWT was determined as the lowest intensity that evoked head-withdrawal responses to five stimuli (duration 1 s). The behavioral testing was conducted under blinded conditions.

Intra-TG administration of Clophosome-A and etanercept

Under deep anesthesia with i.p. butorphanol (2.5 mg/kg), medetomidine (0.375 mg/kg), and midazolam (2.0 mg/kg), a head of rat was placed in a stereotaxic instrument for guidance [4, 16]. The skull was exposed and a small hole (1 mm in diameter) was drilled above the location of the TG (2.8 mm anterior from the posterior fontanelle, 2.7 mm lateral to the sagittal suture) ipsilateral to the location of IANX or sham operation. A guide cannula was extended in the TG (9 mm below the skull surface) and was anchored to the skull bone with dental cement and three stainless-steel screws. To confirm the correct positioning of the tip of the cannula, a trocar was inserted into the cannula as an electrode and multi-unit activities induced by mechanical stimulation of the whisker pad skin were conformed. After implantation of the cannula, rats were allowed to recover for 5 days before performing the IANX or sham operation. Under light anesthesia with 2% isoflurane in oxygen, liposomal clodronate Clophosome-A (LCCA, 6 μl, 7 mg/mL, product code: F70101CA, FormuMax Scientific, Sunnyvale, CA, USA) or plain control liposomes for LCCA (Cont-LCCA, 6 μl, 20 mM, product code: F70101-A, FormuMax Scientific) were administered into the TG through the guide cannula prior to operation and on days 1 to 4 following IANX or sham operation. LCCA has been shown to be effective in successfully depleting proliferated and resident macrophages [17]. Etanercept (1 μg; Pfizer, New York, NY, USA) was dissolved in physiological saline or vehicle alone (physiological saline) and administered (6 μl) into the TG through the guide cannula under light anesthesia with 2% isoflurane in oxygen prior to operation and on days 1 to 4 following IANX or sham operation. The LCCA and etanercept administration were performed immediately after the measurement of the MHWT of whisker pad skin. The MHWT of the whisker pad skin was measured before operation and every other day for 5 days after IANX or sham operation.

Moreover, rats were allowed to recover after implantation of the cannula for 5 days. Under light anesthesia with 2% isoflurane in oxygen, 2 μl of 1,1′-dioctadecyl-3,3,3′,3-tetramethylindocarbocyanine methanesulfonate (DiI, Thermo Fisher Scientific, Waltham, MA) was administered into the TG through the guide cannula. On day 3 after the administration, rats were deeply anesthetized with the above-described solution and transcardially perfused with saline followed by a fixative containing 4% paraformaldehyde in 0.1 M phosphate buffer (PB; pH 7.4). After the perfusion, TGs were removed and immersed in a fixative containing 4% paraformaldehyde for more than 4 h at 4 °C then transferred to 0.01 M phosphate-buffered saline (PBS) for 12 h for cryoprotection. TG from naive rat was also processed in a similar manner. Next, the tissues were embedded in Tissue-Tek (Sakura Finetechnical, Tokyo, Japan) and were cut in 12-μm-thick sections in a horizontal plane along the long axis.

Immunohistochemistry

Under deep anesthesia with i.p. butorphanol (2.5 mg/kg), medetomidine (0.375 mg/kg), and midazolam (2.0 mg/kg), a retrograde labeling tracer, FluoroGold (7 μl dissolved in saline; FG; 4% hydroxystilbamidine; Fluorochrome, Denver, CO, USA), was injected into the skin of the left whisker pad ipsilateral to IANX using a 30-gauge needle before performing the IANX or sham operation. On day 3, rats were deeply anesthetized with the above-described solution and transcardially perfused with saline followed by a fixative containing 4% paraformaldehyde in 0.1 M phosphate buffer (PB; pH 7.4). After the perfusion, TGs were removed and immersed in the same fixative for more than 4 h at 4 °C then transferred to 0.01 M PBS containing 20% sucrose for 12 h for cryoprotection. Next, the tissues were embedded in Tissue-Tek and stored at − 20 °C until cryosectioning. Then, the ganglion tissues were cut in 12-μm-thick sections in a horizontal plane along the long axis. Every 10th section (five sections per rat) was thaw-mounted on a MAS-GP slide glass (Matsunami, Osaka, Japan) and dried overnight at room temperature. The five sections were used for immunohistological analysis. After rinsing with 0.01 M PBS three times for 5 min each, sections were incubated in mouse anti-Iba1 polyclonal antibody (1:200; Abcam, Cambridge, MA, USA) and rabbit anti-TNFα monoclonal antibody (1:200; Abcam) or rabbit anti-glial fibrillary acidic protein (GFAP) polyclonal antibody (1:500; cat.No. ab7260, Abcam) or rabbit anti-F4/80 monoclonal antibody (1:500; cat.No. ab111101, Abcam), or anti-tumor necrosis factor receptor-1 (TNFR1) monoclonal antibody (1:50; Santa Cruz, Santa Cruz, CA, USA), diluted in 0.01 M PBS containing 4% normal donkey serum (Merck, Darmstadt, Germany) in 0.3% Triton X-100 (Merck) overnight at 4 °C. After rinsing with 0.01 M PBS, the sections were incubated in Alexa Fluor 568 anti-rabbit IgG (1:200; Thermo Fisher Scientific) and/or Alexa Fluor 488 anti-mouse IgG (1:200; Thermo Fisher Scientific) in 0.01 M PBS for 2 h at room temperature. After rinsing with 0.01 M PBS, sections were coverslipped in PermaFluor (Thermo Fisher Scientific). The sections were observed using a BZ-9000 system (Keyence, Osaka, Japan). Iba1-IR and TNFα-IR cells in the TGs of the ophthalmic-maxillary division (V1-V2) and mandibular division (V3) were analyzed. The mean relative area (density) of Iba1-IR or TNFα-IR cells were calculated by using a computer-assisted imaging analysis system (ImageJ, NIH, Bethesda, MD, USA). The mean relative area (density) of F4/80- and Iba1-IR area was calculated by using a computer-assisted imaging analysis system (BZ-X analyzer, Keyence, Osaka, Japan). All immunohistochemical measurements were conducted under blinded conditions, performed by observers who were unaware of which treatment the animals received. Using the same conditions, no specific labeling was observed in the absence of primary antibody. Measurement of the area occupied by the immuno-products was made in a region selected identically from V1/V2 and V3 in the TG.

Western blotting

On day 3 following IANX or sham operation, the rats were perfused through the aorta with physiological saline under deep anesthesia as described above. Immediately, the TG was removed and homogenized in ice-cold lysis buffer (137 mM NaCl; 20 mM Tris-HCL, pH 8.0; 1% NP40; 10% glycerol; 1 mM phenylmethylsulfonyl fluoride; 10 μg/ml aprotinin; 1 g/ml leupeptin; 0.05 mM sodium vanadate). The homogenate was centrifuged at 15,000 rpm for 10 min at 4 °C, and the protein concentration of the resulting supernatants was determined using a protein assay kit (Bio-Rad, Hercules, CA, USA). The supernatants were heat-denatured in Laemmli sample buffer solution (Bio-Rad), and 30 μg of each protein sample was subjected to SDS-PAGE using a 10% acrylamide gel. The samples were transferred to a polyvinylidene difluoride membrane (Trans-Blot Turbo Transfer Pack, Bio-Rad) using Trans-Blot Turbo (Bio-Rad). The membrane was rinsed with Tris-buffered saline mixed with 0.1% Tween 20 (TBST) and incubated in 3% bovine serum albumin (BSA; Bovogen, Essendon, Australia). The membrane was then incubated with rabbit anti-TNFα polyclonal antibody (1:200; diluted in TBST and 3% BSA, Abcam) or rabbit anti-Iba1 monoclonal antibody (1:1000; diluted in TBST and 3% BSA, cat.No. ab178847, Abcam) overnight at 4 °C. Next, it was incubated with horseradish peroxidase-conjugated donkey anti-rabbit antibody (Cell Signaling, Danvers, MA, USA) for 2 h at room temperature. Antibody binding was detected using Western Lightning ELC Pro (PerkinElmer, Waltham, MA, USA). Band intensity was analyzed using a ChemiDoc MP system (Bio-Rad) and normalized to β-actin on blots re-probed with the anti-β-actin antibody (1:200; Santa Cruz) after removing bound protein using a stripping reagent (Thermo Scientific).

Statistical analysis

Data were expressed as mean ± standard error. Statistical analyses were performed by Student's *t* test, one-way analysis of variance (ANOVA) with Tukey's multiple-comparison test, and two-way ANOVA with repeated measures followed by Bonferroni's multiple-comparison test where appropriate. A value of $p < 0.05$ was defined as statistically significant.

Results

Mechanical allodynia and Iba1 expression in TG following IANX

The MHWT of the whisker pad skin ipsilateral to IANX was significantly decreased on day 1 following IANX, and this decrease persisted until day 15 when compared with sham-operated animals (Fig. 1a). On day 3 following IANX, Iba1-IR cells were observed in V1/V2 FG-labeled neurons, as well as in V3, in which FG-labeled neurons were absent (Fig. 1b, c). The relative area of Iba1-IR cells in V1/V2 and V3 in TG ipsilateral to IANX was significantly increased on day 3 following IANX compared to that of the sham-operated group (Fig. 1d). The Iba1 protein level was increased in TG ipsilateral to IANX on day 3 following IANX compared to sham-operated animals (Fig. 1e).

Effect of intra-TG LCCA administration on mechanical allodynia and Iba1 expression following IANX

Primarily, it was confirmed that drug administration into the TG through the guide cannula was accurate (Fig. 2a). Daily administration of LCCA into the TG prevented the development and progress of mechanical allodynia in the whisker pad skin ipsilateral to IANX from days 1 to 5 following IANX (Fig. 2b). On day 3 after IANX, Iba1-IR cells in V1/V2, in which FG-labeled neurons were abundant, were observed in the LCCA- and Cont-LCCA-treated groups (Fig. 2c). Moreover, the relative area of Iba1-IR cells in the LCCA-treated group was significantly lower compared to the group treated with Cont-LCCA (Fig. 2d). Before intra-TG LCCA and Cont-LCCA administration, it was confirmed that the guide cannula implantation did not change the mechanical sensitivity (data not shown).

TNFα expression in TG following IANX

TNFα was expressed in activated Iba1-IR cells presented with morphological characteristics such as the bigger cell bodies and thicker ramifications and in activated GFAP-IR cells in V1/V2 on day 3 in the IANX group rather than sham group (Fig. 3a). F4/80 immunoreactivity was observed in the Iba1-IR cells in V1/V2 on day 3 in IANX or sham groups, and the relative F4/80-IR area in the Iba1-IR area was decreased in V1/V2 ipsilateral to IANX compared to that of the sham-operated group (Fig. 3b). The relative area of TNFα immuno-products increased in V1/V2 ipsilateral to IANX compared to that of the sham-operated group (Fig. 3c, d). The TNFα protein level was also increased in TG ipsilateral to IANX on day 3 following IANX compared to naive and sham-operated animals (Fig. 3e). Daily LCCA administration significantly reduced the relative area of TNFα immuno-products in V1/V2 in TG on day 3 following IANX compared to the Cont-LCCA-treated IANX group or sham group (Fig. 4a, b).

Effect of intra-TG etanercept administration in TG on mechanical allodynia following IANX

Daily administration of etanercept into the ipsilateral TG prevented mechanical hypersensitivity in whisker

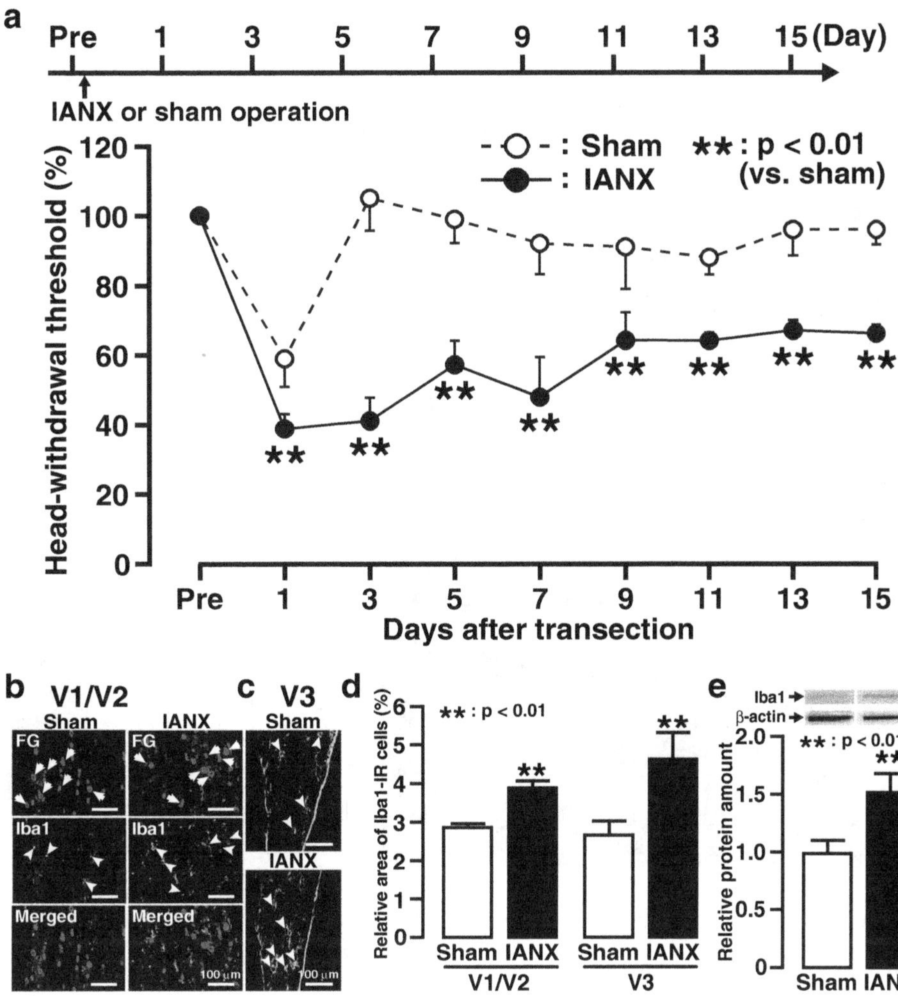

Fig. 1 Mechanical allodynia and Iba1 expression in the TG following IANX. **a** The timing of IANX or sham operation (upper) and the changes in MHWT of the ipsilateral whisker pad skin for 15 days following IANX or sham operation (lower). The MHWT was normalized to the pre-IANX MHWT (100%). Error bars indicate SEM. $^{**}p < 0.01$ vs. sham ($n = 6$ in each; two-way ANOVA with repeated measures followed by Bonferroni's multiple-comparison test). Iba1-IR cells in V1/V2 (**b**) and V3 (**c**) in the ipsilateral TG on day 3 following IANX or sham operation. Arrows indicate FG-labeled neurons. Arrowheads indicate Iba1-IR cells. **d** The relative area of Iba1-IR cells in V1/V2 and V3 in TG on day 3 following IANX and sham operation. Error bars indicate SEM. $^{**}p < 0.01$ vs. sham. ($n = 5$ in each, Student's *t* test). **e** The relative amount of Iba1 protein in TG on day 3 following IANX or sham operation. Error bars indicate SEM. $^{*}p < 0.05$ vs. sham ($n = 10$ in each, Student's *t* test)

pad skin ipsilateral to IANX from days 1 to 5 (Fig. 5a). Immunostaining was performed to examine TNFR1 expression in the TG on day 3 following IANX. TNFR1 expression was observed in FG-labeled neurons, and the mean percentage of FG-labeled TNFR1-IR neurons in TG ipsilateral to IANX was significantly increased compared to the sham-operated group (Fig. 5b).

Discussion

Traumatic injury to the inferior alveolar nerve, which can occur during extraction of an impacted mandibular third molar or mandibular plastic surgery, occasionally causes ectopic pain hypersensitivity in widespread orofacial areas such as the forehead and maxillary regions [1]. In this study, IANX produced long-lasting mechanical allodynia in ipsilateral whisker pad skin, as reported in our previous studies [4, 15, 18]. The long-lasting mechanical allodynia observed in the IANX model mimics ectopic pain hypersensitivity in patients with a history of traumatic injury to the inferior alveolar nerve, indicating that this model may be useful for research into the mechanisms of ectopic orofacial neuropathic pain.

Iba1 expression is known to be widely used as a specific macrophage marker [19]. IANX induced extensive macrophage infiltration in not only V3 but also in V1/V2 and increased Iba1 expression in the ipsilateral TG. Moreover, the infiltrated macrophages showed the bigger cell bodies and thicker ramifications, which

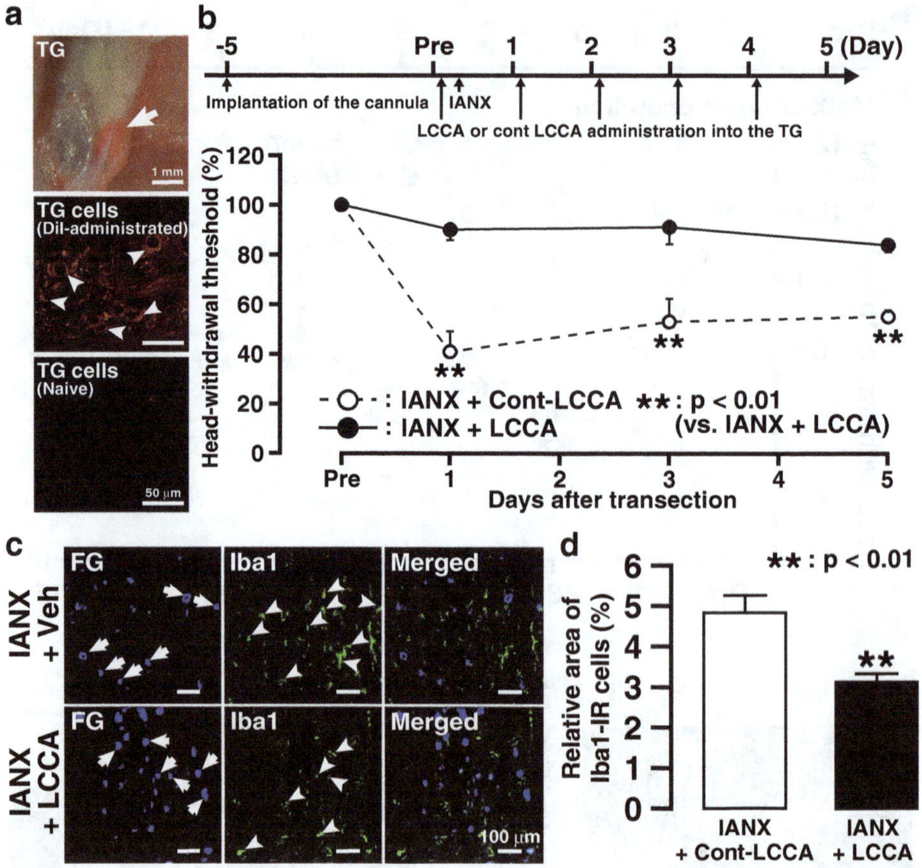

Fig. 2 Effect of intra-TG LCCA administration on mechanical allodynia and Iba1 expression following IANX. **a** Photograph (upper) and photomicrograph (middle) of TG on day 3 following DiI administration into the TG through the guide cannula and photomicrograph (lower) of TG in naive rat. Arrows indicate DiI labeling. **b** The timing of the cannula implantation, LCCA, or Cont-LCCA administration into the TG, IANX, or sham operation (upper) and the changes in MHWT of the ipsilateral whisker pad skin following daily intra-TG LCCA or Cont-LCCA administration following IANX (lower). The MHWT was normalized to the pre-IANX MHWT (100%). Arrows indicate the timing of intra-TG LCCA or Cont-LCCA administration. Error bars indicate SEM. $^{**}p < 0.01$ vs. sham ($n = 6$ in each; two-way ANOVA with repeated measures followed by Bonferroni's multiple-comparison test). **c** Iba1-IR cells and FG-labeled TG neurons in V1/V2 on day 3 following intra-TG LCCA or Cont-LCCA administration in IANX rats. Arrows indicate FG-labeled neurons. Arrowheads indicate Iba1-IR cells. **d** The relative area of Iba1-IR cells in V1/V2 in TG on day 3 following intra-TG LCCA or Cont-LCCA administration in IANX rats. Error bars indicate SEM. $^{**}p < 0.01$ vs. sham. ($n = 5$ in each, Student's *t* test)

indicates their activation [20]. Previous studies have shown that nerve injury increases resident and proliferated macrophages in the sensory ganglion [21–23]. The chemokine C-C motif ligand 2 (CCL2), also referred to as monocyte chemoattractant protein 1, is released from injured neurons and activates the C-C chemokine receptor type 2 (CCR2) in macrophages, which induces macrophage activation and proliferation in the dorsal root ganglion (DRG) following peripheral nerve injury [8, 24]. Moreover, CCL2 hyper-expression and macrophage infiltration in the DRG, induced by peripheral nerve injury, is reduced in Toll-like receptor 2 (TLR2) knock-out mice [25]. Based on these results, we hypothesize that the extensive infiltration of activated macrophages in the TG ipsilateral to IANX observed here was induced by CCL2 released from injured neurons via TLR2 signaling. F4/80 expression is known to be used as tissue-resident macrophage marker [26, 27]. The relative F4/80-IR area in the Iba1-IR area in TG was decreased following IANX in this study, suggesting that the proliferation of the activated macrophages in TG ipsilateral to IANX is mainly caused by exogenous macrophage infiltration into the TG.

The proliferation of activated macrophages was observed in the TG ipsilateral to IANX, and these activated macrophages expressed TNFα. IANX significantly increased TNFα expression in the ipsilateral TG, and macrophage depletion in the TG significantly suppressed the increase in TNFα expression. Macrophages are believed to be the major source of TNFα in the sensory ganglion following peripheral nerve injury [28, 29]. Intracellular signaling cascades such as p38 mitogen-activated protein kinase (MAPK) and extracellular signal-regulated kinase (ERK) cascades result in

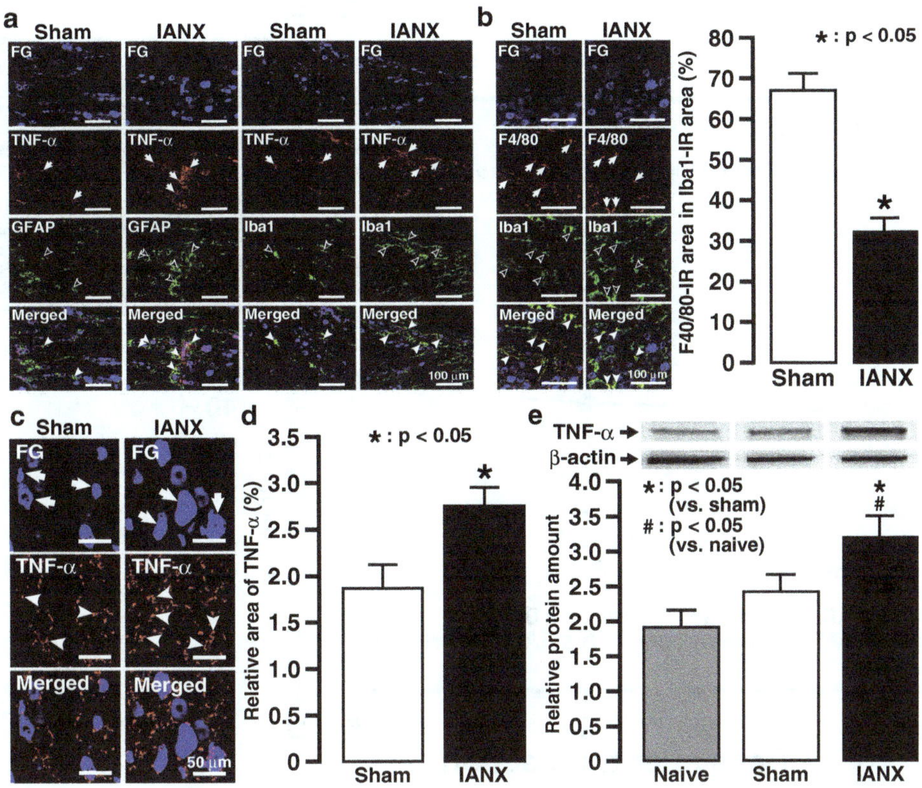

Fig. 3 TNFα expression in TG following IANX. **a** TNFα expression in the Iba1-IR cells or the GFAP-IR cells in ipsilateral TG on day 3 following IANX or sham operation. Arrows indicate TNFα-IR cells, open arrowheads indicate GFAP-IR cells or Iba1-IR cells, and close arrowheads indicate TNFα- and GFAP-IR cells or TNFα- and Iba1-IR cells. **b** F4/80 expression in the Iba1-IR cells in ipsilateral TG on day 3 following IANX or sham operation (left). Arrows indicate F4/80 expression in Iba1-IR cells, open arrowheads indicate Iba1-IR cells, and close arrowheads indicate F4/80- and Iba1-IR cells. The relative area of F4/80 immuno-products in Iba1-IR cells in the TG on day 3 following IANX or sham operation (right). Error bars indicate SEM. ***$p < 0.001$ vs. sham. ($n = 5$ in each, Student's t test). **c** TNFα expression in ipsilateral TG on day 3 following IANX or sham operation. Arrows indicate FG-labeled neurons. Arrowheads indicate TNFα immuno-products. **d** The relative area of TNFα immuno-products in the TG on day 3 following IANX or sham operation. Error bars indicate SEM. *$p < 0.05$ vs. sham ($n = 5$ in each, Student's t test). **e** The relative amount of TNFα protein in TG in naive animals or on day 3 following IANX or sham operation. Error bars indicate SEM. *$p < 0.05$ vs. sham. #$p < 0.05$ vs. naive ($n = 5$ in each, one-way ANOVA with Tukey's multiple-comparison test)

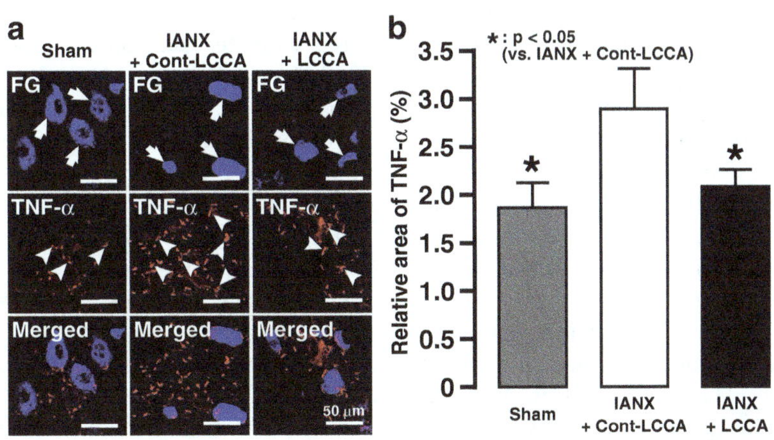

Fig. 4 Changes in TNFα expression in TG following LCCA administration following IANX. **a** TNFα expressed in V1/V2 in the TG on day 3 following intra-TG LCCA or Cont-LCCA administration in IANX rats or in sham-operated rats. Arrows indicate FG-labeled neurons. Arrowheads indicate TNFα immuno-products. **b** Changes in the relative area of TNF-α immuno-products in the TG on day 3 following intra-TG LCCA or Cont-LCCA administration in IANX rats or in sham-operated rats. Error bars indicate SEM. *$p < 0.05$ vs. Cont-LCCA. ($n = 5$ in each, one-way ANOVA with Tukey's multiple-comparison test)

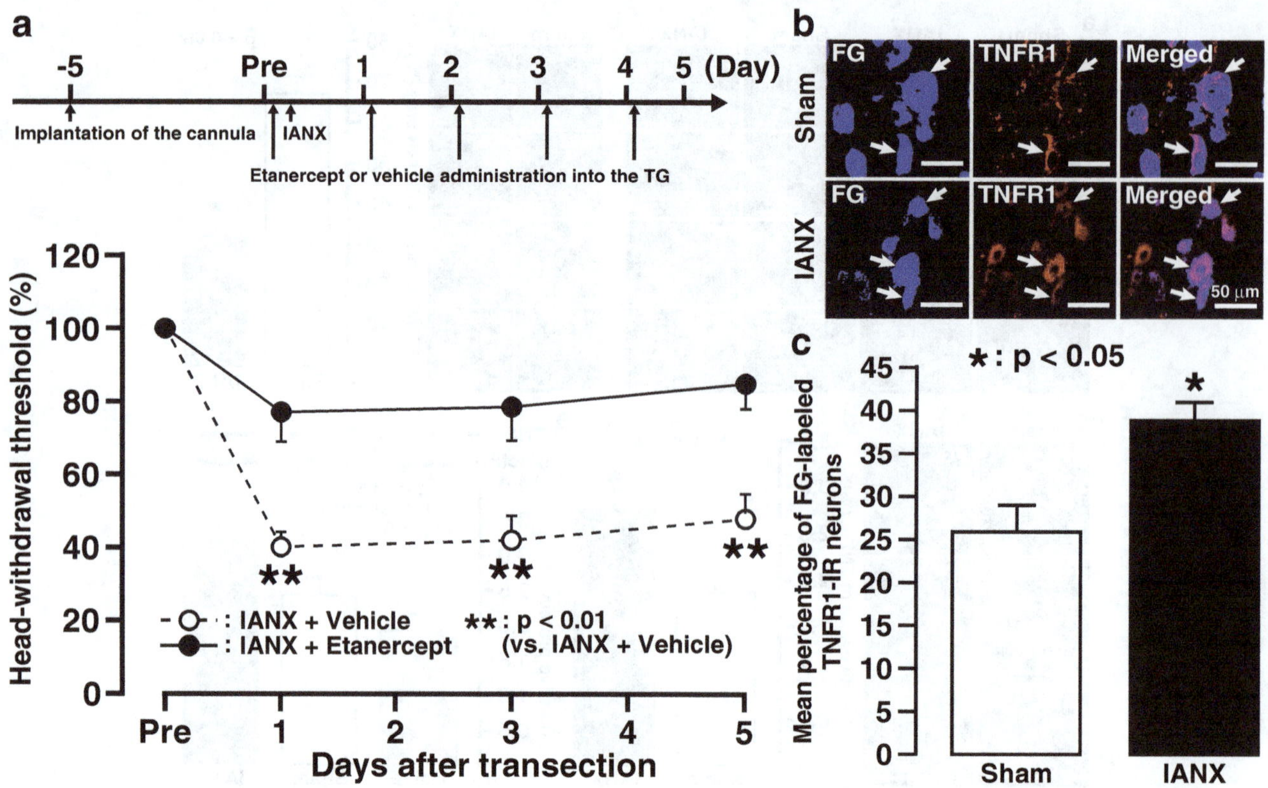

Fig. 5 Effect of intra-TG etanercept administration on mechanical allodynia following IANX. **a** The timing of the cannula implantation, etanercept, or vehicle administration into the TG, IANX, or sham operation (upper) and changes in MHWT of the ipsilateral whisker pad skin by daily etanercept administration into TG following IANX (lower). The MHWT was normalized to the pre-IANX MHWT (100%). Arrows indicate the timing of intra-TG etanercept or vehicle administration. Error bars indicate SEM. **$p < 0.01$ vs. IANX + vehicle ($n = 6$ in each; two-way ANOVA with repeated measures followed by Bonferroni's multiple-comparison test). **b** TNFR1 immunoreactivity in ipsilateral TG on day 3 following IANX or in sham-operated rats. Arrows indicate FG-labeled TNFR1-IR neurons. **c** Changes in the mean percentage of FG-labeled TNFR1-IR neurons on day 3 following IANX. Error bars indicate SEM. *$p < 0.05$ vs. sham ($n = 5$ in each, Student's *t* test)

macrophage activation and TNFα release [30]. The expression of substance P (SP), which is a member of the tachykinin family and a major mediator of neuroimmunomodulation, was found to be enhanced in the sensory ganglion neurons, and SP was released in the early stages after peripheral nerve injury [31]. Neurokinin 1 receptor which is activated by SP is present in macrophage, SP modulates diverse functions of macrophages, and SP signaling activates the ERK 1/2 and p38 MAPK cascades [32–34]. Moreover, the activation of the p38 MAPK cascade and the ensuing TNFα production are induced in macrophages infiltrating into the nerve-injured site [35]. Previous studies have reported that TNFα levels in DRG increased following peripheral nerve injury [36, 37]. Taken together, these results suggest that SP released from TG neurons is transmitted to macrophages, resulting in macrophage activation and TNFα release from activated macrophages via the ERK 1/2 and p38 MAPK signaling cascades. Furthermore, GFAP immunoreactivity which is a marker of the activated satellite glial cells was observed in the TG ipsilateral to IANX, and these activated satellite glial cells also expressed TNFα. Our previous report also indicates that activation of satellite glial cells in the TG was induced after IANX [4], suggesting that the activated satellite glial cells might be another source of TNFα in the TG after IANX. Further studies are needed.

In this study, TNFR1 expression in TG neurons innervating the whisker pad skin and the increase of TNFα in V1/V2 in the TG were observed following IANX. The continuous suppression of TNFα signaling and macrophage depletion in the TG prevented the development and progress of mechanical allodynia in the whisker pad skin ipsilateral to IANX. It was reported that intra-DRG administration of exogenous TNFα depolarizes DRG neurons and increases their neuronal excitability [38]. TNFα signaling in uninjured DRG neurons mediates the activation of voltage-gated sodium channels (Nav) in a dose-dependent manner by upregulating current densities of tetrodotoxin (TTX)-sensitive and TTX-resistant Nav 1.3 and Nav 1.8 in the neurons via p38 MAPK cascade following peripheral nerve injury [36, 39, 40].

TNFα also increases membrane potassium ion conductance in a non-voltage-gated fashion, resulting in the enhancement of neuronal excitability [41, 42]. We have previously reported that satellite glial cells are activated throughout the TG via gap junctions following IANX [4]. Adenosine triphosphate was released from sensory neurons following peripheral nerve injury, and TNFα was released from activated satellite glial cells through $P2X_7$ signaling [43, 44]. Based on the existing reports, this study suggests that TNFα released from proliferated macrophages or satellite glial cells binds to TNFR1 in TG neurons, and TNFα-TNFR1 signaling might contribute to the enhancement of TG neuronal excitability, resulting in mechanical allodynia in the whisker pad skin following IANX, whereas IANX significantly increased TNFα expression in not only the activated macrophages but also in the satellite cells other than the activated macrophages in TG. Some reports indicated that peripheral nerve injury induced TNFα hyper-expression in the satellite cells in DRG, suggesting that TNFα released from the satellite cells following IANX also modulates mechanical sensitivity in the whisker pad skin which occurs as a result of TG neuronal excitability [45, 46].

TNFR1 expression in TG neurons innervating the whisker pad skin was significantly increased following IANX, and neutralizing TNFR1 attenuated thermal and mechanical allodynia following peripheral nerve injury [47]. Moreover, TNFR1 knockout mice do not develop mechanical allodynia induced by peripheral nerve injury [36]. Though these reports indicate that TNFR1 signaling plays a pivotal role in the development of mechanical allodynia and contributor to the enhancement of TNFR1 expression in TG neurons innervating the whisker pad skin following IANX, the detailed mechanism remains to be elucidated.

Conclusions

The signaling cascades induced by TNFα released from infiltrated macrophages in the TG contribute to the development of orofacial neuropathic ectopic pain following IANX. Therefore, TNFα signaling in the TG should be considered as one of the primary targets in the modulation and treatment of ectopic orofacial pain attributed to peripheral trigeminal nerve injury.

Abbreviations

ANOVA: Analysis of variance; BSA: Bovine serum albumin; CCL2: Chemokine C-C motif ligand 2; CCR2: C-C chemokine receptor type 2; Cont-LCCA: Plain control liposomes for LCCA; DRG: Dorsal root ganglion; ERK: Extracellular signal-regulated kinase; FG: FluoroGold; i.p.: Intraperitoneal; IANX: Inferior alveolar nerve transection; IR: Immunoreactive; LCCA: Liposomal clodronate Clophosome-A; MAPK: Mitogen-activated protein kinase; MHWT: Mechanical head-withdrawal threshold; Nav: Voltage-gated sodium channels; PB: Phosphate buffer; PBS: Phosphate-buffered saline; SP: Substance P; TBST: Tris-buffered saline mixed with 0.1% Tween 20; TG: Trigeminal ganglion; TLR2: Toll-like receptor 2; TNFR1: Tumor necrosis factor receptor-1; TNFα: Tumor necrosis factor alpha; TTX: Tetrodotoxin; V1-V2: Ophthalmic-maxillary division; V3: Mandibular division

Acknowledgements

This study was supported in part by research grants from Sato and Uemura Funds from the Nihon University School of Dentistry, a grant from the Dental Research Center in Nihon University School of Dentistry, KAKENHI (Grant-in-Aid for Challenging Exploratory Research 15K15748), Nihon University Multidisciplinary Research Grant for (2016 and 2017), and MEXT-Supported Program for the Strategic Research Foundation at Private Universities 2013–2017.

Authors' contributions

All authors discussed the results and commented on the manuscript. DB, AF, MK, RA, and SY performed experiments and manuscript editing. MS and KI performed results analysis and wrote the manuscript. KH performed results analysis and generation of figures. MS was responsible for the study concept and design, results analysis, and manuscript writing. All authors read and approved the final manuscript.

Consent for publication

Not applicable.

Competing interests

The authors declare that they have no competing interests.

Author details

[1]Department of Oral and Maxillofacial Surgery, Graduate School of Medical and Dental Sciences, Tokyo Medical and Dental University, 1-5-45 Yushima, Bunkyo-ku, Tokyo 113-8549, Japan. [2]Department of Physiology, School of Dentistry, Nihon University, 1-8-13 Kandasurugadai, Chiyoda-ku, Tokyo 101-8310, Japan. [3]Department of Clinical Medicine, School of Dentistry, Nihon University, 1-8-13 Kandasurugadai, Chiyoda-ku, Tokyo 101-8310, Japan. [4]Department of Dentistry, Jikei University School of Medicine, 3-25-8 Nishi-Shimbashi, Minato-ku, Tokyo 105-8461, Japan.

References

1. Renton T, Yilmaz Z, Gaballah K. Evaluation of trigeminal nerve injuries in relation to third molar surgery in a prospective patient cohort. Recommendations for prevention. Int J Oral Maxillofac Surg. 2012;41:1509–18.
2. Khawaja N, Renton T. Case studies on implant removal influencing the resolution of inferior alveolar nerve injury. Br Dent J. 2009;206:365–70.
3. Lin CS, SY W, Huang HY, et al. Systematic review and meta-analysis on incidence of altered sensation of mandibular implant surgery. PLoS One. 2016;11:e0154082.
4. Kaji K, Shinoda M, Honda K, et al. Connexin 43 contributes to ectopic orofacial pain following inferior alveolar nerve injury. Mol Pain. 2016;12: doi:10.1177/1744806916633704.
5. Sugiyama T, Shinoda M, Watase T, et al. Nitric oxide signaling contributes to ectopic orofacial neuropathic pain. J Dent Res. 2013;92:1113–7.
6. Gensel JC, Nakamura S, Guan Z, et al. Macrophages promote axon regeneration with concurrent neurotoxicity. J Neurosci. 2009;29:3956–68.
7. Kwon MJ, Kim J, Shin H, et al. Contribution of macrophages to enhanced regenerative capacity of dorsal root ganglia sensory neurons by conditioning injury. J Neurosci. 2013;33:15095–108.
8. Kwon MJ, Shin HY, Cui Y, et al. CCL2 mediates neuron-macrophage interactions to drive proregenerative macrophage activation following preconditioning injury. J Neurosci. 2015;35:15934–47.
9. Liu T, van Rooijen N, Tracey DJ. Depletion of macrophages reduces axonal degeneration and hyperalgesia following nerve injury. Pain. 2000;86:25–32.
10. Kobayashi Y, Kiguchi N, Fukazawa Y, et al. Macrophage-T cell interactions mediate neuropathic pain through the glucocorticoid-induced tumor necrosis factor ligand system. J Biol Chem. 2015;290:12603–13.

11. Zhang H, Li Y, de Carvalho-Barbosa M, et al. Dorsal root ganglion infiltration by macrophages contributes to paclitaxel chemotherapy-induced peripheral neuropathy. J Pain. 2016;17:775–86.
12. George A, Marziniak M, Schafers M, et al. Thalidomide treatment in chronic constrictive neuropathy decreases endoneurial tumor necrosis factor-alpha, increases interleukin-10 and has long-term effects on spinal cord dorsal horn met-enkephalin. Pain. 2000;88:267–75.
13. Pang M, Yuan Y, Wang D, et al. Recombinant CC16 protein inhibits the production of pro-inflammatory cytokines via NF-kappaB and p38 MAPK pathways in LPS-activated RAW264.7 macrophages. Acta Biochim Biophys Sin Shanghai. 2017;49:435–43.
14. Zimmermann M. Ethical guidelines for investigations of experimental pain in conscious animals. Pain. 1983;16:109–10.
15. Iwata K, Imai T, Tsuboi Y, et al. Alteration of medullary dorsal horn neuronal activity following inferior alveolar nerve transection in rats. J Neurophysiol. 2001;86:2868–77.
16. Katagiri A, Shinoda M, Honda K, et al. Satellite glial cell P2Y12 receptor in the trigeminal ganglion is involved in lingual neuropathic pain mechanisms in rats. Mol Pain. 2012;8:23.
17. Van Rooijen N, Sanders A. Liposome mediated depletion of macrophages: mechanism of action, preparation of liposomes and applications. J Immunol Methods. 1994;174:83–93.
18. Okada-Ogawa A, Nakaya Y, Imamura Y, et al. Involvement of medullary GABAergic system in extraterritorial neuropathic pain mechanisms associated with inferior alveolar nerve transection. Exp Neurol. 2015;267:42–52.
19. Ohsawa K, Imai Y, Kanazawa H, et al. Involvement of Iba1 in membrane ruffling and phagocytosis of macrophages/microglia. J Cell Sci. 2000;113(Pt 17):3073–84.
20. Harvey LD, Yin Y, Attarwala IY, et al. Administration of DHA reduces endoplasmic reticulum stress-associated inflammation and alters microglial or macrophage activation in traumatic brain injury. ASN Neuro. 2015;7(6): doi:10.1177/1759091415618969.
21. Donegan M, Kernisant M, Cua C, et al. Satellite glial cell proliferation in the trigeminal ganglia after chronic constriction injury of the infraorbital nerve. Glia. 2013;61:2000–8.
22. Komori T, Morikawa Y, Inada T, et al. Site-specific subtypes of macrophages recruited after peripheral nerve injury. Neuroreport. 2011;22:911–7.
23. Lu X, Richardson PM. Responses of macrophages in rat dorsal root ganglia following peripheral nerve injury. J Neurocytol. 1993;22:334–41.
24. Abbadie C, Lindia JA, Cumiskey AM, et al. Impaired neuropathic pain responses in mice lacking the chemokine receptor CCR2. Proc Natl Acad Sci U S A. 2003;100:7947–52.
25. Kim D, You B, Lim H, et al. Toll-like receptor 2 contributes to chemokine gene expression and macrophage infiltration in the dorsal root ganglia after peripheral nerve injury. Mol Pain. 2011;7:74.
26. Mass E, Ballesteros I, Farlik M, et al. Specification of tissue-resident macrophages during organogenesis. Science. 2016;353(6304):aaf4238.
27. Hashimoto D, Chow A, Noizat C, et al. Tissue-resident macrophages self-maintain locally throughout adult life with minimal contribution from circulating monocytes. Immunity. 2013;38:792–804.
28. Raghavendra V, Tanga F, Rutkowski MD, et al. Anti-hyperalgesic and morphine-sparing actions of propentofylline following peripheral nerve injury in rats: mechanistic implications of spinal glia and proinflammatory cytokines. Pain. 2003;104:655–64.
29. Wagner R, Myers RR. Endoneurial injection of TNF-alpha produces neuropathic pain behaviors. Neuroreport. 1996;7:2897–901.
30. Wang CL, CY L, Pi CC, et al. Extracellular polysaccharides produced by Ganoderma formosanum stimulate macrophage activation via multiple pattern-recognition receptors. BMC Complement Altern Med. 2012;12:119.
31. Fu C, Yin Z, Yu D, et al. Substance P and calcitonin gene-related peptide expression in dorsal root ganglia in sciatic nerve injury rats. Neural Regen Res. 2013;8:3124–30.
32. Sun J, Ramnath RD, Zhi L, et al. Substance P enhances NF-kappaB transactivation and chemokine response in murine macrophages via ERK1/2 and p38 MAPK signaling pathways. Am J Physiol Cell Physiol. 2008;294: C1586–96.
33. Matsumoto K, Nakajima T, Sakai H, et al. Increased expression of 5-HT3 and NK 1 receptors in 5-fluorouracil-induced mucositis in mouse jejunum. Dig Dis Sci. 2013;58:3440–51.
34. Bardelli C, Gunella G, Varsaldi F, et al. Expression of functional NK1 receptors in human alveolar macrophages: superoxide anion production, cytokine release and involvement of NF-kappaB pathway. Br J Pharmacol. 2005;145:385–96.
35. Nomura H, Furuta A, Tanaka Y, et al. Forced retraction of spinal root injury enhances activation of p38 MAPK cascade in infiltrating macrophages. Neuropathology. 2005;25:37–47.
36. Chen X, Pang RP, Shen KF, et al. TNF-alpha enhances the currents of voltage gated sodium channels in uninjured dorsal root ganglion neurons following motor nerve injury. Exp Neurol. 2011;227:279–86.
37. Miao P, Madec K, Gong Y, et al. Axotomy-induced up-regulation of tumor necrosis factor-alpha in the dorsal root ganglia. Neurol Res. 2008;30:623–31.
38. Schafers M, Lee DH, Brors D, et al. Increased sensitivity of injured and adjacent uninjured rat primary sensory neurons to exogenous tumor necrosis factor-alpha after spinal nerve ligation. J Neurosci. 2003;23:3028–38.
39. He XH, Zang Y, Chen X, et al. TNF-alpha contributes to up-regulation of Nav1.3 and Nav1.8 in DRG neurons following motor fiber injury. Pain. 2010; 151:266–79.
40. Jin X, Gereau RW. Acute p38-mediated modulation of tetrodotoxin-resistant sodium channels in mouse sensory neurons by tumor necrosis factor-alpha. J Neurosci. 2006;26:246–55.
41. Czeschik JC, Hagenacker T, Schafers M, et al. TNF-alpha differentially modulates ion channels of nociceptive neurons. Neurosci Lett. 2008;434:293–8.
42. Leo M, Argalski S, Schafers M, et al. Modulation of voltage-gated sodium channels by activation of tumor necrosis factor receptor-1 and receptor-2 in small DRG neurons of rats. Mediat Inflamm. 2015;2015:124942.
43. Kanno T, Yaguchi T, Nishizaki T. Noradrenaline stimulates ATP release from DRG neurons by targeting beta(3) adrenoceptors as a factor of neuropathic pain. J Cell Physiol. 2010;224:345–51.
44. Zhang X, Chen Y, Wang C, et al. Neuronal somatic ATP release triggers neuron-satellite glial cell communication in dorsal root ganglia. Proc Natl Acad Sci U S A. 2007;104:9864–9.
45. Dubovy P, Jancalek R, Klusakova I, et al. Intra- and extraneuronal changes of immunofluorescence staining for TNF-alpha and TNFR1 in the dorsal root ganglia of rat peripheral neuropathic pain models. Cell Mol Neurobiol. 2006; 26:1205–17.
46. Hatashita S, Sekiguchi M, Kobayashi H, et al. Contralateral neuropathic pain and neuropathology in dorsal root ganglion and spinal cord following hemilateral nerve injury in rats. Spine (Phila Pa 1976). 2008;33:1344–51.
47. Sommer C, Schmidt C, George A. Hyperalgesia in experimental neuropathy is dependent on the TNF receptor 1. Exp Neurol. 1998;151:138–42.

4

Inflammation and blood-brain barrier breach remote from the primary injury following neurotrauma

Nicole M. Smith[1], Marcus K. Giacci[2], Alexander Gough[2], Charlotte Bailey[1], Terence McGonigle[3], Anna M. B. Black[3], Thomas O. Clarke[3], Carole A. Bartlett[2,3], K. Swaminathan Iyer[1], Sarah A. Dunlop[2] and Melinda Fitzgerald[2,3,4*]

Abstract

Background: Following injury to the central nervous system, increased microglia, secretion of pro- and anti-inflammatory cytokines, and altered blood-brain barrier permeability, a hallmark of degeneration, are observed at and immediately adjacent to the injury site. However, few studies investigate how regions remote from the primary injury could also suffer from inflammation and secondary degeneration.

Methods: Adult female Piebald-Viral-Glaxo (PVG) rats underwent partial transection of the right optic nerve, with normal, age-matched, unoperated animals as controls. Perfusion-fixed brains and right optic nerves were harvested for immunohistochemical assessment of inflammatory markers and blood-brain barrier integrity; fresh-frozen brains were used for multiplex cytokine analysis.

Results: Immediately ventral to the optic nerve injury, immunointensity of both the pro-inflammatory biomarker inducible nitric oxide synthase (iNOS) and the anti-inflammatory biomarker arginase-1 (Arg1) increased at 7 days post-injury, with colocalization of iNOS and Arg1 immunoreactivity within individual cells. CD11b+ and CD45+ cells were increased 7 days post-injury, with altered BBB permeability still evident at this time. In the lower and middle optic tract and superior colliculus, IBA1+ resident microglia were first increased at 3 days; ED1+ and CD11b+ cells were first increased in the middle and upper tract and superior colliculus 7 days post-injury. Increased fibrinogen immunoreactivity indicative of altered BBB permeability was first observed in the contralateral upper tract at 3 days and middle tract at 7 days post-injury. Multiplex cytokine analysis of brain homogenates indicated significant increases in the pro-inflammatory cytokines, IL-2 and TNFα, and anti-inflammatory cytokine IL-10 1 day post-injury, decreasing to control levels at 3 days for TNFα and 7 days for IL-2. IL-10 was significantly elevated at 1 and 7 days post-injury with a dip at 3 days post-injury.

Conclusions: Partial injury to the optic nerve induces a complex remote inflammatory response, characterized by rapidly increased pro- and anti-inflammatory cytokines in brain homogenates, increased numbers of IBA1+ cells throughout the visual pathways, and increased CD11b+ and ED1+ inflammatory cells, particularly towards the synaptic terminals. BBB permeability can increase prior to inflammatory cell infiltration, dependent on the brain region.

Keywords: Neurotrauma, Secondary degeneration, Microglia, Macrophages, Cytokines, Blood-brain barrier

* Correspondence: lindy.fitzgerald@curtin.edu.au
[2]Experimental and Regenerative Neurosciences, School of Biological Sciences, The University of Western Australia, Stirling Hwy, Perth, Western Australia 6009, Australia
[3]Curtin Health Innovation Research Institute, Curtin University, Verdun St, Nedlands, Western Australia, Australia
Full list of author information is available at the end of the article

Background

Following an injury to a white matter tract in the central nervous system (CNS), axons located at the primary injury site are lesioned and degenerate [1]. Neurons and glia spatially separated from the site of initial injury to axons undergo further damage and activation due to secondary degeneration [2]. Inflammation following CNS trauma is responsible for both beneficial and detrimental effects, contributing to secondary damage but also facilitating neurorepair [3]. Activation of resident microglia, secretion of immune mediators such as pro- and anti-inflammatory cytokines/chemokines, and infiltration of blood leukocytes characterize this robust inflammatory response [4]. The release of reactive oxygen species (ROS) is a key pro-inflammatory feature, leading to glial activation and oxidative damage in the tissue surrounding the initial injury site [5] early after injury [6, 7]. Protective anti-inflammatory responses include myelin debris phagocytosis [8, 9] and neurotrophic and growth factor secretion [10]. Astrocyte activation leads to a breach of the blood-brain barrier (BBB), with increased monocyte extravasation [11] and associated increases in Ca^{2+} and oxidative cascades of injury to both axons and glia, further contributing to spreading of degeneration [12].

Because macrophages and microglia are key modulator and effector cells in the immune response, much attention has been devoted to defining the dynamics of pro- and anti-inflammatory effects of trauma-induced inflammation within the linear constraints of microglia/macrophage polarization phenotypes, namely anti-inflammatory "M1" vs pro-inflammatory "M2" [5, 13–17]. The in vivo environment is complex and presents a variety of pro- and anti-inflammatory stimuli simultaneously [18–20]. In fact, recent in vivo studies of inflammation following CNS trauma have highlighted the plasticity of these cells where the same cell population is able to switch between polarization states in response to mediators in their surrounding microenvironment, and yet, others report the concurrent expression of both pro- and anti-inflammatory markers by a single cell [21–24]. These findings suggest a lack of exclusivity in microglia/ macrophage activation states in vivo and indicate that the same cell responsible for promoting neuroinflammation can also release factors that promote wound healing. It is likely that the combination and balance of multiple factors (i.e., glial cells, immune cells, pro- and anti-inflammatory cytokines/ chemokine levels, time elapsed after injury, and lesion magnitude) will lead to different degrees of damage, as has been described in a range of injury models including glaucomatous damage at the optic nerve head, partial optic nerve transection, and spared nerve injury [25–27]. Furthermore, it is increasingly understood that specific monocyte, macrophage, and other glial and endothelial cell-derived cytokines play important roles in maintaining or perturbing BBB permeability, thereby further modulating the injury response [28]. Characterizing the magnitude, timing, and duration of expression of these mediators has the potential to offer mechanistic insight and aid in the development of novel therapeutics.

Despite the plethora of research on trauma-induced inflammation at the site of a primary injury and immediately adjacent, relatively few studies investigate how regions remote from the primary injury site could also suffer from secondary degeneration and inflammation following neurotrauma [29–31]. Clinical studies suggest a link between remote damage and symptomatology, a phenomenon termed "diaschisis," which contributes to functional impairments [32–34]. Previous studies in the spinal cord have shown that remote injury induces substantial changes in microglia and astrocytes, which contribute to central inflammatory responses [35, 36]. In addition, peripheral nerve injury evokes trafficking of immune cells from the circulation into the spinal cord parenchyma [37]. Using our in vivo partial optic nerve transection model of secondary degeneration in adult Piebald-Viral-Glaxo (PVG) female hooded rats, we have previously demonstrated that a remote injury in the CNS (optic nerve) can cause a transient opening of the BBB in the visual pathways of the brain as early as 1 day following injury, with Evans blue fluorescence visible around the optic chiasm, optic tract, lateral geniculate nucleus, and superior colliculus. BBB permeability was maximal at 3 days following injury and decreased to levels not significantly different from uninjured controls at 7 days [38]. An initial analysis of the inflammatory response early (1 day) following injury indicated that ED1 + and IBA1+ microglia/macrophage activation occurred along the length of the injured optic nerve, in the optic chiasm, and adjacent to the cerebral ventricles [38], and earlier studies have shown increases in these cells immediately adjacent to the injury at 3 days [25]. However, a quantitative assessment of a range of inflammatory cell subtypes along the optic tract and into the superior colliculus is lacking. Furthermore, the spatiotemporal relationship between inflammation and blood-brain barrier breach remote to an injury is unknown. Specifically, it is not yet clear whether inflammatory cells that rapidly infiltrated the injury site spread along the optic nerve and tract into the brain, thereby initiating BBB breakdown. Alternative hypotheses include axonal degeneration and compromise of axonal transport initiating remote inflammation and BBB breakdown close to synaptic terminals in the superior colliculus or systemic changes contributing to a widespread inflammatory response. Here, we assess microglia and macrophage dynamics together with indicators of BBB breach and cytokine profiles, at various sites distal to a partial optic nerve transection injury, focusing on identifying the time at which changes are first observed in order to determine in a region-specific manner, whether blood-brain barrier breach precedes inflammation.

Methods

Animal procedures

Adult female PVG hooded rats (160–180 g) were bred at the Animal Resources Centre (Murdoch, WA, Australia), housed under a standard 12-h light/dark cycle and fed standard rat chow and water ad libitum. Procedures adhered to the National Health and Medical Research Council Australian Code of Practice for the care and use of animals for scientific purposes and were approved by the University of Western Australia's Animal Ethics Committee, approval numbers RA3/100/1201, RA3/100/673, and RA3/100/1485. The rats were anesthetized intraperitoneally with a combination of xylazine (Ilium Xylazil, Troy Laboratories, 10 mg/kg) and ketamine (Ketamil, Troy Laboratories, 50 mg/kg), and euthanized with an intraperitoneal injection of Euthal (pentobarbitone sodium 850 mg/kg; phenytoin sodium 125 mg/kg; Virbac).

The partial optic nerve transection procedure was similar to that described previously [25]. Briefly, anesthetized rats were shaved along the skull towards the right eye. Under aseptic conditions, the skin was incised and retracted, and the right optic nerve accessed by deflecting the Harderian lachrymal gland immediately behind the right eye. The nerve parenchyma was exposed about 1 mm behind the eye by making a slit in the dura mater with ophthalmic scissors. A controlled 200-μm cut was made in the dorsum of the right optic nerve using a diamond radial keratotomy knife (Geuder), with the depth determined by the protrusion of the blade beyond a surrounding guard. Care was taken not to stretch the optic nerve or damage major ophthalmic blood vessels. The deflected tissue was replaced, and the skin was sutured with 4/0 non-absorbable silk suture. The eyes were lubricated with Luxyal eye drops, and the rats were placed on a warming blanket for recovery with subcutaneous injections of analgesic (Carprieve, 5 mg kg^{-1} in sterile water, Norbrook Australia, Pty. Ltd.; Victoria, Australia) and sterile PBS (1 ml). No postoperative infections were observed.

The right optic nerves from normal, age-matched, unoperated animals were used as controls, as sham-operated animals have been shown to be not different to normal in terms of a range of relevant cellular and oxidative stress outcomes [25]. Three cohorts of animals were used, with animals within each cohort being randomized into groups reflecting the number of days post-injury, for details see Table 1. In brief, cohort 1 was used for immunohistochemical studies assessing microglia/macrophages in the right optic nerves of animals at 3, 7, and 28 days post-injury and in uninjured controls. For cohort 1, three groups of uninjured controls collected at days 3, 7, and 28 were compared and found to be not different (ANOVA, $p > 0.05$); the 3-day controls were used for statistical comparisons. Cohort 2 was used for BBB analyses in the optic tracts and superior colliculus of animals at 3, 7, 14, and 28 days post-injury and in uninjured controls, assessing the presence of Evans blue dye. Once it was established that no Evans blue dye was visible in the optic tracts and superior colliculus, a subset of cohort 2 was randomly selected for immunohistochemical studies assessing microglia and macrophages as well as fibrinogen and caveolin-1 immunoreactivity with increases being surrogate markers for BBB breach in these brain regions ($n = 5–6$/group). Cohort 3 was used for cytokine analyses in the homogenized brains of animals at 1, 3, and 7 days post-injury and in uninjured controls.

Immunohistochemistry, microscopy and analysis

Animals for BBB analyses (cohort 2) were administered a 2% (*w*/*v*) sterile solution of Evans blue (Sigma, E2129_10G) in PBS (2.8 ml/kg) via tail vein injection 1 h prior to euthanasia. Immediately following euthanasia, the animals for cohorts 1 and 2 (BBB and immunohistochemical assessments) were transcardially perfused-fixed with 0.9% (*w*/*v*) saline followed by 4% (*w*/*v*)

Table 1 Summary of cohorts and numbers of animals per group

	Uninjured	Day 1	Day 3	Day 7	Day 14	Day 28
Cohort 1						
- Microglia/macrophages in the optic nerve	$n = 10$*		$n = 10$	$n = 10$		$n = 10$
Cohort 2						
- BBB analyses	$n = 9–12$ EB		$n = 9–12$ EB	$n = 9–12$ EB	$n = 9–12$ EB	$n = 9–12$ EB
- Microglia/macrophages in the optic tract	$n = 9$	$n = 6$ no EB	$n = 6$	$n = 5–6$	$n = 4–5$	$n = 4$
Cohort 3						
- Cytokines	$n = 8$	$n = 8$	$n = 8$	$n = 8$		

Day is the day after partial optic nerve transection injury. * For cohort 1, three groups of uninjured controls collected at days 3, 7, and 28 were compared and found to be not different ($p \leq 0.05$); the 3-day controls were used for statistical comparisons. EB denotes intravenous injection of Evans blue for the specified animals. Numbers of animals per group are presented as a range if suitable sections were not available for specific brain regions. BBB analyses encompass assessments of Evans blue, caveolin, and fibrinogen immunoreactivity paraformaldehyde (Sigma-Aldrich; St. Louis, Missouri, USA) in 0.1 M phosphate buffer, pH 7.2–7.4. The right optic nerves and brains were harvested and post-fixed in 4% paraformaldehyde for 1 h (nerves) or overnight (brains) and then cryoprotected in 15% sucrose in PBS and stored at 4 °C. The optic nerves were cryosectioned transversely (14 µm thickness), and the brains were cryosectioned coronally (20 µm thickness) and collected onto a series of slides so that each slide had a representative section from each area of interest. Sections for Evans blue analysis were collected onto Superfrost® Plus slides, air dried for an hour, and only briefly rinsed in PBS to reduce leakage of the dye from the sections before mounting using Fluoromount-G (Southern Biotech). The sections for immunohistochemistry were collected onto Superfrost® Plus slides and stored at – 80 °C.

Immunohistochemical analyses were conducted according to the previously described procedures [39]. Primary antibodies used for immunohistochemical assessments of the optic nerves detected inducible nitric oxide synthase (iNOS) (1:400, BD Biosciences, ab3523), Arginase-1 (Arg-1) (1:400, Santa Cruz Biotechnology, sc-18355), CD45 (1:200, BD Pharmingen, 555482), and CD11b (1:400, 553310, BD Pharmingen). Primary antibodies used for immunohistochemical assessments of the brains (optic tracts and superior colliculus) recognized CD45 (1:500, Abcam, ab10558), CD11b (1:300, Sapphire Bioscience, ab2910), ionized calcium-binding adapter molecule 1 (IBA1) (1:1000, Abcam, ab5076), CD68 (ED1) (1:1000, Millipore Corporation, MAB1435), Caveolin-1 (1:400, Sapphire Bioscience, Ab2910), and Fibrinogen (1:500, HiTech Group Australia, A008002). Secondary antibodies were species-specific AlexaFluor 488-, 555-, and 647-conjugated antibodies (1:500, Invitrogen Australia). All tissue sections for a particular immunohistochemical outcome were processed at the same time.

Fluorescence imaging was performed using a Nikon Si1 inverted microscope (Nikon Corporation, Japan) for the right optic nerve and optic tract assessments of microglia and macrophages and a Leitz Diaplan microscope with an Olympus DP70 camera controlled by DP controller (version 2.1.1.183) for superior colliculus; a confocal Nikon C2 mounted on an upright Ni-E microscope, for assessments of BBB integrity (Evans blue fluorescence, fibrinogen, and caveolin-1 immunoreactivity), or for immunohistochemical assessments of microglia and macrophages in the brain (optic tracts and superior colliculus). Images from the Nikon microscopes were captured in a stack of 13 optical slices at 0.5 µm increments along the *z*-axis, obtained from the middle 6 µm of the section, controlled by NIS elements 4.3 software. All images for assessment of each outcome measure were captured at a constant exposure, using consistent microscope settings.

A single section was selected for optic nerves that showed the dorsal injury site and the ventral nerve. The fields of view imaged were located in the ventral portion of the right optic nerve of that section, directly below the dorsal primary injury site. The intensities of iNOS and Arg-1 immunoreactivity were assessed on the single central optical slice most in focus from the relevant 13 image z-stack. Mean fluorescence intensities were quantified on the whole image of ventral optic nerve and were normalized by subtracting the average of three randomly selected background regions of interest per animal. The numbers of CD45+ and CD11b+ cells were assessed within similar regions of interest. This non-stereological technique does not allow for an estimate of total cell numbers within the nerve but does allow for comparative assessment between time points after injury. Similarly for the brains, assessments of the numbers of CD45+, CD11b+, IBA1+, and ED1+ cells were conducted in single visual slices from images of single sections capturing either the lower, middle, or upper regions of both the ipsilateral and contralateral optic tracts and at the rostral end of the superior colliculus for each animal (Fig. 1). While sampling of more than one section may have been preferable, the brain regions of interest were often only clearly present in one section per slide. The optic tract is relatively small and was only apparent in one section per region of interest per slide along the rostrocaudal plane. Similarly, the optic nerve injury site, and therefore the ventral region directly under the injury, is only clearly apparent in one or two sections per slide. Not all markers were assessed for all regions at all time points; analyses were based on identifying the first time at which significant increases were observed and at times were constrained by the availability of sections containing the precise region of interest (e.g., superior colliculus at day 1). The numbers of positively stained cells within each field of view were expressed per unit area. Assessments of Evans blue fluorescence were conducted qualitatively, scanning multiple sections of the right optic nerves and regions throughout the brain including optic tracts, ventricles, choroid plexus, and the superior colliculus and applying a score to fluorescence; representative images are shown. Caveolin-1 immunoreactivity of endothelial cells lining the ventricles in the brain was quantified by measuring the length of immunoreactive cells expressed as a percentage of the total length of the lining of the ventricle that was visible in the single image used for analysis; the choice of section for imaging was based upon ventricle size and shape to ensure consistency of the region of analysis for all animals. Assessment of fibrinogen immunofluorescence was performed throughout the optic tracts, on single central visual slices from the relevant 13 image z-stack. Fibrinogen was quantified as mean fluorescent intensity and the area above the threshold as a percentage of the total area of interest. Threshold values were

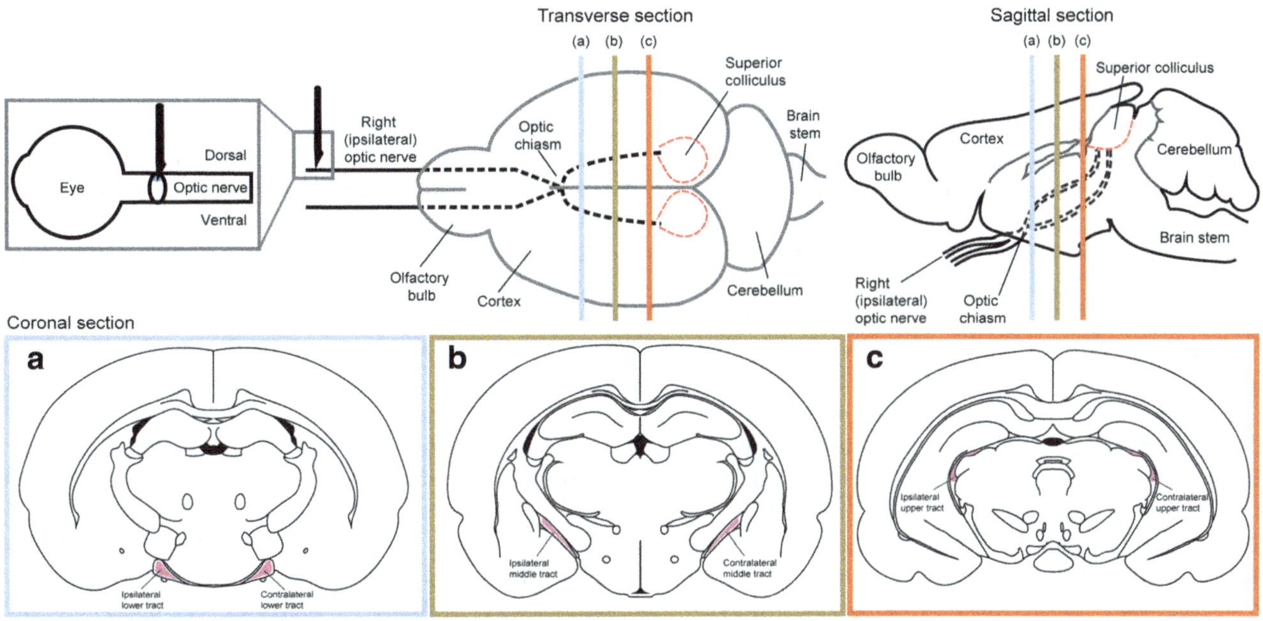

Fig. 1 Schematic overview of the regions of interest used for quantification of the inflammatory response following partial injury to the optic nerve. The ventral aspect of the optic nerve (gray box) was used to quantify Arg1 and iNOS immunoreactivity and CD11b and CD45 cell density. The lower (blue box), middle (yellow box), and upper (red box) tracts were used to quantify the density of CD11b-, IBA1-, ED1-, CD45-, and CD11b/IBA1/ED1-positive cells

normalized to the background of each image by dividing the average of three random background measurements by the average background of a control image then multiplying the original threshold value by this transformation factor. Average intensities above the threshold were normalized by subtracting the background from the mean fluorescence intensity.

Cytokine measurements—multiplex assay

Rats from cohort 3 ($n = 8$ per group) were euthanized and transcardially perfused with ice-cold 0.9% saline, after which the brains were harvested, washed with ice-cold PBS, and homogenized in ice-cold RIPA buffer (Sigma Aldrich) supplemented with 1× protease inhibitor cocktail (Sigma Aldrich) (10 ml). Brain homogenates were incubated on ice for 20 min to aid protein solubilization, after which they were centrifuged at 12000*g* for 20 min at 4 °C, and the lysates were stored at − 80 °C until use. Total protein concentration of the brain lysates from each animal was determined using the Pierce BCA Protein Assay Kit (Thermo Fisher Scientific Pty Ltd.) according to the manufacturer's instructions.

The concentration of ten cytokines (GM-CSF, Interleukin (IL)-12, Interferon (IFN)-γ, IL-1α, IL-1β, IL-2, IL-4, IL-6, IL-10, tumor necrosis factor (TNF)-α) in brain lysates was determined using the Cytokine Rat Magnetic 10-Plex Panel kit (Life Technologies) according to the manufacturer's instructions using the Luminex® 200™ system (CMCA). Briefly, brain lysates were thawed, clarified by centrifugation (1000*g* for 10 min at 4 °C), and standardized at 500 μg/ml protein using assay diluent provided in the Rat Cytokine 10-Plex kit. Lyophilized cytokine standards (Rat Cytokine 10-Plex kit) were reconstituted in assay diluent (Rat Cytokine 10-Plex kit), and 1:3 serial dilutions were performed with assay diluent as instructed (Rat Cytokine 10-Plex kit) to give seven standard solutions. Colored magnetic beads conjugated with cytokine antibodies (Rat Cytokine 10-Plex kit) were reconstituted in 1× wash solution (Rat Cytokine 10-Plex kit) to give a 1× antibody bead solution, which was then pipetted into 80 wells of a 96-well plate (25 μl/well). The antibody beads were washed twice with 1× wash solution (200 μl/well). Following washing, prepared incubation buffer (Rat Cytokine 10-Plex kit) was added to each of the 80 wells (50 μl/well). Seven cytokine standard solutions were added in duplicate to wells designated for standards (100 ul/well), assay diluent was added in duplicate to wells designated for blanks (100 μl/well), and the 32 brain lysate samples from each animal (500 μg/ml) were added in duplicate to wells designated for samples (50 μl of sample + 50 μl of assay diluent), following which the plate was incubated at room temperature on a shaking platform (2 h) to enable cytokines to bind to their respective antibody beads. Following incubation, the wells were washed twice with 1× wash solution (200 μl/well), and subsequently, a 1× biotinylated antibody solution (Rat Cytokine 10-Plex kit) containing a mixture of biotinylated antibodies against each cytokine was added to each of the 80 wells (100 μl/well) and incubated at room temperature on a shaking platform (1 h). Following incubation, the wells were washed twice with 1× wash solution (200 μl/well), and subsequently, a 1× streptavidin-phycoerythrin solution (Rat Cytokine 10-Plex kit) was added to each of the 80 wells (100 μl/well) and incubated at room temperature on a shaking platform (30 min). Following incubation, the wells were washed thrice with 1× wash solution (200 μl/well) and stored in 1× wash solution (125 μl/well) overnight at 4 °C. The following day, working wash solution was decanted, and fresh 1× working wash solution was added (125 μl/well). The plate was then placed on a shaking platform (3 min) and inserted into an XY platform on the Luminex® 200™ system (CMCA) to measure cytokine concentrations for each sample calculated against the standard curve. Each well was sampled using a volume of 75 μl and a bead count of 100 per analyte before advancing to the next well.

Data analysis and statistics

Data are presented as mean ± standard error of mean. Statistical analyses of activated microglia and macrophage densities, Arg1 and iNOS immunointensities, and caveolin-1 and fibrinogen immunoreactivity were performed on SPSS (IBM) software, using one-way ANOVA or two-way ANOVAs to compare regions at a particular time point. For two-way ANOVAs, overall *p*, *F*, and df values are provided, with *p*, *F*, and df values provided for subsets where significance was reached. Tukey post hoc tests were used for optic nerve data and Sidak post hoc tests for optic tract data. If Levene's test indicated inequality of variances, data were log or square root transformed for two-way ANOVAs or Games-Howell post hoc tests employed for one-way ANOVAs. Post hoc *p* values were provided where significance was reached using ANOVAs. Statistical analyses of cytokine data were performed on GraphPad Prism 6 software using

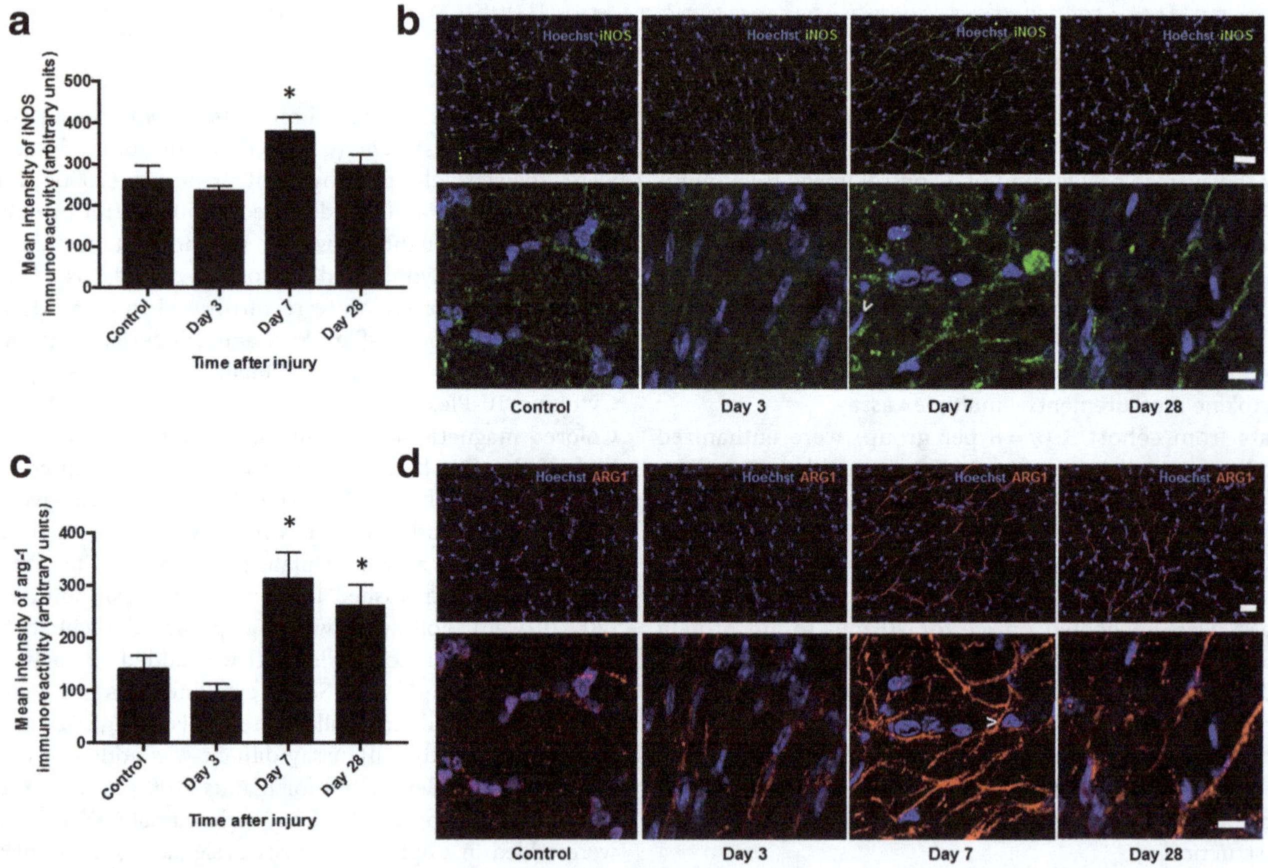

Fig. 2 Semi-quantification of iNOS and Arg1 immunoreactivity in ventral ON vulnerable to secondary degeneration. Mean ± SEM fluorescence intensity of **a** iNOS and **c** Arg1 in the control optic nerve and at 3, 7, and 28 days following partial optic nerve transection, in ventral optic nerve vulnerable to secondary degeneration are shown. * indicates significantly different from normal ($p \le 0.05$), $n = 10$/group. Representative low- and high-magnification images of **b** iNOS and **d** Arg1 in the ventral aspect of the optic nerve are shown in control uninjured, 3, 7, and 28 days after injury. Examples of iNOS- and Arg1-positive cells are indicated by ">." Scale bar of **b** and **d**: 40 μm top images and 10 μm bottom images for each

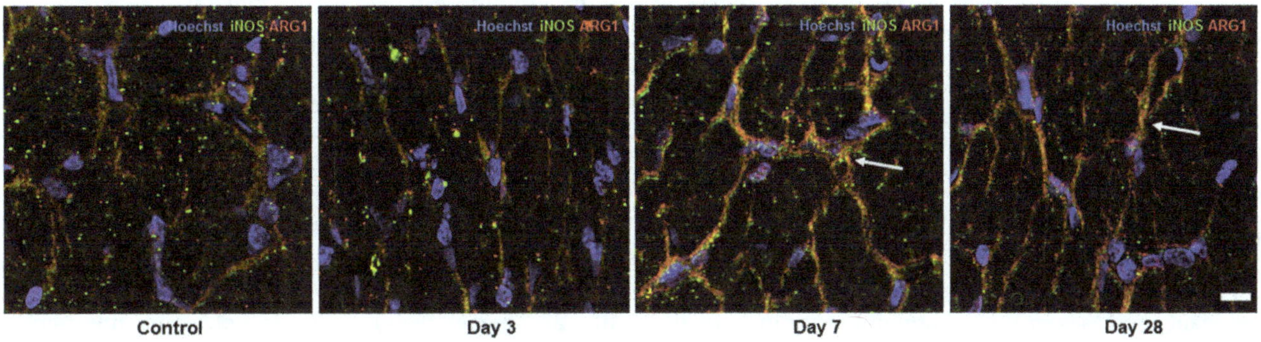

Fig. 3 Representative images of iNOS and Arg-1 colocalization in ventral ON vulnerable to secondary degeneration. iNOS+/Arg1+cells are yellow and indicated by white arrows, particularly apparent 7 and 28 days after injury to the optic nerve, $n = 6$/group. Scale bar: 10 μm

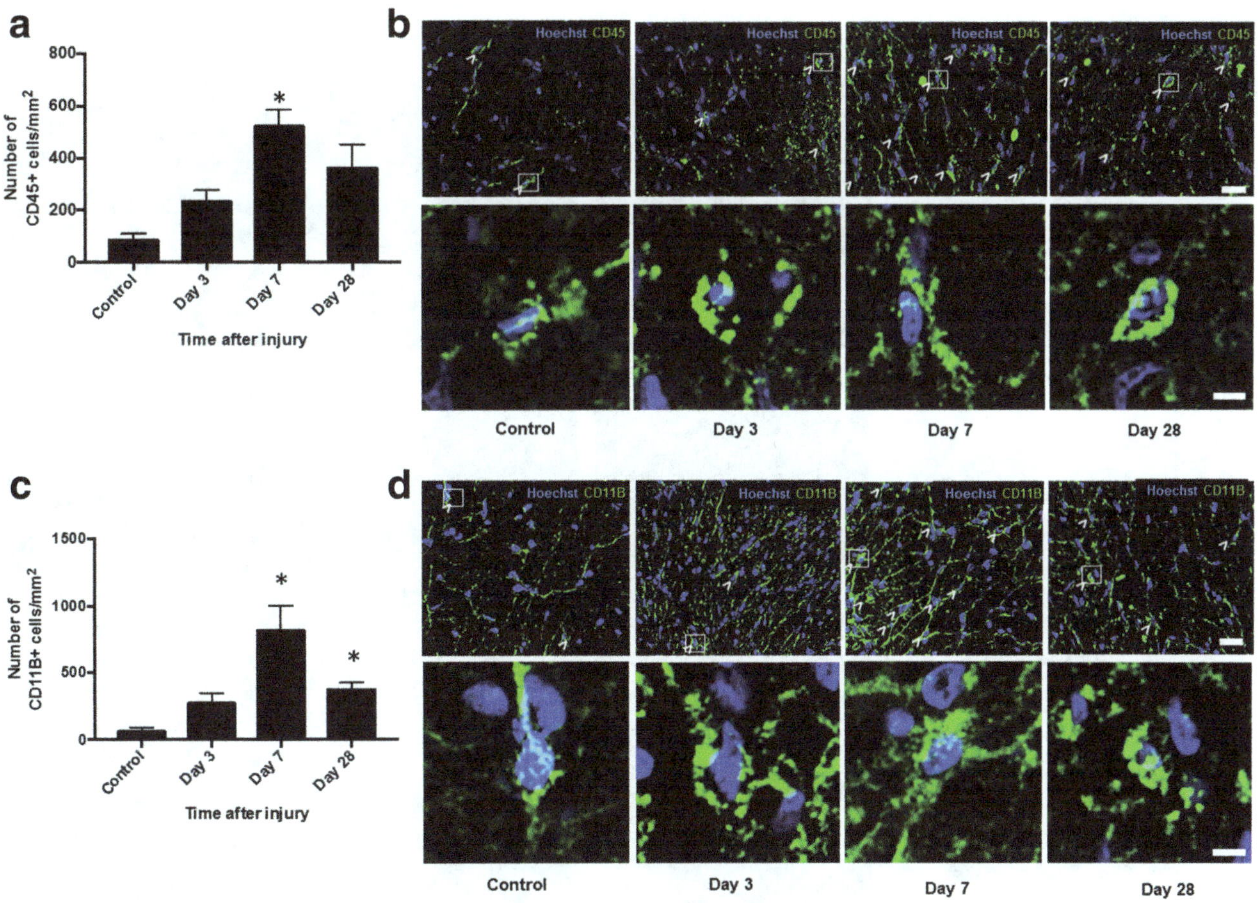

Fig. 4 Quantification of CD11B+ and CD45+ cells in ventral ON vulnerable to secondary degeneration. Mean ± SEM numbers of **a** CD45+ and **c** CD11b+ cells in control, uninjured optic nerve and at 3, 7, and 28 days following partial optic nerve transection, in ventral optic nerve vulnerable to secondary degeneration are shown. * indicates significantly different from normal ($p \leq 0.05$), $n = 6$/group. Representative low- and high-magnification images of **b** CD45 and **d** CD11b in the ventral aspect of the optic nerve are shown in control uninjured, 3, 7, and 28 days after injury. Examples of CD45+ and CD11b+ cells, boxed cells at low magnification, are shown in high magnification. Scale bar of **b** and **d**: 20 μm top images and 3 μm bottom images for each

one-way ANOVA to compare means of $n = 8$ animals at each time point, conducted individually for each cytokine, using Tukey post hoc tests.

Results

Inflammatory responses in optic nerve immediately adjacent to the primary injury

Semi-quantitative assessment 3, 7, and 28 days after injury in the ventral portion of the right optic nerve directly below the dorsal primary injury site revealed significant increases in the immunointensity of both the pro-inflammatory biomarker inducible nitric oxide synthase (iNOS) (Fig. 2a, b) and anti-inflammatory biomarker arginase-1 (Arg-1) (Fig. 2c, d) at 7 days ($p \leq 0.05$, $F = 5.04$, df = 38 and $p \leq 0.05$, $F = 7.41$, df = 38, respectively). Immunointensity of iNOS returned to control levels 28 days after injury ($p > 0.05$), while arg-1 remained elevated ($p \leq 0.05$). Contrary to the microglia/macrophage "polarization" phenotype previously described [40], we demonstrate colocalization of iNOS and Arg1 immunoreactivity within individual cells, evident 7 and 28 days after injury (Fig. 3).

The numbers of cells expressing CD11b (complement 3 receptor) a constitutive marker of leukocytes and CD45 which is expressed on all nucleated hematopoietic cells was assessed in the ventral portion of the right optic nerve. Quantification of CD45+ and CD11b+ microglia and macrophages demonstrated significant increases in the numbers of both CD45+ and CD11b+ cells 7 days after injury ($p \leq 0.05$, $F = 4.74$, df = 23 and $p \leq 0.05$, $F = 9.15$, df = 23, respectively) (Fig. 4a, c). The numbers of CD11b+ cells remained significantly higher than in uninjured controls at 28 days post-injury ($p \leq 0.05$) (Fig. 4c, d), whereas CD45+ cells returned to levels not different from control at this time point ($p > 0.05$) (Fig. 4a, b).

Inflammatory cell responses in the brain

Changes in densities of inflammatory cell populations were assessed in the lower, middle, and upper optic tracts (i.e., progressing from juxta-chiasmal = lower;

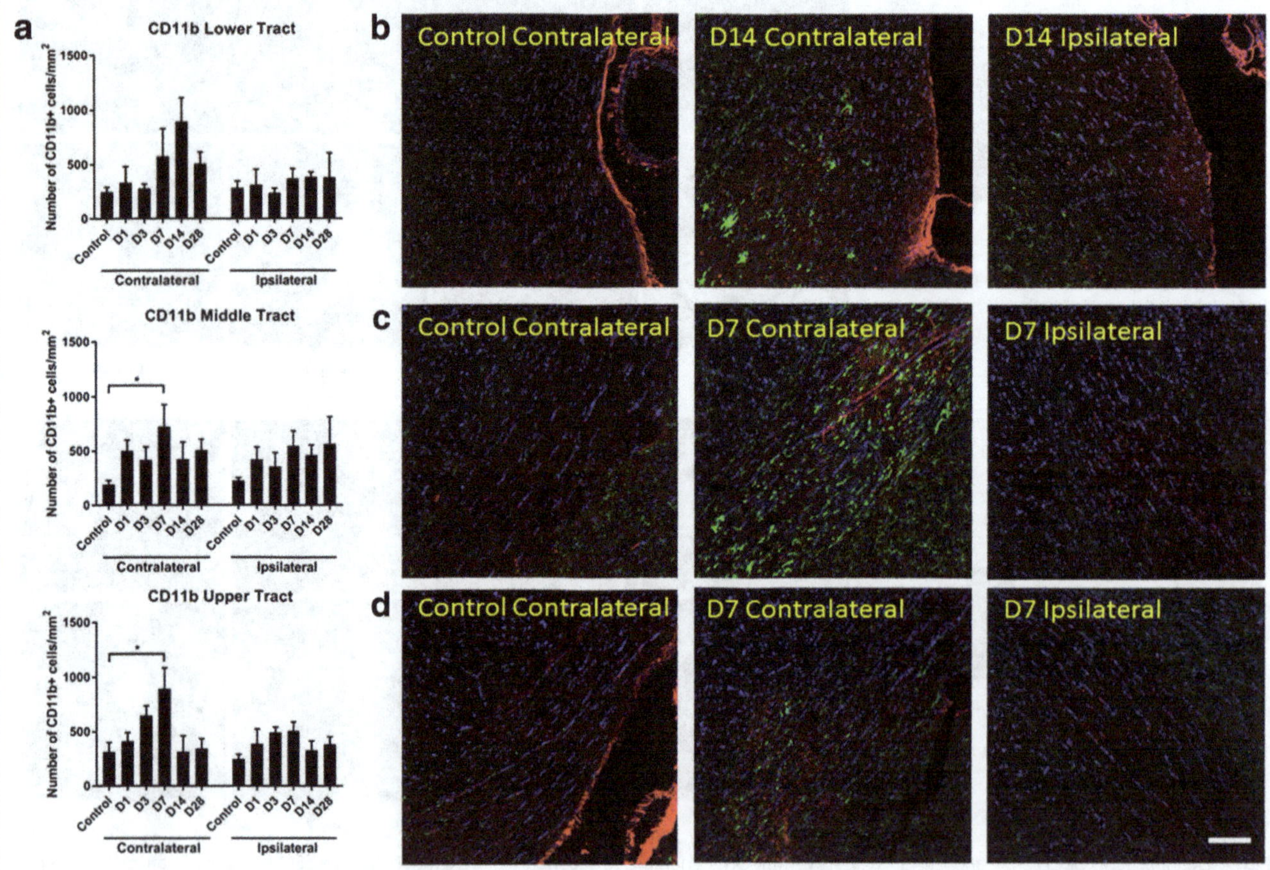

Fig. 5 Quantification of CD11b+ cells in the optic tract of the brain. Mean ± SEM numbers of **a** CD11b+ cells in the lower, middle, and upper regions of the optic tract in control uninjured optic nerve, compared to 1, 3, 7, 14, and 28 days following partial optic nerve transection, assessed separately for the right and left hand sides of the brain, $n = 5$–6/group. *$p \leq 0.05$, **$p \leq 0.01$, ***$p \leq 0.001$, ****$p \leq 0.0001$. Representative images of infiltrating CD11b+ cells in the **b** lower, **c** middle, and **d** upper optic tract, in control uninjured, and 7–14 days following partial optic nerve transection: D is day. Scale bar of **b**–**d**: 100 μm

mid-way between the chiasm and the superior colliculus = middle; pre-superior colliculus = upper) of the brain at 1, 3, 7, 14, and 28 days following partial injury to the optic nerve. Time points were chosen to complement the optic nerve analyses of the present study together with published work assessing microglia and macrophages in the partial optic nerve cut model [25, 39]. CD11b+ cells were assessed on both the left and right optic tracts, corresponding to the contralateral and ipsilateral sides to the injury, respectively. Two-way ANOVA revealed no significant changes in the densities of CD11b+ leukocytes in the lower tracts, compared to uninjured controls ($p = 0.17$, $F = 1.63$, df = 5) (Fig. 5a). There were changes in the number of CD11b+ cells/mm^2 in the middle (two-way ANOVA: $p = 2 \times 10^{-3}$, $F = 4.53$, df = 5; contralateral: $p = 0.02$, $F = 3.09$, df = 5; ipsilateral: $p = 0.17$, $F = 1.69$, df = 5) and upper tracts (two-way ANOVA: $p = 1 \times 10^{-4}$, $F = 6.217$, df = 5; contralateral: $p = 9 \times 10^{-3}$, $F = 3.95$, df = 5; ipsilateral: $p = 0.051$, $F = 2.561$, df = 5), with post hoc analysis revealing a significant increase relative to uninjured controls 7 days post-injury on the contralateral side ($p = 0.03$, middle tract; $p = 0.01$, upper tract), returning to control levels at day 14 (Fig. 5b, c).

Additional analyses were conducted focusing on the contralateral optic tract, to investigate first increases in further microglial/ macrophage subpopulations in a subset of sections of the optic tract at 1, 3, and 7 days following partial injury to the optic nerve. CD11b+ cells that also colocalized with IBA1 (a microglia/ macrophage marker which recognizes both resident and activated microglia/ macrophages) and ED1 (a marker of resident and infiltrating activated macrophages) were unchanged in the lower tract at the measured time points ($p = 0.14$, $F = 2.29$, df = 2) but significantly increased at 7 days compared to uninjured controls in the middle ($p = 6 \times 10^{-4}$, $F = 13.54$, df = 2) and upper tract ($p = 0.03$, $F = 20.33$, df = 2) (Fig. 6a, b), indicating that

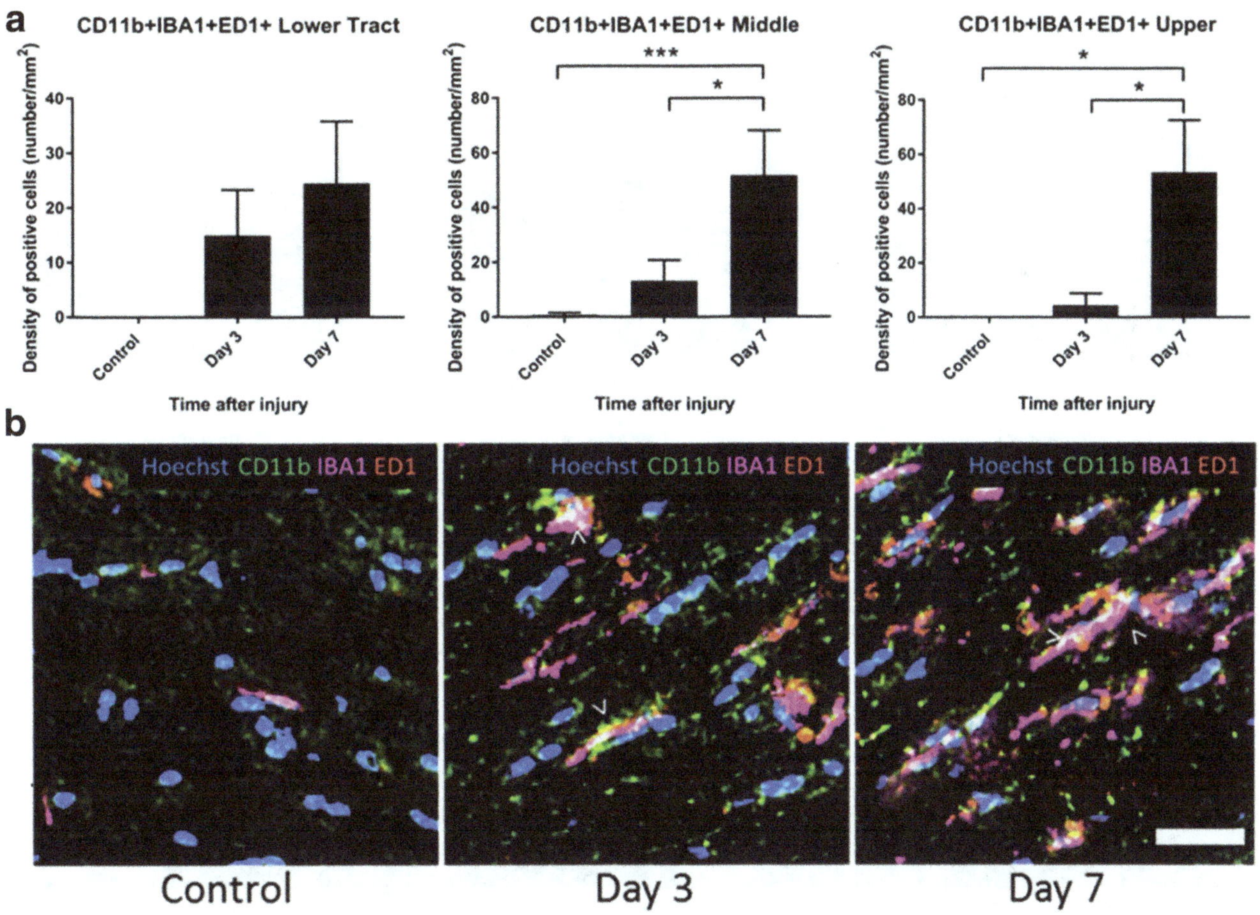

Fig. 6 Quantification of CD11b+/IBA1+/ED1+ cells in the optic tract of the brain. Mean ± SEM numbers of **a** CD11b+/IBA1+/ED1+ cells across the lower, middle, and upper regions of the optic tract in control uninjured optic nerve, compared to 3 and 7 days following partial optic nerve transection. $n = 6$ for control, $n = 5$ for 3 and for 7 days. *$p \leq 0.05$, **$p \leq 0.01$, ***$p \leq 0.001$, ****$p \leq 0.0001$. Representative images of **b** CD11b+/IBA1+/ED1+ cells, indicated by ">," in the lower region of the optic tract in control uninjured, 3 and 7 days following partial optic nerve transection. Scale bar of **b**: 5 μm

activation was enhanced in these regions. In contrast to outcomes within the optic nerve, there were no changes in the density of $CD45^{+}$-positive cells in the contralateral optic tract. Quantification of CD45+ microglia and macrophages did not reveal any significant changes at 3 or 7 days following injury in any of the optic tract regions analyzed ($p = 0.57$, $F = 0.59$, df = 2 for lower; $p = 0.41$, $F = 0.96$, df = 2 for middle; and $p = 0.60$, $F = 0.53$, df = 2 for upper optic tract) (Fig. 7a, b).

Cells positive for the markers IBA1 and ED1 in isolation were also quantified in the contralateral optic tract at 3 and 7 days post-injury. Density of IBA1+ cells significantly increased from uninjured controls at 3 days post-injury, with a further increase at 7 days post-injury in the lower ($p = 1 \times 10^{-4}$, $F = 20.08$, df = 2; 3 days $p = 0.01$, 7 days $p = 0.01$) and middle ($p = 7 \times 10^{-6}$, $F = 33.48$, df = 2; 3 days $p = 3 \times 10^{-3}$, 7 days $p = 4 \times 10^{-3}$) regions of the optic tract. Increases in the upper tract only reached significance at 7 days ($p = 3 \times 10^{-5}$, $F = 28.38$, df = 2; 7 days $p = 2 \times 10^{-5}$) (Fig. 8a, b, e; high and low magnification representative images, respectively). The densities of ED1+ cells increased at 7 days following injury in the lower, middle, and upper tracts ($p = 7 \times 10^{-5}$, $F = 23.33$, df = 2; $p = 0.00$, $F = 77.39$, df = 2 ;and $p = 0.00$, $F = 87.61$, df = 2, respectively; 7 days $p = 6 \times 10^{-3}$, $p = 1 \times 10^{-4}$, $p = 0.00$, respectively) (Fig. 8c, d, e; high and low magnification representative images, respectively).

IBA1+ and ED1+ cells were also quantified in the superior colliculus at 1, 3, and 7 days post-injury, assessing both the contralateral and ipsilateral sides. IBA1+ cells did not significantly change relative to control uninjured nerve on either the contralateral or ipsilateral sides ($p = 0.057$, $F = 4.21$, df = 3; ipsilateral: $p = 0.25$, $F = 1.46$, df = 3) (Fig. 9a). However, post hoc tests revealed that ED1+ cells were significantly increased at day 7 on the contralateral side ($p = 0.002$) (contralateral: $p = 2 \times 10^{-4}$, $F = 10.47$, df = 3; ipsilateral: $p = 0.50$, $F = 0.80$, df = 3) (Fig. 9b).

Blood-brain barrier integrity

Extravasation of Evans blue dye into the brains of rats following partial optic nerve injury was assessed qualitatively,

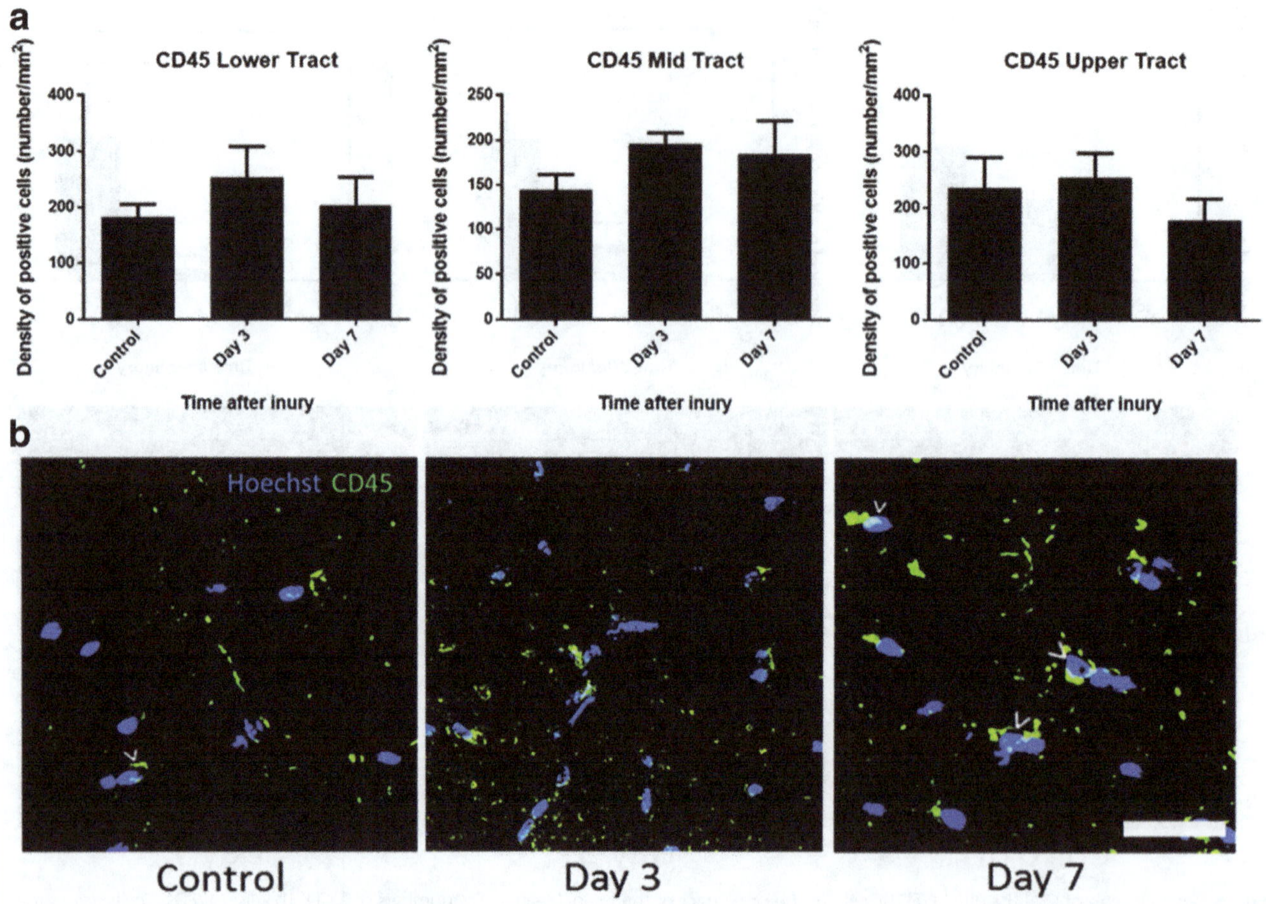

Fig. 7 Quantification of CD45+ cells in the optic tract of the brain. Mean ± SEM numbers of CD45+ cells **a** across the lower, middle, and upper regions of the optic tract in control uninjured optic nerve, compared to 3 and 7 days following partial optic nerve transection. $n = 6$ for control, $n = 5$ for 3/7 days. Representative images of CD45+ cells (**b**), indicated by ">" in the lower region of the optic tract in control uninjured optic nerve, and 3 and 7 days following partial ON transection. Scale bar for **b**: 3 μm

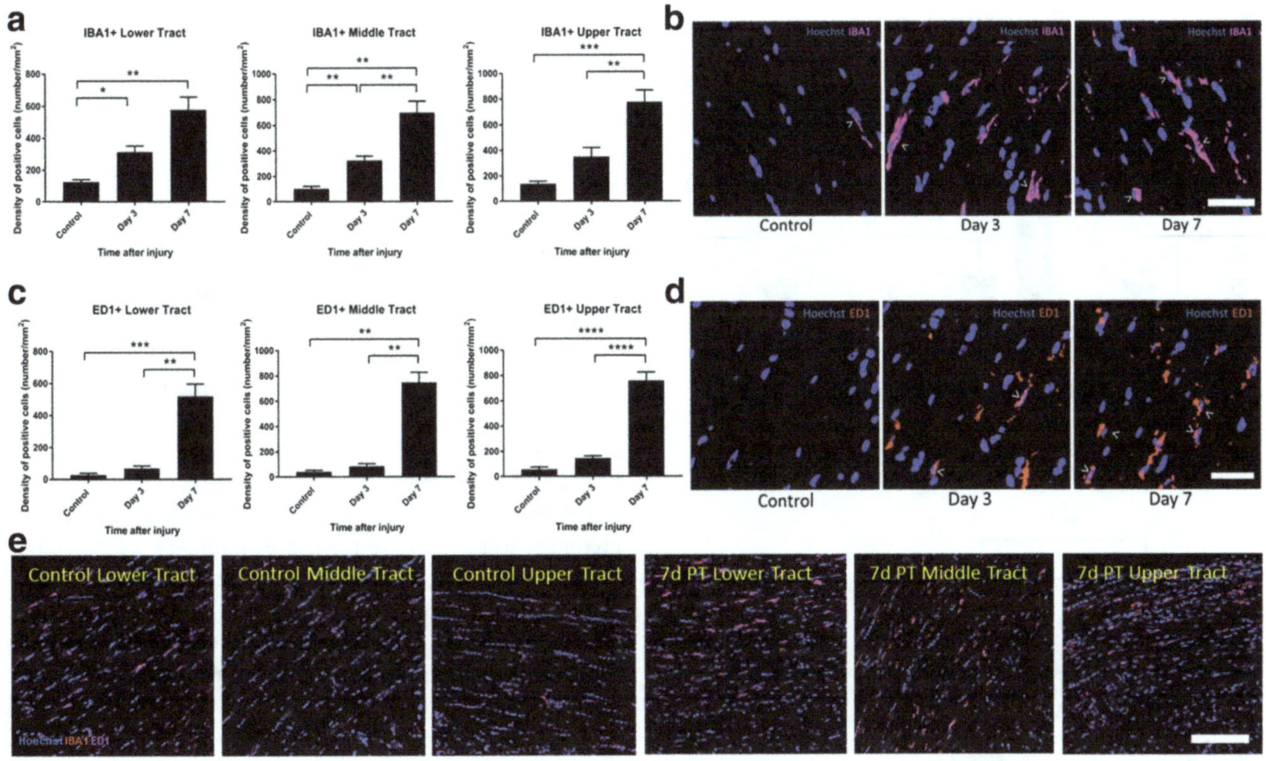

Fig. 8 Quantification of IBA1+ and ED1+ cells in the optic tract of the brain. Mean ± SEM numbers of **a** IBA1+ and **c** ED1+ cells across the lower, middle, and upper regions of the optic tract in control uninjured optic nerve, compared to 3 and 7 days following partial optic nerve transection. $n = 6$ for control, $n = 5$ for 3 and for 7 days. $^{*}p \leq 0.05$, $^{**}p \leq 0.01$, $^{***}p \leq 0.001$, $^{****}p \leq 0.0001$. Representative images of **b** IBA1+ and **d** ED1+ cells at high magnification, indicated by ">," in the lower region of the optic tract in control uninjured optic nerve, and 3 and 7 days following partial optic nerve transection. Scale bar for **b**–**d**: 5 μm. **e** Representative images of IBA1+ and ED1+ cells at low magnification, in the lower middle and upper regions of the optic tract in control uninjured optic nerve, and 7 days following partial optic nerve transection. Scale bar: 100 μm

being mindful of the caveats of this technique for assessing BBB integrity [41]. Despite our earlier observations of Evans blue dye in the brain at days 1 and 3 following this injury using multispectral imaging and quantitative assessment of extravasated Evans blue respectively [38], we did not observe Evans blue fluorescence at above background levels in cryosections of the brain viewed by confocal microscopy in the current study (Fig. 10a). The lack of Evans blue fluorescence in the brain sections in the current study may have been due to storage in sucrose and PBS prior to sectioning, and the single washing of the brain sections required to remove the OCT prior to section mounting. Previously, we observed Evans blue dye in the optic nerve at days 1 and 3 following injury [38]. In the current study, assessment of later time points indicated the presence of intense Evans blue staining at the optic nerve injury site and low-intensity diffuse staining ventral to the site of injury at 7 days post-injury (Fig. 10b). However, Evans blue fluorescence was not different to control at 28 days after partial transection (Fig. 10c, d), indicating closure of the BBB in the optic nerve at this time point after injury.

Caveolin-1 is a structural component of caveolae, mediates transcytosis through endothelial cells via interactions with claudin [42], and can be used as an indicator of BBB integrity [38]. Caveolin-1 immunoreactivity surrounding the third ventricle was assessed at 3, 7, 14, and 28 days following injury, to provide insight regarding the time of closure of the BBB following remote injury. The percentage of the third ventricle lined with caveolin-1+ cells was not different to control at 3, 7, and 28 days following partial optic nerve transection but was significantly reduced at 14 days (ANOVA: $p = 5 \times 10^{-4}$, $F = 6.52$, df = 4; 14 days $p = 5 \times 10^{-3}$) (Fig. 10e, f), indicating a transient compromise of caveolin-1-mediated junctions at this later time point.

Given the potential for washout of Evans blue dye from the tissue sections, immunoreactivity of fibrinogen was used as an additional measure of BBB integrity. Fibrinogen is a blood-derived protein whose accumulation in the brain indicates loss of BBB integrity [43]. The area of fibrinogen immunoreactivity, indicative of the size of the breach of the BBB, did not change with injury in the optic chiasm (two-way ANOVA: $p = 0.24$, $F = 1.41$,

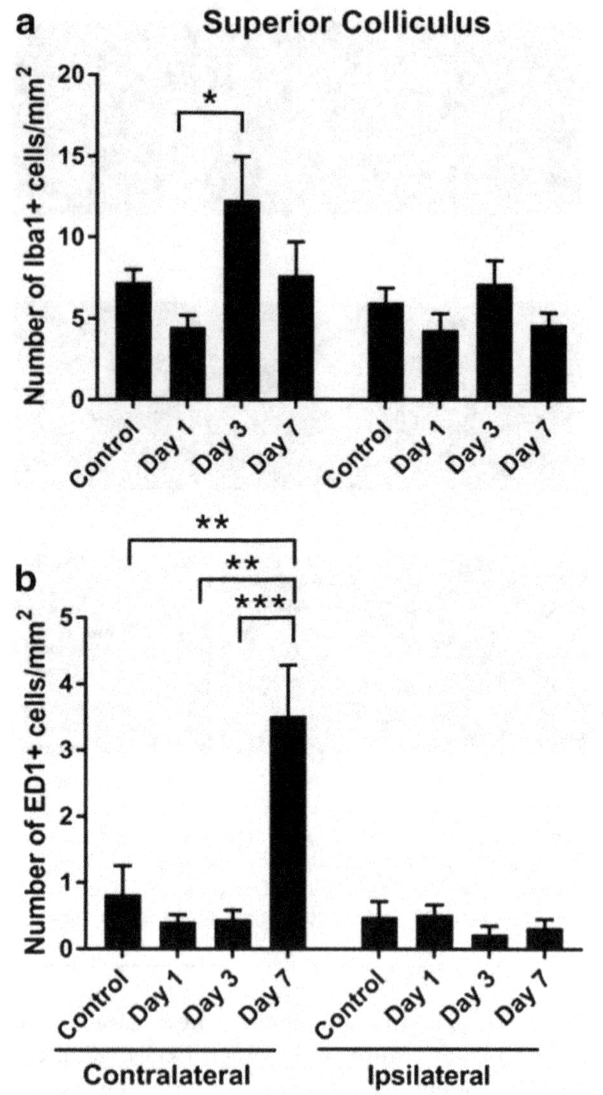

Fig. 9 Quantification of IBA1+ and ED1+ cells in the superior colliculus. Mean ± SEM numbers of **a** IBA1+ and **b** ED1+ cells across the lower, middle, and upper regions of the optic tract in control uninjured optic nerve, compared to 3 and 7 days following partial optic nerve transection. $n = 6$ for control, $n = 5$ for 3 and for 7 days. $^{*}p \leq 0.05$, $^{**}p \leq 0.01$, $^{***}p \leq 0.001$, $^{****}p \leq 0.0001$

df = 4) (Fig. 11a). However, the intensity of staining in the chiasm, perhaps indicating a focal breach, did change with injury (contralateral: $p = 0.03$, $F = 3.10$, df = 4; ipsilateral: $p = 2 \times 10^{-3}$, $F = 5.18$, df = 4), with post hoc analysis revealing that increases in signal intensity relative to control were confined to the ipsilateral side at 7 days post-injury ($p = 0.03$) (Fig. 11b). Changes in the area of fibrinogen immunoreactivity in the lower tract were seen on both sides (contralateral: $p = 0.02$, $F = 3.33$, df = 4; ipsilateral: $p = 0.03$, $F = 2.98$, df = 4); however, post hoc tests only revealed differences between 7 and 28 days, rather than relative to control (contralateral: $p = 0.03$; ipsilateral: $p = 0.04$) (Fig. 11a). No differences in the intensity of fibrinogen immunoreactivity were observed in the lower tract (contralateral: $p = 0.10$, $F = 2.09$, df = 4; ipsilateral: $p = 0.27$, $F = 1.35$, df = 4). In the middle tract, changes in the area of fibrinogen immunoreactivity were confined to the contralateral side (contralateral: $p = 3 \times 10^{-4}$, $F = 7.12$, df = 4; ipsilateral: $p = 0.06$, $F = 2.48$, df = 4), with post hoc analysis revealing differences relative to control 7 days post-injury ($p = 4 \times 10^{-3}$). There were no significant differences in the intensity of fibrinogen immunoreactivity in the middle tract (contralateral: $p = 0.24$, $F = 1.45$, df = 4; ipsilateral: $p = 0.06$, $F = 2.55$, df = 4). Changes in the upper tract were similar to the middle tract but occurred earlier (contralateral: $p = 0.001$, $F = 5.98$, df = 4; ipsilateral: $p = 0.69$, $F = 0.56$, df = 4) with post hoc tests showing that area of the breach increased at day 3 on the contralateral side ($p = 0.004$) (Fig. 11a, c). No changes were observed in the intensity of fibrinogen immunoreactivity in the upper tract (contralateral: $p = 0.086$, $F = 2.26$, df = 4; ipsilateral: $p = 0.10$, $F = 2.10$, df = 4) (Fig. 11b). Finally, in the superior colliculus, no significant changes in fibrinogen immunoreactivity were observed for area (contralateral: $p = 0.058$, $F = 2.95$, df = 3; ipsilateral: $p = 0.06$, $F = 2.82$, df = 3) or intensity of immunoreactivity (contralateral: $p = 0.32$, $F = 1.23$, df = 3; ipsilateral: $p = 0.16$, $F = 1.88$, df = 3) (Fig. 11a, b).

Cytokine expression is altered in rat brains in a time-dependent manner following partial injury to the optic nerve

The inflammatory response in the whole brain homogenates following partial injury to the optic nerve was determined by measuring changes in cytokine protein levels in homogenized rat brains at 1, 3, and 7 days post-injury compared to uninjured controls (Fig. 12). While it would perhaps have been preferable to assess the cytokines in the individual optic tract regions of interest, the volume of tissue required for these assays precluded these assessments. In these experiments, ten cytokines were measured: IL-6, IL-1β, TNFα, IL-2, IL-4, IL-10, IL-12, GMCSF, IL-1α, INFγ; however, differences between injured and control rat brains were only detected for three of them, TNFα, IL-2, and IL-10. The pro-inflammatory cytokine, IL-1β, and the anti-inflammatory cytokine, IL-4, remained unaltered in injured rat brains compared to controls, and five cytokines were below the detection limit of the multiplex assay, IL-6, IL-12, GMCSF, IL-1α, and INFγ. Tumor necrosis factor (TNFα) is a multifunctional cytokine most often referred to as a potent pro-inflammatory cytokine, produced by microglia and astrocytes. There was a significant increase in TNFα protein levels in rat brains in the early time point, 1 day post-injury (1.6-fold increase ± 0.14) compared to uninjured controls ($p < 0.0001$, $F = 4.13$, df = 3) (Fig. 12). At 3 days post-injury, the concentration of TNFα

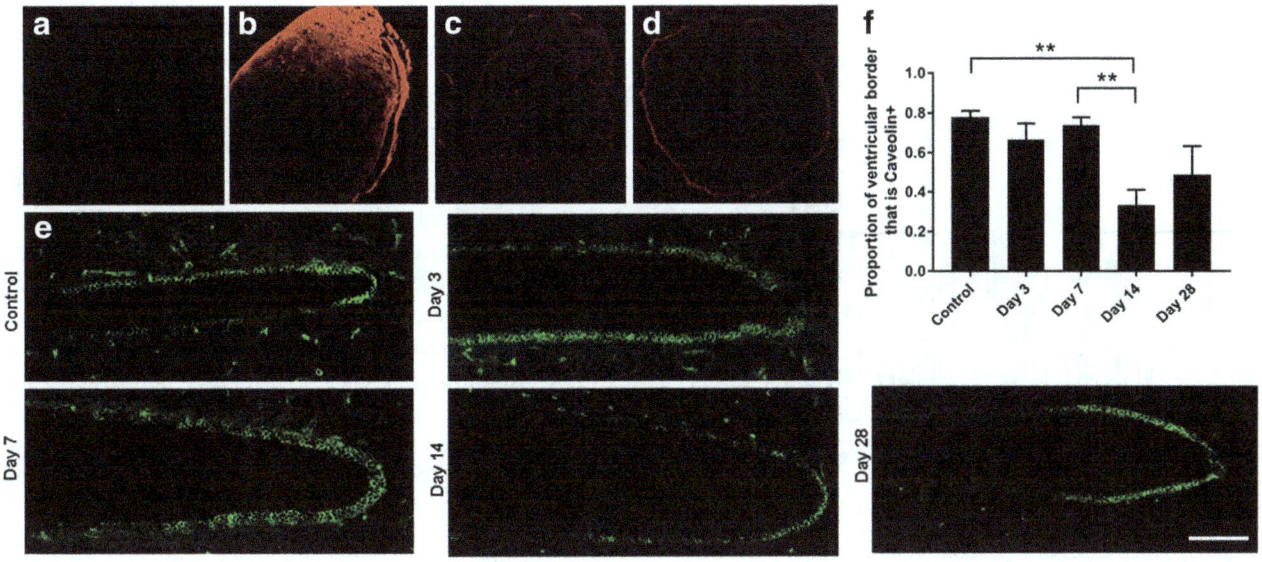

Fig. 10 Evans blue fluorescence and caveolin immunoreactivity in the brain following partial optic nerve transection. Lack of Evans blue fluorescence in a representative image of the periventricular region of the brain at 3 days after partial optic nerve transection (**a**), compared to strongly positive fluorescence at the partial optic nerve injury site 7 days after injury (**b**). Evans blue fluorescence in optic nerve 28 days after injury (**c**) was not different from uninjured controls injected with Evans blue (**d**). Caveolin immunoreactivity in endothelial cells lining the ventricles at 3, 7, 14, and 28 days after injury (**e**), scale = 100 μm. Mean ± SEM proportion of the ventricle lined with caveolin-1+ cells (**f**). $n = 7$–12. $^*p \leq 0.05$, $^{**}p \leq 0.01$, $^{***}p \leq 0.001$, $^{****}p \leq 0.0001$

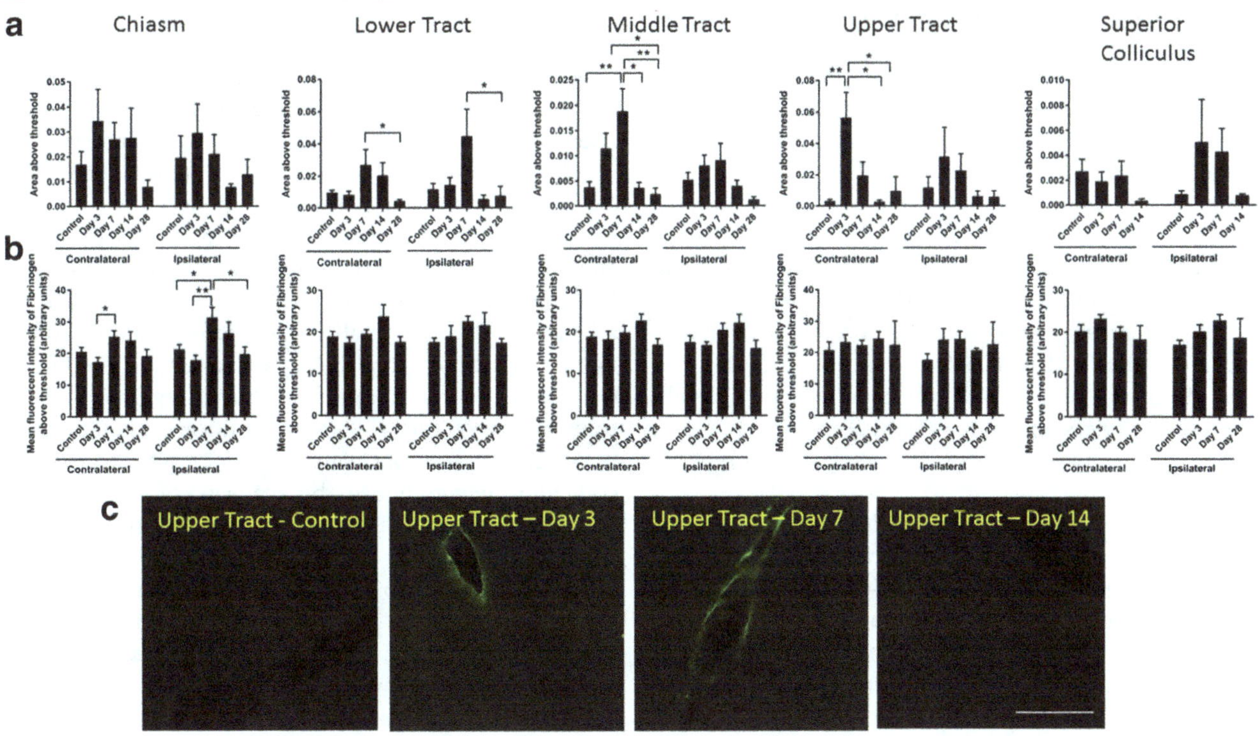

Fig. 11 Fibrinogen immunoreactivity in the brain following partial optic nerve transection. Mean ± SEM fibrinogen immunoreactivity assessing **a** area and **b** intensity above a constant set threshold in control uninjured optic nerve, compared to 1, 3, 7, 14, and 28 days, assessed separately for the right- and left-hand sides of the brain. Lower, middle, and upper regions of the optic tract were assessed separately. $n = 5$–6/group. $^*p \leq 0.05$, $^{**}p \leq 0.01$, $^{***}p \leq 0.001$, $^{****}p \leq 0.0001$. Representative images of the upper tract (**c**) show breaches in the BBB indicated by increased areas of diffuse fibrinogen immunoreactivity (bracketed), 3 days after injury, compared to control uninjured, and 7 and 14 days following partial optic nerve transection. Scale bar for **c**: 100 μm

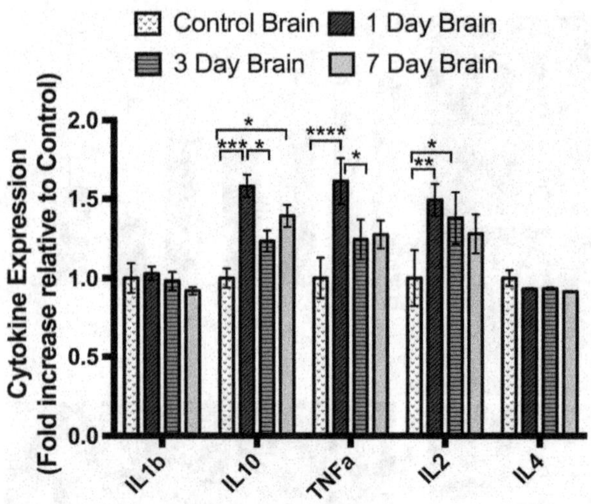

Fig. 12 Multiplex analysis of cytokines in the brain following injury. Data are expressed as mean ± standard error of mean. $^*p \leq 0.05$, $^{**}p \leq 0.01$, $^{***}p \leq 0.001$, $^{****}p \leq 0.0001$, one-way ANOVA (Tukey's correction)

returned to levels that were not significantly different from uninjured controls ($p > 0.05$), and these levels were maintained at 7 days post-injury (Fig. 12). The pro-inflammatory cytokine IL-2 was significantly elevated in the rat brains at an early time point following injury, 1 day (1.4-fold increase, $p < 0.05$, $F = 2.12$, df = 3), remained elevated at 3 days post-injury (1.4-fold increase, $p < 0.05$, $F = 2.12$, df = 3), and decreased to levels not significantly different from controls at 7 days post-injury (Fig. 12). IL-10 is regarded primarily as an anti-inflammatory cytokine, having a potent inhibitory effect on the production of several pro-inflammatory mediators including TNFα and IL-1β. IL-10 levels were biphasic, being significantly elevated from control levels at both an early time point, 1 day (1.6-fold increase, $p < 0.001$, $F = 13.28$, df = 3), and a later time point, 7 days (1.4-fold increase, $p < 0.05$, $F = 13.28$, df = 3) post-injury, with a decline to control levels in between at 3 days post-injury (Fig. 12).

Discussion

The current study has provided evidence that an injury to the optic nerve instigates a remote response in the brain in a time-dependent manner, with production of both pro- and anti-inflammatory cytokines and increases in resident and infiltrating inflammatory cells (for summary of outcomes including relevant published data in this model, see Fig. 13). Cytokines were rapidly increased in the brain, prior to changes in the measured inflammatory cell populations in the ventral portion of the optic nerve, immediately adjacent to the injury. Inflammatory cell infiltration was evident in well-defined regions of the brain with significant accumulation being limited to the contralateral side of the brain. Specific populations of inflammatory cells were increased in a region-specific manner. Increases in the density of resident IBA1+ cells were seen in the lower and middle regions of the contralateral optic tract and the superior colliculus as early as 3 days post-injury. However, increases in the number of leukocytes and activated microglia and macrophages relative to control, indicated by CD11b+ and ED1+ cells, were only evident 7 days post-injury in the upper tract regions and in the contralateral side of the superior colliculus, indicating progression of damage both towards and from the synaptic terminals. This progression of activated inflammatory cells was further confirmed by an increase in triple-positive CD11b/IBA1/ED1 cells in both the middle and upper regions of the contralateral optic tract at 7 days post-injury. Increases in microglia and macrophages in the ipsilateral optic tract were minimal and not significant. Importantly, breaches to the BBB can precede inflammation, particularly apparent in the upper tract in this study. Taken together, the data indicate that an injury to the optic nerve results in rapid changes towards the synaptic terminals of affected retinal ganglion cells, which initiate localized inflammatory cell infiltration perhaps potentiated by early increases in selected cytokines. Further studies will be required to determine whether similar changes also occur in an anterograde trans-synaptic fashion, for example, in cortically connected regions [44, 45].

Delayed secondary damage often occurs to remote brain regions that are anatomically connected to the primary infarct by axonal projections. Studies in rats using middle cerebral artery occlusion as an ischemia model consistently show that distinct regions of the thalamus with axonal connections to the primary infarct develop gliosis, inflammation, and significant neuronal loss at delayed post-stroke time points [29]. In our current study, a commonality among all observations of altered inflammatory cell density and BBB permeability in the brain is the axonal connectedness of these regions with the primary injury site, i.e., most significant alterations are observed in the contralateral optic tract and superior colliculus, which house the majority of injured axons that cross over at the optic chiasm, suggesting a role for axonal degeneration and potential white matter pathology, suggested to be of functional relevance for post-stroke recovery [33]. Our findings indicate that remote damage is limited to areas connected to the primary injury site. However, it is important to note some limitations of the current study. Only one section per brain region was analyzed, and we did not examine all visual projections, such as the lateral geniculate nucleus. In addition, the analyses of cytokines used whole brain homogenates and thus were not confined to axonally connected pathways. Nevertheless, we observed a

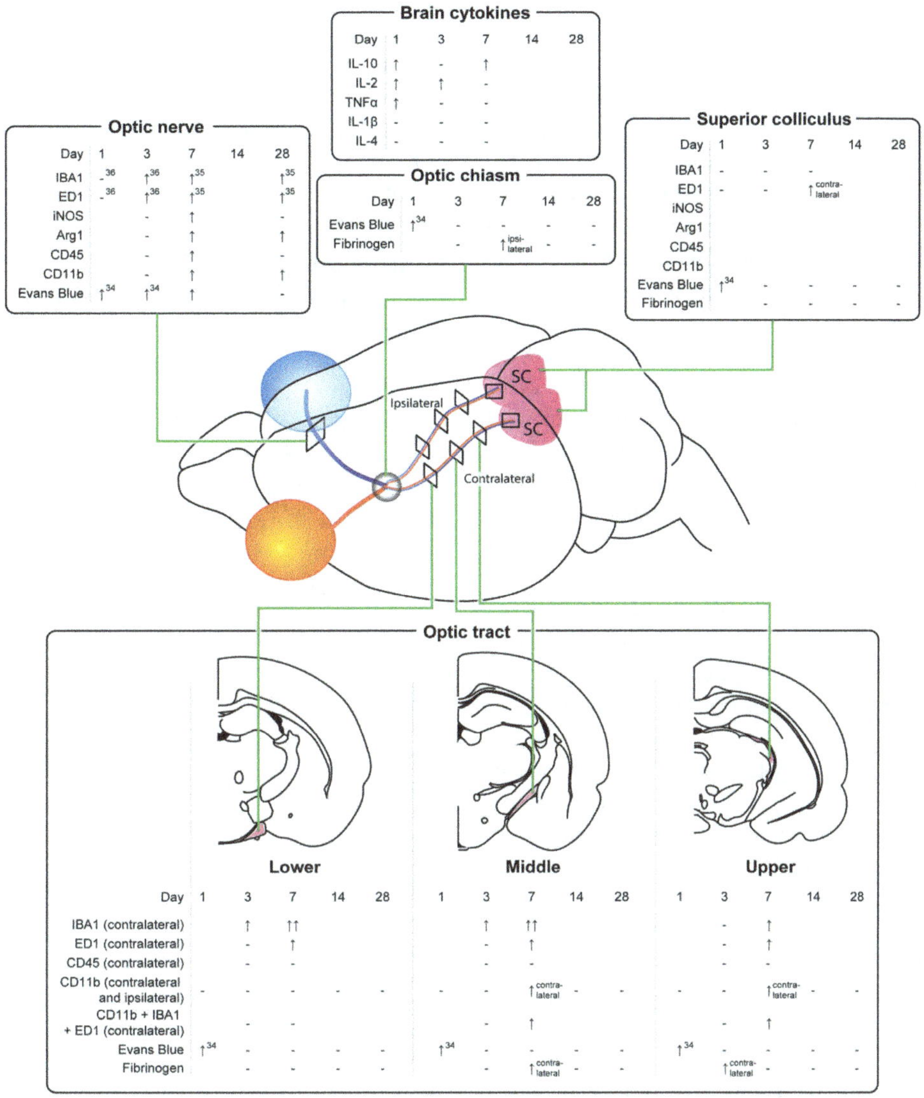

Fig. 13 Summary of study outcomes. ↑ indicates a significant increase relative to uninjured control, ↑↑ indicates a further increase, and ↓ indicates a significant decrease ($p \leq 0.05$) in a measured marker relative to control; "-" indicates no change relative to control. A space indicates not yet tested. Note that data for the optic tract are referring to the contralateral left-hand side, unless specifically indicated. Small numbers refer to references to published literature

significant increase in the anti-inflammatory cytokine, IL-10, at 7 days post-injury, which coincided with increased numbers of microglia in the brain, perhaps indicating a concerted response by anti-inflammatory cell subtypes at this time. Depletion of CD11b+ cells worsens damage 24 h following ischemic injury, associated with increased pro-inflammatory indicators, and similar mechanisms may act here [46]. Further, more focused assessments may provide additional insight. It is also important to note that PVG rats have particular susceptibilities to immune challenges [47]. Indeed, there are strain-specific differences for many outcomes in rats [48]. PVG rats were initially chosen for our studies using the partial optic nerve transection model of secondary degeneration, as they are not albino and therefore have better vision for assessments of visual function following injury. Female rats were chosen for ease of housing and to provide much needed and oft-missing information on injury outcomes in female animals.

Using Evans blue dye, we have observed breaches in the BBB in the brain as early as 1 day after this partial optic nerve injury [38], at the same time as both the current observed increases in both pro- (IL-2, TNFα) and anti- (IL-10) inflammatory cytokines in whole brain homogenates. While IL-2 and TNFα can cross the BBB [49, 50], and IL-10 cannot [51] the breached BBB may have facilitated entry of cytokines, elevated as a result of optic nerve injury, into the brain from the circulation.

The delayed increases in inflammatory cell numbers observed in the middle contralateral optic tract at 7 days post-injury coincided with a significant increase in the area of fibrinogen-positive signal in this brain region, indicating associated alterations in BBB permeability. Increases in microglia- and macrophage-derived cytokines including TNFα correlate with immune cell infiltration and have been implicated in the modulation of endothelial cell function [28] and changes in BBB permeability [52]. Reactive oxygen species generated by macrophages [7] also compromise BBB integrity [50]. Thus, while BBB breaches in the upper tract precede, and may contribute to increases in inflammatory cells, multiple factors may be contributing to a feed forward system exacerbating the damage. While it is clear from our earlier published work that infiltration of microglia and macrophages also occurs at the partial optic nerve injury site and spreads in an efferent direction towards the brain along the nerve vulnerable to secondary degeneration [38, 39], it now becomes apparent that as time passes, inflammation may also move from degeneration in the upper tract and synaptic terminals back towards the injury. The anti-inflammatory cytokine IL-10 increases in brain homogenates in a biphasic pattern, being elevated at 1 day, returning to control levels at 3 days and elevated at 7 days after injury, likely as a compensatory response, associated with the later changes in microglia/ macrophage activation and phagocytosis. Further studies assessing cytokines in specific brain regions identified in this study as sites of inflammatory cell infiltration, pooling tissue from multiple animals, will be required to determine the direct relationships between cytokine changes, cellular infiltrations, and BBB breach. At later times after injury, there is a disruption to caveolin-1 immunoreactivity lining the ventricles, indicating that compromise of the BBB is not swiftly resolved and that injury to the optic nerve has persisting remote consequences in the brain.

While the increase in CD45+ cells in the optic nerve was transient, decreasing to control levels at 28 days following injury, the number of CD11b+ cells in the ventral optic nerve remained elevated at 28 days following injury. Similarly, iNOS and Argl expression were significantly increased within the ventral optic nerve 7 days after injury compared to uninjured controls, with only iNOS levels decreasing to control at 28 days post-injury. Interestingly, cells showed concurrent expression of iNOS and Argl indicating that these immunoreactive cells exhibit a mixed phenotype, as previously shown following traumatic brain injury [18]. Similar findings have also been reported in the cortex following spared nerve injury to the sciatic nerve [26]. As both microglia and infiltrating non-myeloid-derived leukocytes express CD11b and CD45 markers, but differ in the levels of expression of these markers, i.e., infiltrating leukocytes have high CD45 expression compared to resident microglia, we were unable to differentiate microglia from macrophages and leukocytes in general in this instance. Interestingly, CD45+ cells were not elevated in the optic tract, indicating differences in the features of the adjacent and remote inflammatory responses.

Conclusion

In summary, our study demonstrates that a partial injury to the optic nerve induces transient changes in whole brain cytokine expression and increased inflammatory cell density and BBB permeability remotely along the visual pathways in the brain. Significant alterations are restricted to the contralateral side of the brain, suggesting that, at least in this traumatic injury model, inflammatory and BBB damage is confined to regions that are "axonally connected" to the primary injury site, although it remains to be determined whether such damage also extends trans-synaptically.

Abbreviations

ANOVA: Analysis of variance; Arg1: Arginase 1; BBB: Blood-brain barrier; CNS: Central nervous system; df: Degrees of freedom; GMCSF: Granulocyte-macrophage colony-stimulating factor; IFN: Interferon; IL : Interleukin; iNOS: Inducible nitric oxide synthase; OCT: Optimal cutting temperature; TNFα: Tumor necrosis factor alpha

Acknowledgements

We are grateful to Dr. Diwei Ho for generating the scientific illustrations.

Funding

National Health and Medical Research Council (NHMRC), Australia (APP1082403), and Neurotrauma Research Program, WA. MF is supported by an NHMRC Career Development Fellowship (APP1087114). The funding bodies played no part in the conduct of the study.

Authors' contributions

NS, MG, AG, CB, and CAB conducted the experiments. NS, MG, AG, CB, TM, AB, TC, and MF analyzed the data. NS, MF, and MG wrote the manuscript. NS, MG, CAB, SI, SD, and MF designed the study, provided intellectual input, and edited the manuscript. All authors approved the final manuscript.

Consent for publication

Not applicable

Competing interests

The authors declare that they have no competing interests.

Author details

[1]School of Molecular Sciences, The University of Western Australia, Stirling Hwy, Perth, Western Australia 6009, Australia. [2]Experimental and Regenerative Neurosciences, School of Biological Sciences, The University of Western Australia, Stirling Hwy, Perth, Western Australia 6009, Australia. [3]Curtin Health Innovation Research Institute, Curtin University, Verdun St, Nedlands, Western Australia, Australia. [4]Perron Institute for Neurological and Translational Science, Sarich Neuroscience Research Institute, Verdun St, Nedlands, Western Australia 6009, Australia.

References

1. Jia Z, Zhu H, Li J, Wang X, Misra H, Li Y. Oxidative stress in spinal cord injury and antioxidant-based intervention. Spinal Cord. 2012;50:264–74.
2. Oyinbo CA. Secondary injury mechanisms in traumatic spinal cord injury: a nugget of this multiply cascade. Acta Neurobiol Exp. 2011;71:281–99.
3. David S, Kroner A. Repertoire of microglial and macrophage responses after spinal cord injury. Nat Rev Neurosci. 2011;12:388–99.
4. Perez-Polo JR, Rea HC, Johnson KM, Parsley MA, Unabia GC, Xu G, Infante SK, DeWitt DS, Hulsebosch CE. Inflammatory consequences in a rodent model of mild traumatic brain injury. J Neurotrauma. 2013;30:727–40.
5. Loane DJ, Byrnes KR. Role of microglia in neurotrauma. Neurotherapeutics. 2010;7:366–77.
6. Banati RB, Gehrmann J, Schubert P, Kreutzberg GW. Cytotoxicity of microglia. GLIA. 1993;7:111–8.
7. Doig RLOH, Bartlett CA, Maghzal GJ, Lam M, Archer M, Stocker R, Fitzgerald M. Reactive species and oxidative stress in optic nerve vulnerable to secondary degeneration. Exp Neurol. 2014;261:136–46.
8. Ruckh JM, Zhao J-W, Shadrach JL, PvPV W, Rao TN, Wagers AJ, RJM F. Rejuvenation of regeneration in the aging central nervous system. Cell Stem Cell. 2011;10:96–103.
9. Kotter MR, Li W-W, Zhao C, Franklin RJM. Myelin impairs CNS remyelination by inhibiting oligodendrocyte precursor cell differentiation. J Neurosci. 2006; 26:328–32.
10. Kotter MR, Zhao C, Nv R, Franklin RJM. Macrophage-depletion induced impairment of experimental CNS remyelination is associated with a reduced oligodendrocyte progenitor cell response and altered growth factor expression. Neurobiol Dis. 2005;18:166–75.
11. Persidsky Y, Ghorpade A, Rasmussen J, Limoges J, Liu XJ, Stins M, Fiala M, Way D, Kim KS, Witte MH, et al. Microglial and astrocyte chemokines regulate monocyte migration through the blood-brain barrier in human immunodeficiency virus-1 encephalitis. Am J Pathol. 1999;155:1599–611.
12. Bock MD, Wang N, Decrock E, Ml B, Gadicherla AK, Culot M, Cecchelli R, Bultynck G, Leybaert L. Endothelial calcium dynamics, connexin channels and blood–brain barrier function. Prog Neurobiol. 2013;108:1–20.
13. Edwards JP, Zhang X, Frauwirth KA, Mosser DM. Biochemical and functional characterization of three activatedmacrophage populations. J Leukoc Biol. 2006;80:1298–307.
14. Hsieh CL, Kim CC, Ryba BE, Niemi EC, Bando JK, Locksley RM, Liu J, Nakamura MC, Seaman WE. Traumatic brain injury induces macrophage subsets in the brain. Eur J Immunol. 2013;43:2010–22.
15. Wang G, Zhang J, Hu X, Zhang L, Mao L, Jiang X, Liou AK-F, Leak RK, Gao Y, Chen J. Microglia/macrophage polarization dynamics in white matter after traumatic brain injury. J Cereb Blood Flow Metab. 2013;33:1864–74.
16. Orihuela R, McPherson CA, Harry GJ. Microglial M1/M2polarization and metabolic states. Br J Pharmacol. 2016;173:649–65.
17. Turtzo LC, Lescher J, Janes L, Dean DD, Budde MD, Frank JA. Macrophagic and microglial responses after focal traumatic brain injury in the female rat. J Neuroinflammation. 2014;11:1742–2094.
18. Morganti JM, Riparip L-K, Rosi S. Call off the dog(ma): M1/M2 polarization is concurrent following traumatic brain injury. PLoS One. 2016;11:e0148001.
19. Pettersen JS, Fuentes-Duculan J, Suárez-Fariñas M, Pierson KC, Pitts-Kiefer A, Fan L, Belkin DA, Wang CQF, Bhuvanendran S, Johnson-Huang LM, et al. Tumor-associated macrophages in the cutaneous SCC microenvironment are heterogeneously activated. J Invest Dermatol. 2011;131:1322–30.
20. Vogel DY, Vereyken EJ, Glim JE, Heijnen PD, Moeton M, Pvd V, Amor S, Teunissen CE, Jv H, Dijkstra CD. Macrophages in inflammatory multiple sclerosis lesions have an intermediate activation status. J Neuroinflammation. 2013;10:1742–2094.
21. Kim CC, Nakamura MC, Hsieh CL. Brain trauma elicits non-canonical macrophage activation states. J Neuroinflammation. 2016;13:117.
22. Ransohoff RM. A polarizing question: do M1 and M2 microglia exist? Nat Neurosci. 2016;19:987–91.
23. Martinez FO, Gordon S. The M1 and M2 paradigm of macrophage activation: time for reassessment. F1000Prime Reports. 2014;6:13.
24. Perego C, Fumagalli S, Simoni M-GD. Temporal pattern of expression and colocalization of microglia/macrophage phenotype markers following brain ischemic injury in mice. J Neuroinflammation. 2011;8:174.
25. Fitzgerald M, Bartlett CA, Evill L, Rodger J, Harvey AR, Dunlop SA. Secondary degeneration of the optic nerve following partial transection: the benefits of lomerizine. Exp Neurol. 2009;216:219–30.
26. Xu N, Tang X-H, Pan W, Xie Z-M, Zhang G-F, Ji M-H, Yang J-J, Zhou M-T, Zhou Z-Q. Spared nerve injury increases the expression of microglia M1 markers in the prefrontal cortex of rats and provokes depression-like behaviors. Front Neurosci. 2017;11. Article 209.
27. Evangelho K, Mogilevskaya M, Losada-Barragan M, Vargas-Sanchez JK. Pathophysiology of primary open-angle glaucoma from a neuroinflammatory and neurotoxicity perspective: a review of the literature. Int Ophthalmol. 2017. https://doi.org/10.1007/s10792-017-0795-9.
28. Daneman R, Prat A. The blood-brain barrier. Cold Spring Harb Perspect Biol. 2015;7:a020412.
29. Block F, Dihné M, Loos M. Inflammation in areas of remote changes following focal brain lesion. Prog Neurobiol. 2005;75:342–65.
30. Weishaupt N, Zhang A, Deziel RA, AndrewTasker R, Whitehead SN. Prefrontal ischemia in the rat leads to secondary damage and inflammation in remote gray and white matter regions. Front Neurosci. 2016;10:81.
31. Viscomi MT, Molinari M. Remote neurodegeneration: multiple actors for one play. Mol Neurobiol. 2014;50:368–89.
32. Demeurisse G, Capon A, Verhas M, Attig E. Pathogenesis of aphasia in deep-seated lesions: likely role of cortical diaschisis. Eur Neurol. 1990;30:67–74.
33. Thiel A, Radlinska BA, Paquette C, Sidel M, Soucy J-P, Schirrmacher R, Minuk J. The temporal dynamics of poststroke neuroinflammation: a longitudinal diffusion tensor imaging–guided PET study with 11C-PK11195 in acute subcortical stroke. The Journal of Nuclear Medicine. 2010;51:1404–12.
34. Finger S, Koehler PJ, Jagella C. The Monakow concept of diaschisis: origins and perspectives. Arch Neurol. 2004;61:283–8.
35. Hausmann ON. Post-traumatic inflammation following spinal cord injury. Spinal Cord. 2003;41:369–78.
36. Mietto BS, Mostacada K, Martinez AMB. Neurotrauma and inflammation: CNS and PNS responses. Mediat Inflamm. 2015;2015. article 251204.
37. Echeverry S, Shi XQ, Rivest S, Zhang J. Peripheral nerve injury alters blood–spinal cord barrier functional and molecular integrity through a selective inflammatory pathway. J Neurosci. 2011;31:10819–28.
38. Smith NM, Gachulincova I, Ho D, Bailey C, Bartlett CA, Norret M, Murphy J, Buckley A, Rigby PJ, House MJ, et al. An unexpected transient breakdown of the blood brain barrier triggers passage of large intravenously administered nanoparticle. Sci Rep. 2016;6. article 22595.
39. Fitzgerald M, Bartlett CA, Harvey AR, Dunlop SA. Early events of secondary degeneration after partial optic nerve transection: an immunohistochemical study. J Neurotrauma. 2010;27:439–52.
40. Miron VE, Boyd A, Zhao J-W, Yuen TJ, Ruckh JM, Shadrach JL, Pv W, Wagers AJ, Williams A, Franklin RJM, ffrench-Constant C. M2 microglia and macrophages drive oligodendrocyte differentiation during CNS remyelination. Nat Neurosci. 2013;16:1211–8.
41. Saunders NR, Dziegielewska KM, Møllgård K, Habgood MD. Markers for blood-brain barrier integrity: how appropriate is Evans blue in the twenty-first century and what are the alternatives? Front Neurosci. 2015;9:385.
42. Liu J, Jin X, Liu KJ, Liu W. Matrix metalloproteinase-2-mediated occludin degradation and caveolin-1-mediated claudin-5 redistribution contribute to blood-brain barrier damage in early ischemic stroke stage. J Neurosci. 2010;32:3044–57.
43. Ryu JK, Petersen MA, Murray SG, Baeten KM, Meyer-Franke A, Chan JP, Vagena E, Bedard C, Machado MR, Coronado PER, et al: Blood coagulation protein fibrinogen promotesautoimmunity and demyelination via chemokine release and antigen presentation. Nat Commun 2015, 6. 42.
44. Chan KC, Kancherla S, Fan S-J, Wu EX: Long-term effects of neonatal hypoxia-ischemia on structural and physiological integrity of the eye and visual pathway by multimodal MRI. Invest Ophthalmol Vis Sci 2015, 56:1–9.
45. Lawlor M, Danesh-Meyer H, Levin LA, Davagnanam I, De Vita E, Plant GT: Glaucoma and the brain: trans-synaptic degeneration, structural change, and implications for neuroprotection. Surv Ophthalmol 2017, In Press:1–11.
46. Perego C, Fumagalli S, Zanier ER, Carlino E, Panini N, Erba E, Simoni M-GD. Macrophages are essential for maintaining a M2 protective response early after ischemic brain injury. Neurobiol Dis. 2016;96:284–93.
47. Leenaerts PL, Stad RK, Hall BM, Van Damme BJ, Vanrenterghem Y, Daha MR. Hereditary C6 deficiency in a strain of PVG/c rats. Clin Exp Immunol. 1994; 97:478–82.
48. Harvey AR, Hu Y, Leaver SG, Mellough CB, Park K, Verhaagen J, Plant GW, Cui Q. Gene therapy and transplantation in CNS repair: the visual system. Prog Retin Eye Res. 2006;25:449–89.
49. Banks WA, Kastin AJ, Broadwell RD. Passage of cytokines across the blood-brain barrier. Neuroimmunomodulation. 1995;2:241–8.
50. Waguespack PJ, Banks WA, Kastin AJ. Interleukin-2 does not cross the blood-brain barrier by a saturable transport system. Brain Res Bull. 1994;34:103–9.

5

Combined effect of non-bacteriolytic antibiotic and inhibition of matrix metalloproteinases prevents brain injury and preserves learning, memory and hearing function in experimental paediatric pneumococcal meningitis

Lukas Muri[1,2], Denis Grandgirard[1], Michelle Buri[1], Michael Perny[1] and Stephen L. Leib[1*]

Abstract

Background: Pneumococcal meningitis is associated with high mortality and morbidity rates. Up to 50% of survivors show neurologic sequelae including hearing loss, cognitive impairments and learning disabilities, being particularly detrimental in affected infants and children where adjuvant therapy with dexamethasone has no proven beneficial effect. We evaluated the effect of concomitantly targeting specific pathophysiological mechanisms responsible for brain damage—i.e. matrix-metalloproteinase (MMP) activity and the exacerbated cerebral inflammation provoked through antibiotic-induced bacterial lysis. Here, we combined adjunctive therapies previously shown to be neuroprotective when used as single adjuvant therapies.

Methods: Eleven-day-old Wistar rats were infected intracisternally with $6.44 \pm 2.17 \times 10^3$ CFU *Streptococcus pneumoniae* and randomised for treatment with ceftriaxone combined with (a) single adjuvant therapy with daptomycin ($n = 24$), (b) single adjuvant therapy with Trocade ($n = 24$), (c) combined adjuvant therapy ($n = 66$) consisting of daptomycin and Trocade, or (d) ceftriaxone monotherapy ($n = 42$). Clinical parameters and inflammatory CSF cytokine levels were determined during acute meningitis. Cortical damage and hippocampal apoptosis were assessed 42 h after infection. Morris water maze and auditory brainstem responses were used to assess neurofunctional outcome 3 weeks after infection.

(Continued on next page)

* Correspondence: stephen.leib@ifik.unibe.ch
[1]Neuroinfection Laboratory, Institute for Infectious Diseases, University of Bern, Friedbühlstrasse 51, 3001 Bern, Switzerland
Full list of author information is available at the end of the article

(Continued from previous page)

Results: We found significantly reduced apoptosis in the hippocampal subgranular zone in infant rats receiving adjuvant Trocade ($p < 0.01$) or combined adjuvant therapy ($p < 0.001$). Cortical necrosis was significantly reduced in rats treated with adjuvant daptomycin ($p < 0.05$) or combined adjuvant therapy ($p < 0.05$) compared to ceftriaxone monotherapy. Six hours after treatment initiation, CSF cytokine levels were significantly reduced for TNF-α ($p < 0.01$), IL-1β ($p < 0.01$), IL-6 ($p < 0.001$) and IL-10 ($p < 0.01$) in animals receiving combined adjuvant intervention compared to ceftriaxone monotherapy. Importantly, combined adjuvant therapy significantly improved learning and memory performance in infected animals and reduced hearing loss (77.14 dB vs 60.92 dB, $p < 0.05$) by preserving low frequency hearing capacity, compared to ceftriaxone monotherapy.

Conclusion: Combined adjuvant therapy with the non-bacteriolytic antibiotic daptomycin and the MMP inhibitor Trocade integrates the neuroprotective effects of both single adjuvants in experimental paediatric pneumococcal meningitis by reducing neuroinflammation and brain damage, thereby improving neurofunctional outcome. This strategy represents a promising therapeutic option to improve the outcome of paediatric patients suffering from pneumococcal meningitis.

Keywords: Pneumococcal meningitis, Brain injury, Neurologic sequelae, Neuroinflammation, Hearing loss, Combined adjuvant therapy

Background

Pneumococcal meningitis (PM) causes considerable mortality and leads to long-lasting neurofunctional deficits in survivors [1, 2]. Neurofunctional sequelae from PM include hearing loss, epilepsy, cerebral palsy but also behavioural problems and cognitive deficits. Especially in affected children, these deficits negatively influence neurointegrative function, schooling performance and quality of life and may persist into adulthood [1–5]. Central nervous system (CNS) injury during PM is characterised by cortical necrosis and apoptosis of dentate gyrus granular cell progenitors in the hippocampus representing the histomorphologic correlates of behavioural and learning deficits [6–9] found in humans [10] and animal models [11, 12]. PM affects the peripheral nervous system (PNS) by damaging hair cells and spiral ganglion neurons in the inner ear leading to sensorineural hearing loss [13, 14]. Within the brain, neural cell death is caused by multiple factors including bacterial toxins and the excessive inflammatory host reaction [15–17]. Pneumolysin and hydrogen peroxide—produced by the pneumococci—are responsible for caspase-independent cell death in mature and immature dentate gyrus granular neurons [15–18]. Stimulated by pneumococcal components, leukocytes release soluble factors inducing a caspase-dependent apoptosis of immature neurons in the subgranular zone of the dentate gyrus [11, 15, 16]. Brain-resident immune cells, including microglia and leptomeningeal macrophages, are potently activated via TLR 2, 4 and 9 by pneumolysin, bacterial cell wall components and bacterial CpG DNA [15, 19, 20]. Together with the recruited neutrophils, activated microglia are able to produce large quantities of pro-inflammatory cytokines, reactive oxygen and nitrogen species, helping to eradicate the causative pathogen of PM but also contributing to the development of neuronal damage [15, 20, 21]. In addition, PM induces damage to hair cells and spiral ganglion neurons in the inner ear [13, 14, 22], provoking hearing impairments in up to 30% of survivors [2, 4, 23]. Increased levels of CSF TNF-α during acute PM has been positively correlated to increased hearing threshold in infant rat PM [13].

In clinical studies, adjunctive dexamethasone—an anti-inflammatory corticosteroid—was shown to improve the outcome of adults with PM in high-income countries and children with meningitis caused by *Haemophilus influenzae* type b [24]. To date, scientific evidence for the use of dexamethasone in children with PM is lacking. Moreover, in experimental models of PM, adjunctive dexamethasone aggravated mortality and acute hippocampal injury with subsequent learning performance deficits [9, 25–27]. Increased hippocampal apoptosis with adjuvant dexamethasone was also found independently in a rabbit model of *Escherichia coli* meningitis [28]. Adjuvant therapies targeting relevant pathophysiologic mechanisms in PM—such as non-bacteriolytic antibiotics, matrix metalloproteinase (MMP) inhibitors or antioxidants—have shown promising neuroprotective benefits in infant animal models [29–32]. Until now, most adjuvant therapies have been evaluated exclusively in the modality of single adjuvant therapies or combined with dexamethasone [33, 34], with very limited data on combined adjuvant interventions [35]. Based on present knowledge of the pathophysiology, we propose herein to combine complementary approaches targeting different pathophysiological mechanisms of PM, with the aim to more efficiently reduce CNS and PNS damage and improve the disease outcome. In this study, we evaluated a combination therapy consisting of daptomycin, a non-bacteriolytic antibiotic, with Trocade (Ro-32-3555, cipemastat), an orally active matrix metalloproteinase (MMP) inhibitor, originally designed to prevent cartilage breakdown in arthritis [36–39]. Single antibiotic therapy with daptomycin has previously been shown to clear pneumococci from CSF more rapidly than ceftriaxone without inducing bacterial lysis [40, 41]. In infant rat PM, adjunctive daptomycin with ceftriaxone reduced neuroinflammatory cytokine expression in the cerebrospinal fluid (CSF) and decreased brain injury compared to ceftriaxone monotherapy [29]. Trocade is an inhibitor of collagenases (MMP-1, -8 and -13) and gelatinase B (MMP-9) [36]. Adjuvant Trocade therapy in infant rat PM inhibited collagenase activity, decreased CSF levels of TNF-α and IL-1β, improved survival and reduced cerebral damage [30]. To our knowledge, this is the first study assessing behavioural outcomes after adjuvant daptomycin or Trocade therapy in experimental paediatric PM.

By targeting multiple pathophysiological mechanisms responsible for brain injury during acute bacterial meningitis with a combined adjunctive therapy regimen, we aim to integrate the neuroprotective effect of both substances and improve the neurofunctional outcome and quality of life after paediatric PM.

Methods

Infecting organism

A clinical isolate of *Streptococcus pneumoniae* (serotype 3) from a patient with bacterial meningitis was cultured overnight in brain heart infusion (BHI) medium, diluted 10-fold in fresh, pre-warmed BHI medium and grown for 5 h to reach the logarithmic phase as reported earlier [29, 42]. The bacteria were centrifuged for 10 min at 3100×*g*, washed twice and re-suspended in sterile, pyrogen-free saline (NaCl 0.85%). Bacteria were further diluted in saline to the desired density by measuring the optical density at 570 nm (OD_{570}). Inoculum accuracy was determined by serial dilutions and plating on Columbia sheep blood agar (CSBA) plates.

Infant rat model of pneumococcal meningitis

All animal studies were approved by the Animal Care and Experimentation Committee of the Canton of Bern, Switzerland (licence BE 129/14) and followed the Swiss national guidelines for the performance of animal experiments. A well-established infant rat model of PM was used for the experiments as previously described [29, 42]. Eleven-day-old Wistar rats together with their dams were obtained from Charles River Laboratories (Sulzfeld, Germany). The dams were provided with tap water and pellet diet at libitum. Litters were kept in rooms at a controlled temperature of 22 ± 2 °C. During the acute phase of the disease, animals were housed in conventional cages in a room with natural light. For long-term experiments after bacterial curing, animals were transferred to individually ventilated cages (IVC) in a room with controlled 12-h light/dark cycles. Intracisternal infections were performed by injection of 10 μl saline containing 6.44 ± 2.17 × 10^5 CFU/ml living *S. pneumoniae*. Control animals received an equivalent volume of saline. Pneumococcal meningitis was confirmed 18 h post infection (hpi) by quantitative analysis of bacterial titres in CSF samples, when the animals developed symptomatic disease. For this, 5 μl of CSF were collected by puncture of the cisterna magna, followed by serial dilution and cultivation on a CSBA plates.

A total of 180 infant, mixed-sex rats were included in this study, representing 15 independent experiments with 12 infant rats per experiment (10 acute infection experiments plus 5 experiments to assess neurofunctional outcome). Specifically, 120 animals were included in the acute PM study to assess neuroinflammation and brain damage and an additional 60 animals were studied to investigate neurofunctional outcomes. Infected animals were randomised for treatment with ceftriaxone (CRO, 100 mg/kg, bid, i.p. Rocephine, Roche) combined with different adjuvant treatment groups: (a) single adjuvant therapy with daptomycin (DAP, $n = 24$, 10 mg kg^{-1} day^{-1}, s.c. in saline, single application; Cubicin, Cubist Pharmaceuticals); (b) single adjuvant therapy with Trocade ($n = 24$, 2 × 75 mg kg^{-1} day^{-1}, i.p in succinylated gelatine [Physiogel®, University Hospital Bern, Switzerland]); (c) combined adjuvant therapy using both DAP and Trocade ($n = 66$); (d) CRO monotherapy ($n = 42$, single s.c. saline application and i.p. succinylate gelatine, bid). Animals in the adjuvant daptomycin group received vehicle injections with Physiogel® (i.p.); animals in the adjuvant Trocade group received one saline vehicle injection (s.c.); and animals in the CRO monotherapy group received both vehicles. All animals received the same amount of fluids during the course of the experiment. All therapies were started at 18 hpi. Therapies involving DAP were started by the application of DAP followed by a 15-min delayed application (i.e. at 18:15 hpi) of all other therapies, similar to the currently recommended application sequence for adjuvant dexamethasone in adult PM [43]. Mock-infected animals either received combined adjuvant therapy ($n = 12$) or CRO monotherapy with vehicles ($n = 12$).

The rats were weighted and examined clinically at 0, 18, 24 hpi and before sacrificing at 42 hpi, as previously described [42]. Activity scores range from 1 = coma; 2 = does not turn upright; 3 = turns upright within 30 s; 4 = minimal ambulatory activity, turns upright in < 5 s; to 5 = normal.

Investigators were blinded for treatment modalities. Spontaneous mortality was documented. Punctures of the cisterna magna were performed using a 30-gauge needle to obtain CSF samples at 18, 24, and 42 hpi. CSF samples not used for bacterial titre determination were centrifuged (16,000×*g* at 4 °C for 10 min), and supernatants were frozen at – 80 °C until further use.

Animals were sacrificed with an overdose of pentobarbital at 42 hpi and perfused with 4% paraformaldehyde (PFA) in phosphate-buffered saline (PBS) before their brains were removed and fixed in 4% PFA for histological analysis.

Histomorphometric assessment of cortical damage and hippocampal apoptosis

In all animals sacrificed at 42 hpi, damage to cerebral structures was quantified as previously described by us and other independent research groups [11, 28, 30, 44–46]. Briefly, brains were fixed in 4% PFA and cryopreserved in 18% sucrose in PBS at 4 °C overnight. Coronal brain cryosections (45 μm thick) obtained by systematic uniform sampling were stained for Nissl substance with cresyl violet. Cortical damage was defined as areas of decreased neuronal density. Dead cells with histological features of apoptosis were quantified in 48 visual fields (× 400 magnification) spanning the hippocampus of both hemispheres. To prevent inter-rater confounding, histologic assessment was performed and evaluated by one single person blinded to treatment modalities of the individual animals.

Quantitative analysis of cytokine expression in the CSF

A panel of cytokines previously found to be upregulated in PM [15, 47]—i.e. IL-1β, IL-6, TNF-α, IL-10 and IFN-γ—was assessed using a magnetic multiplex assay (Rat Magnetic Luminex® Assay, Rat Premixed Multi-Analyte Kit, R&D Systems, Bio-Techne) on a Bio-Plex 200 station (Bio-Rad Laboratories) as previously described [13, 30]. Five microlitres of CSF harvested and centrifuged at 18, 24 and 42 hpi was diluted to a final volume of 50 μl using the provided assay buffer. At least 50 beads were measured for each analyte. Calibration curves from recombinant standards were calculated with Bio-Plex Manager software (version 4.1.1) using a five-parameter logistic curve fitting. For samples below the detection limit, a value corresponding to the detection limit provided by the manufacturer (TNF-α, 22.1 pg/ml; IL-6, 56.0 pg/ml; IL-1β, 26.7 pg/ml; IL-10, 18.6 pg/ml; IFN-γ, 70.5 pg/ml) multiplied by the dilution factor was assigned.

Assessment of learning and memory function by Morris water maze

Learning and memory performance was evaluated 3 weeks after infection using Morris water maze as previously described [48]. Swimming patterns of rats were recorded and evaluated with the video tracking system EthoVision XT-11 (Noldus Information Technology, Wageningen, Netherlands). The water was made turbid by addition of nontoxic black colour, and the water maze arena was virtually divided into four quadrants. An adjustable black platform measuring 16 × 13 cm was placed in the centre of the first quadrant 0.5 cm below the water surface, invisible to the swimming rat. Extra-maze distal cues were placed on the walls surrounding the water maze arena. Over 5 days, the animals performed five training trials per day with a hidden platform in a fixed position. Facing the tank wall, the rats were transferred into the water at one of the three entry zones determined by randomisation. When an animal found the platform within 90 s, it could stay on it for 15 s before starting the next training trial. If the rat did not find the platform within 90 s, it was guided to the platform by hand and could stay on it for 15 s. During training trials, latency to platform, distance to reach platform and velocity were recorded. On day 5 of the experiment, a probe trial without the platform was performed before and after the training trial session to assess long-term and short-term memory. Mean distance of rats to the centre of the virtual platform and percent of time spent in the quadrant that used to contain the platform were evaluated. Additionally, the first training trial per day was used as a measure of memory performance. On day 1, the first training trial was termed "day 0" for the learning curve (Fig. 4b). Investigators were blinded for treatment modalities of the individual animals. All measurements for swimming path were automatically recorded and computed by the video tracking system.

Determination of hearing capacity by click and pure tone evoked auditory brainstem response

Auditory brainstem responses (ABRs) were recorded in response to click stimulations and pure tones on both ears using the SmartEP system (Intelligent Hearing Systems, Miami, USA), as previously described [13]. Animals were anesthetised with isoflurane (5% for induction and 2% for maintenance) using the Combi-Vet Vaporizer System equipped with a digital flowmeter (Rothacher Medical, Switzerland). One hundred-microsecond click stimuli and 5-ms pure tone pips (Blackman envelope; polarity alternating) were presented at a rate of 21.1 s^{-1}, ranging from 100 to 20 dB SPL in 10 dB decrements (5 dB decrements close to threshold). Responses were measured at 4, 8, 16 and 32 kHz. A total of 1024 responses were averaged at each sound level and filtered between 100 and 1500 Hz. The hearing threshold was defined as the lowest intensity that induced the appearance of a visually detectable first peak. ABRs were recorded after water maze experiments (at postnatal day

P37 to P39). Hearing thresholds were independently analysed by multiple blinded investigators.

Statistical analysis

Statistical analyses were performed with GraphPad Prism (Prism 7; GraphPad Software Inc., San Diego, USA). If not stated otherwise, results are presented as mean values ± standard deviations. To compare data between two groups, an unpaired Student *t* test was used for parametric data and a Mann-Whitney for non-parametric data. Mortality rates were calculated using a log rank (Mantel-Cox) test for significance. For repeated measures (pure-tone hearing threshold, learning and memory performance in Morris water maze), a two-way ANOVA was performed to analyse differences between treatment modalities over time (for water maze data) or according to pure-tone frequencies (for ABRs). A two-tailed p value of < 0.05 was considered statistically significant, with $p < 0.05$ (*), $p < 0.01$ (**), $p < 0.001$ (***) and $p < 0.0001$ (****).

For exploratory data analysis, a multivariate linear regression model was used to estimate predictors and determinants for bacterial meningitis-induced hearing loss. The linear coefficients and a 95% confidence interval were calculated for each variable. These statistical analyses were performed using STATA 12 (STATA Corp., College Station, TX).

Results

A total of 180 infant Wistar rats were included in the study. All animals infected with *S. pneumoniae* ($n = 156$) developed meningitis, as proven by growth of bacteria ($\geq 10^7$ CFU/ml) in CSF samples obtained at 18 hpi and the appearance of disease symptoms (clinical score < 5, weight loss, changes in posture).

Weight loss, clinical score and survival

Survival was significantly reduced in infected animals (Fig. 1a) compared to mock-infected controls. Adjuvant therapies did not significantly improve survival compared to CRO monotherapy. Relative weight change in infected animals was not significantly altered by any of the treatment groups (Fig. 1b). However, the combined adjuvant therapy showed a strong trend towards improved weight gain at 42 hpi compared to CRO monotherapy ($p = 0.0503$). Upon infection, clinical scores in all infected animals decreased and reached a minimum at 24 hpi with subsequent improvement at 42 hpi. Clinical scores of infected infant rats treated with the combined adjuvant therapy were significantly improved compared to CRO monotherapy at 24 hpi ($p < 0.01$). At 42 hpi, all infected animals receiving adjuvant therapies demonstrated a significantly improved clinical score compared to

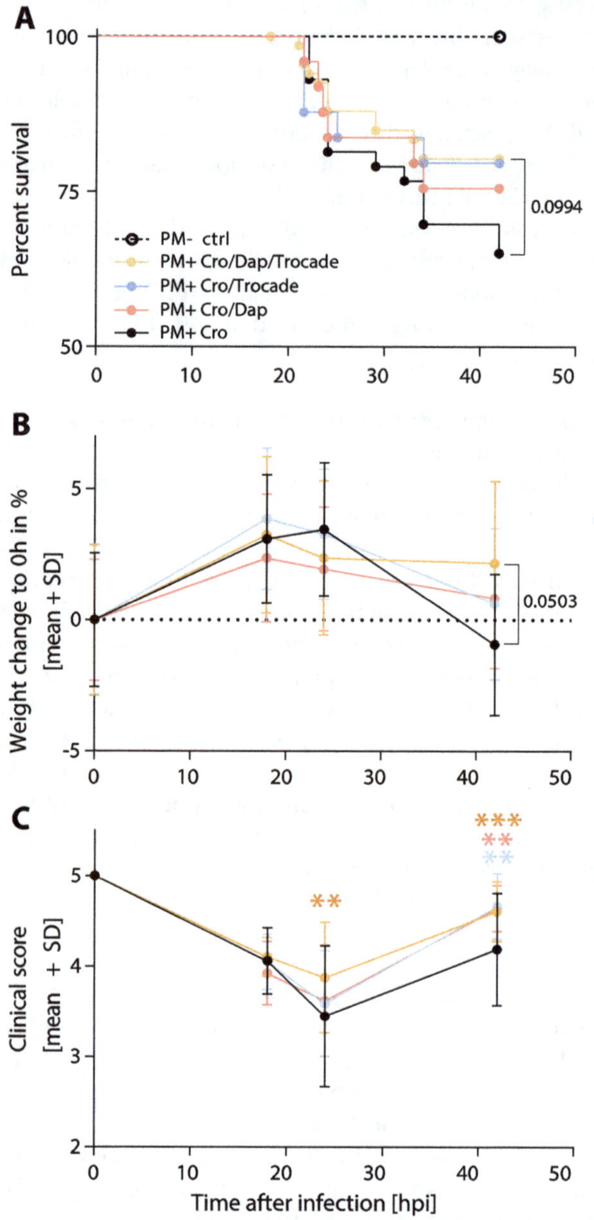

Fig. 1 Survival, relative weight change and clinical scores of infant rats with acute pneumococcal meningitis. (**a**) Survival analysis revealed a significant difference of infected rats compared to mock-infected controls. Within the treatment groups, no significant differences in survival were found. Combined adjuvant therapy showed a non-significant trend ($p = 0.0994$) towards better survival compared to infant rats receiving CRO monotherapy. (**b**) Relative weight change during acute infections showed a slight increase within the first 18 hpi and a decrease of weight with the onset of clinical symptoms and treatment initiation until 42 hpi. In the combined adjuvant therapy group (Cro/Dap/Trocade), a strong trend points towards increased weight gain compared to animals receiving CRO monotherapy (Cro) at 42 hpi. (**c**) Clinical scores decrease upon infection until 24 hpi where the animals start to recover until 42 hpi. At 24 hpi, infant rats treated with combined adjuvant therapy displayed significantly higher clinical scores than animals treated with CRO monotherapy. Significance levels are always indicated as compared to CRO monotherapy

CRO monotherapy, independent of the treatment regimen ($p < 0.001$ for CRO/DAP/Trocade; $p < 0.01$ for CRO/DAP; $p < 0.01$ for CRO/Trocade, Fig. 1c). Data on acute clinical parameters are summarised in Table 1.

Combined adjuvant therapy reduces hippocampal apoptosis and cortical necrosis

In mock-infected animals (PM-), hippocampal apoptosis was found to occur at physiologic levels and no cortical damage was detectable (Fig. 2a, c), as previously described [9]. The highest amount of apoptotic neurons in the subgranular zone of the dentate gyrus was found in animals receiving CRO monotherapy (9.26 ± 6.06 apoptotic cells per visual field, $n = 9$). Hippocampal apoptosis was significantly reduced in infant rats receiving adjuvant Trocade (3.41 ± 2.97 apoptotic cells per visual field, $n = 19$, $p < 0.01$) and in animals receiving the combined adjuvant therapy (3.307 ± 3.70 apoptotic cells per visual field, $n = 35$, $p < 0.001$, Fig. 2a) compared to animals treated with CRO monotherapy. Adjuvant therapy with DAP did not significantly reduce hippocampal apoptosis (4.75 ± 7.52 apoptotic cells per visual field, $n = 18$, $p = 0.131$).

The highest extent of cortical necrosis was found in the animals receiving CRO monotherapy (2.70% [IQR 0.97–4.49]). Cortical necrosis was significantly reduced in infant rats treated with adjuvant DAP (0.13% [IQR 0–1.75], $p < 0.05$) and in animals receiving the combined adjuvant therapy (0.25% [IQR 0–2.19], $p < 0.05$, Fig. 2c). In this study, adjuvant Trocade did not significantly decrease the amount of cortical necrosis in infant rats with pneumococcal meningitis. The range of hippocampal apoptosis and cortical necrosis were found at levels of previously published studies [29, 30, 48].

As only the combined adjuvant therapy was able to protect from both acute cerebral damages, further analysis therefore focused on comparing the combined treatment modality to CRO monotherapy.

Combined adjuvant therapy decreases inflammation and clears bacteria faster in CSF

Inflammatory cytokines were measured immediately before, 6 and 24 h after treatment initiation (representing 18, 24 and 42 hpi). At treatment start, there was no significant difference in the cytokine profile between infected animals receiving CRO monotherapy or combined adjuvant therapy, indicating a comparable severity of inflammation between these two groups (Fig. 3a–e). Six hours after treatment initiation, levels of TNF-α ($p < 0.01$), IL-1β ($p < 0.01$), IL-6 ($p < 0.001$) and IL-10 ($p < 0.01$) were significantly reduced in animals receiving combined adjuvant therapy ($n = 14$) compared to CRO monotherapy ($n = 15$). Thereafter, all CSF cytokine levels decreased and no differences in CSF cytokine concentrations were found between the two groups 24 h after starting the therapy. Similar bacterial CSF concentrations were found in both groups before treatment initiation ($1.46 \pm 1.29 \times 10^8$ CFU/ml for CRO ($n = 38$) vs. $1.31 \pm 0.86 \times 10^8$ CFU/ml for CRO/DAP/Trocade ($n = 38$), $p = 0.566$, Fig. 3f), confirming a comparable severity of infection. Six hours after therapy start, bacterial CSF concentrations were efficiently reduced in both treatment groups. While none of the animals with combined adjuvant therapy showed detectable bacteria in the CSF (< 10^2 CFU/ml, $n = 11$), the majority of animals treated receiving CRO monotherapy still presented living bacteria in the CSF (median of 1.00×10^3 CFU/ml vs. 1.00×10^2 CFU/ml, $n = 10$, $p < 0.001$), indicating faster bacterial clearance in the CSF in animals receiving combined adjuvant therapy compared to monotherapy with CRO.

Combined adjuvant therapy improves learning and memory performance

Neurofunctional outcome after pneumococcal meningitis was evaluated using a Morris water maze test (Fig. 4a) 3 weeks after infection. Learning ability was observed in all animal groups, as indicated by a steady decrease of total distance swum until reaching the platform during

Table 1 Relative weight change, clinical scores and bacterial CSF titres in infant rats with pneumococcal meningitis ($n = 156$) and uninfected controls ($n = 24$) during the acute phase of the disease. Activity scores represent 1 = coma; 2 = does not turn upright; 3 = turns upright within 30 s; 4 = minimal ambulatory activity, turns upright in < 5 s; and 5 = normal. Weight change describes percentage of weight gain compared to weight at time of infection. Bacterial titre depicts colony-forming units (CFU) per millilitre CSF at 18 hpi. Data represent mean ± SD. hpi hours post infection, PM pneumococcal meningitis, Cro ceftriaxone, Dap daptomycin

	18 hpi			24 hpi		42 hpi	
	Activity	Weight change	Bacterial titre	Activity	Weight change	Activity	Weight change
PM+ Cro ($n = 42$)	4.1 ± 0.4	3.1 ± 2.4	$1.46 \pm 1.29 \times 10^8$	3.4 ± 0.8	3.5 ± 2.5	4.2 ± 0.6	− 0.9 ± 2.7
PM+ Cro+Dap ($n = 24$)	4.1 ± 0.3	3.8 ± 2.7	$1.03 \pm 0.72 \times 10^8$	3.6 ± 0.6	3.3 ± 2.9	4.6 ± 0.3	0.6 ± 2.9
PM+ Cro+Trocade ($n = 24$)	3.9 ± 0.3	2.4 ± 2.4	$0.96 \pm 0.56 \times 10^8$	3.6 ± 0.6	2.0 ± 2.4	4.7 ± 0.4	0.8 ± 2.7
PM+ Cro+Dap+Trocade ($n = 66$)	4.1 ± 0.3	3.3 ± 3.0	$1.15 \pm 0.76 \times 10^8$	3.9 ± 0.6	2.4 ± 3.0	4.7 ± 0.3	2.2 ± 3.1
PM− ctrl ($n = 24$)	5.0 ± 0	13.8 ± 2.6	Undetectable	5.0 ± 0	21.8 ± 2.8	4.98 ± 0.1	31.1 ± 5.8

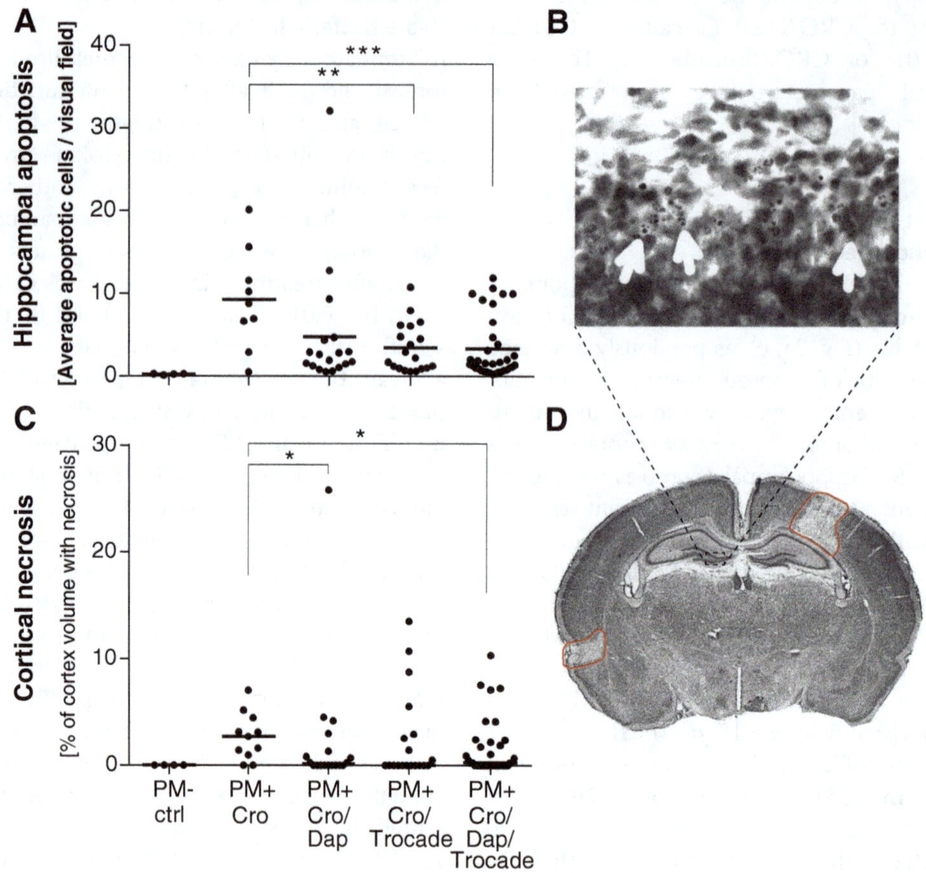

Fig. 2 Hippocampal apoptosis and cortical damage during acute pneumococcal meningitis. Hippocampal apoptosis was most abundant in infant rats receiving CRO monotherapy. (**a**) Treatment with adjuvant Trocade and with combined adjuvant therapy significantly reduced hippocampal apoptosis. (**b**) Apoptotic cells in the subgranular zone of the dentate gyrus show condensed nuclei or formation of apoptotic bodies (white arrows). (**c**) Cortical necrosis was most prominently observed in animals receiving CRO monotherapy. Adjuvant daptomycin and combined adjuvant therapy significantly reduced cortical necrosis. (**d**) Cortical necrosis with reduced neuronal density is visible on cresyl violet stained brain sections. Foci of cortical necrosis are indicated by red lines. In **a**, the horizontal line depicts the sample mean and an unpaired *t* test was used for single comparison. In **c**, the horizontal line represents the sample median and a Mann-Whitney test was used for single comparison

the training trials over the 5 days (Fig. 4b). Mock-infected animals (PM− ctrl, $n = 20$) showed significant better learning performance than infected animals receiving CRO monotherapy (PM+ CRO, $n = 12$, $p < 0.001$) and infected animals receiving combined adjuvant therapy (PM+ CRO/DAP/Trocade, $n = 13$, $p < 0.05$). Animals receiving combined adjuvant therapy performed significantly better in the learning assessment than infected animals with CRO monotherapy ($p = 0 < 0.05$). Analysing latency to reach platform during training trials revealed similar findings for learning performance (data not shown).

Mock-infected animals showed the best performance for memory formation over the 5 days of testing, as assessed by separate analysis of the first training trial per day (Fig. 4c). These animals displayed significant better memory compared to infected animals receiving CRO ($p < 0.0001$) and to infected animals receiving combined adjuvant therapy ($p < 0.05$). Infected animals receiving combined adjuvant therapy showed significantly improved memory performance compared infected animals receiving CRO monotherapy ($p < 0.01$). On days 1 and 5, spatial memory was further assessed using probe trials performed without platform by evaluating the average distance of the animal's swimming path to the virtual platform location. Two-way ANOVA tests revealed impaired performance of infected animals receiving CRO monotherapy to mock-infected animals ($p < 0.05$) and to infected animals receiving combined adjuvant therapy ($p < 0.01$, Fig. 4d). For the second probe trial performed on day 5—representing short-term memory formation—a significant better performance of infected animals receiving the combined adjuvant therapy compared to infected animals receiving only CRO ($p < 0.01$) was documented. Analysing probe trial memory formation by time spent in the quadrant that used to harbour the platform revealed similar findings (data not shown).

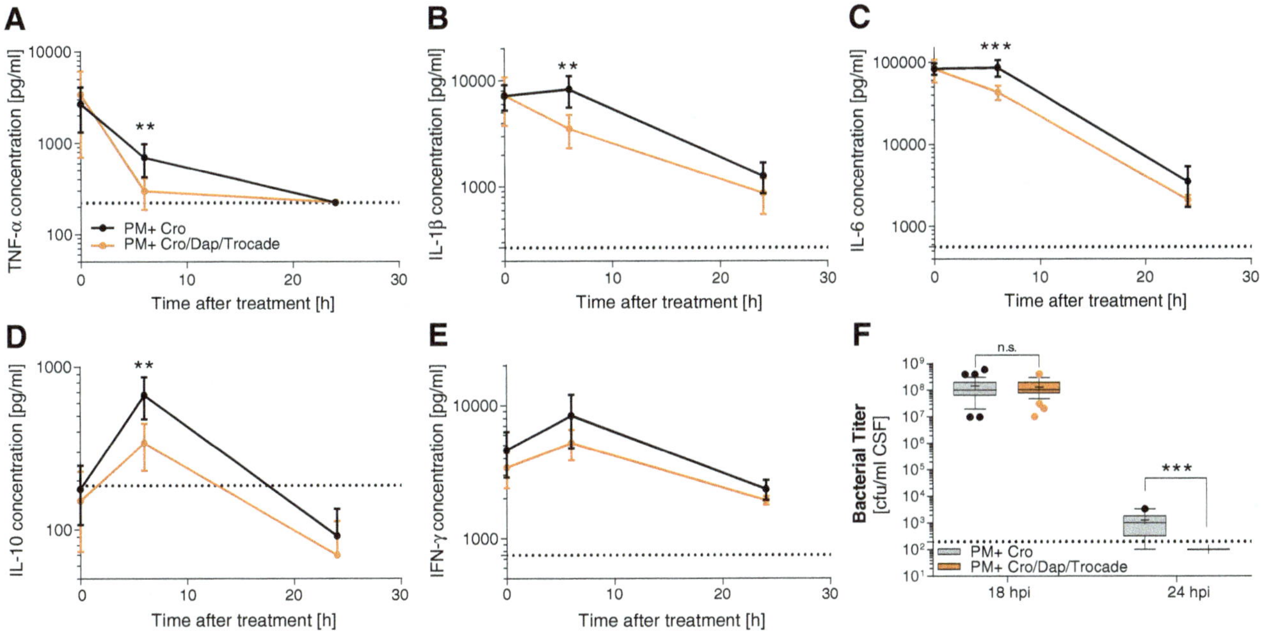

Fig. 3 Inflammatory cytokines and bacterial clearance in the CSF during the acute pneumococcal meningitis. Cytokine levels are represented by mean ± 95% confidence interval starting before treatment initiation, 6 h and 24 h after treatment start (representing 18, 24 and 42 hpi) for TNF-α (**a**), IL-1β (**b**), IL-6 (**c**), IL-10 (**d**) and IFN-γ (**e**). Six hours after treatment initiation, TNF-α, IL-1β, IL-6 and IL-10 were significantly reduced in infected animals receiving the combined adjuvant therapy compared to infected animals with CRO monotherapy. Bacterial titres in the CSF were similar in both treatment groups before starting therapy (at 18 hpi) with a faster bacterial clearance in animals receiving the combined adjuvant therapy (**f**). Statistical differences were assessed using an unpaired t-test for cytokines and bacterial titre at 18 hpi. For bacterial titre at 24 hpi, a Mann-Whitney test was used as data were not normally distributed

Combined adjuvant therapy reduces hearing loss

Hearing thresholds were determined 4 weeks after infection using broadband click stimuli and pure tones. We found significantly increased hearing thresholds in infected animals compared to their respective mock-infected control animals (CRO-treated animals 77.14 ± 16.84 dB vs. 28.38 ± 1.67 dB in mock-infected controls, $p < 0.0001$; combined adjuvant therapy-treated animals 60.92 dB ± 20.82 vs. 27.85 ± 3.55 dB in mock-infected controls, $p < 0.0001$, Fig. 5a). In infected rats, combined adjuvant therapy significantly improved average hearing capacity compared to CRO monotherapy ($p < 0.05$). Pure tone ABR testing revealed higher thresholds for all assessed frequencies in infected animals compared to mock-infected animals ($p < 0.0001$, two-way ANOVA, independent of therapeutic modality, Fig. 5b). Infected animals that received combined adjuvant therapy demonstrated significantly better pure tone hearing capacity than those treated with CRO monotherapy ($p < 0.05$, Fig. 5b). Frequency-specific analysis disclosed that at lower frequencies (4 kHz and 8 kHz), hearing was improved in animals treated with combined adjuvant therapy (Fig. 5c) 60.25 ± 17.9 dB vs 78.46 ± 14.49 dB for 4 kHz ($p < 0.01$) and 64.92 ± 16.99 dB vs 82.69 ± 17.24 dB for 8 kHz ($p < 0.05$). No significant difference was found at 16 kHz and 32 kHz.Univariate linear regression analysis (Table 2) revealed significantly increased hearing thresholds with increasing bacterial titres in CSF (29.5 dB per additional log of CSF titres at 18 hpi, $p < 0.01$). Treatment with combined adjuvant therapy (– 16.8 dB compared to infected animals treated with CRO monotherapy, $p < 0.05$) and better clinical score at 24 hpi (– 21.7 dB per additional score, $p < 0.01$) were predictive for reduced hearing loss. The multivariate linear regression analysis—including bacterial titres in the CSF at 18 hpi and treatment regimen—presented a significant contribution of bacterial titres to higher hearing threshold (35.1 dB per additional log of CSF titre at 18 hpi, $p < 0.001$) and a significant benefit of treating infected animals with combined adjuvant therapy (– 21.7 dB compared to infected animals receiving CRO monotherapy, $p < 0.001$).

Discussion

The results of the present study demonstrate that a combined adjuvant therapy consisting of DAP and Trocade was able to integrate the beneficial effects of both compounds in experimental paediatric PM. Moreover, the adjuvant combination therapy significantly improved the neurofunctional outcome in experimental infant rat PM compared to CRO monotherapy.

Brain damage caused by PM is associated with an exacerbated CSF inflammation and results in an

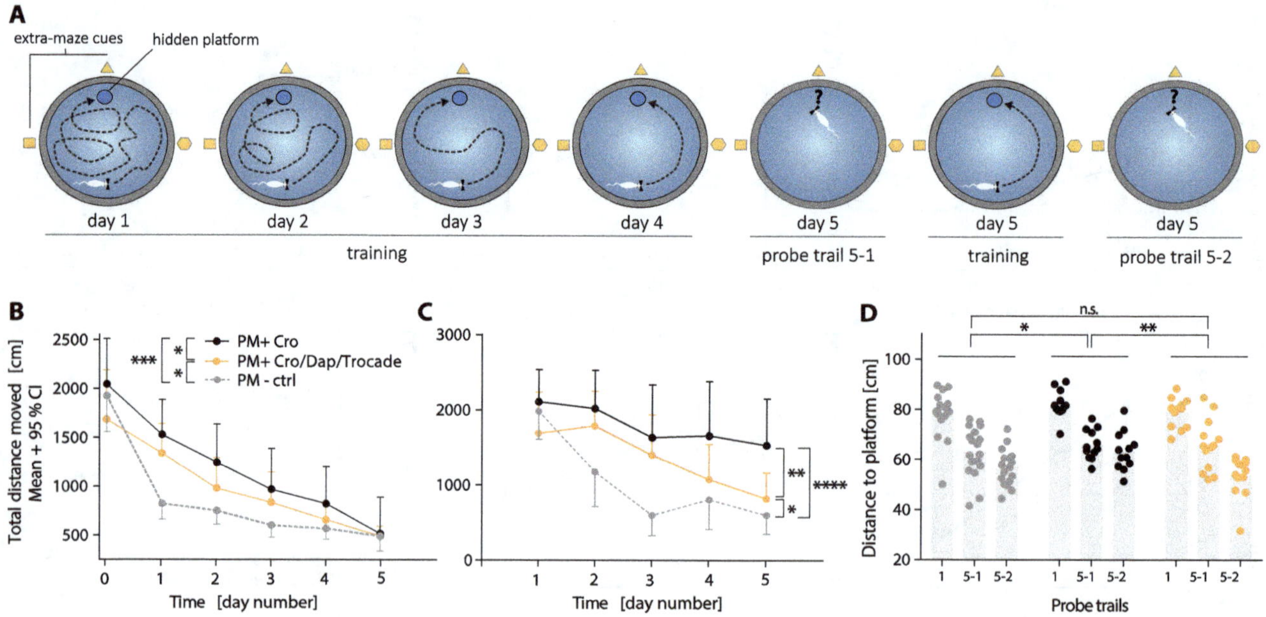

Fig. 4 Learning and memory performance 3 weeks after acute pneumococcal meningitis assessed by Morris water maze. (**a**) Schematic representation of our Morris water maze protocol used during these experiments (scheme sketch inspired by Kipnis et al. [35]). Learning performance assessed on five consecutive days revealed impaired learning of infected animals compared to mock-infected animals. Infected animals treated with combined adjuvant therapy revealed significantly improved learning behaviour compared to their infected counterparts receiving CRO monotherapy (**b**). Memory assessment—by analysing the first training trial for each day separately—showed significantly reduced memory performance in infected animals compared to mock-infected animals. Infected animals treated with combined adjuvant therapy showed significantly improved memory compared to their infected counterparts treated with CRO monotherapy (**c**). Memory formation assessed with probe trials after removing the platform further demonstrated the impaired performance of infected animals with CRO monotherapy to infected animals receiving combined adjuvant therapy and to mock-infected animals (**d**). Statistical differences were assessed by two-way ANOVAs to compare learning and memory performance between groups over repeated time points

unfavourable neurofunctional outcome of the disease [15, 49–51]. The initial unrestricted growth of *S. pneumoniae* in CSF produces large amounts of pathogen-associated molecular patterns (PAMPs), a situation that is aggravated by treatment with bacteriolytic antibiotics, causing release of bacterial components into the CSF and inducing an even more severe inflammatory reaction [49, 50]. Based on these observations, the use of adjunctive therapies is meant to attenuate this cerebral hyperinflammatory reaction. In adults and children with PM, dexamethasone is currently recommended as adjuvant therapy in high-income countries based on a Cochrane meta-analysis [24, 43]. The beneficial effect of corticosteroids in paediatric bacterial meningitis was, however, exclusively

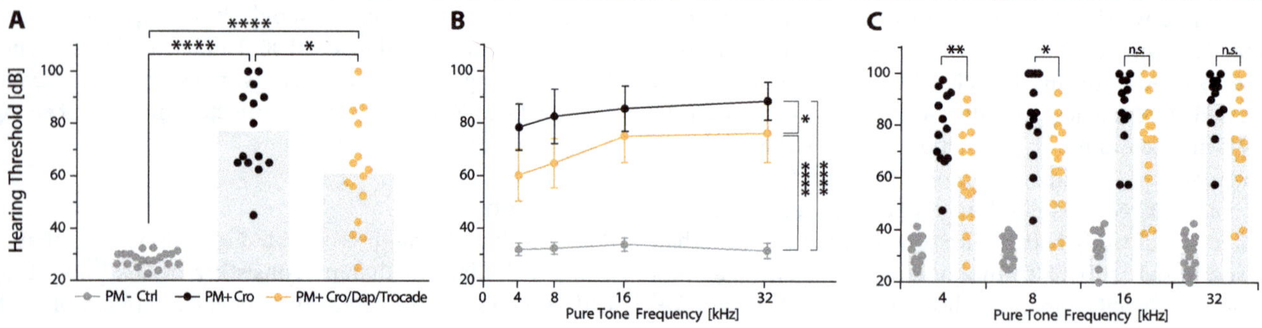

Fig. 5 Hearing capacity assessed 3 weeks after acute pneumococcal meningitis. ABR recordings using broadband click stimuli disclosed significantly increased hearing threshold in infected rats. Combined adjuvant therapy significantly improved hearing capacity in infected rats compared to CRO monotherapy (**a**). Pure tone ABR threshold (mean ± 95% confidence interval) demonstrated significantly impaired hearing in infected animals but improved hearing function in infected rats receiving the combined adjuvant therapy (**b**). Frequency-specific hearing threshold in infected rats revealed preservation of low frequency hearing (4 kHz and 8 kHz) in rats receiving the combined adjuvant therapy (**c**). Statistical differences were assessed by single comparison using an unpaired *t* test in **a** and **c** and by two-way ANOVA in **b**

Table 2 Univariate and multivariate linear regression for click hearing threshold in infant rats ($n = 29$) 4 weeks after surviving an episode of pneumococcal meningitis measured by click stimuli

	Hearing threshold					
	Univariate			Multivariate		
	Coef.	95% CI	*p*	Coef.	95% CI	*p*
Log bacterial CSF titre at 18 hpi	29.5	11.13–47.8	0.003	35.1	20.1–50.0	< 0.001
Treatment with combined adjuvant therapy	− 16.8	− 31.3 to − 2.2	0.026	− 21.7	− 32.7 to − 10.7	< 0.001
Female sex	1.8	− 15.5–19.1	0.832	–	–	–
Relative weight gain (per add. percent)	− 1.03	− 2.4–0.4	0.141	–	–	–
Clinical score at 24 hpi	− 21.7	− 35.4 to − 7.9	0.003	–	–	–

demonstrated for meningitis caused by *Haemophilus influenzae* and not for PM or other causative pathogens [24]. In animal models for infant PM, the outcome after adjunctive dexamethasone therapy was aggravated with regard to survival, weight loss, hippocampal apoptosis and memory performance [9, 25, 26]. Since this present study was performed in a model of infant PM, we did not compare treatment regimens to adjunctive dexamethasone, which has previously been shown to impair the outcome in comparison to CRO monotherapy [9, 25–28].

Daptomycin, a non-bacteriolytic and bactericidal lipopeptide antibiotic, is used for treatment of serious Gram-positive infections [52]. Insertion of the lipophilic tail of daptomycin into the bacterial cell membrane causes a rapid membrane depolarisation, thereby stopping biosynthesis and causing bacterial death [52–54]. Treatment with daptomycin has been shown to minimise antibiotic-induced cell wall lysis compared to ceftriaxone in experimental pneumococcal meningitis in rabbits [40]. In previous work, we showed that daptomycin in infant rat PM led to a faster bacterial clearance from the CSF, thereby reducing inflammatory parameters and decreasing cortical injury compared to CRO treatment [41, 55]. Addition of daptomycin to CRO in infant rats reduced PM-associated cerebral damage, inflammatory cytokine levels in the CSF and improved hearing capacity [29]. In adult rats with PM, daptomycin treatment attenuated cognitive impairment compared to CRO [56]. Although *S. pneumoniae* and group B streptococci (GBS) are very frequent causes of paediatric and neonatal bacterial meningitis, recent European data reported that *Neisseria meningitidis* and *Haemophilus influenzae* account for 55% of all paediatric cases beyond neonatal age [43]. Thus, for empiric therapy, daptomycin needs to be combined with a broad spectrum antibiotic targeting Gram-negative bacteria (e.g. CRO as an expanded-spectrum cephalosporin), to cover potential infection with *N. meningitidis* or *H. influenzae* [29].

Brain injury in acute PM involves an upregulation of MMP activity, measurable in the CSF of infected patients [15, 57] with higher MMP-9 level being associated with the development of hearing impairment or secondary epilepsy in infected children [57]. MMP-9 weakens the blood-brain barrier (BBB) by degrading collagen, e.g. in the basal lamina [42, 58], thereby facilitating leukocyte extravasation and BBB leakage [30, 59]. Moreover, MMPs are potent sheddases and convertases able to cleave and activate inflammatory cytokines and chemokines, thereby contributing to the hyperinflammatory reaction driving the development of brain damage [30, 60–62]. In previous work, we showed that MMP inhibition with adjunctive Trocade treatment in infant rats with PM increased survival and significantly reduced the collagenase activity of MMPs, the intrathecal concentrations of pro-inflammatory cytokines and the level of cortical necrosis and hippocampal apoptosis [30].

Combining adjuvant daptomycin and Trocade reduces CSF inflammation and neuropathology in experimental paediatric PM

During acute PM, combining adjuvant daptomycin and Trocade improved clinical scores of infant rats at 24 and 42 hpi and showed a non-significant trend ($p = 0.0503$) towards improved weight gain at 42 hpi compared to CRO monotherapy (Fig. 1b). Single adjuvant therapies with either daptomycin or Trocade also improved the clinical scoring at 42 hpi. In the present study, no significant difference in survival could be found between groups. In an earlier report with adjuvant Trocade therapy, survival was improved [30]. In this earlier study, however, adjuvant Trocade therapy was initiated at an earlier time point after infection (at 5 hpi), whereas in the present study, it was applied concomitantly with the appearance of the clinical symptoms (at 18 hpi) and the initiation of antibiotic treatment.

All tested adjuvant therapies protected the subjects from at least one form of neuronal damage observed during pneumococcal meningitis (Fig. 2). Adjuvant Trocade significantly reduced the amount of apoptosis in the dentate gyrus of the hippocampus. On the other hand, adjuvant daptomycin significantly reduced cortical necrosis. The adjuvant combination therapy was superior to single adjuvants by reducing both forms of cerebral damage. Thereby, we could validate our hypothesis that adjuvant therapies targeting different pathophysiological mechanisms during acute PM generate additive protective effects on brain damage. The neuroprotective effects of single adjunctive Trocade and daptomycin have already been reported previously [29, 30]. Since only the combined adjuvant therapy was able to significantly reduce both forms of brain injury during acute PM, we further focused on comparing the combination therapy to the CRO monotherapy. Combining adjuvant daptomycin and Trocade with CRO reduced CSF levels of TNF-α, IL-1β, IL-6 and IL-10 6 hours after treatment initiation and caused a faster bacterial clearance in the CSF (Fig. 3). Faster bacterial clearance might be attributed to adjuvant daptomycin, as reported earlier [40, 41, 55]. Overall reduction in neuroinflammatory parameters is mostly likely caused by a combined effect of faster bacterial clearance and limited release of bacterial cell wall components due to daptomycin [40, 41, 55] plus reduced collagenase-induced BBB leakage and reduced cytokine and chemokine shedding by Trocade [30, 60–62]. In the present study, we found no statistically significant reduction of IFN-γ CSF levels in infected animals treated with combined adjuvant therapy compared to CRO monotherapy. This is in agreement with findings from previous studies on single adjuvant Trocade therapy and single antibiotic therapy with daptomycin that did not show significantly reduced IFN- γ levels [30, 55]. Differences in inflammatory cytokine reduction, bacterial clearance and clinical parameters are in accordance to what has been previously reported for single adjuvant therapies [13, 29, 30, 40, 41, 55].

Combining adjuvant daptomycin and Trocade improves the neurofunctional outcome in experimental paediatric PM

Hippocampal apoptosis during acute pneumococcal meningitis correlates with impaired learning performance and memory formation [6–9], in turn preservation of the dentate gyrus is associated with intact learning and memory performance [9, 48]. Combining adjuvant daptomycin and Trocade preserved learning and memory performance assessed by Morris water maze testing (Fig. 4b). Compared to uninfected control animals, infected rats, independently of the treatment regimen, showed significantly decreased learning performance. However, infected rats receiving combined adjuvant therapy showed significantly improved learning performance compared to their infected counterparts receiving CRO monotherapy. Memory performance testing revealed that infected animals treated with CRO monotherapy presented markedly impaired spatial memory compared to uninfected animals (Fig. 4c). Animals receiving combined adjuvant therapy showed significantly improved memory performance compared to infected rats receiving CRO monotherapy, although demonstrating significant memory impairments compared to uninfected controls. Probe trials performed on day 5 confirmed that infected animals treated with CRO monotherapy had impaired memory formation compared to uninfected animals. These memory impairments were prevented by adjuvant combination therapy (Fig. 4d). Short term memory—assessed with the second probe trial—was especially improved in animals receiving combined adjuvant therapies. By reducing hippocampal apoptosis, combined adjuvant therapy thus improved learning and memory formation. As long-term memory consolidation and retrieval is a complex procedure and also involves cortical structures [63–65], reduction of cortical necrosis during acute PM possibly also contributed to the improved learning and memory performance found in animals receiving combined adjuvant therapy.

During acute PM, pneumococci and leukocytes infiltrate the cochlea from the CSF via the cochlear aqueduct [2, 4, 13, 23, 66], causing damage to the spiral ganglion neurons and sensory hair cells, resulting in sensorineural hearing loss [13, 14, 22, 25, 67–69]. Previous studies showed that TNF-α levels during acute experimental PM positively correlate with the severity of hearing loss [13] and that a reduction in inflammatory cytokines improved hearing capacity [29, 55, 67]. Here, combining daptomycin with Trocade during acute PM significantly reduced inflammatory cytokines and improved hearing capacity 4 weeks after infection (Fig. 5). Frequency-dependent analysis showed that hearing at low frequencies was preserved, which would correspond to a protection of cochlear sensory hair cells and spiral ganglion neurons in the cochlear apex. As bacteria from the CSF enter the inner ear via the cochlear aqueduct, we would expect a gradient of ototoxic substances with highest concentrations at the base and decreasing towards the apex—a hypothesis supported by previous animal and human studies [13, 70]. Our results suggest that faster bacterial clearance together with overall reduction of inflammatory parameters may reduce the concentration of ototoxic substances particularly in the apex thereby preserving hearing capacity at low frequencies. This finding is in line with an earlier study showing that the severity of infection modulates the extent of hearing loss, with moderately infected animals having a preserved hearing capacity for low frequencies perceived at the cochlear apex, whereas severely infected animals lost hearing capacity at all frequencies [13]. Multivariate linear regression confirmed a beneficial effect of the combination therapy on hearing loss after adjusting for severity of infection based on bacterial CSF titre at 18 hpi. Combined adjuvant therapy was able to significantly preserve 21.7 dB hearing capacity compared to CRO monotherapy (Table 2).

Limitations of this study include lack of comparison to single adjuvants in long-term experiments. As only combined adjuvant therapy was able to reduce both forms of cerebral damage, i.e. cortical necrosis and hippocampal apoptosis, behavioural tests were only conducted in infected animals receiving combined adjuvant therapy or CRO monotherapy. Thus, we do not have a direct comparison to single adjuvant therapies for neurofunctional outcomes. The proven superiority of combined adjuvant therapy to single adjuvant therapies is therefore based on data gathered from the acute phase of the disease. Furthermore, we did not include a direct comparison to adjuvant dexamethasone, as there is no clear evidence for its beneficial effect on the outcome of paediatric PM in the clinics [24, 71] nor animal models [9, 25–28].

Conclusion

Combined adjuvant therapy with non-bacteriolytic daptomycin and the matrix-metalloproteinase inhibitor Trocade reduces CSF cytokine levels, known to be mediators of brain damage during acute PM. Neuroprotective effects of single adjuvants were integrated by combined adjuvant intervention and attenuated neurologic sequelae by preserving learning and memory performance and preventing hearing loss. Based on these results, we conclude that combining adjuvant daptomycin and Trocade with ceftriaxone is a promising therapeutic option to improve the outcome of paediatric PM.

Abbreviations

ABR: Auditory brainstem response; BBB: Blood-brain barrier; BHI: Brain heart infusion; CFU: Colony-forming units; CNS: Central nervous system; CRO: Ceftriaxone; CSF: Cerebrospinal fluid; DAP: Daptomycin; GBS: Group B streptococci; MMP: Matrix-metalloproteinase; MWM: Morris water maze; PM: Pneumococcal meningitis; PNS: Peripheral nervous system

Acknowledgements

We acknowledge Roche Pharma, Basel, Switzerland, for providing Ro 32-3555. We thank Franziska Simon for excellent technical support. Productive discussions and inputs from the Cluster of Regenerative Neurosciences (Department of BioMedical Research, University of Bern) and the ESCMID Study Group for Infectious Diseases of the Brain (ESGIB) were highly appreciated.

Funding

This work was supported by a grant from the Swiss National Science Foundation (Grant 310030-162583).

Authors' contributions

LM, DG and SLL conceived and designed the study. LM, MB and MP performed experiments. LM, MP, MB, DG and SLL analysed the data. LM, DG, MB, MP and SLL contributed to writing of the manuscript. All authors read and approved the final manuscript.

Consent for publication

Not applicable

Competing interests

The authors declare that they have no competing interests.

Author details

[1]Neuroinfection Laboratory, Institute for Infectious Diseases, University of Bern, Friedbühlstrasse 51, 3001 Bern, Switzerland. [2]Graduate School for Cellular and Biomedical Sciences (GCB), University of Bern, Freiestrasse 1, 3012 Bern, Switzerland.

References

1. Koedel U, Scheld WM, Pfister H-W. Pathogenesis and pathophysiology of pneumococcal meningitis. Lancet Infect Dis. 2002;2:721–36.
2. Edmond K, Clark A, Korczak VS, Sanderson C, Griffiths UK, Rudan I. Global and regional risk of disabling sequelae from bacterial meningitis: a systematic review and meta-analysis. Lancet Infect Dis. 2010;10:317–28.
3. Brouwer MC, Tunkel AR, van de Beek D. Epidemiology, diagnosis, and antimicrobial treatment of acute bacterial meningitis. Clin Microbiol Rev. 2010;23:467–92.
4. Chandran A, Herbert H, Misurski D, Santosham M. Long-term sequelae of childhood bacterial meningitis: an underappreciated problem. Pediatr Infect Dis J. 2011;30:3–6.
5. Baraff LJ, Lee SI, Schriger DL. Outcomes of bacterial meningitis in children: a meta-analysis. Pediatr Infect Dis J. 1993;12:389–94.
6. Wellmer A, Noeske C, Gerber J, Munzel U, Nau R. Spatial memory and learning deficits after experimental pneumococcal meningitis in mice. Neurosci Lett. 2000;296:137–40.
7. Loeffler JM, Ringer R, Hablützel M, Täuber MG, Leib SL. The free radical scavenger α-phenyl-tert-butyl nitrone aggravates hippocampal apoptosis and learning deficits in experimental pneumococcal meningitis. J Infect Dis. 2001;183:247–52.
8. Nau R, Brück W. Neuronal injury in bacterial meningitis: mechanisms and implications for therapy. Trends Neurosci. 2002;25:38–45.
9. Leib SL, Heimgartner C, Bifrare Y-D, Loeffler JM, Täuber MG. Dexamethasone aggravates hippocampal apoptosis and learning deficiency in pneumococcal meningitis in infant rats. Pediatr Res. 2003;54:353–7.
10. Nau R, Soto A, Bruck W. Apoptosis of neurons in the dentate gyrus in humans suffering from bacterial meningitis. J Neuropathol Exp Neurol. 1999; 58:265–74.
11. Grandgirard D, Steiner O, Täuber MG, Leib SL. An infant mouse model of brain damage in pneumococcal meningitis. Acta Neuropathol. 2007;114: 609–17.
12. Bifrare Y-D, Gianinazzi C, Imboden H, Leib SL, Täuber MG. Bacterial meningitis causes two distinct forms of cellular damage in the hippocampal dentate gyrus in infant rats. Hippocampus. 2003;13:481–8.
13. Perny M, Roccio M, Grandgirard D, Solyga M, Senn P, Leib SL. The severity of infection determines the localization of damage and extent of sensorineural hearing loss in experimental pneumococcal meningitis. J Neurosci. 2016;36:7740–9.
14. Perny M, Solyga M, Grandgirard D, Roccio M, Leib SL, Senn P. Streptococcus pneumoniae-induced ototoxicity in organ of Corti explant cultures. Hear Res. 2017;350:100–9.
15. Mook-Kanamori BB, Geldhoff M, van der Poll T, van de Beek D. Pathogenesis and pathophysiology of pneumococcal meningitis. Clin Microbiol Rev. 2011; 24:557–91.
16. Mitchell L, Smith SH, Braun JS, Herzog K, Weber JR, Tuomanen EI. Dual phases of apoptosis in pneumococcal meningitis. J Infect Dis. 2004;190: 2039–46.
17. Agyeman P, Grandgirard D, Leib S, Chapter 23: Pathogenesis and pathophysiology of bacterial infections. In: Scheld MW, Whitley RJ, Marra CM. (Eds.). Infect Cent Nerv Syst, fourth ed. Philadelphia: Lippincott Williams & Wilkins. 2014.
18. Braun JS, Sublett JE, Freyer D, Mitchell TJ, Cleveland JL, Tuomanen EI, Weber JR. Pneumococcal pneumolysin and H2O2 mediate brain cell apoptosis during meningitis. J Clin Invest. 2002;109:19–27.
19. Ebert S, Gerber J, Bader S, Mühlhauser F, Brechtel K, Mitchell TJ, Nau R. Dose-dependent activation of microglial cells by toll-like receptor agonists alone and in combination. J Neuroimmunol. 2005;159:87–96.
20. Iliev AI, Stringaris AK, Nau R, Neumann H. Neuronal injury mediated via stimulation of microglial toll-like receptor-9 (TLR9). FASEB J. 2003;18:412–4.

21. Marques CP, Cheeran MC-J, Palmquist JM, Hu S, Lokensgard JR. Microglia are the major cellular source of inducible nitric oxide synthase during experimental herpes encephalitis. J Neuro-Oncol. 2008;14:229–38.
22. Klein M, Koedel U, Pfister H-W, Kastenbauer S. Morphological correlates of acute and permanent hearing loss during experimental pneumococcal meningitis. Brain Pathol. 2006;13:123–32.
23. van de Beek D, de Gans J, Spanjaard L, Weisfelt M, Reitsma JB, Vermeulen M. Clinical features and prognostic factors in adults with bacterial meningitis. N Engl J Med. 2004;351:1849–59.
24. Brouwer MC, McIntyre P, Prasad K, van de Beek D. Corticosteroids for acute bacterial meningitis. In: van de Beek D, editor. Cochrane database Syst. Chichester: Rev. John Wiley & Sons, Ltd; 2015. p. CD004405.
25. Coimbra RS, Loquet G, Leib SL. Limited efficacy of adjuvant therapy with dexamethasone in preventing hearing loss due to experimental pneumococcal meningitis in the infant rat. Pediatr Res. 2007;62:291–4.
26. Bally L, Grandgirard D, Leib SL. Inhibition of hippocampal regeneration by adjuvant dexamethasone in experimental infant rat pneumococcal meningitis. Antimicrob Agents Chemother. 2016;60:1841–6.
27. Zysk G, Brück W, Gerber J, Brück Y, Prange HW, Nau R. Anti-inflammatory treatment influences neuronal apoptotic cell death in the dentate gyrus in experimental pneumococcal meningitis. J Neuropathol Exp Neurol. 1996;55:722–8.
28. Spreer A, Gerber J, Hanssen M, Schindler S, Hermann C, Lange P, Eiffert H, Nau R. Dexamethasone increases hippocampal neuronal apoptosis in a rabbit model of Escherichia coli meningitis. Pediatr Res. 2006;60:210–5.
29. Grandgirard D, Burri M, Agyeman P, Leib SL. Adjunctive daptomycin attenuates brain damage and hearing loss more efficiently than rifampin in infant rat pneumococcal meningitis. Antimicrob Agents Chemother. 2012;56:4289–95.
30. Liechti FD, Grandgirard D, Leppert D, Leib SL. Matrix metalloproteinase inhibition lowers mortality and brain injury in experimental pneumococcal meningitis. Infect Immun. 2014;82:1710–8.
31. Leib SL, Clements JM, Lindberg RLP, Heimgartner C, Loeffler JM, Pfister L-A, Täuber MG, Leppert D. Inhibition of matrix metalloproteinases and tumour necrosis factor α converting enzyme as adjuvant therapy in pneumococcal meningitis. Brain. 2001;124:1734–42.
32. Auer M, Pfister LA, Leppert D, Täuber MG, Leib SL. Effects of clinically used antioxidants in experimental pneumococcal meningitis. J Infect Dis. 2000; 182:347–50.
33. Kasanmoentalib ES, Valls Seron M, Morgan BP, Brouwer MC, van de Beek D. Adjuvant treatment with dexamethasone plus anti-C5 antibodies improves outcome of experimental pneumococcal meningitis: a randomized controlled trial. J Neuroinflammation. 2015;12:149.
34. Mook-Kanamori BB, Rouse MS, Kang C-I, van de Beek D, Steckelberg JM, Patel R. Daptomycin in experimental murine pneumococcal meningitis. BMC Infect Dis. 2009;9:50.
35. Masouris I, Klein M, Dyckhoff S, Angele B, Pfister HW, Koedel U. Inhibition of DAMP signaling as an effective adjunctive treatment strategy in pneumococcal meningitis. J Neuroinflammation. 2017;14:214.
36. Whittaker M, Floyd CD, Brown P, Gearing AJ. Design and therapeutic application of matrix metalloproteinase inhibitors. Chem Rev. 1999;99:2735–76.
37. Lewis EJ, Bishop J, Bottomley KMK, et al. Ro 32-3555, an orally active collagenase inhibitor, prevents cartilage breakdown *in vitro* and *in vivo*. Br J Pharmacol. 1997;121:540–6.
38. Brewster M, Lewis JE, Wilson KL, Greenham AK, Bottomley KMK. Ro 32-3555, an orally active collagenase selective inhibitor, prevents structural damage in the STR/ORT mouse model of osteoarthritis. Arthritis Rheum. 1998;41:1639–44.
39. Hemmings FJ, Farhan M, Rowland J, Banken L, Jain R. Tolerability and pharmacokinetics of the collagenase-selective inhibitor Trocade in patients with rheumatoid arthritis. Rheumatology (Oxford). 2001;40:537–43.
40. Stucki A, Cottagnoud M, Winkelmann V, Schaffner T, Cottagnoud P. Daptomycin produces an enhanced bactericidal activity compared to ceftriaxone, measured by [3H] choline release in the cerebrospinal fluid, in experimental meningitis due to a penicillin-resistant pneumococcal strain without lysing its cell wall. Antimicrob Agents Chemother. 2007;51:2249–52.
41. Grandgirard D, Schürch C, Cottagnoud P, Leib SL. Prevention of brain injury by the nonbacteriolytic antibiotic daptomycin in experimental pneumococcal meningitis. Antimicrob Agents Chemother. 2007;51:2173–8.
42. Leib SL, Leppert D, Clements J, Tauber MG. Matrix metalloproteinases contribute to brain damage in experimental pneumococcal meningitis. Infect Immun. 2000;68:615–20.
43. van de Beek D, Cabellos C, Dzupova O, et al. ESCMID guideline: diagnosis and treatment of acute bacterial meningitis. Clin Microbiol Infect. 2016;22:S37–62.
44. Gianinazzi C, Grandgirard D, Imboden H, Egger L, Meli DN, Bifrare Y-D, Joss PC, Täuber MG, Borner C, Leib SL. Caspase-3 mediates hippocampal apoptosis in pneumococcal meningitis. Acta Neuropathol. 2003;105: 499–507.
45. Gehre F, Leib SL, Grandgirard D, Kummer J, Bhlmann A, Simon F, Gumann R, Kharat AS, Tuber MG, Tomasz A. Essential role of choline for pneumococcal virulence in an experimental model of meningitis. J Intern Med. 2008; 264:143–54.
46. Gerber J, Pohl K, Sander V, Bunkowski S, Nau R. Rifampin followed by ceftriaxone for experimental meningitis decreases lipoteichoic acid concentrations in cerebrospinal fluid and reduces neuronal damage in comparison to ceftriaxone alone. Antimicrob Agents Chemother. 2003; 47:1313–7.
47. van Furth AM, Roord JJ, van Furth R. Roles of proinflammatory and anti-inflammatory cytokines in pathophysiology of bacterial meningitis and effect of adjunctive therapy. Infect Immun. 1996;64:4883–90.
48. Liechti FD, Studle N, Theurillat R, Grandgirard D, Thormann W, Leib SL. The mood-stabilizer lithium prevents hippocampal apoptosis and improves spatial memory in experimental meningitis. PLoS One. 2014;9:17–9.
49. Bewersdorf JP, Grandgirard D, Koedel U, Leib SL. Novel and preclinical treatment strategies in pneumococcal meningitis. Curr Opin Infect Dis. 2018;31:85–92.
50. van de Beek D, Brouwer M, Hasbun R, Koedel U, Whitney CG, Wijdicks E. Community-acquired bacterial meningitis. Nat Rev Dis Prim. 2016;2:16074.
51. Gerber J, Nau R. Mechanisms of injury in bacterial meningitis. Curr Opin Neurol. 2010;23:312–8.
52. Steenbergen JN, Alder J, Thorne GM, Tally FP. Daptomycin: a lipopeptide antibiotic for the treatment of serious Gram-positive infections. J Antimicrob Chemother. 2005;55:283–8.
53. Sauermann R, Rothenburger M, Graninger W, Joukhadar C. Daptomycin: a review 4 years after first approval. Pharmacology. 2008;81:79–91.
54. Baltz RH. Daptomycin: mechanisms of action and resistance, and biosynthetic engineering. Curr Opin Chem Biol. 2009;13:144–51.
55. Grandgirard D, Oberson K, Bühlmann A, Gäumann R, Leib SL. Attenuation of cerebrospinal fluid inflammation by the nonbacteriolytic antibiotic daptomycin versus that by ceftriaxone in experimental pneumococcal meningitis. Antimicrob Agents Chemother. 2010;54:1323–6.
56. Barichello T, Gonçalves JCN, Generoso JS, Milioli GL, Silvestre C, Costa CS, Coelho da Rosa J, Comim CM, Quevedo J. Attenuation of cognitive impairment by the nonbacteriolytic antibiotic daptomycin in Wistar rats submitted to pneumococcal meningitis. BMC Neurosci. 2013;14:42.
57. Leppert D, Leib SL, Grygar C, Miller KM, Schaad UB, Hollander GA. Matrix metalloproteinase (MMP)-8 and MMP-9 in cerebrospinal fluid during bacterial meningitis: association with blood-brain barrier damage and neurological sequelae. Clin Infect Dis. 2000;31:80–4.
58. Rosenberg GA. Matrix metalloproteinases in neuroinflammation. Glia. 2002; 39:279–91.
59. Sellner J, Leib SL. In bacterial meningitis cortical brain damage is associated with changes in parenchymal MMP-9/TIMP-1 ratio and increased collagen type IV degradation. Neurobiol Dis. 2006;21:647–56.
60. Leppert D, Lindberg RLP, Kappos L, Leib SL. Matrix metalloproteinases: multifunctional effectors of inflammation in multiple sclerosis and bacterial meningitis. Brain Res Rev. 2001;36:249–57.
61. Khokha R, Murthy A, Weiss A. Metalloproteinases and their natural inhibitors in inflammation and immunity. Nat Rev Immunol. 2013;13:649–65.
62. Song J, Wu C, Zhang X, Sorokin LM. In vivo processing of CXCL5 (LIX) by matrix metalloproteinase (MMP)-2 and MMP-9 promotes early neutrophil recruitment in IL-1-induced peritonitis. J Immunol. 2013;190:401–10.
63. Josselyn SA, Köhler S, Frankland PW. Finding the engram. Nat Rev Neurosci. 2015;16:521–34.
64. Preston AR, Eichenbaum H. Interplay of hippocampus and prefrontal cortex in memory. Curr Biol. 2013;23:R764–73.
65. D'Hooge R, De Deyn PP. Applications of the Morris water maze in the study of learning and memory. Brain Res Rev. 2001;36:60–90.
66. Møller MN, Brandt C, Østergaard C, Caye-Thomasen P. Bacterial invasion of the inner ear in association with pneumococcal meningitis. Otol Neurotol. 2014;35:e178–86.
67. Meli DN, Coimbra RS, Erhart DG, Loquet G, Bellac CL, Täuber MG, Neumann U, Leib SL. Doxycycline reduces mortality and injury to the brain and cochlea in experimental pneumococcal meningitis. Infect Immun. 2006;74:3890–6.

68. Brandt CT, Cayé-Thomasen P, Lund SP, Worsøe L, Østergaard C, Frimodt-Møller N, Espersen F, Thomsen J, Lundgren JD. Hearing loss and cochlear damage in experimental pneumococcal meningitis, with special reference to the role of neutrophil granulocytes. Neurobiol Dis. 2006;23:300–11.
69. Demel C, Hoegen T, Giese A, Angele B, Pfister H-W, Koedel U, Klein M. Reduced spiral ganglion neuronal loss by adjunctive neurotrophin-3 in experimental pneumococcal meningitis. J Neuroinflammation. 2011;8:7.
70. Senn P, Rostetter C, Arnold A, Kompis M, Vischer M, Häusler R, Ozdoba C, Mantokoudis G, Caversaccio M. Retrograde cochlear implantation in postmeningitic basal turn ossification. Laryngoscope. 2012;122:2043–50.
71. Peltola H, Roine I, Fernandez J, et al. Hearing impairment in childhood bacterial meningitis is little relieved by dexamethasone or glycerol. Pediatrics. 2010;125:e1–8.

6

Suppression of MyD88-dependent signaling alleviates neuropathic pain induced by peripheral nerve injury in the rat

Fan Liu[1†], Zhiyao Wang[1†], Yue Qiu[2], Min Wei[2], Chunyan Li[1], Yikuan Xie[1], Le Shen[2], Yuguang Huang[2*] and Chao Ma[1*]

Abstract

Background: MyD88 is the adaptor protein of MyD88-dependent signaling pathway of TLRs and IL-1 receptor and regulates innate immune response. However, it was not clear whether and how MyD88 and related signaling pathways in the dorsal root ganglion (DRG) and spinal dorsal horn (SDH) are involved in neuropathic pain.

Methods: Chronic constriction injury (CCI) was used to induce neuropathic pain in the rat. The expression of MyD88, TRIF, IBA1, and GFAP was detected with immunofluorescent staining and Western blot. The expression of interleukin-1 beta (IL-1β), high mobility group box 1 (HMGB1), NF-κB-p65, phosphorylated NF-κB-p65, ERK, phosphorylated ERK, and tumor necrosis factor-alpha (TNF-α) was detected with Western blot. Pain-related behavioral effects of MyD88 homodimerization inhibitory peptide (MIP) were accessed up to 3 weeks after intrathecal administration.

Results: Peripheral nerve injury significantly increased the protein level of MyD88 in the DRG and SDH, but had no effect on TRIF. MyD88 was found partly distributed in the nociceptive neurons in the DRGs and the astrocytes and microglia in the SDH. HMGB1 and IL-1β were also found upregulated in nociceptive pathways of CCI rats. Intrathecal application of MIP significantly alleviated mechanical and thermal hyperalgesia in the CCI rats and also reversed CCI-induced upregulation of MyD88 in both DRG and SDH. Further investigation revealed that suppression of MyD88 protein reduced the release of TNF-α and glial activation in the SDH in the CCI rats.

Conclusions: MyD88-dependent TIR pathway in the DRG and SDH may play a role in CCI-induced neuropathic pain. MyD88 might serve as a potential therapeutic target for neuropathic pain.

Keywords: MyD88, TRIF, Dorsal root ganglion, Spinal dorsal horn, CCI, Neuropathic pain

Background

Neuropathic pain is associated with sensory abnormalities and altered stimulus-response function, such as allodynia, hyperalgesia, and loss of sensation in some areas [1, 2]. The International Association for the Study of Pain defined neuropathic pain as "pain caused by a lesion or disease of the somatosensory nervous system" (www.iasp-pain.org/Taxonomy#Neuropathicpain).

Neuropathic pain poses a heavy burden on the quality of life of patients while currently available treatments are often ineffective. The underlying molecular and cellular mechanisms of neuropathic pain remain poorly elucidated. There are increasing evidences indicating a role of neuroimmune processes in the development of neuropathic pain [3–6].

The myeloid differentiation factor-88 adaptor protein (MyD88) is involved in Toll-like receptors (TLRs, except for TLR3) signaling and interleukin-1 receptor (IL-1R) signaling [7–10]. MyD88 mediates activation of TLRs or IL-1R and leads to NF-κB activation, inflammatory cytokines such as tumor necrosis factor-alpha (TNF-α) in immune cells [8–10]. TLRs are danger-associated and pathogen-associated molecular pattern receptors that

* Correspondence: garybeijing@163.com; machao@ibms.cams.cn
[†]Equal contributors
[2]Department of Anesthesiology, Peking Union Medical College Hospital, Chinese Academy of Medical Sciences, Peking Union Medical College, Beijing 100730, China
[1]Department of Human Anatomy, Histology and Embryology, Institute of Basic Medical Sciences, Chinese Academy of Medical Sciences, School of Basic Medicine, Peking Union Medical College, Beijing 100005, China

regulate innate immunity via activated NF-κB-dependent and mitogen-activated protein kinase (MAPK)-dependent cytokine production [11, 12]. TLRs and IL-1R are not only expressed on immune cells but also found on sensory neurons in dorsal root ganglions (DRGs) and glial cells (microglia and astrocytes) in the spinal cord [5, 13–17]. A number of previous studies have found that TLRs in the spinal cord played an important role in the model of neuropathic pain and nerve injury, in which microglia and astrocytes produced proinflammatory cytokines by activating TLRs [18–20]. Nociceptors of DRG that express TLRs or IL-1R are also activated by LPS or inflammatory cytokine interleukin-1β, inducing pain hypersensitivity [5, 18–22]. Recent publications show that MyD88, adaptor protein of TLRs and IL-1R, is also found in the expression in DRG and spinal cord [18–20].We hypothesized that suppressed MyD88 adaptor protein in the DRG and spinal cord could alleviate peripheral nerve injury-induced neuropathic pain. Our findings reveal MyD88 adaptor protein involved in the neuropathic pain and may provide potential therapeutic strategies for treatment of neuropathic pain.

Methods

Animals

The adult male Sprague-Dawley rats (120–180 g) were used in our study. All animals were housed (4–5 rats per cage) in a standard 12-h light/dark cycle. These experiments were approved by the Institutional Animal Care and Use Committee in Chinese Academy of Medical Sciences, Institute of Basic Medical Sciences. Animals were randomly assigned to treatment or control groups.

Animal model of neuropathic pain

In accordance with the study of Bennett and Xie [23], we performed chronic constriction injury (CCI) in the rats anesthetized through intraperitoneal injection of sodium pentobarbital (40 mg/kg) under aseptic condition. After the sciatic nerve of the mid-thigh level on right side was exposed, four snug ligatures of chromic gut suture were loosely tied around the nerve with about 1 mm space between the knots. The sciatic nerves of sham animals were exposed without ligation.

Intrathecal catheterization and drug delivery

A PE10 catheter (length, 18 cm) was implanted intrathecally according to the protocol as described previously [24, 25]. Briefly, rats were anesthetized with sodium pentobarbital (40 mg/kg) and a 2-cm longitudinal incision was made above vertebrae L5–6.The catheter with guide wire was inserted in the hole that was made by a 23-gauge needle between lumbar vertebrae L5 and 6. The catheter was pushed through the intervertebral space until a sudden movement of tail or the hindlimb was observed and then passed gently 2 cm upward to reach the lumbar enlargement. The tip of the catheter was fixed on the neck area of the rats. After implantation, catheter localization was verified by intrathecal injection of lidocaine and all rats were observed for a minimum of 5 days before being performed with CCI surgery as described above. Rats showing motor weakness or without catheter in spinal space were excluded from the research. An intrathecal injection of 500 μM of MyD88 homodimerization inhibitory peptide (MIP, Novus Biologicals, CO, USA) or control peptide (Novus Biologicals, CO, USA) resolved in PBS was administrated on preoperative and postoperative days. A previous report showed that application of similar dose of MIP did not induce any significant change in locomotor function in the rats [18].

Behavioral assessment of pain

All the behavioral measurements were carried out by an experimenter blinded to schedule during 10 am–3 pm. Mechanical allodynia was assessed by the up-down method using calibrated Electronic von Frey (Electronic von Frey 2393:II TC, USA). Rats were acclimated in suspended cages with wire mesh floor. The probe was applied perpendicularly to the paw with no acceleration at a force and held for approximately 6–8 s. An acute withdrawal of the paw was considered a positive response. Thermal hypersensitivity was tested using plantar test as described previously [24, 25]. The three measurements of mechanic threshold or thermal latency per side were averaged.

Western blot analysis

The L4–6 spinal dorsal horn and DRGs were harvested from rats that were deeply anesthetized with sodium pentobarbital (40 mg/kg) and snap-frozen in liquid nitrogen. Tissues were homogenized on ice in RIPA buffer (20 mM Tris-HCl, 150 mM NaCl, 1% NP40, 1 mM EDTA, 0.5% Na deoxycholate, and 0.1% sodium dodecyl sulfate (SDS)) mixed with proteases inhibitor cocktail and phosphatases inhibitor cocktail (Sigma-Aldrich, MO, USA). After centrifuging, supernatants were collected and denatured with SDS-PAGE loading buffer consisting of 0.25 M Tris-HCl, 52% glycerol, 6% SDS, 5% β-mercaptoethanol, and 0.1% bromophenol blue for 5 min at 95 °C. Equal concentrations of lysates (30 μg) were separated by SDS-polyacrylamide gel electrophoresis gels and transferred to a PVDF membrane (GE Healthcare life science). After blocking with 5% BSA in TBST (Tris-buffered saline with 0.1%Tween 20) for 1 h at room temperature, membranes were incubated in TBST overnight at 4 °C with primary antibodies. The membranes were washed with TBST and then incubated with secondary antibodies diluted with 5% skim milk in

TBST for 1 h at room temperature (Table 1 lists the primary and secondary antibodies used for Western blot analysis). Bands were detected with enhanced chemiluminescence reagents eECL Kit (CWBio, Beijing, China) using an ImageQuant LAS 4000 mini Chemiluminescence imaging analysis system (GE Healthcare life science, PA, USA), and the band densities were analyzed using ImageJ software (NIH, USA). For the detecting of total extracellular signal-regulated protein kinase (ERK) or total NF-κB protein, we again blocked the same member that was washed by Western blot antibody Stripping Buffer (CWbio, Beijing, China) with 5% BSA in TBST for 1 h at room temperature after detecting the phosphorylated ERK or phosphorylated NF-κB protein, incubated the member with primary antibodies (anti-total ERK or total NF-κB protein) overnight at 4 °C, and then incubated with secondary antibodies for 1 h at room temperature. Members that were re-incubated by primary and secondary antibodies were detected with enhanced chemiluminescence reagents eECL Kit using ImageQuant LAS4000 mini Chemiluminescence imaging analysis system.

Immunofluorescence staining

Rats were deeply anesthetized with sodium pentobarbital (40 mg/kg) and then perfused with warm saline followed by fresh 4% paraformaldehyde through the ascending aorta. The L4–6 spinal dorsal horn (SDH) and DRGs were collected, fixed in 4% paraformaldehyde for 4 h, and then dehydrated in 30% sucrose overnight at 4 °C. Tissues were mounted and finally cut to a thickness of 15 μm in a cryostat for immunofluorescent staining. After blocking in 10% normal donkey serum and 0.2% Triton X-100 in PBS for 1 h at room temperature, the tissue sections were incubated overnight at 4 °C in 10% normal donkey serum in PBS containing primary antibodies and then incubated with the proper secondary antibodies or Alexa Fluor 594-conjugated isolectin B4 (IB4) (1:100, Invitrogen/Thermo Fisher Scientific, USA) for 1 h. The slides were then washed in PBS and coverslipped with VECTASHIELD Mounting Medium with DAPI. Table 2 lists the primary and secondary antibodies used for the immunofluorescence staining analyses. The percentages of positive neurons to total neurons were calculated and statistically analyzed. Images were captured using a confocal laser scanning microscope (FV1000, Olympus) and Olympus FluoView software. At least 12 fields of view (×200) from three sections on each ganglion were examined. DRG neurons were classified according to the cross-sectional areas of soma as small- (area <636 μm^2), medium- (area 637–1431 μm^2) and large-sized (area >1431 μm^2). This classification is based on the criteria as previously described [26].

Statistical analysis

Values were expressed as group mean and standard errors (mean ± SEM) and analyzed using GraphPad Prism 6 and SPSS software (version 17.0). For analysis of Western blot, data were analyzed with one-way ANOVA followed by Student-Newman-Keuls test. Behavioral data were analyzed with two-way ANOVA. Chi-square tests

Table 1 List of primary and secondary antibodies used for Western blot analysis

Antibody	Host	Company	Catalog number	Dilution	incubation conditions
MyD88 [a]	rabbit	Abcam	ab2064	1:500	Overnight 4 °C
TRIF [b]	rabbit	Abcam	ab13810	1:1000	Overnight 4 °C
IL-1β	rabbit	Proteintech	16806-1-AP	1:500	Overnight 4 °C
IBA1	rabbit	Proteintech	10904-1-AP	1:500	Overnight 4 °C
TNF-α	rabbit	Sino Biological	80045-RP02	1:500	Overnight 4 °C
GFAP	rabbit	Cell signaling technology	#12389	1:1000	Overnight 4 °C
HMGB1	rabbit	Cell signaling technology	#6893	1:1500	Overnight 4 °C
ERK	rabbit	Cell signaling technology	#4695	1:2000	Overnight 4 °C
pERK	rabbit	Cell signaling technology	#4370	1:1000	Overnight 4 °C
NF-κB	rabbit	Cell signaling technology	#8242	1:1000	Overnight 4 °C
pNF-κB	mouse	Cell signaling technology	#13346	1:1000	Overnight 4 °C
β-actin	mouse	Santa Cruz Biotechnology	TA-09	1:1000	Overnight 4 °C
Anti-rabbit IgG horseradish peroxidase (HRP)	Goat	ZSGB-BIO	ZDR-5306	1:3000	1 h RT
Anti-mouse IgG horseradish peroxidase (HRP)	Goat	ZSGB-BIO	ZDR-5307	1:3000	1 h RT

[a] MyD88 antibody (Abcam, catalog #ab2064) was used for IHC or WB in 18 research articles (PubMed ID: 27389279, 26191134, 25446227, 26224622, 24307174, 24410883, 24477912, 24719558, 25187650, 23479602, 21278343, 20212458, 20837465, 20456021, 19553541, 17503341, 17114422, 16517734, 16461741)

[b] TRIF antibody (Abcam, catalog #ab13810) was used for IHC or WB in 11 research articles (PubMedID: 27389279, 26191134, 24146036, 22361049, 20511556, 19265160, 19648648, 19389833, 17503341, 17314314, 17000866)

Table 2 List of primary and secondary antibodies used for Immunofluorescence staining

Antibody	Host	Company	Catalog ID	Dilution	incubation conditions
MyD88	rabbit	Abcam	ab2064	1:100	Overnight 4 °C
TRIF	rabbit	Abcam	ab13810	1:200	Overnight 4 °C
IBA1	goat	Abcam	ab107159	1:200	Overnight 4 °C
GFAP	goat	Abcam	ab53554	1:100	Overnight 4 °C
CGRP	goat	LifeSpan BioSciences	LS-C122785	1:500	Overnight 4 °C
anti-rabbit IgG Alexa Fluor 488	donkey	Jackson ImmunoResearch	711-545-152	1:400	1 h RT
anti-goat IgG Alexa Fluor 594	donkey	Jackson ImmunoResearch	705-585-147	1:400	1 h RT

were used to compare between two or more incidence of events. $P < 0.05$ was considered statistically significant.

Results

Up-regulation of MyD88 in nociceptive pathways after CCI

First, we determined the time course of expression levels of MyD88 in DRGs and SDH after CCI in rats. Our Western blot results showed that CCI produced gradually rapid (in 3 days) and long-lasting (over 21 days) increase in the protein levels of in DRGs. MyD88 started increase from 3 days, peaked at 7 days, and maintained to the highest level at 21 days after CCI (Fig. 1a) in DRGs. And the protein levels of MyD88 were found produced and later increased to a high level from 14 to 21 days in the SDH after CCI operation (Fig. 1b).

Similar to the result of Western blot, we found that MyD88 were present at only very low levels in DRG and SDH of naïve and sham operation rats with immunofluorescence staining. Furthermore, by using immunofluorescence, the MyD88 protein immunoreactivity was found to be distributed in the three categories of neurons: large-sized, medium-sized, and small-sized neurons in DRG. We found a significant increase in the

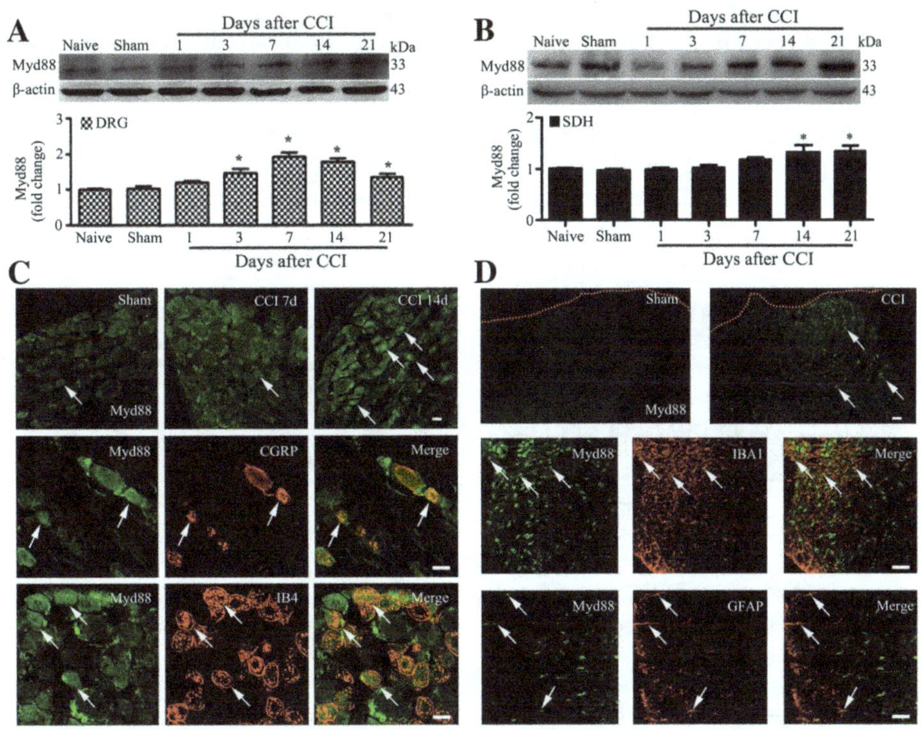

Fig. 1 CCI increase expression MyD88 in rat DRG and SDH. **a** and **b** Western blot analyses the time course for MyD88 expression in DRG **(a)** and SDH **(b)** ($n = 4$ in each). Western blot analysis is shown on the top; quantification of protein levels (relative to naive group) is shown on the bottom. One-way ANOVA, $*P < 0.05$ versus naive and sham. **c** Cellular distribution of MyD88 in DRGs. MyD88 was expressed in the large-, medium-, and small-sized neurons (white arrows) sham to the CCI (top row). Double immunostaining shows coexpression of MyD88 with CGRP- and IB4-positive neurons, respectively (*middle and bottom rows*). **d** Distribution and cellular of MyD88 in the SDH. MyD88 was distributed predominantly in the superficial layers (*top row*). MyD88 was coexpression with astrocytes (GFAP, red) and microglial cells (IBA1, red) (*middle and bottom rows*). Scale bar: 20 μm (**c**, **d**)

expression of MyD88 in DRG neurons (sham: 47.04%, 1049/2230; CCI 7 day: 67.30%, 1844/2740; CCI 14 day: 65.79%, 1579/2400) especially in small-sized neurons (sham: 55.34%, 974/1760; CCI 7 day: 77.86%, 1744/2240; CCI 14 day: 80.44%, 1448/1800) on days 7 and 14 after CCI in DRGs (Fig. 1c and Additional file 1: Figure S1A-B). The cellular localization of MyD88 in small neurons of DRGs was determined by double immunofluorescence. In the nociceptive small neurons, staining of MyD88 was colocalized in calcitonin gene-related peptide (CGRP)-positive and nonpeptidergic isolectin B4 (IB4)-positive nociceptive neurons of DRGs (Fig. 1c). As shown in the result of immunofluorescence, the expression of MyD88 was significantly upregulated in response to CCI operation in the SDH of rats. And the MyD88 protein was dominated and distributed in the superficial layers of the SDH. We also found that within 7 days after CCI, MyD88 immunoreactivity was colocalized with astrocytes (GFAP) and microglial cells (IBA1) (Fig. 1d). These results suggest that MyD88 signaling was activated in neurons of DRGs as well as SDH astrocytes and microglial cells after nerve injury.

CCI increases expression of IL-1β and HMGB1 in nociceptive pathways

MyD88 is the downstream signaling adaptor protein of Toll/interleukin-1 receptor (TIR) signaling and is expressed in DRG and SDH. TLRs and IL-1R were also found to express on primary sensory neurons of DRG and glial cells in SDH [4, 5, 17, 21, 27, 28]. To define the mechanism of MyD88-dependent TIR signaling in CCI, we examined the expression of TLR2 and TLR4 endogenous ligand, high mobility group box 1 (HMGB1) and IL-1R endogenous ligand, interleukin-1 beta (IL-1β).

Western blot showed CCI significantly increased protein levels of both pro-IL-1β and IL-1β in the DRG (Fig. 2a). In the SDH, CCI induced significant upregulation of the protein levels (from day 3 to day 7 after CCI) of IL-1β, not pro-IL-1β (Fig. 2b). We then examined the protein levels of HMGB. After CCI, protein expression levels of HMGB1 in the DRG increased rapidly and significantly from 1 day to lasting 21 days (Fig. 2c). The levels of HMGB1 also greatly increased in the SDH of CCI rat model (Fig. 2d).

Regulation and activation of NF-κB signal and ERK signal in nociceptive pathways of CCI rats

The protein levels of both total NF-κB p65 and activated phospho-NF-κB p65, in L4 and L5 DRGs, increased significantly compared with naïve and sham groups. We detected rapid and long lasting increase of the expression of total and activated phospho-NF-κB p65 in DRG (Fig. 3a-b). Both total NF-κB p65 and activated phospho-NF-κB p65 levels were found to peak at 3 days after CCI and remained elevated to the 21 days, and did not recover to the control level of naïve and sham after CCI. Similar to the changes on DRGs, activated phospho-NF-κB p65 as well as total NF-κB p65 also significantly increased in SDH after CCI. Phospho-NF-κB p65 were found to increase significantly and persistent on all time points from 1 day to 21 days of CCI-induced nerve injure compare with control group. Our results demonstrated that total NF-κB p65 did not increase rapidly but showed an obvious increase at 7 to 21 days

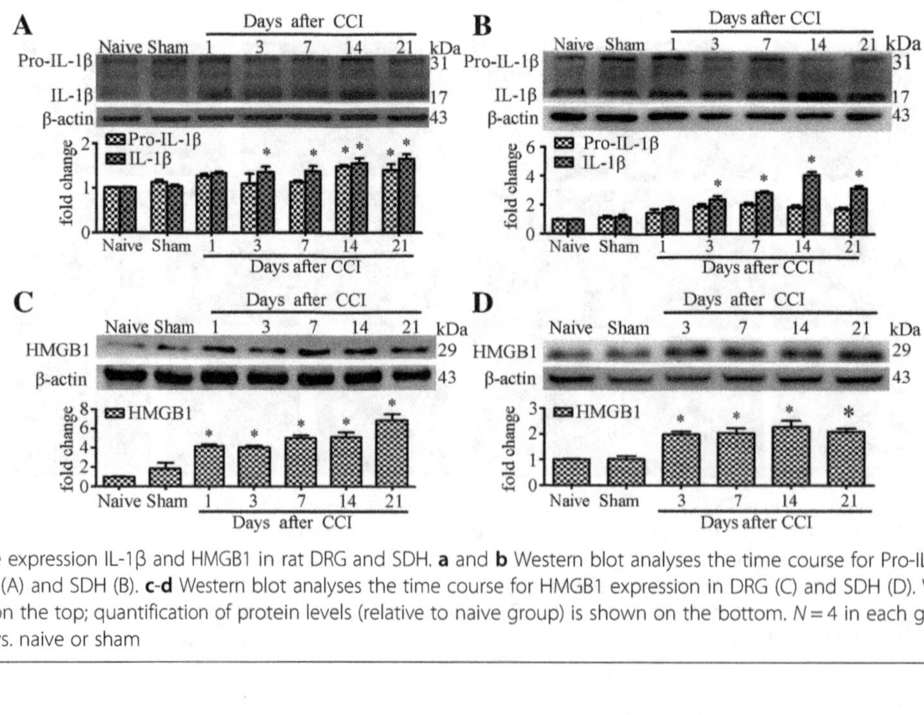

Fig. 2 CCI increase expression IL-1β and HMGB1 in rat DRG and SDH. **a** and **b** Western blot analyses the time course for Pro-IL-1β and IL-1β expression in DRG (A) and SDH (B). **c-d** Western blot analyses the time course for HMGB1 expression in DRG (C) and SDH (D). Western blot analysis is shown on the top; quantification of protein levels (relative to naive group) is shown on the bottom. $N = 4$ in each group, One-way ANOVA, $^*P < 0.05$ vs. naive or sham

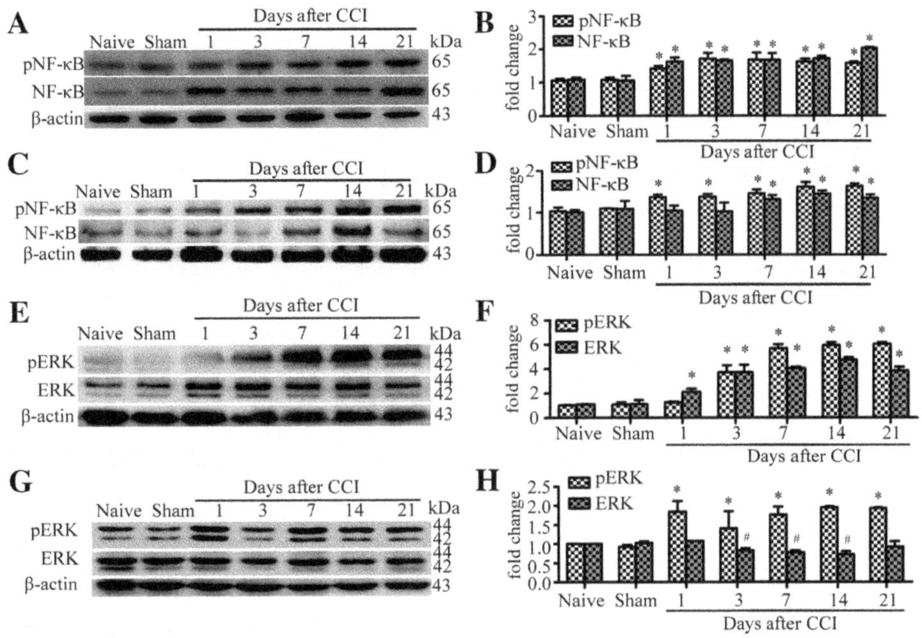

Fig. 3 CCI induce NF-κB p65 and ERK signaling activation in rat DRG and SDH. **a-b** Western blot analysis shows time course for the expression of total NF-κB p65 and activated phospho-NF-κB p65 in DRG (A). Quantification of protein levels of total NF-κB p65 and activated phospho-NF-κB p65 in DRG (B). One-way ANOVA, $^*P < 0.05$ versus naive and sham. **c-d** Western blot analysis shows time course for the expression of total NF-κB p65 and activated phospho-NF-κB p65 in SDH (C). Quantification of protein levels of total NF-κB p65 and activated phospho-NF-κB p65 in SDH (D). **e-f** Western blot analysis shows time course for the expression of total ERK and activated pERK in DRG (E). Quantification of protein levels of total ERK and activated pERK in DRG (F). **g-h** Western blot analysis shows time course for the expression of total ERK and activated pERK in SDH (G). Quantification of protein levels of total ERK and activated pERK in SDH (H). $N = 4$ in each group, One-way ANOVA, $^*P < 0.05$ vs. naive or sham

compared with naïve and sham groups in SDH after CCI (Fig. 3c-d). The expression of total NF-κB p65 on SDH maximized at day 14 and maintained elevated to day 21after CCI-induced nerve injury.

Extracellular signal-regulated protein kinase 1/2 (ERK) signal pathway was involved in TLR-mediated proinflammatory response. We found the protein levels of both ERK1 (p44 MAPK, 44 kDa) and ERK2 (p42 MAPK, 42 kDa) increased significantly on all time points from 1 to 21 days after CCI in DRG (Fig. 3e, f). Western blot analysis also revealed activation of ERK in DRG and SDH after CCI. A marked and persistent increase of both phospho-ERK1 and phospho-ERK2 were observed in DRG (3 to 21 days) and SDH (1 to 21 days) after CCI (Fig. 3e–h).

MIP treatment relieve neuropathic pain after CCI

Compared with sham group, rats with CCI showed a decrease in paw mechanical withdrawal threshold at postoperative day (POD) + 3, achieving a significant difference at POD7, getting maximal at POD14 and thus maintained throughout POD21 (Fig. 4a). The paw thermal withdrawal latency of CCI group rats also decreased significantly at POD7 and POD14 compared to that of sham group (Fig. 4b). To determine the role of MyD88-dependent signaling of TIR in CCI, we used MIP to inhibit MyD88 dependent signaling. MIP was delivered into the cerebrospinal fluid of lumbar enlargement by intrathecal injection (500 μM in a volume of 20 μl in rats).

We intrathecally administrated MIP and control peptide daily from preoperative day −3 to day −1 (before CCI). The results showed that MIP administration on preoperative period delayed CCI-induced mechanical allodynia and thermal hyperalgesia, with no effects in sham operative rats (Fig. 4c, d). Then we injected MIP and control peptide intrathecally daily for three consecutive days (POD 3–5). We found that MIP administration reversed the CCI-induced neuropathic pain and produced long-lasting alleviative effects (POD 7–21) on the mechanical allodynia and thermal hyperalgesia (Fig. 4e, f).

MIP treatment decrease expression level of MyD88 protein after CCI

Given that MyD88 expression increased significantly and MyD88-NF-κB p65 signaling pathways activated postoperatively, we examined whether MyD88-dependent signaling pathways could be suppressed by MIP treatment, which relieved neuropathic pain in the CCI rats. Our Western blot and immunofluorescent results showed that the expression of MyD88 was significantly

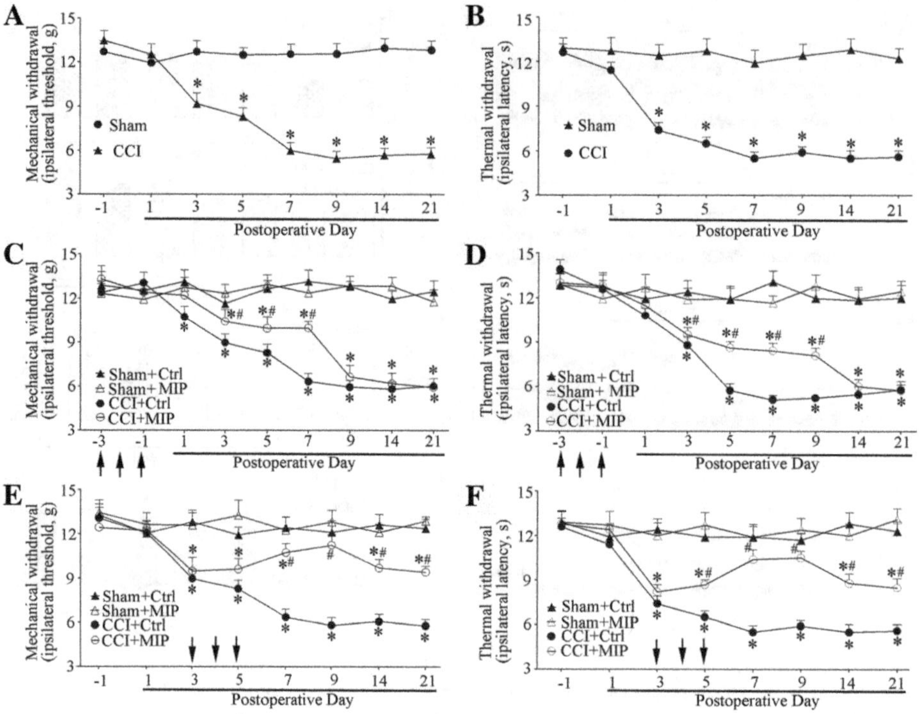

Fig. 4 Attenuated neuropathic pain by of MIP after CCI treatment. **a-b** CCI-induced mechanical allodynia (**a**) and thermal hyperalgesia (**b**). Two-way ANOVA, $^{*}P < 0.05$ versus sham. **c-d** Pre-intrathecal injection of MIP attenuated CCI-induced mechanical allodynia (**c**) and thermal hyperalgesia (**d**) (each administration is indicated by an arrow on the 3, 2, and 1 days before CCI). **e-f** Mechanical allodynia (**e**) and thermal hyperalgesia (**f**) is attenuated by MIP in the early phase of CCI operation (each administration is indicated by an arrow on the 3, 4, and 5 days after CCI). MIP (500 mM) was administrated i.t.in a volume of 20 μl; The control peptide was used in the control (Ctrl) group. Nine rats were included in each group. Two-way ANOVA, $^{*}P < 0.05$ vs. Sham + Ctrl or Sham + MIP, $\#P < 0.05$ vs. Sham + Ctrl, Sham + MIP or CCI + Ctrl

decreased in the L4–5 DRGs and SDH at day 14 after intrathecally administered MIP to the CCI rats in comparison to rats that received the control peptide (Fig. 5a–e and Additional file 1: Figure S1C).

Inhibition MyD88 suppresses activation of NF-κB signal and ERK signal after CCI

NF-κB p65 and ERK signaling pathways were activated at postoperation, we examined whether suppressed MyD88 by MIP treatment could alter the activated situation of NF-κB p65 and ERK proteins in rats of CCI-induced nerve injury. Our Western blot results showed that the MIP treatment significantly decreased the phosphorylation of NF-κB p65 and ERK proteins in CCI-rat SDH at day 14 after intrathecally administered MIP on CCI rats in comparison to rats that received the control peptide (Fig. 6a–d).

Inhibition MyD88-dependent pathway suppresses the production of TNF-α and activation of astrocyte and microglial cell

Glial cells, including astrocytes and microglial cells, play a critical role in the initiation and maintenance of neuropathic pain [4, 15, 29]. Nerve injury-induced activation of astrocytes and microglial cells act as modulators in the maintenance of central sensitization. GFAP is an astrocyte-specific marker that distinguishes from other glial cells and also activation marker of astrocytes in the CNS. IBA1 play as specific activated marker of microglia in the CNS. Immunofluorescent results showed CCI-induced activation of astrocytes (GFAP) and microglia (IBA1) were suppressed by intrathecal injection of MIP (500 μM on POD 3–5) (Fig. 7a). CCI-induced increased expression of GFAP and IBA1 protein in the spinal cord SDH were also reduced by the administration of MIP (Fig. 7b, c).

We also examined the expression of proinflammatory cytokines TNF-α of SDH. After nerve injury, the TNF-α was upregulated and played an important role in the maintenance of neuropathic pain [30]. The significantly increased protein levels of TNF-α induced CCI were suppressed greatly by intrathecal injection of MIP in the SDH (Fig. 7b, c). These results suggested that MyD88-dependent TIR signaling played an essential role in the development of neuropathic pain.

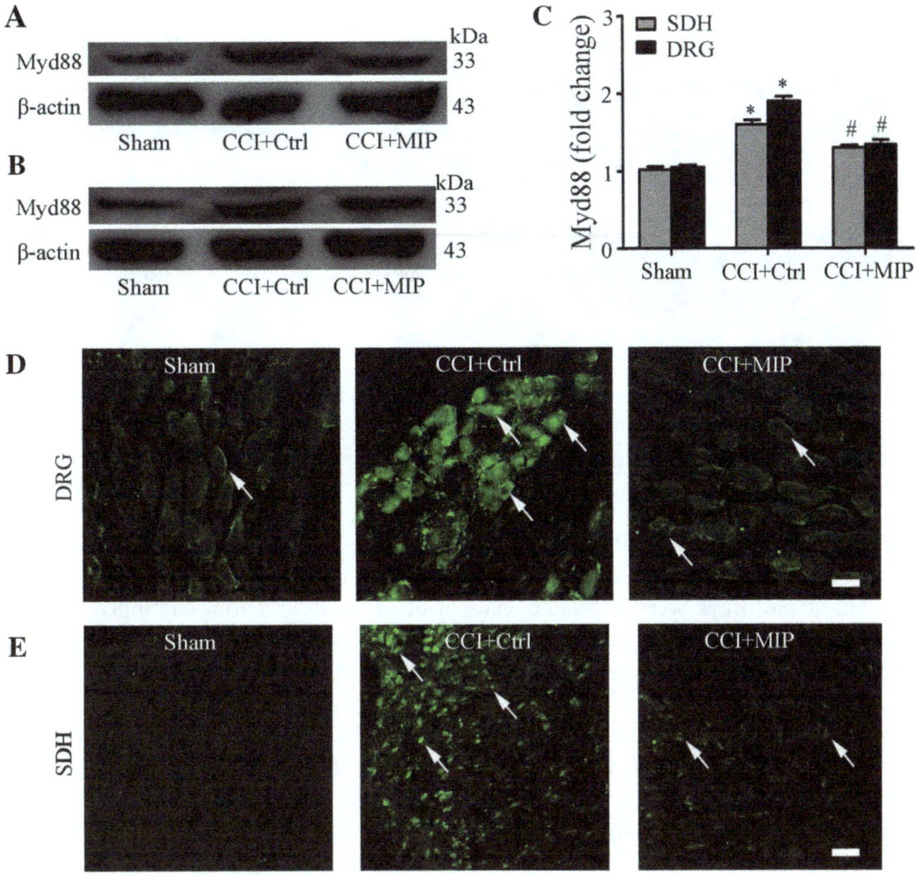

Fig. 5 Intrathecal administration of MIP decreases MyD88 protein expression in rat DRG and SDH after CCI. **a-b** Western blot showing inhibitory effects of MIP on CCI-increased protein level of MyD88 in DRG (A) and SDH (B). **c** Data summary of B. **d-e** Immunofluorescence showing inhibitory effects of MIP on expression of MyD88 in DRG (D) and SDH (E). Scale bar: 20 μm (**d**, **e**). MIP (i.t., in a volume of 20 μl, 500 mM) was given once a day on postoperative days 3, 4, and 5, respectively. The control peptide was used in the control (Ctrl) group. Tissues were collected on postoperative days 14 (n = 4 each group). One-way ANOVA, *$P < 0.05$ vs. Sham, #$P < 0.05$ vs. CCI + Ctrl

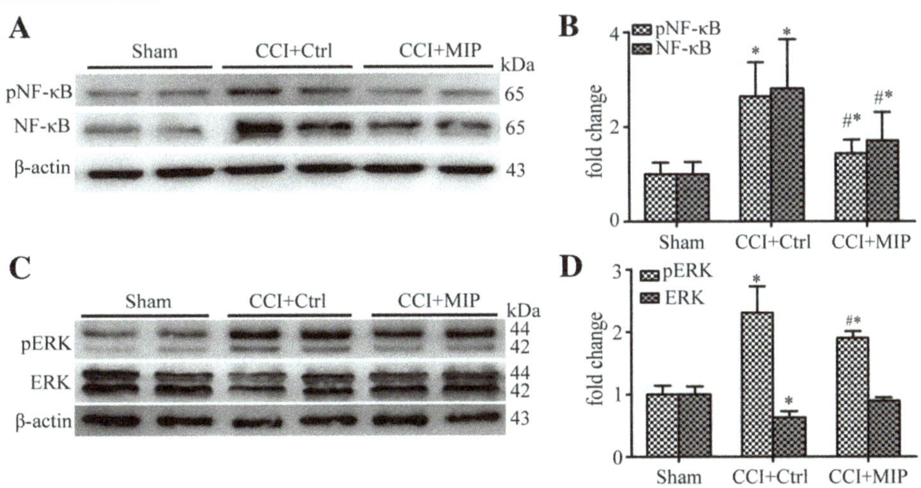

Fig. 6 Suppressed of NF-κB p65, ERK signal by inhibition of Myd88 in rat SDH after CCI. **a** Western blot showing inhibitory effects of MIP on CCI-induced increased protein level of NF-κB p65 and pNF-κB p65. **b** Data summary of A. **c** Western blot showing inhibitory effects of MIP on CCI-induced increased protein level of ERK and pERK. **d** Data summary of C. Others are the same as Fig. 5

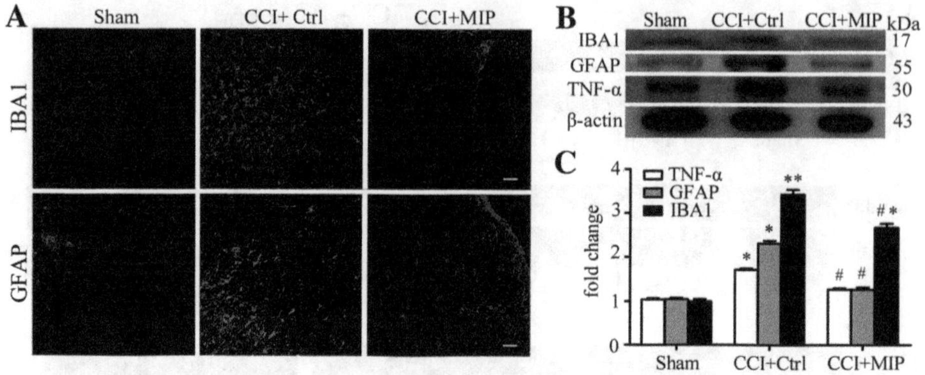

Fig. 7 Suppressed activation of glial cells and TNF-α production by inhibition of MyD88 in rat SDH after CCI. **a** Immunostaining showing inhibitory effects of MIP on activation of microglial cells (IBA1), and astrocytes (GFAP). Scale bar: 20 μm. **b** Western blot showing inhibitory effects of MIP on CCI-induced increased protein level of IBA1, GFAP, and TNF-α. **c** Data summary of B. Others are the same as Fig. 5

Unchanged expression and distributions of TRIF in DRG and SDH after CCI

Toll-like receptor signaling pathways were activated via MyD88-dependent signaling transduction and MyD88-independent signaling transduction pathway [8, 13]. Toll-receptor-associated activator of interferon (TRIF) was the adaptor protein of MyD88-independent signaling transduction pathway [7]. The results of Western blot were observed that CCI had no effect on the protein level of TRIF compared with naïve and sham operation in L4–5 DRGs and SDH of rats (Additional file 1: Figure S2A-B and Additional file 1: Figure S4A-B). The protein presented in the neurons of DRGs and co-expressed partly with CGRP and IB4-positive neurons (Additional file 1: Figure S2C). In SDH, we found that TRIF distributed in the superficial layers. And astrocytes and microglial cells partly expressed TRIF protein on SDH (Additional file 1: Figure S2D). After CCI, unchanged TRIF protein of DRGs and SDH may indicate that MYD88-independent signaling transduction of DRGs and SDH was not activated.

In addition, we performed experiments to test whether MIP treatment could also decrease the expression of TRIF in DRG and SDH. However, our Western blot and immunofluorescent data showed that the expression of TRIF was not affected in the DRG and SDH at POD 14 in MIP treatment CCI rats (Additional file 1: Figure S3A-E and Figure S4C).

Discussion

In the present study, we explored the role of MyD88-dependent TIR signaling pathways in the DRG and SDH in a rat model of CCI-induced neuropathic pain. We found that CCI induced a rapid and long-term upregulation of MyD88 in the DRG and SDH of rat. Meanwhile, the proinflammatory cytokine IL-1β and HMGB1 were upregulated in the DRG and SDH. We also found that phospho-NF-κB p65 and phospho-p44/42 MAPK of Toll/interleukin-1 receptor downstream signal protein were rapidly and long-lastingly upregulated in the DRG and SDH after CCI. In contrast, CCI did not cause any significant change in TRIF. Intrathecal injection of MyD88 inhibitor MIP attenuated CCI-induced pain and decreased MyD88 expression in DRG and SDH. Inhibition of MyD88 suppressed the phospho-NF-κB p65, phospho-p44/42 MAPK, the production of TNF-α, and the activation of astrocytes and microglial cells in SDH. These results suggested that MyD88-dependent TIR/NF-κB p65 and p44/42 MAPK pathway, activated by IL-1β and HMGB1, was involved in CCI-induced neuroinflammation and neuropathic pain. In this study, we administrated MIP on preoperative days −3 to −1 (before CCI) to achieve a maximum and sustaining effect of the drug. Previous studies used a similar strategy of MIP application to inhibit MyD88 in vitro or in vivo [31–33].

HMGB1 is a proinflammation mediator and endogenous ligand of TLRs such as TLR2 and TLR4 [34]. HMGB1 can be induced in the DRG and/or SDH in multiple animal models of pain [34–36]. IL-1β is a potent proinflammatory cytokine and endogenous ligand of IL-1R [21]. HMGB1 and IL-1β can activate calcium mobilization in DRG neurons and stimulate astrocytes or microglia cells to produce proinflammatory mediators or cytokines such as TNF-α via activation of NF-kappa-B, MAPK, or other pathways [35, 37]. Previous studies showed that intrathecal injection of HMGB1 or IL-1β induced pain hypersensitivity including heat hyperalgesia and mechanical allodynia [34, 37]. Release of HMGB1 and IL-1β in the nociceptive pathway may play a crucial role for the development of pain via influencing adjacent neurons and glia [38]. In this study, we also found that HMGB1 and IL-1β was robustly produced and sustained through POD 21 in the DRG and SDH of CCI rats.

TLRs play a pivotal role in innate immune responses. Increasing evidence suggests that TLRs are expressed in primary sensory neurons in DRG and TG [5]. TLR4 mainly express in small-diameter sensory neurons of DRG and TG, which are mostly nociceptive sensor and regulate nociceptive sensation such as pain [16, 20, 21]. Functional TLRs including TLR2 and TLR4 also express in microglia and astrocytes that modulate glial activation and spinal inflammatory of the spinal injury or chronic pain-induced central sensitization [17, 39]. TLR4 mediates the hyperalgesia and neuroinflammation by damage/pathogen-associated molecular pattern components such as heat shock protein 90 (HSP90), HMGB1, and LPS [16, 21, 34, 35, 40]. Peripheral neurons of DRG or glial cells of spinal cord may directly produce HMGB1 and/or HSP90 when peripheral and/or central nervous system are damaged or administrated with drugs [18, 34, 35]. In this study, we measured total HMGB1 by Western blots, while only disulfide HMGB1 is known to be a TLR4 agonist [41, 42]. This problem will be addressed in future studies. In addition, a recent study also found that HMGB1 activates pro-inflammatory signaling via TLR5, leading to allodynia [43]. Further experiments using specific TLR2 or TLR4 antagonists or knockout mice could be performed to determine their roles in the MyD88-dependent signaling pathway.

IL-1R was an important receptor for regulating immune responses and inflammation [44]. It expresses in nociceptive neurons of DRG and glial cells of SDH and mediates interleukin-1 including interleukin-1β-induced activation of cell [27, 28, 45]. IL-1β can act directly on primary sensory neurons to evoke excitatory action on nociceptor neurons by IL-1R [28]. IL-1β also activates IL-1R to contribute to hyperalgesia and the establishment of peripheral and central sensitization [28, 46].

Two distinct signaling transduction pathways of TLRs were found [13]. Activated TLRs and/or IL-1R signaling are involved in the recruitment of adaptor molecules such as MYD88 or TRIF, then phosphorylate NF-kappa-B or MAPK via IL-1 receptor-associated kinasel (IRAK1) and TNF receptor-associated factors6 (TRAF6) [7, 9, 10, 13]. MyD88 is the adaptor protein of Toll/interleukin-1 receptor (TIR) and plays an important role in the trafficking of TIR signal pathway [7, 10]. MyD88 is expressed in DRG neurons and glial cells and could be significantly increased in the DRG from rat models of chronic pain induced by chemotherapy [18]. SNL lesions produce chronic pain is approximately 50% reduced in MyD88-deficient mice [19, 47]. Consistently, intrathecal administration of MyD88 inhibitor suppresses pain of paclitaxel-induced peripheral neuropathy when applied 14 days after paclitaxel administration [18]. TRIF is an adaptor protein of the MyD88-independent signaling transduction pathways of TLRs and shares mostly by TLR3 and TLR4 signaling [13]. The SNL-induced allodynia was significantly alleviated in the MyD88 knock-out mice with reduced glial activation in SDH and ATF3 expression in the DRG, but these effects were not observed in the TRIF deficient mice [47]. TRIF expression was found not significantly changed in the SDH in a rat model of paclitaxel-induced peripheral neuropathic pain [18]. Our results also showed a lack of change in TRIF protein in the DRG and SDH of CCI rats. Detailed mechanisms for the upregulation and activation of MyD88 without increases in TRIF with TLR signaling should be further investigated in the future.

Conclusions

In this study, we found that peripheral nerve injury triggered the upregulation of IL-1β and HMGB1, which could bind to their receptors in the DRG and SDH and transmit signals via adaptor protein MyD88. MyD88 may subsequently act through phosphorylated NF-κB and ERK to regulate the expression of proinflammation

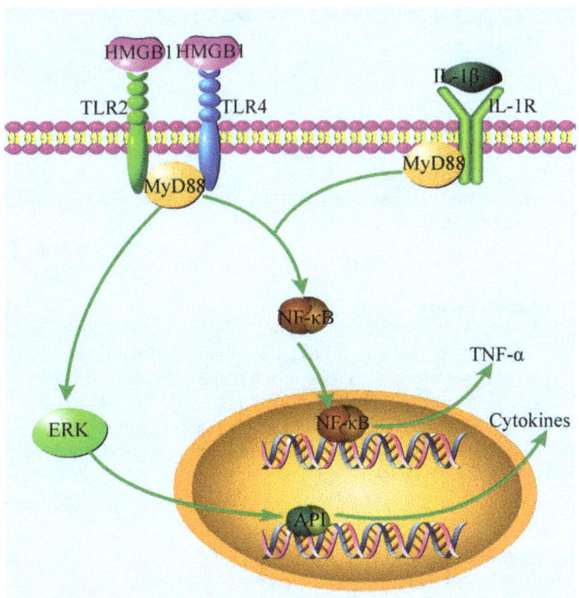

Fig. 8 Schematic illustration demonstrates MyD88-dependent signaling pathways of neuropathic pain induced by CCI. Nerve injury produces abundant HMGB1and IL-1β in the DRG and SDH. The binding of HMGB1 and IL-1β to their receptors (TLR2/4 andIL-1R, respectively) activates MyD88 in the DRG and SDH, which phosphorylate NF-κB p65 and ERK. Phosphorylated NF-κB p65 subsequently enter the nucleus to regulate the expression of proinflammation cytokines such as TNF-α. Phosphorylated ERK enter the nucleus to induce transcription factors such as AP-1, which regulates the expression of certain cytokines and activates glial cells. All these signaling events consequently result in central and peripheral sensitizations that produce neuropathic pain

cytokines and activate glia cells. MyD88-dependent TIR pathway may play a role in CCI-induced neuroinflammation and neuropathic pain. A schematic illustration for the proposed MyD88-dependent signaling pathways of neuropathic pain was provided in Fig. 8 This study might suggest a potential strategy for the treatment of neuropathic pain targeting MyD88.

Abbreviations

CCI: Chronic constriction injury; CGRP: Calcitonin gene-related peptide; CNS: Central nervous system; DRG: Dorsal root ganglion; ERK: Extracellular signal-regulated protein kinase; GFAP: Glial fibrillary acidic protein; HMGB1: High mobility group box 1; IB4: Isolectin B4; IBA1: Allograft inflammatory factor 1; IL-1β: Interleukin-1 beta; IRAK1: IL-1 receptor-associated kinase1; MAPK: Mitogen-activated protein kinase; MIP: MyD88 homodimerization inhibitory peptide; MyD88: Myeloid differentiation primary response protein 88; NF-κB: Transcription factors of the nuclear factor κB; POD: Postoperative day; SDH: Spinal dorsal horn; TIR: Toll/interleukin-1 receptor; TLR: Toll-like receptor; TNF-α: Tumor necrosis factor-alpha; TRAF6: TNF receptor-associated factors 6; TRIF: TIR-domain-containing adaptor-inducing beta interferon

Acknowledgements

We thank Dr. Wenyin Qiu, Xiaojin Qian, and Yongmei Chen in the Department of Anatomy, Histology and Embryology, Institute of Basic Medical Sciences, Chinese Academy of Medical Sciences for their technical assistance in immunohistochemistry. We thank Dr. Xiaojing Liu, Department of Dermatology, Peking University People's Hospital, China, for their generous help in providing the mouse anti-pNF-κB-p65 antibody.

Funding

This work was supported by grants from National Science Foundation of China #81271239 (C.M.) and #31070930 (Y.H.), the IBMS/CAMS Dean's Fund #2011RC01 (C.M.), the PUMC Youth Fund #201211 (C.M.) and the PUMC Innovation Fund for Postgraduate #2016 (F.L.), and the CAMS Innovation Fund for Medical Sciences (CIFMS).

Authors' contributions

FL and ZW drafted the manuscript. FL performed the immunofluorescence staining. ZW and MW performed the CCI and behavioral assessment of pain. ZW, YQ and CL performed the Western blot and analysis. ZW and YQ performed the Intrathecal catheterization and drug delivery. CM, YH and LS conceived of the study, participated in its design and coordination and helped to draft the manuscript. All authors read and approved the final manuscript.

Competing interests

The authors declare that they have no competing interests.

Consent for publication

Not applicable.

References

1. Campbell JN, Meyer RA. Mechanisms of neuropathic pain. Neuron. 2006;52(1):77–92.
2. Denk F, McMahon SB. Chronic pain: emerging evidence for the involvement of epigenetics. Neuron. 2012;73(3):435–44.
3. Reichling DB, Green PG, Levine JD. The fundamental unit of pain is the cell. Pain. 2013;154:S2–9.
4. McMahon SB, Cafferty WB, Marchand F. Immune and glial cell factors as pain mediators and modulators. Exp Neurol. 2005;192(2):444–62.
5. Nicotra L, Loram LC, Watkins LR, Hutchinson MR. Toll-like receptors in chronic pain. Exp Neurol. 2012;234(2):316–29.
6. Moalem G, Tracey DJ. Immune and inflammatory mechanisms in neuropathic pain. Brain Res Rev. 2006;51(2):240–64.
7. O'Neill LAJ, Bowie AG. The family of five: TIR-domain-containing adaptors in Toll-like receptor signalling. Nat Rev Immunol. 2007;7(5):353–64.
8. Muzio M, Ni J, Feng P, Dixit VM. IRAK (Pelle) family member IRAK-2 and MyD88 as proximal mediators of IL-1 signaling. Science. 1997;278 (5343):1612–5.
9. Burns K, Martinon F, Esslinger C, Pahl H, Schneider P, Bodmer JL, Di Marco F, French L, Tschopp J. MyD88, an adapter protein involved in interleukin-1 signaling. J Biol Chem. 1998;273(20):12203–9.
10. Medzhitov R, Preston-Hurlburt P, Kopp E, Stadlen A, Chen CQ, Ghosh S, Janeway CA. MyD88 is an adaptor protein in the hToll/IL-1 receptor family signaling pathways. Mol Cell. 1998;2(2):253–8.
11. Peroval MY, Boyd AC, Young JR, Smith AL. A critical role for MAPK signalling pathways in the transcriptional regulation of toll like receptors. PloS one. 2013;8(2):e51243.
12. Walker-Caulfield ME, Guo Y, Johnson RK, McCarthy CB, Fitz-Gibbon PD, Lucchinetti CF, Howe CL. NFκB signaling drives pro-granulocytic astroglial responses to neuromyelitis optica patient IgG. J Neuroinflammation. 2015;12(1):1–15.
13. Takeda K, Kaisho T, Akira S. Toll-like receptors. Annu Rev Immunol. 2003;21:335–76.
14. Kigerl KA, Lai W, Rivest S, Hart RP, Satoskar AR, Popovich PG. Toll-like receptor (TLR)-2 and TLR-4 regulate inflammation, gliosis, and myelin sparing after spinal cord injury. J Neurochem. 2007;102(1):37–50.
15. Inoue K, Tsuda M. Microglia and neuropathic pain. Glia. 2009;57(14):1469–79.
16. Due MR, Piekarz AD, Wilson N, Feldman P, Ripsch MS, Chavez S, Yin H, Khanna R, White FA. Neuroexcitatory effects of morphine-3-glucuronide are dependent on Toll-like receptor 4 signaling. J Neuroinflammation. 2012;9:12.
17. Heiman A, Pallottie A, Heary RF, Elkabes S. Toll-like receptors in central nervous system injury and disease: a focus on the spinal cord. Brain Behav Immun. 2014;42:232–45.
18. Li Y, Zhang H, Zhang H, Kosturakis AK, Jawad AB, Dougherty PM. Toll-like receptor 4 signaling contributes to Paclitaxel-induced peripheral neuropathy. J Pain. 2014;15(7):712–25.
19. Stokes JA, Cheung J, Eddinger K, Corr M, Yaksh TL. Toll-like receptor signaling adapter proteins govern spread of neuropathic pain and recovery following nerve injury in male mice. J Neuroinflammation. 2013;10(1):1–14.
20. Liu XJ, Liu T, Chen G, Wang B, Yu XL, Yin C, Ji RR. TLR signaling adaptor protein MyD88 in primary sensory neurons contributes to persistent inflammatory and neuropathic pain and neuroinflammation. Sci Rep. 2016;6:28188.
21. Diogenes A, Ferraz CC, Akopian AN, Henry MA, Hargreaves KM. LPS sensitizes TRPV1 via activation of TLR4 in trigeminal sensory neurons. J Dent Res. 2011;90(6):759–64.
22. Braun TP, Grossberg AJ, Veleva-Rotse BO, Maxson JE, Szumowski M, Barnes AP, Marks DL. Expression of myeloid differentiation factor 88 in neurons is not requisite for the induction of sickness behavior by interleukin-1β. J Neuroinflammation. 2012;9(1):1–13.
23. Bennett GJ, Xie YK. A peripheral mononeuropathy in rat that produces disorders of pain sensation like those seen in man. Pain. 1988;33(1):87–107.
24. Xue ZJ, Shen L, Wang ZY, Hui SY, Huang YG, Ma C. STAT3 inhibitor WP1066 as a novel therapeutic agent for bCCI neuropathic pain rats. Brain Res. 2014;1583:79–88.
25. Qiu Y, Chen WY, Wang ZY, Liu F, Wei M, Ma C, Huang YG. Simvastatin Attenuates Neuropathic Pain by Inhibiting the RhoA/LIMK/Cofilin Pathway. Neurochem Res. 2016;41(9):2457–69.
26. Qu L, Zhang P, LaMotte RH, Ma C. Neuronal Fc-gamma receptor I mediated excitatory effects of IgG immune complex on rat dorsal root ganglion neurons. Brain Behav Immun. 2011;25(7):1399–407.
27. Gangadharan V, Kuner R. Pain hypersensitivity mechanisms at a glance. Dis Model Mech. 2013;6(4):889–95.
28. Binshtok AM, Wang H, Zimmermann K, Amaya F, Vardeh D, Shi L, Brenner GJ, Ji RR, Bean BP, Woolf CJ, et al. Nociceptors are interleukin-1beta sensors. J Neurosci. 2008;28(52):14062–73.
29. Zhuo M, Wu G, Wu LJ. Neuronal and microglial mechanisms of neuropathic pain. Mol Brain. 2011;4:31.
30. Leung L, Cahill CM. TNF-α and neuropathic pain - a review. J Neuroinflammation. 2010;7(1):1–11.
31. Funderburg N, Lederman MM, Feng Z, Drage MG, Jadlowsky J, Harding CV,

Weinberg A, Sieg SF. Human -defensin-3 activates professional antigen-presenting cells via Toll-like receptors 1 and 2. Proc Natl Acad Sci U S A. 2007;104(47):18631–5.
32. Benedetti F, Davinelli S, Krishnan S, Gallo RC, Scapagnini G, Zella D, Curreli S. Sulfur compounds block MCP-1 production by Mycoplasma fermentans-infected macrophages through NF-kappaB inhibition. J Transl Med. 2014;12:145.
33. Lin X, Kong J, Wu Q, Yang Y, Ji P. Effect of TLR4/MyD88 signaling pathway on expression of IL-1beta and TNF-alpha in synovial fibroblasts from temporomandibular joint exposed to lipopolysaccharide. Mediat Inflamm. 2015;2015:329405.
34. Maeda T, Ozaki M, Kobayashi Y, Kiguchi N, Kishioka S. HMGB1 as a Potential Therapeutic Target for Neuropathic Pain. J Pharmacol Sci. 2013;123(4):301–5.
35. Agalave NM, Larsson M, Abdelmoaty S, Su J, Baharpoor A, Lundback P, Palmblad K, Andersson U, Harris H, Svensson CI. Spinal HMGB1 induces TLR4-mediated long-lasting hypersensitivity and glial activation and regulates pain-like behavior in experimental arthritis. Pain. 2014;155(9):1802–13.
36. Allette YM, Due MR, Wilson SM, Feldman P, Ripsch MS, Khanna R, White FA. Identification of a functional interaction of HMGB1 with Receptor for Advanced Glycation End-products in a model of neuropathic pain. Brain Behav Immun. 2014;42:169–77.
37. Wolf G, Yirmiya R, Goshen I, Iverfeldt K, Holmlund L, Takeda K, Shavit Y. Impairment of interleukin-1 (IL-1) signaling reduces basal pain sensitivity in mice: genetic, pharmacological and developmental aspects. Pain. 2003;104(3):471–80.
38. Kim JB, Sig Choi J, Yu YM, Nam K, Piao CS, Kim SW, Lee MH, Han PL, Park JS, Lee JK. HMGB1, a novel cytokine-like mediator linking acute neuronal death and delayed neuroinflammation in the postischemic brain. J Neurosci. 2006;26(24):6413–21.
39. Freria CM, Bernardes D, Almeida GL, Simões GF, Barbosa GO, Oliveira ALR. Impairment of toll-like receptors 2 and 4 leads to compensatory mechanisms after sciatic nerve axotomy. J Neuroinflammation. 2016;13(1):1–15.
40. Swaroop S, Sengupta N, Suryawanshi AR, Adlakha YK, Basu A. HSP60 plays a regulatory role in IL-1β-induced microglial inflammation via TLR4-p38 MAPK axis. J Neuroinflammation. 2016;13(1):1–19.
41. Li G, Liang X, Lotze MT. HMGB1: The Central Cytokine for All Lymphoid Cells. Front Immunol. 2013;4:68.
42. Li G, Tang D, Lotze MT. Ménage à Trois in stress: DAMPs, redox and autophagy. Semin Cancer Biol. 2013;23(5):380–90.
43. Das N, Dewan V, Grace Peter M, Gunn Robin J, Tamura R, Tzarum N, Watkins Linda R, Wilson Ian A, Yin H. HMGB1 Activates Proinflammatory Signaling via TLR5 Leading to Allodynia. Cell Rep. 2016;17(4):1128–40.
44. Dinarello CA. Immunological and Inflammatory Functions of the Interleukin-1 Family. In: Annual Review of Immunology, vol. 27. Palo Alto: Annual Reviews; 2009. p. 519–50.
45. Li M, Shi J, Tang JR, Chen D, Ai B, Chen J, Wang LN, Cao FY, Li LL, Lin CY, et al. Effects of complete Freund's adjuvant on immunohistochemical distribution of IL-1beta and IL-1R I in neurons and glia cells of dorsal root ganglion. Acta Pharmacol Sin. 2005;26(2):192–8.
46. Gougeon PY, Lourenssen S, Han TY, Nair DG, Ropeleski MJ, Blennerhassett MG. The pro-inflammatory cytokines IL-1beta and TNFalpha are neurotrophic for enteric neurons. J Neurosci. 2013;33(8):3339–51.
47. Stokes JA, Corr M, Yaksh TL. Spinal toll-like receptor signaling and nociceptive processing: regulatory balance between TIRAP and TRIF cascades mediated by TNF and IFNbeta. Pain. 2013;154(5):733–42.

7

Macrophage migration inhibitory factor facilitates production of CCL5 in astrocytes following rat spinal cord injury

Yue Zhou[1,2†], Wei Guo[3†], Zhenjie Zhu[1], Yuming Hu[1], Yingjie Wang[2], Xuejie Zhang[2], Wenjuan Wang[2], Nan Du[2], Tiancheng Song[2], Kaini Yang[4], Zongyu Guan[4], Yongjun Wang[2*] and Aisong Guo[1*]

Abstract

Background: Astrocytes act as immune effector cells with the ability to produce a wide array of chemokines and cytokines in response to various stimuli. Macrophage migration inhibitory factor (MIF) is inducibly expressed in injured spinal cord contributing to excessive inflammation that affects motor functional recovery. Unknown is whether MIF can facilitate inflammatory responses through stimulating release of chemokines from astrocytes following spinal cord injury.

Methods: Following the establishment of the contusion spinal cord injury rat model, the correlation of chemokine (C-C motif) ligand 5 (CCL5) expression with that of MIF was assayed by Western blot, ELISA, and immunohistochemistry. Immunoprecipitation was used to detect MIF interaction with membrane CD74 receptor. Intracellular signal transduction of MIF/CD74 axis was analyzed by transcriptome sequencing of primary astrocytes and further validated by treatment of various inhibitors. The effects of CCL5 released by astrocytes on macrophage migration were performed by transwell migration assay. The post-injury locomotor functions were assessed using the Basso, Beattie, and Bresnahan (BBB) locomotor scale.

Results: The protein levels of chemokine CCL5/RANTES were remarkably increased in the astrocytes of rat injured spinal cord, in parallel with the expression of MIF. Treatment of MIF inhibitor 4-IPP in the lesion sites resulted in a significant decrease of CCL5 protein levels. In vitro study revealed MIF was capable of facilitating CCL5 production of astrocytes through interaction with CD74 membrane receptor, and knockdown of this receptor attenuated such effects. Production of CCL5 in astrocytes was significantly blocked by inhibitor of c-Jun N-terminal kinase, rather than by those of ERK and P38. Recombinant CCL5 protein was found to be more effective in promoting migration of M2- compared to M1-type macrophages.

Conclusion: Collectively, these data reveal a novel function of MIF in regulation of CCL5 release from astrocytes, which in turn favors for recruitment of inflammatory cells to the injured site of the spinal cord, in association with activation of excessive inflammation.

Keywords: MIF, CCL5, Spinal cord, Astrocyte, Inflammation, Chemokines

* Correspondence: wyjbs@ntu.edu.cn; 15851300188@163.com
[†]Yue Zhou and Wei Guo contributed equally to this work.
[2]Key Laboratory of Neuroregeneration of Jiangsu and Ministry of Education, Co-innovation Center of Neuroregeneration, Nantong University, Nantong 226001, People's Republic of China
[1]Department of Rehabilitation Medicine, Affiliated Hospital of Nantong University, Nantong 226001, People's Republic of China
Full list of author information is available at the end of the article

Background

The central nervous system (CNS) can activate innate immune responses by sensing pathogens or tissue damages [1]. Upon acute traumatic spinal cord injury, the resident immune and glial cells are rapidly motivated to release various cytokines and chemokines, which further induce leukocyte infiltration to the injury sites [2, 3]. Astrocytes are the most abundant glial cell contributing to the functional homeostasis of the healthy CNS. They can also receive and integrate information from synapses, other glial cells, and the blood vessels and as a consequence generate complex outputs that control the neural circuitry and coordinate it with the local microcirculation [4]. Astrocytes have been shown to participate in local inflammatory responses [5–8]. In the context of inflammatory or otherwise pathological conditions, the activated astrocytes proliferate and produce a wide variety of cytokines and chemokines, including CCL2 (monocyte chemotactic protein-1), CCL5 (RANTES), and CXCL8 (IL-8), which are associated with the recruitment of immune cells of alternative activation status [5, 9]. These recruited microglia/macrophages play either a pro-inflammatory (M1) or anti-inflammatory (M2) role as seen in a spinal cord injury model or neuroinflammatory diseases like multiple sclerosis (MS) [10]. Chemokine (C-C motif) ligand 5 (CCL5) may serve to amplify inflammatory responses by facilitating the recruitment of inflammatory cells into autoimmune lesions [6, 11, 12]. As such, astrocyte-released cytokines and chemokines which contribute to inflammatory responses will inevitably exacerbate the neuropathological changes following CNS injury.

Macrophage migration inhibitory factor (MIF) is a pro-inflammatory cytokine produced by a variety of cells and tissues, including monocytes, the anterior pituitary gland, T-lymphocytes, hepatocytes, and keratinocytes [13, 14]. MIF has been found to be constitutively or inducibly expressed in astrocytes, neurons, microglia, ependymal cells, and epithelial cells of the choroid plexus in the CNS [14–17]. Besides its roles of inducing neuronal death and activating inflammatory episodes in microglia, MIF is capable of promoting proliferation and inflammatory cytokine production of astrocytes [16, 18]. Deletion of MIF has been shown to promote functional recovery after compression-induced spinal cord injury [17], suggesting that MIF plays key roles in the neuropathogenesis of injured spinal cord. Astrocytes are the main sources of chemokines involved in recruitment of inflammatory cells; whether MIF is able to induce the release of chemokines from the cells remains unclear.

Astrocytes are endowed with the ability to secrete cytokines through expressing an array of receptors involved in innate immunity, such as Toll-like receptors and nucleotide-binding oligomerization domains [19, 20]. Also, the cells express CD74 surface receptor which can interact with MIF to elicit inflammatory responses after spinal cord injury (SCI) [18]. As MIF/CD74 axis has been found to activate intracellular MAPKs of astrocytes, an intermediate signaling essential for regulation of CCL5 and other chemokines [21, 22], MIF/CD74 axis is therefore postulated to mediate the production of CCL5 in astrocytes, which has been identified to promote inflammatory cell recruitment. In the present study, we analyzed the correlations between expression of MIF and CCL5 in the injured spinal cord of rat. We further investigated MIF-induced production of CCL5 in the astrocytes, as well as the underlying molecular mechanism. Our results have revealed that MIF affects pathological changes of the injured spinal cord through not only activation of astrocyte inflammatory responses, but also promoting release of chemokines.

Methods

Animals

Adult male Sprague–Dawley (SD) rats, weighing 180–220 g, were provided by the Center of Experimental Animals, Nantong University. All animal care, breeding, and testing procedures were approved according to the Animal Care and Use Committee of Nantong University and the Jiangsu Province Animal Care Ethics Committee. All animals were housed in individual cages in a temperature and light/dark cycle controlled environment with free access to food and water.

Establishment of the contusion SCI rat model

The number of animals subjected to surgical treatment was calculated by six per experimental group in triplicate. The contusion SCI rat model was prepared as the previous description [23]. Briefly, rats were anesthetized with an intraperitoneal injection of 10% chloral hydrate (3 mg/kg). The fur was shaved from the surgical site and the skin was disinfected with chlorhexidine. A 15-mm midline skin incision was made to expose the vertebral column. After the spinal thoracic region was exposed by separation of the dorsal muscles to the side, the spinous processes of T8–T10 vertebrae were exposed. A laminectomy was performed at vertebral level T9, exposing the dorsal cord surface with the dura remaining intact. The exposed spinal cord segment (about 3 mm in length) received a 150-kilodyne spinal contusion injury using the IH-0400 Impactor (Precision Systems and Instrumentation) injury device. The impact rod was removed immediately, and the wound was irrigated. Muscles and incisions were sutured using silk threads. Postoperative care included butorphanol administration twice a day for a 5-day period, as well as vitamins, saline, and enrofloxacin twice a day for a 7-day period. Manual expression of the bladders was performed twice a day until animals recovered spontaneous voiding.

Cell culture

Astrocytes were prepared from the spinal cord of newborn Sprague–Dawley rats, 1–2 days after birth, and the astrocytes were isolated and cultured according to previously described methods [24]. Briefly, the cells were enzymatically dissociated using 0.25% trypsin (Gibco-BRL) for 6 min at 37 °C, and the suspension was then centrifuged at 1200 rpm for 5 min and cultured in 1:1 Dulbecco's modified Eagle's medium to Ham's F-12 medium supplemented with 10% fetal bovine serum (FBS), 0.224% $NaHCO_3$, and 1% penicillin/streptomycin in the presence of 5% CO_2. A monolayer of astrocytes was obtained 12–14 days after the plating. Non-astrocytes were detached from the flasks by shaking and were removed by changing the medium. Third or fourth passage cells were rendered quiescent through incubation in the medium containing 0.5% FBS for 4 days prior to the experiments. Astrocyte phenotype was confirmed by cells exhibiting a characteristic morphology and positive staining for the astrocytic marker glial fibrillary acid protein (GFAP).

Western blot

Protein was extracted from cells with a buffer containing 1% SDS, 100 mM Tris-HCl, 1 mM PMSF, and 0.1 mM β-mercaptoethanol, following treatment with 0.5 μg/ml rat recombinant MIF (ProSpec) for 15 min, 30 min, and 60 min, respectively. Alternatively, protein was extracted from 1-cm spinal segments of the injured site at 0 day, 1 day, 4 days, and 1 week following contusion ($n = 8$ in each time point). Protein concentration of each specimen was detected by the Bradford method to maintain the same loads. Protein extracts were heat-denatured at 95 °C for 5 min, electrophoretically separated on 10% SDS-PAGE, and transferred to PVDF membranes. The membranes were subjected to the reaction with a 1:1000 dilution of primary antibodies in TBS buffer at 4 °C overnight, followed by a reaction with the secondary antibody conjugated with goat anti-rabbit or goat anti-mouse HRP dilution 1:1000 (Santa Cruz) at room temperature for 2 h. After the membrane was washed, the HRP activity was detected using an ECL kit. The image was scanned with a GS800 Densitometer Scanner (Bio-Rad), and the data were analyzed using PDQuest 7.2.0 software (Bio-Rad). β-actin (1:5000) was used as an internal control. The antibodies used in Western blot are as follows: MIF (Abcam); p65NFκB (Cell Signaling Technology, CST), p-ERK1/2, and ERK1/2 (CST); and CD74 (Biorbyt) and β-actin (Proteintech).

ELISA

Primary astrocytes were treated with 0–2.5 μg/ml rat recombinant MIF for 24 h, or tissue samples of spinal segments were prepared as mentioned ($n = 6$ in each time point). Cell supernatants were harvested, and cells were lysed in the buffer containing 1% SDS, 100 mM Tris-HCl, 1 mM PMSF, and 0.1 mM β-mercaptoethanol. The lysates were centrifuged at 12,000*g* for 15 min. Levels of CCL5 were assessed using the appropriate ELISA kits (BD Biosciences, R&D Systems) according to the manufacturer's directions. Plates were read using a 96-well plate reader (Biotek Synergy2) at a 450-nm wavelength.

Tissue immunohistochemistry

The vertebra segments were harvested from six experimental models of each time point, post-fixed, and sectioned. Sections were allowed to incubate with monoclonal MIF antibody (1:200 dilution), rabbit anti-IBA-1 antibody (1:400 dilution, Wako), polyclonal rabbit anti-CCL5 antibody (1:200 dilution, novusbio), or monoclonal mouse anti-human GFAP antibody (1:400 dilution, Sigma) at 4 °C for 36 h. The sections were further reacted with the FITC-labeled secondary antibody goat anti-mouse IgG (1:400 dilution, Gibco) or the TRITC-labeled secondary antibody donkey anti-rabbit IgG (1:400 dilution, Gibco) at 4 °C overnight, followed by observation under a confocal laser scanning microscope (Leica, Heidelberg, Germany).

Immunoprecipitation

The primary astrocytes were washed twice with cold phosphate-buffered saline and then extracted with lysis buffer (20 mM Tris-HCl, pH 7.5, 150 mM NaCl, 1 mM EDTA, 1 mM EGTA, 1% Triton X-100, 2.5 mM sodium pyrophosphate, 1 mM β-glycerolphosphate, 1 mM Na_3VO_4, 1 mM phenylmethylsulfonyl fluoride, and Roche Applied Science's complete protease inhibitors). Whole-cell extracts were centrifuged at 14,000 rpm for 20 min to remove the debris. The proteins in the supernatant were measured using a Protein Assay Kit II (Bio-Rad). For immunoprecipitation analysis, 500 μg of total cell lysates was precleared with protein A plus G-Sepharose before incubation with specific antibodies, followed by addition of protein A plus G-Sepharose. The precipitated proteins were resolved in 2× SDS-PAGE sample buffer and separated by electrophoresis on 10–12% SDS-PAGE. After being transferred onto a polyvinylidene difluoride membrane (Millipore Corp.), they were incubated with anti-MIF or anti-CD74 antibody and further with horseradish peroxidase-conjugated secondary antibody (Santa Cruz).

Transwell migration assay

Migration of RAW264.7 cells were measured using 6.5-mm transwell chambers with 8-μm pores (Costar, Cambridge, MA) as described previously [25]. A total of

100 μl of RAW264.7 cells (2×10^5 cells/ml) was transferred into the top chamber of the transwells and allowed to migrate at 37 °C in 5% CO_2. Meanwhile, 600 μl of astrocytes (1×10^5 cells/ml) was seeded into the lower chambers. After migration for 48 h, the upper surface of each membrane was cleaned with a cotton swab. Cells attached to the bottom surface of each membrane were stained with 0.1% crystal violet, imaged, and counted using a DMR inverted microscope (Leica Microsystems, Bensheim, Germany). Assays were performed in triplicate for three times. To determine the effect of CCL5 on astrocyte-stimulated RAW264.7 migration, astrocytes were stimulated with 0.5 μg/ml recombinant MIF following CCL5 siRNA interference for 24 h prior to a transwell assay. For M2 macrophage transition, RAW264.7 cells were treated with or without 20 ng/ml rat recombinant IL-13 for 2 days.

Sequencing of mRNA

Total RNA of astrocytes following treatment with CD74-siRNA [18] or scramble for 48 h, and then with 2.0 μg/ml recombinant MIF for 12 h and 24 h, respectively, was extracted using the mirVana miRNA Isolation Kit (Ambion, Austin, TX) according to the manufacturer's instructions. They were then selected by RNA Purification Beads (Illumina, San Diego, CA) and undergone library construction and RNA-seq analysis. The library was constructed by using the Illumina TruSeq RNA sample Prep Kit v2 and sequenced by the Illumina HiSeq-2000 for 50 cycles. High-quality reads that passed the Illumina quality filters were kept for the sequence analysis.

Bioinformatics analysis

Differentially expressed mRNA was designated in a criterion of greater than twofold or less than twofold change in comparison with control. Function of genes was annotated by Blastx against the NCBI database or the AGRIS database (https://agris-knowledgebase.org/) with E value threshold of 10^{-5}. Gene ontology (GO) classification was obtained by WEGO (http://wego.genomics.org.cn/) via GO id annotated by Perl and R program. Kyoto Encyclopedia of Genes and Genomes (KEGG) pathways were assigned to the sequences using KEGG Automatic Annotation Server (KAAS) online. For all heatmaps, genes were clustered by Jensen-Shannon divergence.

A reconstructed gene network was created using the Ingenuity Pathway Analysis (IPA) Software on the basis of differentially expressed genes (fold change < 0.5 for down-regulated genes at 12 h and 24 h following CD74 knockdown) to investigate their regulatory pathways and cellular functions [26].

Behavioral tests

The hindlimb locomotor function recovery was evaluated using the Basso, Beattie, and Bresnahan (BBB) locomotor scale as previously described [27], after MIF or CCL5 treatment on 0, 7, 14, and 21 days after surgery. Three well-trained investigators who were blind to the study observed the behavior of rats for 5 min. The BBB score ranged from 0 to 21 according to the rating scale. Every rat had a BBB score of 21 before surgery. The BBB score would become 0 to 1 after a successful SCI.

Statistical analysis

Statistical significance of differences between groups was analyzed by one-way analysis of variance (ANOVA) followed by Bonferroni's post hoc comparisons tests with SPSS 15.0 (SPSS, Chicago, IL, USA). Normality and homoscedasticity of the data were verified before any statistical analysis using Levene's test. Statistical significance was set at $P < 0.05$.

Results

MIF facilitated expression of chemokine CCL5 in the astrocytes of injured rat spinal cord

To uncover the potential function of MIF in CCL5 expression, we firstly determined the protein levels of MIF and CCL5 in the contused spinal cord at different time points. Results revealed that CCL5 protein levels, assayed by ELISA, were synchronously increased with elevation of MIF assayed by Western blot (Fig. 1a–c). While treatment of 8 μl of 100 mM MIF inhibitor 4-IPP in the lesion site resulted in the remarkable reduction of CCL5 production (Fig. 1c). The data indicate that MIF efficiently regulates CCL5 production following SCI.

Next, we sought to understand whether MIF-induced CCL5 expression was astrocyte-related. Immunostaining showed that CCL5 was exclusively colocalized with GFAP-positive, rather than with NeuN-, IBA-1-, or Olig2-positive cells (Additional file 1). CCL5 production was significantly increased in the GFAP-positive cells at 4 days following SCI (Fig. 1d, e). Whereas injection of 8 μl 4-IPP (100 mM) at the lesion site markedly decreased the expression of CCL5 in astrocytes (Fig. 1e). The results indicate that MIF is involved in regulation of CCL5 production in astrocytes after SCI.

Expression of CCL5 was regulated by MIF/CD74 axis in astrocytes

MIF has been shown to interact with CD74 surface receptor, which forms a receptor complex with CXCR2 and CXCR4 to elicit intracellular signaling [28, 29]. To elucidate whether MIF/CD74 couple also exists in astrocytes, the rat astrocytes were firstly isolated and cultured with purity more than 95% (Fig. 2a, b). Co-immunoprecipitation was then carried out using anti-His or anti-CD74 antibody. As

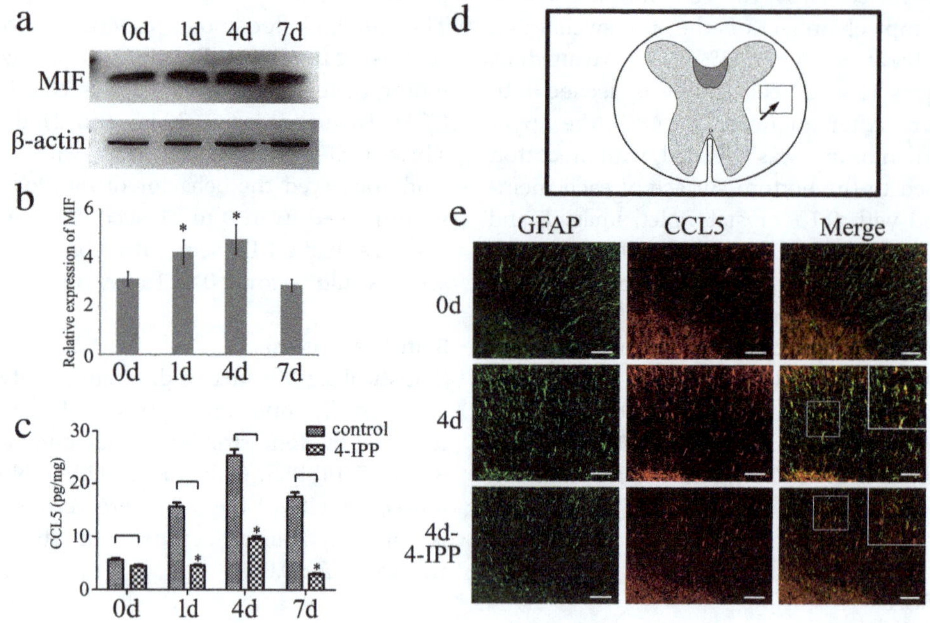

Fig. 1 Determination of MIF and CCL5 expression following spinal cord injury. **a** Western blot analysis of MIF expression following spinal cord contusion at 0d, 1d, 4d, and 7d, respectively. **b** Quantification data as shown in **a**; quantities were normalized to endogenous β-actin. **c** CCL5 protein levels were assayed by ELISA for the injured cord at different time points with or without injection of 8 μl 4-IPP (100 mM) at the lesion sites. **d** Illustration of section sites showing immunostaining. **e** Immunostaining of CCL5 in the cross sections of rat contused spinal cord showed colocalization with GFAP-positive cells at 0d and 4d, with or without injection of 4-IPP, respectively. The rectangle indicates region magnified. Error bars represent the standard deviation ($P < 0.05$). Scale bars, 100 μm

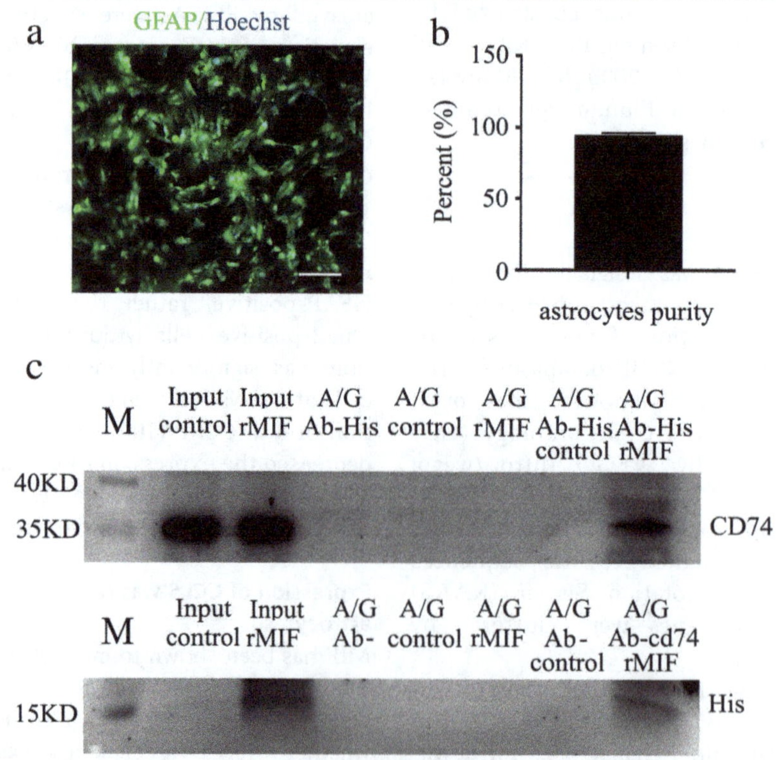

Fig. 2 Binding assay of MIF with CD74 receptor in the primary astrocytes. **a** Purified primary astrocytes stained with GFAP and Hoechst 33342. **b** Statistical analysis of primary astrocyte purity. **c** Immunoprecipitation using anti-His or anti-CD74 antibody and detection of the components of the rMIF- or CD74-associated complexes with anti-CD74 or anti-His antibody. M marker, A/G protein A/G magnetic beads. Scale bars, 50 μm

shown in Fig. 2c, recombinant His-tagged MIF was present in the CD74-associated complexes immunoprecipitated with anti-CD74 antibody, so was CD74 in the His-associated complexes. The results indicate that MIF can bind with CD74 surface receptor of astrocytes.

To understand whether CCL5 expression is under regulation of MIF/CD74 axis, we performed transcriptome analysis on primary astrocytes interfered by effective CD74 siRNA or scramble for 48 h [18], followed by stimulation with 2.0 μg/ml recombinant MIF protein for 12 and 24 h, respectively. A total of 456 and 255 differentially expressed genes (DEGs; siRNA versus scramble) were identified at the two time points, with defined criteria of $P < 0.05$ and a greater than twofold or less than twofold change (Fig. 3a). We further integrated the DEGs and characterized 175 functional genes (Fig. 3a). KEGG pathway enrichment analysis of these integrated DEGs revealed that chemotaxis signaling, inflammatory responses, and related ERK1/2 cascades were included in the significantly enriched functional pathway (Fig. 3b). Such pathways account for 48 of all 175 DEGs.

To shed light on the mechanism of molecular changes following blockade of CD74, the Ingenuity Pathway Analysis (IPA) was performed for the DEGs integrated at 12 and 24 h. The weight value of each gene in the network was calculated, representing the effect of MIF on the downstream targets. A reconstructed gene network showed that CCL5 and CCL12 with the highest weight value were highlighted as the important chemokines regulated by MIF/CD74 axis (Fig. 3c). As CCL12 has only been described in mice, we thus focus our attention on regulation of CCL5 [30].

All the genes displayed dynamic alteration following CD74 siRNA knockdown, as shown by the heatmap and cluster dendrogram (Fig. 4).

MIF inhibitor attenuated CCL5 expression of astrocytes in vitro

To substantiate inference drawn from transcriptome analysis, the primary astrocytes were stimulated with recombinant MIF protein at a concentration of 0–2.5 μg/ml for 24 h, with or without addition of 100 μM 4-IPP. ELISA results showed that MIF was able to facilitate CCL5 production of astrocytes in a concentration-dependent manner. Treatment of astrocytes with 0.5 μg/ml MIF led to remarkable synthesis and secretion of CCL5, while addition of 100 μM 4-IPP to the culture significantly reduced CCL5 protein levels in both supernatant and lysate (Fig. 5a, b). It

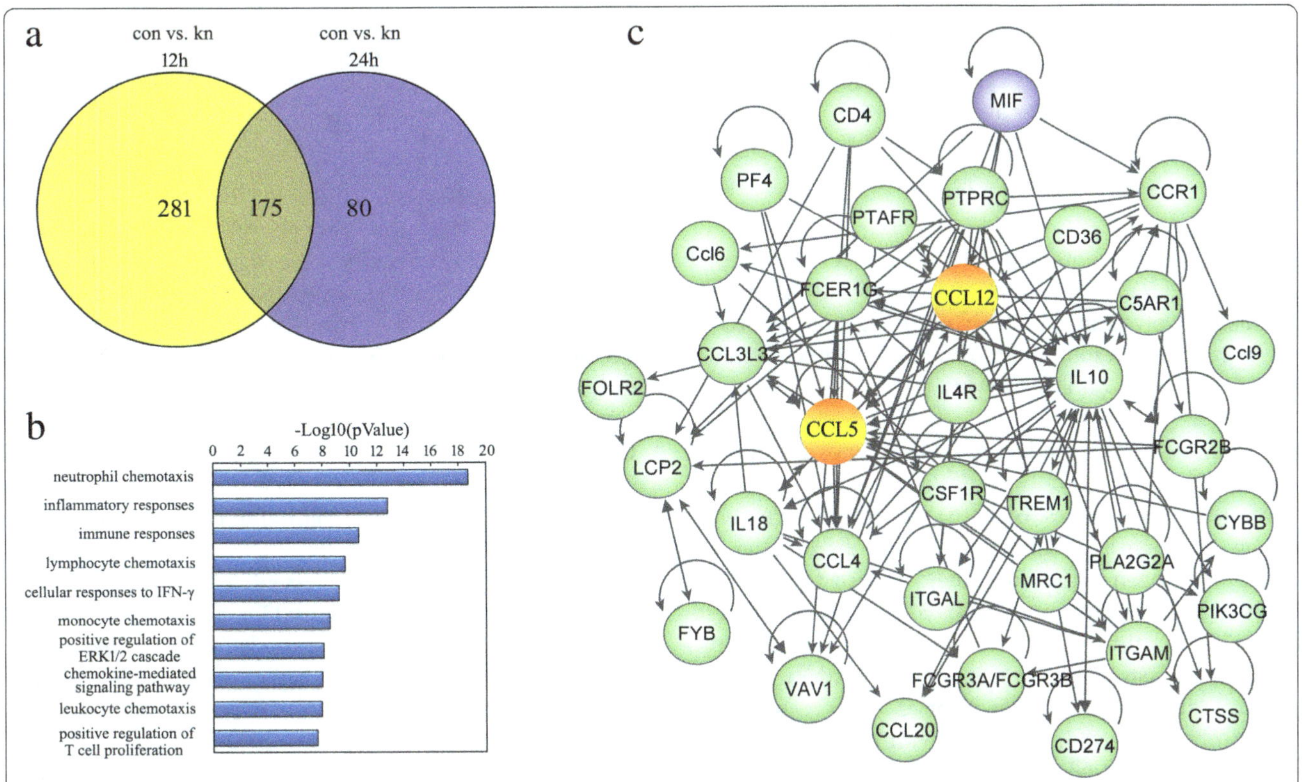

Fig. 3 Functional annotations of DEGs and the inferred gene network in the astrocytes. **a** Integration of DEGs following knockdown of CD74 receptor for 48 h and then treated with 2 μg/ml recombinant rat MIF at 12 h and 24 h, respectively. **b** Most significantly enriched groups for the integrated DEGs relating to pathways. **c** A reconstructed gene network was created using the Ingenuity Pathway Analysis (IPA) Software on the basis of integrated DEGs

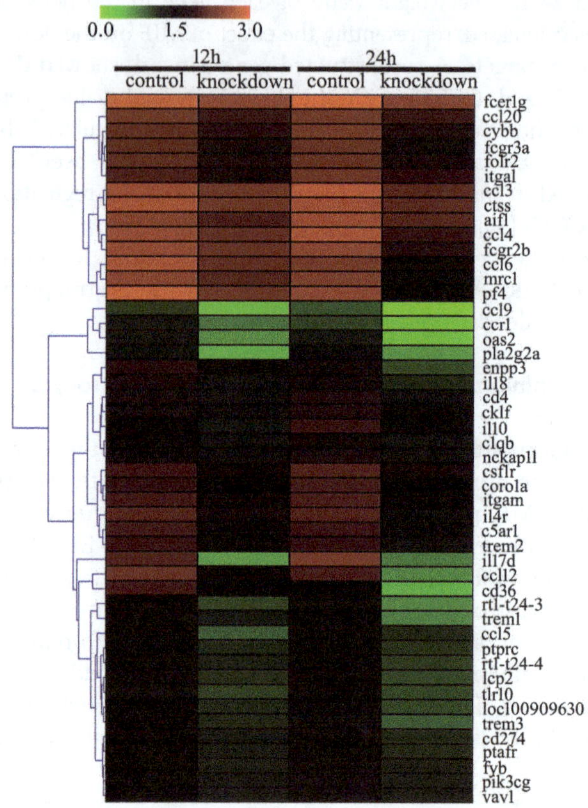

Fig. 4 Heatmap and cluster dendrogram of integrated DEGs following knockdown of CD74 receptor for 48 h and stimulated astrocytes with 2 μg/ml recombinant rat MIF for 12 h and 24 h, respectively. The color scale shown at the top illustrates the relative expression level of the indicated mRNA across all samples: red denotes expression > 0 and green denotes expression < 0

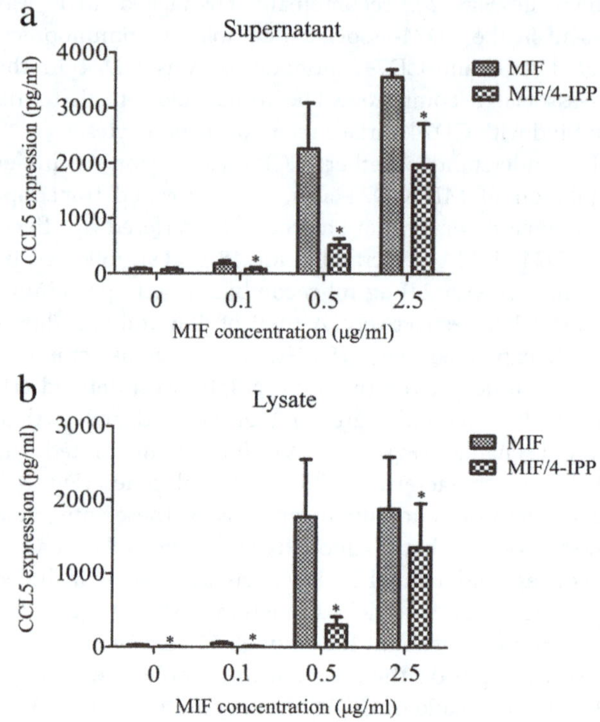

Fig. 5 Examination of CCL5 production in astrocytes following stimuli with gradient recombinant MIF in the presence of 4-IPP. Cell supernatants (**a**) and lysates (**b**) were tested by ELISA for the chemokine CCL5, following astrocyte treatment with 0–2.5 μg/ml recombinant MIF for 24 h in the presence of 100 μM 4-IPP. Experiments were performed in triplicates. Error bars represent the standard deviation ($P < 0.05$)

was interesting to note that 4-IPP even decreased protein levels of CCL5 in lysate in the absence of MIF stimulation, probably involved in inhibition of endogenous CCL5 expression. These results indicate that MIF directly induces the CCL5 expression in astrocytes.

MIF promoted CCL5 production of astrocytes through JNK signaling

Several virus, cytokines, or natural chemicals are able to induce CCL5 production in immune cells or glial cells through mitogen-activated protein kinase (MAPK) and NFκB signaling pathways [21, 31, 32]. To clarify the relevant pathway through which MIF facilitates CCL5 production of astrocytes, we interfered with the signal pathway through knockdown of CD74 receptor. The siRNA oligonucleotide (siRNA2) with nearly 60% knockdown efficiency of CD74 was chosen for the next experiments (Fig. 6a). CD74 receptor of astrocyte was knocked down by siRNA2 for 48 h, followed by the cell treatment with 0.5 μg/ml recombinant MIF protein for 15 min, 30 min, and 60 min, respectively. Determination of ERK, P38, and c-Jun N-terminal kinase (JNK) phosphorylation demonstrated that the phosphorylated level of these kinases and NFkB activity were significantly reduced in astrocytes (Fig. 6b, c). However, CCL5 production in the cells stimulated with recombinant MIF for 24 h was exclusively attenuated by treatment of JNK (SP600125), rather than by ERK (PD98059) or P38 (SB203580) inhibitor (Fig. 6d). These data indicate that MIF induces CCL5 production of astrocytes through JNK signaling.

CCL5 primarily potentiated migration of IL-13-treated macrophages

Chemokines are known to be essential for macrophage migration towards the site of injury [33]. To elucidate chemotactic function of astrocyte-released CCL5, we performed transwell assay to observe migration of macrophage RAW 264.7 cells in the presence of astrocytes with or without siRNA knockdown of CCL5 expression (Fig. 7a). Of three siRNA oligonucleotides, siRNA1 with a 72% CCL5 knockdown efficiency was selected (Fig. 7b). Astrocytes were stimulated with 0.5 μg/ml recombinant MIF following CCL5 siRNA1 interference for 24 h prior to macrophage migration for 48 h. Addition of recombinant MIF promoted

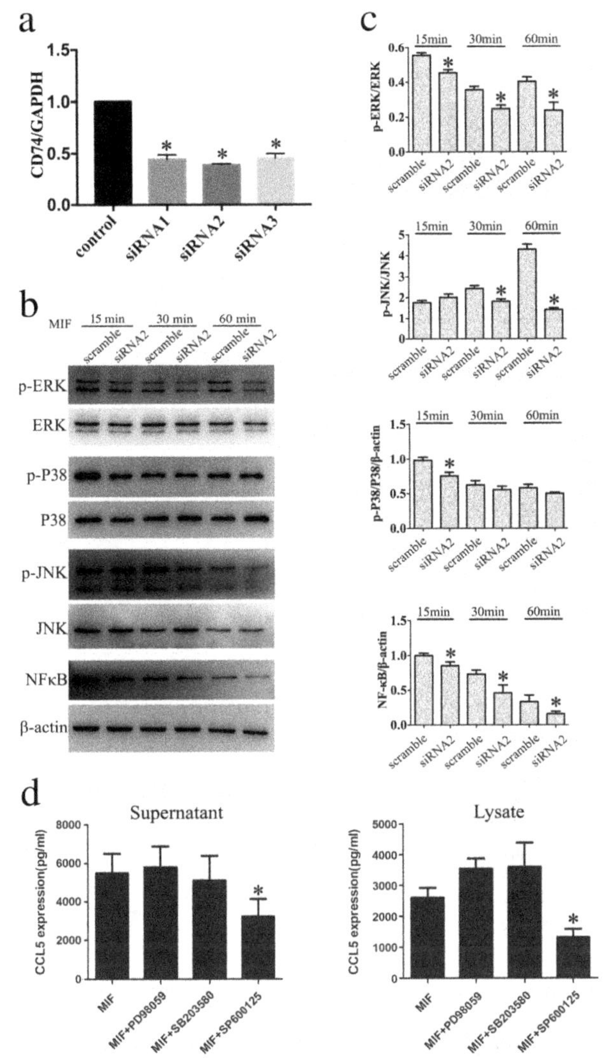

Fig. 6 Determination of intracellular signaling associated with regulation of CCL5 expression. **a** Interference efficiency of three siRNA oligonucleotides for CD74 was measured by RT-PCR, and siRNA2 was used for the knockdown experiments. **b** Western blot analysis of pERK, p-P38, pJNK, and p65NFκB following astrocytes treated with siRNA oligonucleotides or scramble for 48 h and then with 2 μg/ml recombinant MIF for 15 min, 30 min, and 60 min, respectively. **c** Quantification data as shown in **a**. **d** Cell supernatants and lysates were tested by ELISA for the production of CCL5 following astrocyte treatment with inhibitor of ERK (PD98059), P38 (SB203580), or JNK (SP600125). Experiments were performed in triplicates. Error bars represent the standard deviation ($P < 0.05$)

a moderate migration of the unmodified macrophages, and such effect could be slightly attenuated by CCL5 siRNA1 interference, suggesting other factors in action (Fig. 7c, d). However, when the macrophages were incubated in 20 ng/ml recombinant rat IL-13 protein for 2 days, a transition from M1- to M2-phenotype identified by iNOS and Arginase1 expression [34], MIF was found to significantly facilitate the migration of these IL-13-modified cells (Fig. 7c–e). CCL5 knockdown of astrocytes remarkably reduced migratory cell numbers (Fig. 7c, d). The data indicate that CCL5 produced by astrocytes is primarily involved in promoting migration of M2 macrophages.

To observe the effects of MIF-induced CCL5 on migration of microglia in vivo, we detected the temporal distribution of microglia following spinal cord injury. Immunostaining with IBA-1 antibody displayed that SCI resulted in significant accumulation of microglia in the injured cord, with a peak at 4 days (Fig. 8a, c). Injection of 8 μl of 100 μg/ml recombinant MIF or 4 μl of 100 μg/ml recombinant CCL5 protein at the lesion site aggravated the amounts of IBA-1-positive cells. However, treatment with 8 μl of 100 mM 4-IPP resulted in a significant reduction of microglia migration (Fig. 8a–e).

To assess the influences of MIF or CCL5 on the functional recovery, BBB scores were measured during 3 weeks after the spinal cord injury. Injection of 8 μl of 100 μg/ml recombinant MIF or 4 μl of 100 μg/ml recombinant CCL5 significantly aggravated the hindlimb motor function compared with the vehicle. However, treatment of 4-IPP demonstrated a significant improvement (Fig. 8f). The results indicate that MIF-induced CCL5 release from astrocytes is sufficient to potentiate migration of microglia in the injured spinal cord, which is involved in the neuropathogenesis.

Discussion

Emerging evidence has shown that MIF plays a role as a neuroimmuno-modulator in the CNS. Multiple cell types in CNS express this protein, such as microglia, fibroblasts, pituitary cells, endothelial cells, neurons, and neural stem cell progenitors [35]. Aberrant expression of MIF has shown to result in several pathological diseases of the CNS including Alzheimer's disease, autism spectrum disorders, encephalomyelitis, and tumorigenesis [35–38]. In the acute phase of spinal cord injury, MIF contributes to neuropathological impairments through promoting neuronal death and inflammatory activation [14, 16]. It has been thought that microglia and other leukocytes are main resources of inflammatory cytokines in response to MIF stimuli [13, 39]. However, inflammatory signal pathway in astrocytes can also be activated by MIF through phosphorylation of ERK [18]. Here, we revealed a novel role of MIF in facilitating CCL5 production of astrocytes through activation of JNK, suggesting that MIF-induced releases of cytokines and chemokines are associated with multiple intracellular signals. Previous reports have shown that M1 and M2 macrophages populate the injury site with relatively equal distribution within the first week after SCI [40, 41]. MIF-induced CCL5 release from astrocytes is primarily implicated in the cell events of M2 macrophages.

MIF regulates distinct intracellular signaling in a cell type-dependent way. This factor has been shown to interact

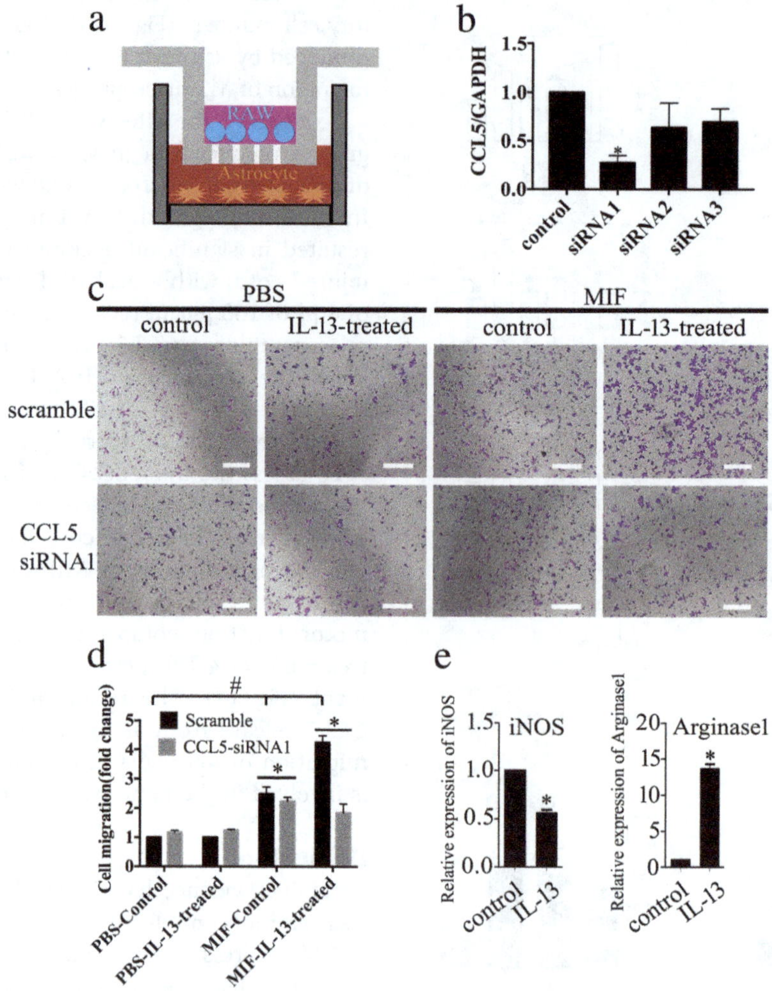

Fig. 7 Effects of CCL5 on macrophage migration in vitro. **a** Transwell assay using cell co-culture model. **b** Interference efficiency of three siRNA oligonucleotides for CCL5 was measured by RT-PCR, and siRNA1 was used for the knockdown experiments. **c** Migration assay of macrophages co-cultured with astrocytes with or without knockdown of CCL5. Astrocytes were stimulated with 0.5 μg/ml recombinant MIF following CCL5 siRNA interference for 24 h prior to macrophage migration for 48 h. For a transition of macrophages from M1- to M2-phenotype, the cells were incubated in 20 ng/ml recombinant rat IL-13 protein for 2 days. **d** Quantification data as shown in **c**. **e** The expression of M1 and M2 macrophage markers, *iNOS* and *Arginase1*, was determined by RT-PCR. Quantities were normalized to endogenous β-actin. Error bars represent the standard deviation. $^{*}P < 0.05$, $^{\#}P < 0.05$. Scale bars, 100 μm

with CD74 receptor on macrophages, astrocytes, fibroblasts, tumor cells, or B lymphocytes, resulting in sustained activation of ERK1/2 kinase that brings in various effects [13, 18, 42]. Activation of MIF on JNK signaling has been identified in fibroblasts and T cell lines, in which phosphorylation of JNK is regulated by kinases PI3K and SRC [43]. In the CD11b^{+}Gr-1^{+} myeloid cells, MIF is capable of potentiating chemotaxis, differentiation, and pro-angiogenesis through activation of p38/MAPK and PI3K/AKT signal pathways [44]. In the present study, we demonstrated that MIF/CD74 axis was able to regulate activities of ERK, P38, and JNK in astrocytes, suggesting a multifunctionality of MIF on astrocytes.

CCL5 induces the migration and recruitment of a wide variety of cells including T cells, dendritic cells, NK cells, eosinophils, basophils, mast cells, and endothelial progenitor cells [9, 45]. Interestingly, its effects on chemotaxis of macrophages are found to have tissue specificity. For examples, CCL5 is involved in recruitment and survival of macrophages in human adipose tissue [46] and in accumulation of macrophage in the kidney, liver, and peripheral nervous tissues [47–49]. In the CNS, however, the role of CCL5 in recruitment of inflammatory cells is controversial. In the hippocampi of mice, CCL5 has been shown to be not critical for accumulation of microglia [2]. We revealed that CCL5 primarily facilitates migration of IL-13-incubated macrophages, in consistency with that of IL-4-treated M2 macrophages [10]. The discrepancy may be attributed to the distinct phenotypes of microglia, either a greater recruitment of monocyte-derived macrophages in

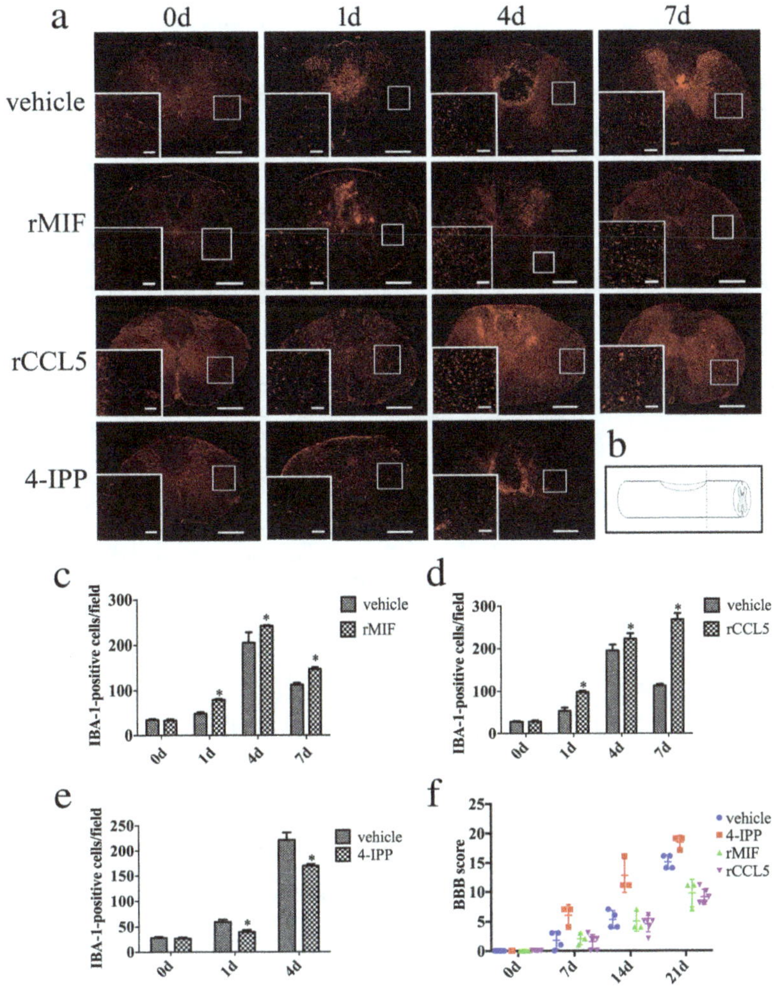

Fig. 8 Immunostaining of microglia after rat spinal cord injury. **a** Immunostaining of IBA-1-positive cells following spinal cord contusion at 0d, 1d, 4d, and 7d, following injection of 8 μl of 100 μg/ml recombinant MIF, 4 μl of 100 μg/ml recombinant CCL5, or 8 μl of 100 mM 4-IPP, respectively. The rectangle indicates region magnified. **b** Illustration of section sites for immunostaining in the contused cord. **c–e** Statistic analysis of IBA-1-positive cells in **a** from 15 fields each. **f** BBB scores for hindlimb motor function in each group at different time points. Six rats/group were evaluated at 0d after injury, and four rats in the vehicle-treated group and three rats in the 4-IPP- or rMIF-treated group were evaluated from 7 days onwards due to sacrifice for immunostainings following significant difference ($n = 3–6$). Error bars represent the standard deviation ($P < 0.05$). Scale bars, 500 μm in section, and 100 μm in magnification

SCI or the alternative activation status stimulated by specific milieu [10, 50]. These results indicate that CCL5 alternatively facilitates accumulation of macrophages, depending on the cell subtype.

CCL5 is inducibly produced by invading pathogens or proinflammatory cytokines through activation of intracellular signals in a cell-specific manner [9, 31]. HIV-1 induces CCL5 primarily by transcriptional activation, while bacterial lipopolysaccharide (LPS) induces CCL5 in microglia via activation of TLR4 receptor [51]. Cytokine IL-1 is able to induce expression of CCL5 in astrocytes through phosphorylation of P38 or JNK, but not of ERK [31]. In the present study, we displayed that MIF induced CCL5 production in astrocytes through activation of JNK signaling. These results indicate that the regulatory mechanism of CCL5 expression is differential in different cell types.

Conclusions

Protein levels of MIF were increased in response to SCI, which interacted with CD74 receptor of astrocytes to promote CCL5 production through activation of JNK. CCL5 in turn facilitated migration of macrophages to the lesion site, which affected repair of injured spinal cord.

Abbreviations

ANOVA: Analysis of variance; MIF: Macrophage migration inhibitory factor; CCL5: Chemokine (C-C motif) ligand 5; PBS: Phosphate-buffered saline; MS: Multiple sclerosis; SCI: Spinal cord injury; GFAP: Glial fibrillary acid protein; ELISA: Enzyme-linked immunosorbent assay; KEGG: Kyoto Encyclopedia of

Genes and Genomes; IPA: Ingenuity Pathway Analysis; DEGs: Differentially expressed genes

Funding
This study was supported by the the National Key Research and Development Program of China (2018YFC1105603), and the National Natural Science Foundation of China (No. 31471011; 31640042; 31871211).

Authors' contributions
YjunW and AG designed this work. YjunW wrote the paper. YZ, YjunW, and WG performed the experiments. YZ, YjunW, WG, AG, ZZ, YH, YjieW, XZ, WW, ND, KY, ZG, and TS analyzed the data. AG joined discussions. All authors have approved the final version of the manuscript and have agreed to be accountable for all aspects of the work regarding questions related to the accuracy or integrity of any part of the work.

Consent for publication
Not applicable.

Competing interests
The authors declare that they have no competing interests.

Author details
[1]Department of Rehabilitation Medicine, Affiliated Hospital of Nantong University, Nantong 226001, People's Republic of China. [2]Key Laboratory of Neuroregeneration of Jiangsu and Ministry of Education, Co-innovation Center of Neuroregeneration, Nantong University, Nantong 226001, People's Republic of China. [3]School of Basic Medical Sciences, Nanjing Medical University, Nanjing, People's Republic of China. [4]Medical College, Nantong University, Nantong 226001, People's Republic of China.

References
1. Gadani SP, Walsh JT, Lukens JR, Kipnis J. Dealing with danger in the CNS: the response of the immune system to injury. Neuron. 2015;87:47–62.
2. Babcock AA, Kuziel WA, Rivest S, Owens T. Chemokine expression by glial cells directs leukocytes to sites of axonal injury in the CNS. J Neurosci. 2003; 23:7922–30.
3. Hausmann ON. Post-traumatic inflammation following spinal cord injury. Spinal Cord. 2003;41:369–78.
4. Rossi D. Astrocyte physiopathology: at the crossroads of intercellular networking, inflammation and cell death. Prog Neurobiol. 2015;130:86–120.
5. Luo Y, Berman MA, Zhai Q, Fischer FR, Abromson-Leeman SR, Zhang Y, Kuziel WA, Gerard C, Dorf ME. RANTES stimulates inflammatory cascades and receptor modulation in murine astrocytes. Glia. 2002;39:19–30.
6. Meeuwsen S, Persoon-Deen C, Bsibsi M, Ravid R, van Noort JM. Cytokine, chemokine and growth factor gene profiling of cultured human astrocytes after exposure to proinflammatory stimuli. Glia. 2003;43:243–53.
7. Carpentier PA, Begolka WS, Olson JK, Elhofy A, Karpus WJ, Miller SD. Differential activation of astrocytes by innate and adaptive immune stimuli. Glia. 2005;49:360–74.
8. Falsig J, Porzgen P, Lund S, Schrattenholz A, Leist M. The inflammatory transcriptome of reactive murine astrocytes and implications for their innate immune function. J Neurochem. 2006;96:893–907.
9. Marques RE, Guabiraba R, Russo RC, Teixeira MM. Targeting CCL5 in inflammation. Expert Opin Ther Targets. 2013;17:1439–60.
10. Vogel DY, Heijnen PD, Breur M, de Vries HE, Tool AT, Amor S, Dijkstra CD. Macrophages migrate in an activation-dependent manner to chemokines involved in neuroinflammation. J Neuroinflammation. 2014;11:23.
11. Glabinski AR, Tuohy VK, Ransohoff RM. Expression of chemokines RANTES, MIP-1alpha and GRO-alpha correlates with inflammation in acute experimental autoimmune encephalomyelitis. Neuroimmunomodulation. 1998;5:166–71.
12. Oh JW, Schwiebert LM, Benveniste EN. Cytokine regulation of CC and CXC chemokine expression by human astrocytes. J Neuro-Oncol. 1999;5:82–94.
13. Calandra T, Roger T. Macrophage migration inhibitory factor: a regulator of innate immunity. Nat Rev Immunol. 2003;3:791–800.
14. Chalimoniuk M, King-Pospisil K, Metz CN, Toborek M. Macrophage migration inhibitory factor induces cell death and decreases neuronal nitric oxide expression in spinal cord neurons. Neuroscience. 2006;139:1117–28.
15. Ogata A, Nishihira J, Suzuki T, Nagashima K, Tashiro K. Identification of macrophage migration inhibitory factor mRNA expression in neural cells of the rat brain by in situ hybridization. Neurosci Lett. 1998;246:173–7.
16. Koda M, Nishio Y, Hashimoto M, Kamada T, Koshizuka S, Yoshinaga K, Onodera S, Nishihira J, Moriya H, Yamazaki M. Up-regulation of macrophage migration-inhibitory factor expression after compression-induced spinal cord injury in rats. Acta Neuropathol. 2004;108:31–6.
17. Nishio Y, Koda M, Hashimoto M, Kamada T, Koshizuka S, Yoshinaga K, Onodera S, Nishihira J, Okawa A, Yamazaki M. Deletion of macrophage migration inhibitory factor attenuates neuronal death and promotes functional recovery after compression-induced spinal cord injury in mice. Acta Neuropathol. 2009;117:321–8.
18. Su Y, Wang Y, Zhou Y, Zhu Z, Zhang Q, Zhang X, Wang W, Gu X, Guo A, Wang Y. Macrophage migration inhibitory factor activates inflammatory responses of astrocytes through interaction with CD74 receptor. Oncotarget. 2017;8:2719–30.
19. Dong Y, Benveniste EN. Immune function of astrocytes. Glia. 2001;36:180–90.
20. Farina C, Aloisi F, Meinl E. Astrocytes are active players in cerebral innate immunity. Trends Immunol. 2007;28:138–45.
21. Lin MS, Hung KS, Chiu WT, Sun YY, Tsai SH, Lin JW, Lee YH. Curcumin enhances neuronal survival in N-methyl-d-aspartic acid toxicity by inducing RANTES expression in astrocytes via PI-3K and MAPK signaling pathways. Prog Neuro-Psychopharmacol Biol Psychiatry. 2011;35:931–8.
22. Gangwani MR, Noel RJ Jr, Shah A, Rivera-Amill V, Kumar A. Human immunodeficiency virus type 1 viral protein R (Vpr) induces CCL5 expression in astrocytes via PI3K and MAPK signaling pathways. J Neuroinflammation. 2013;10:136.
23. Chehrehasa F, Cobcroft M, Young YW, Mackay-Sim A, Goss B. An acute growth factor treatment that preserves function after spinal cord contusion injury. J Neurotrauma. 2014;31:1807–13.
24. Liu J, Du L. PERK pathway is involved in oxygen-glucose-serum deprivation-induced NF-kB activation via ROS generation in spinal cord astrocytes. Biochem Biophys Res Commun. 2015;467:197–203.
25. Zhao Y, Wang Y, Gong J, Yang L, Niu C, Ni X, Wang Y, Peng S, Gu X, Sun C, Yang Y. Chitosan degradation products facilitate peripheral nerve regeneration by improving macrophage-constructed microenvironments. Biomaterials. 2017;134:64–77.
26. Kramer A, Green J, Pollard J Jr, Tugendreich S. Causal analysis approaches in Ingenuity Pathway Analysis. Bioinformatics. 2014;30:523–30.
27. Basso DM, Beattie MS, Bresnahan JC. A sensitive and reliable locomotor rating scale for open field testing in rats. J Neurotrauma. 1995;12:1–21.
28. Leng L, Metz CN, Fang Y, Xu J, Donnelly S, Baugh J, Delohery T, Chen Y, Mitchell RA, Bucala R. MIF signal transduction initiated by binding to CD74. J Exp Med. 2003;197:1467–76.
29. Bernhagen J, Krohn R, Lue H, Gregory JL, Zernecke A, Koenen RR, Dewor M, Georgiev I, Schober A, Leng L, et al. MIF is a noncognate ligand of CXC chemokine receptors in inflammatory and atherogenic cell recruitment. Nat Med. 2007;13:587–96.
30. DeLeon-Pennell KY, Iyer RP, Ero OK, Cates CA, Flynn ER, Cannon PL, Jung M, Shannon D, Garrett MR, Buchanan W, et al. Periodontal-induced chronic inflammation triggers macrophage secretion of Ccl12 to inhibit fibroblast-mediated cardiac wound healing. JCI Insight. 2017;2:14.
31. Kim MO, Suh HS, Brosnan CF, Lee SC. Regulation of RANTES/CCL5 expression in human astrocytes by interleukin-1 and interferon-beta. J Neurochem. 2004; 90:297–308.
32. Nakamichi K, Saiki M, Sawada M, Takayama-Ito M, Yamamuro Y, Morimoto K, Kurane I. Rabies virus-induced activation of mitogen-activated protein kinase and NF-kappaB signaling pathways regulates expression of CXC and CC chemokine ligands in microglia. J Virol. 2005;79:11801–12.
33. Tanuma N, Sakuma H, Sasaki A, Matsumoto Y. Chemokine expression by astrocytes plays a role in microglia/macrophage activation and subsequent neurodegeneration in secondary progressive multiple sclerosis. Acta Neuropathol. 2006;112:195–204.

34. Murray PJ, Allen JE, Biswas SK, Fisher EA, Gilroy DW, Goerdt S, Gordon S, Hamilton JA, Ivashkiv LB, Lawrence T, et al. Macrophage activation and polarization: nomenclature and experimental guidelines. Immunity. 2014;41:14–20.
35. Leyton-Jaimes MF, Kahn J, Israelson A. Macrophage migration inhibitory factor: a multifaceted cytokine implicated in multiple neurological diseases. Exp Neurol. 2018;301:83–91.
36. Bacher M, Schrader J, Thompson N, Kuschela K, Gemsa D, Waeber G, Schlegel J. Up-regulation of macrophage migration inhibitory factor gene and protein expression in glial tumor cells during hypoxic and hypoglycemic stress indicates a critical role for angiogenesis in glioblastoma multiforme. Am J Pathol. 2003;162:11–7.
37. An JH, Lee SY, Jeon JY, Cho KG, Kim SU, Lee MA. Identification of gliotropic factors that induce human stem cell migration to malignant tumor. J Proteome Res. 2009;8:2873–81.
38. Benedek G, Meza-Romero R, Jordan K, Keenlyside L, Offner H, Vandenbark AA. HLA-DRalpha1-mMOG-35-55 treatment of experimental autoimmune encephalomyelitis reduces CNS inflammation, enhances M2 macrophage frequency, and promotes neuroprotection. J Neuroinflammation. 2015;12:123.
39. Calandra T, Bernhagen J, Mitchell RA, Bucala R. The macrophage is an important and previously unrecognized source of macrophage migration inhibitory factor. J Exp Med. 1994;179:1895–902.
40. David S, Kroner A. Repertoire of microglial and macrophage responses after spinal cord injury. Nat Rev Neurosci. 2011;12:388–99.
41. Thawer SG, Mawhinney L, Chadwick K, de Chickera SN, Weaver LC, Brown A, Dekaban GA. Temporal changes in monocyte and macrophage subsets and microglial macrophages following spinal cord injury in the Lys-Egfp-ki mouse model. J Neuroimmunol. 2013;261:7–20.
42. Shi X, Leng L, Wang T, Wang W, Du X, Li J, McDonald C, Chen Z, Murphy JW, Lolis E, et al. CD44 is the signaling component of the macrophage migration inhibitory factor-CD74 receptor complex. Immunity. 2006;25:595–606.
43. Lue H, Dewor M, Leng L, Bucala R, Bernhagen J. Activation of the JNK signalling pathway by macrophage migration inhibitory factor (MIF) and dependence on CXCR4 and CD74. Cell Signal. 2011;23:135–44.
44. Zhu G, Tang Y, Geng N, Zheng M, Jiang J, Li L, Li K, Lei Z, Chen W, Fan Y, et al. HIF-alpha/MIF and NF-kappaB/IL-6 axes contribute to the recruitment of CD11b+Gr-1+ myeloid cells in hypoxic microenvironment of HNSCC. Neoplasia. 2014;16:168–79.
45. Ishida Y, Kimura A, Kuninaka Y, Inui M, Matsushima K, Mukaida N, Kondo T. Pivotal role of the CCL5/CCR5 interaction for recruitment of endothelial progenitor cells in mouse wound healing. J Clin Invest. 2012;122:711–21.
46. Keophiphath M, Rouault C, Divoux A, Clement K, Lacasa D. CCL5 promotes macrophage recruitment and survival in human adipose tissue. Arterioscler Thromb Vasc Biol. 2010;30:39–45.
47. Keepers TR, Gross LK, Obrig TG. Monocyte chemoattractant protein 1, macrophage inflammatory protein 1 alpha, and RANTES recruit macrophages to the kidney in a mouse model of hemolytic-uremic syndrome. Infect Immun. 2007;75:1229–36.
48. Liou JT, Yuan HB, Mao CC, Lai YS, Day YJ. Absence of C-C motif chemokine ligand 5 in mice leads to decreased local macrophage recruitment and behavioral hypersensitivity in a murine neuropathic pain model. Pain. 2012; 153:1283–91.
49. Lee CM, Peng HH, Yang P, Liou JT, Liao CC, Day YJ. C-C chemokine ligand-5 is critical for facilitating macrophage infiltration in the early phase of liver ischemia/reperfusion injury. Sci Rep. 2017;7:3698.
50. Zhang B, Gensel JC. Is neuroinflammation in the injured spinal cord different than in the brain? Examining intrinsic differences between the brain and spinal cord. Exp Neurol. 2014;258:112–20.
51. Si Q, Kim MO, Zhao ML, Landau NR, Goldstein H, Lee S. Vpr- and Nef-dependent induction of RANTES/CCL5 in microglial cells. Virology. 2002; 301:342–53.

Splenic involvement in umbilical cord matrix-derived mesenchymal stromal cell-mediated effects following traumatic spinal cord injury

Anna Badner[1,2], Justin Hacker[1], James Hong[1,2], Mirriam Mikhail[1], Reaz Vawda[1] and Michael G. Fehlings[1,2,3*]

Abstract

Background: The spleen plays an important role in erythrocyte turnover, adaptive immunity, antibody production, and the mobilization of monocytes/macrophages (Mφ) following tissue injury. In response to trauma, the spleen initiates production of inflammatory cytokines, which in turn recruit immune cells to the inflamed tissue, exacerbating damage. Our previous work has shown that intravenous mesenchymal stromal cell (MSC) infusion has potent immunomodulatory effects following spinal cord injury (SCI), associated with the transplanted cells homing to and persisting within the spleen. Therefore, this work aimed to characterize the relationship between the splenic inflammatory response and SCI pathophysiology, emphasizing splenic involvement in MSC-mediated effects.

Methods: Using a rodent model of cervical clip-compression SCI, secondary tissue damage and functional recovery were compared between splenectomised rodents and those with a sham procedure. Subsequently, 2.5 million MSCs from the term human umbilical cord matrix cells (HUCMCs) were infused via tail vein at 1-h post-SCI and the effects were assessed in the presence or absence of a spleen.

Results: Splenectomy alone had no effect on lesion volume, hemorrhage, or inflammation. There was also no significant difference between the groups in functional recovery and those in lesion morphometry. Yet, while the infusion of HUCMCs reduced spinal cord hemorrhage and increased systemic levels of IL-10 in the presence of a spleen, these effects were lost with splenectomy. Further, HUCMC infusion was shown to alter the expression levels of splenic cytokines, suggesting that the spleen is an important target and site of MSC effects.

Conclusions: Our results provide a link between MSC function and splenic inflammation, a finding that can help tailor the cells/transplantation approach to enhance therapeutic efficacy.

Keywords: Spleen, Spinal cord injury, Mesenchymal stromal cells

Background

Even with recent strides in patient care, spinal cord injury (SCI) remains a devastating and debilitating condition, where motor and sensory impairments hamper patient quality of life and present a major economic burden. While there is a significant need for better treatment options, few therapies succeed in clinical translation [1]. For this reason, greater understanding of injury pathophysiology, especially in relation to treatment application, will be imperative for progress to occur.

Traumatic SCI, initiated by mechanical insult known as the primary injury, involves a secondary cascade of further damage. Specifically, the disruption of local vasculature results in hemorrhage, tissue ischemia, and permeability of the blood spinal cord barrier, thereby allowing for the infiltration of peripheral immune cells and release of inflammatory cytokines [2]. Through a positive feedback loop, chemoattractants and activated immune cells further contribute to a pro-inflammatory

* Correspondence: Michael.Fehlings@uhn.ca
[1]Division of Genetics and Development, Krembil Research Institute, University Health Network, 60 Leonard Ave, Toronto, Ontario M5T 2S8, Canada
[2]Institute of Medical Science, University of Toronto, 1 King's College Circle, Toronto, Ontario M5S 1A8, Canada
Full list of author information is available at the end of the article

state, which exacerbates cell death and increases tissue damage. Yet, beyond localized spinal cord changes, increasing attention has been placed on the contribution of peripheral immune organs in SCI pathophysiology [3], with considerable focus on the spleen.

Briefly, the spleen plays an important role in erythrocyte turnover, adaptive immunity, antibody production, and, more recently revealed, the mobilization of monocytes/macrophages (Mϕ) following tissue injury [4]. In the context of high-level SCI, several studies have evaluated dysfunctional antibody synthesis following loss of splenic sympathetic preganglionic innervation [5–7] and the production of autoantibodies against spinal cord tissue [8]. Yet, equally important is the acute response to trauma-induced inflammation, where the spleen initiates production of tumor necrotic factor-α (TNFα), mostly by resident Mϕs, and in turn influences the recruitment of immune cells to the inflamed tissue [9]. Relatedly, acute splenic atrophy and changes in the activation of residing Mϕs as well as T cells have been reported in models of acute brain ischemia [10–12], as well as SCI [13]. Further, targeting this peripheral inflammatory response, via splenectomy, has been shown to significantly reduce the number of infiltrating blood-derived Mϕs, thereby improving functional recovery following thoracic SCI [14]. In contrast, despite promising effects, splenectomy studies in brain injury have had mixed results [15, 16].

Notably, the application of mesenchymal stromal cells (MSCs) has further highlighted a link between the spleen and central nervous system injury. Intravenously infused MSCs have been shown to localize in the spleen following stroke [17, 18], traumatic brain injury [19, 20], and SCI [21, 22]. Although this distribution may vary with source and recipient age [23], these studies have reported dramatic changes in splenic gene expression [21], cytokine production [18, 22], and the proportion of CD4+ T cells [20] following MSC infusion. Therefore, expanding on these results, this study aimed to characterize the acute splenic cytokine response to SCI and determine its role in MSC-mediated recovery. Here, we demonstrate that cervical SCI induces a unique splenic inflammatory response, with significantly greater expression of TNFα, as early as 1 h following trauma, which is followed by a pronounced influx of other pro-inflammatory cytokines, including IL-17, IL-13, IL-1 β, and CXCL10. Despite these implications, there was no difference detected in secondary tissue damage or long-term functional recovery when compared between splenectomised rodents and those with a sham procedure. However, while the infusion of term human umbilical cord matrix (HUCMCs) reduced spinal cord hemorrhage and increased systemic levels of interleukin-10 (IL-10) in the presence of a spleen, these effects were lost with splenectomy. Further, the HUCMCs were also shown to alter splenic cytokine expression levels following SCI, suggesting that the spleen is an important target and site of MSC effects (when systemically infused). Taken together, these results highlight splenic involvement in acute pathophysiology and demonstrate that peripheral immune tissue may be a minimally invasive therapeutic target for SCI, with important clinical implications.

Methods

Clip-compression spinal cord injury (SCI)

All animal experiments were approved by the animal care committee at the University Health Network (Toronto, Ontario, Canada) in compliance with the Canadian Council on Animal Care. Adult female (approximately 250 g; 10–11 weeks old) Wistar rats (Charles River Laboratories, Wilmington, MA) were given buprenorphine (0.05 mg/kg) and 5 mL of saline prior to surgery. All rats were anesthetized with isoflurane (delivered in a 1:1 mixture of O_2/N_2O) and received a C7-T1 laminectomy. Next, a 35-g aneurysm clip was applied to the C7 level (1 min), modeling traumatic cervical SCI. Buprenorphine, amoxicillin trihydrate/clavulanate potassium, and subcutaneous saline injections (5 mL) were administered postoperatively. Animals were housed at 26 °C in a 12-h light/dark cycle, and their bladders were manually expressed twice a day.

Cytokine array for splenic response to SCI & MSC infusion

The spleens of naive, laminectomy-only, and SCI animals were collected at 1 h as well as 24 h following surgery. The tissue was snap-frozen on dry ice after transcardial perfusion (with 250 ml of phosphate buffer solution; PBS) and stored for later use. When all samples were collected, the spleens were homogenized using radioimmunoprecipitation assay (RIPA) buffer (20-188, EMD Millipore) with proteinase inhibitors (Thermo Fisher Scientific), according to the manufacturer's instructions. Total protein levels were determined using a BCA Protein Assay Kit (Thermo Fisher Scientific). The homogenate was diluted, and 100 μg of protein assessed with the cytokine R&D ELISA Proteome Profiler array (ARY008, R&D Systems Inc.) as per manufacturer's instructions. To increase detection sensitivity, IRDye 800CW Streptavidin (926-32230, LI-COR) was used at a 1:2000 dilution (30 min, room temperature) as replacement for the kit's streptavidin-horseradish peroxidase. The array membranes were scanned on an Odyssey Imager CLx (LI-COR), and images quantified as previously described with a semi-automated ImageJ macro [22]. The same approach was applied for the splenic cytokine profile following MSC infusion.

Splenectomy

All Wistar rats received amoxicillin trihydrate/clavulanate potassium in water prior to the procedure. In a clean surgical space and under isoflurane anesthesia, the abdomen was accessed through a midline laparotomy. The spleen was pulled through the incision, and splenic vessels ligated prior to removal. In sham splenectomies, the spleen was returned to the abdominal cavity and the incision was closed via muscle and skin layers. Buprenorphine (0.05 mg/kg) and 5 mL of saline were administered postoperatively.

In vivo very high-resolution ultrasound and Power Doppler imaging

In vivo very high-resolution ultrasound (VHRUS) and Power Doppler imaging was performed as previously described [24]. Briefly, a customized stabilization frame was used to fix the animal position on an imaging platform (Vevo Imaging Station, VisualSonics, Toronto, Ontario). The injury was exposed and ultrasound gel (scanning gel, Medi-Inn, Cameron, Ontario) placed on the dura mater. The VHRUS probe (44 MHz, Vevo 770, VisualSonics, Toronto, Ontario) was used to scan the spinal cord in three-dimensional (3D) B-Mode. The acute lesion and 8-week cavity volume were assessed with the TrakEM2 plugin on ImageJ software [22].

Drabkin's assay for intraparenchymal hemorrhage

As previously described [25], intraparenchymal hemorrhage post-SCI was assessed with Drabkin's assay. In short, a 5-mm segment of the injured spinal cord was collected after transcardial perfusion with 250 mL of PBS. The samples were subsequently homogenized in 100 µl of distilled water and spun down at 13000 rpm for 15 min. The supernatant was collected and 20 µl added to 80 µl of Drabkin's reagent (Drabkin's Reagent powder [D5941] Sigma-Aldrich, in 1000 ml of distilled H_2O and 0.5 ml of 30% Brij 35 Solution) in a clear 96-well plate. The reaction was incubated for 15 min and absorbance read at 560 nm (Wallac 1420 VICTOR2; PerkinElmer).

Long-term neurobehavioral assessment

All neurobehavioral assessments were performed weekly (for 8 weeks) following SCI by two independent observers blinded to the experimental groups ($n = 10$ per group). As previously described, forelimb motor function was measured with a grip strength meter (SDI Grip Strength System, model DFM-10; San Diego Instruments, San Diego, CA) [26], trunk stability was evaluated with the inclined plane test [27], and hind limb locomotion was assessed by using the 22-point (0–21) Basso, Beattie, and Bresnahan (BBB) locomotor rating scale [28]. When animals reached consistent weight bearing ability (week 5–6), the CatWalk multivariate system (Noldus, Version 7.1) was used to determine detailed parameters of paw and limb function during locomotion. No food restriction or reward was used to motivate the animals to walk, and successful performance required three complete crossings with at least three consecutive step cycles for analysis. Prints were labeled by an observer blinded to the experimental groups (at week 6 and 8 post-SCI).

Lesion morphometry

Under isoflurane anesthesia, animals were transcardially perfused with 180 mL of PBS and another 60 mL of chilled 4% paraformaldehyde (PFA). A 1-cm-length spinal cord segment (spanning the lesion epicenter) was isolated, postfixed for 1 day, and then cryoprotected in 30% sucrose before embedding in OCT medium (Thermo Fisher Scientific, Oakwood Village, OH). The spinal cord was cut into 30-µm transverse sections and stained with luxol fast blue (LFB) and hematoxylin-eosin (H&E) as previously described [29]. Lesional tissue, gray matter, and white matter percent area (sampled at every 240 µm over a distance of 2400 µm) were quantified by an observer blinded to the experimental groups using the Cavalieri probe on Stereo Investigator (MBF Bioscience, Williston, VT).

Cell isolation, culture, immunophenotypic antigen profiling, and intravenous delivery

Umbilical cord tissue was obtained postpartum (Chelsea and Westminster Hospital, London, UK), and the veins/arteries removed under aseptic conditions. Subsequently, the Wharton's jelly (also known as umbilical cord matrix) was diced, incubated with collagenases I and II (1 mg/ml, Thermo Fisher Scientific, Oakwood Village, OH) for 2 h (at 37 °C), and centrifuged at 2000 rpm for 10 min. The obtained human umbilical cord matrix cells (HUCMCs) were plated on culture T175 flasks (Greiner Bio-One, Monroe, NC) in minimum essential medium Eagle α modification (α-MEM) with 10% fetal bovine serum (FBS) (Wisent Bioproducts, St. Bruno, Quebec) and 0.1% gentamycin (Sigma-Aldrich, St. Louis, MO). HUCMCs were grown to 80% confluence and used at passages 7–8. Prior to in vivo application, immunophenotypic cell antigen profiling was completed with a mesenchymal cell characterization kit (1:500; SCR067, EMD Millipore, Billerica, MA) in addition to mouse anti-human CD13 (1:500; C8589, Sigma-Aldrich) and 4′,6-diamidino-2-phenylindole (DAPI; 1:1000) as nuclear counterstain. HUCMCs expressed mesenchymal cell markers sCD73, CD146, CD44, CD13, and PDGFR (Fig. 5b). For in vivo experiments, 2.5 million passage-matched (7–8) HUCMCs in 1 ml of Hanks' buffer/2 mM EDTA (HE) were slowly infused (200 µl/minute) via the tail vein at 1 h following SCI.

Interleukin-10 (IL-10) enzyme-linked immunosorbent assay (plasma)

Plasma levels of IL-10 were evaluated at 24 h following SCI and in SCI with HUCMC infusion. Blood samples were collected via cardiac puncture, prior to transcardial perfusion, into EDTA-coated Vacutainer tubes (K2 EDTA Plus Blood Collection Tubes, BD Biosciences, San Jose, CA). The samples were subsequently centrifuged at 3000 rpm (centrifuge 5810R, Eppendorf) for 10 min (4 °C), and the plasma was collected. The plasma samples were applied for the rat interleukin-10 (IL-10) enzyme-linked immunosorbent assay (ELISA) kit (AB100765, Abcam) per the manufacturer's instructions, and the absorbance was read at 450 nm (Wallac 1420 VICTOR2; PerkinElmer, Waltham, MA).

Statistical analysis

Quantitative data are expressed as the mean ± standard error of the mean (SEM). The R&D ELISA Proteome Profiler array results were normalized to laminectomy-only surgeries assessed by multiple t tests with Holm-Sidak correction for multiple comparisons. Other differences between groups were assessed by unpaired t test as well as two-way analysis of variance (ANOVA) with Tukey's post hoc tests (statistically significant at $p \leq 0.05$). All data were analyzed with GraphPad Prism (GraphPad Software Inc., La Jolla, CA, USA, http://www.graphpad.com).

Results

The spleen is a site of a SCI-induced inflammation

Splenic cytokine changes were evaluated with the R&D ELISA Proteome Profiler array (Fig. 1). Within the first hour following SCI, a significant ($p = 0.002$) rise in splenic TNFα levels was detected when compared to laminectomy-only surgery animals ($n = 4$ per group, multiple t tests, Holm-Sidak correction for multiple comparisons). This was followed by a pronounced influx in the expression of IL-17 ($p = 0.04$), IL-13 ($p = 0.02$), IL-1β ($p = 0.03$), CXCL10 ($p = 0.002$), and sICAM ($p = 0.003$) at 24-h post-SCI. Similarly, although the levels of IL-6 and thymus chemokine/CXCL7 were relatively lower than those in time-matched naive animals, expression also increased 24 h following injury. There

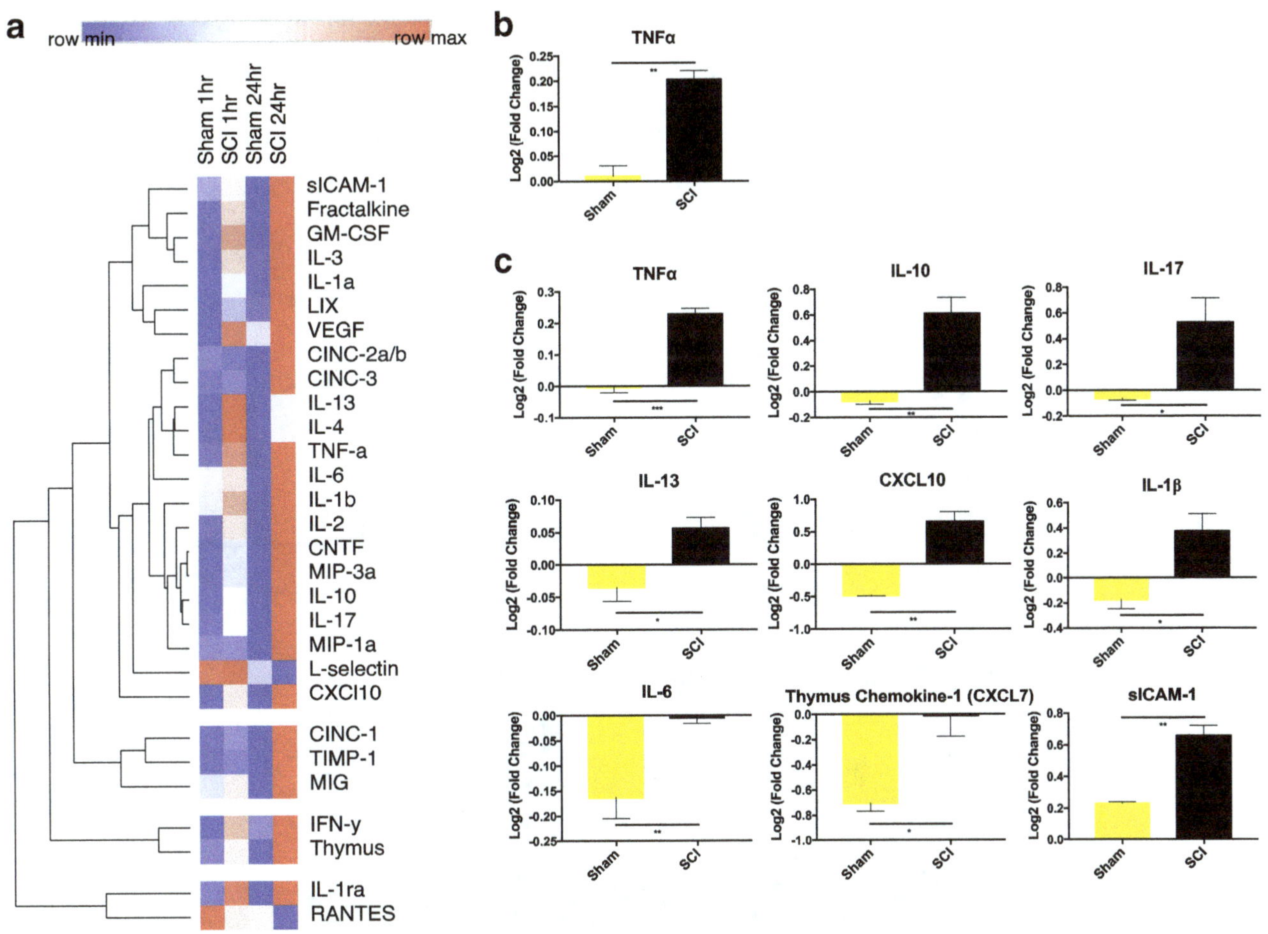

Fig. 1 The spleen is a site of cervical SCI-induced inflammation within hours of trauma. Splenic tissue was collected at 1 and 24 h following cervical SCI and laminectomy-only surgeries. Cytokines were assessed using the rat cytokine R&D ELISA Proteome Profiler array (ARY008), and a representative heat map was generated using the BROAD Institute's R implementation of Morpheus with Euclidean distance hierarchical clustering (**a**). Data are expressed as mean Log2 (fold change) relative to aged-matched naive spleen tissue ($n = 4$ per group). Statistically significant differences in cytokine expression (multiple t tests with Holm-Sidak correction for multiple comparisons) are shown at 1 h (**b**) and 24 h (**c**) following SCI between time-matched laminectomy-only surgery and injured groups

was no significant difference in spleen weight or length (Additional file 1: Figure S1).

Splenectomy does not reduce parenchymal hemorrhage and lesion volume following SCI

In order to understand how the spleen contributes to secondary pathology, parenchymal hemorrhage and lesion volume were compared between splenectomised rodents versus those with a sham procedure (Fig. 2). Although SCI prompted splenic inflammation, there was no significant difference in spinal cord blood volume at 1 ($p = 0.71$), 3 ($p = 0.25$), and 7 ($p = 0.36$) days post-injury (unpaired *t* tests). Similarly, the lesion volume, quantified via in vivo VHRUS imaging, was also unaffected by splenectomy at 1 ($p = 0.34$), 3 ($p = 0.82$), and 7 ($p = 0.07$) days post-SCI.

Splenectomy does not result in long-term functional recovery and tissue preservation following SCI

Long-term functional recovery ($n = 10$ per group) was assessed with a battery of standardized neurobehavioral tests (Fig. 3). Consistent with the acute study, splenectomy did not lead to changes in grip strength ($p = 0.07$, two-way ANOVA), the inclined plane test ($p = 0.92$, two-way ANOVA), or the BBB locomotor score ($p = 0.79$, two-way ANOVA) as well as sub-score ($p = 0.62$, two-way ANOVA). Animal gait parameters were also evaluated with the CatWalk system at 6 and 8 weeks post-SCI (Fig. 3c, d). No significant differences were detected in forelimb/hind limb print area ($p = 0.67$ for forelimbs and $p = 0.85$ for hind limbs, two-way ANOVA), swing speed ($p = 0.56$ for forelimbs and $p = 0.18$ for hind limbs, two-way ANOVA), stride length ($p = 0.28$ for forelimbs and $p = 0.07$ for hind limbs, two-way ANOVA), and stand time ($p = 0.78$ for forelimbs and $p = 0.93$ for hind limbs, two-way ANOVA).

The absence of changes at 8 weeks with splenectomy was further confirmed with histomorphometric analysis ($n = 4$ per group, two-way ANOVA) of LFB- and H&E-stained sections (Fig. 4). There was no effect on lesional tissue ($p = 0.11$), gray ($p = 0.44$), or white ($p = 0.14$) matter sparing. Similarly, cavity volume was unchanged ($p = 0.78$, unpaired

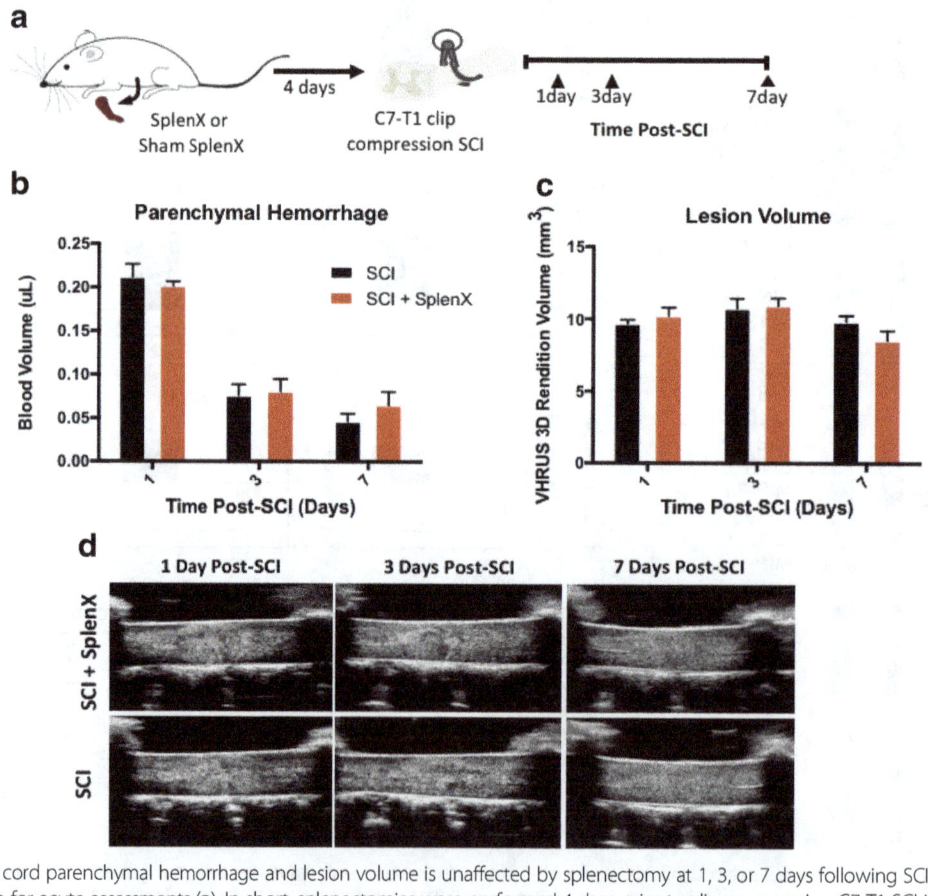

Fig. 2 Acute spinal cord parenchymal hemorrhage and lesion volume is unaffected by splenectomy at 1, 3, or 7 days following SCI. Schematic of experimental design for acute assessments (**a**). In short, splenectomies were performed 4 days prior to clip-compression C7-T1 SCI in Wistar rats. Drabkin's assay was applied to quantify parenchymal hemorrhage at 1 ($n = 5$ per group), 3 ($n = 7$ per group), and 7 ($n = 5$ per group) days post-SCI between the animals with or without a spleen (**b**). Very high-resolution ultrasound (VHRUS) imaging in B mode was also applied to quantify lesion volume (**c**). The representative sagittal view VHRUS images are shown at 1, 3, and 7 days post-SCI (**d**). Data are expressed as mean ± SEM, and unpaired *t* tests were performed at each time point with no significant differences found

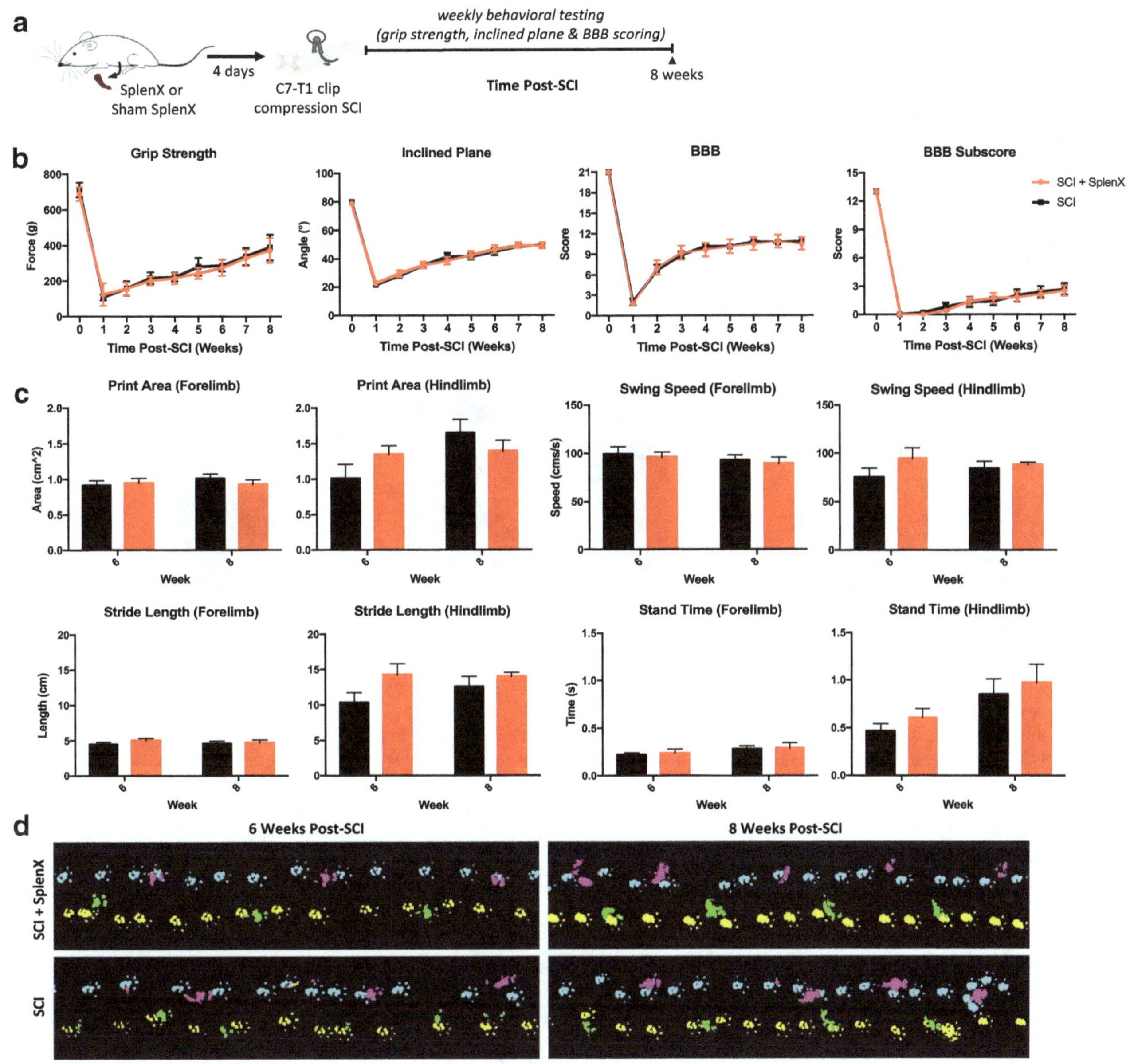

Fig. 3 Long-term functional recovery following SCI was unaffected by splenectomy. Schematic of experimental design for long-term assessment (**a**). Briefly, splenectomies were performed 4 days prior to clip-compression C7-T1 SCI, and the Wistar rats followed for 8-weeks with weekly standard behavioral testing. There was no significant difference ($n = 10$ per group) in grip strength, inclined plane trunk stability, BBB locomotor scale, and BBB sub-score (**b**). Data are expressed as percent mean ± SEM, and two-way ANOVA analysis was performed. There was also no difference in animal gait parameters analyzed by CatWalk at 6 and 8 weeks post-SCI (**c**). Representative gait images are shown (**d**). Data are expressed as percent mean ± SEM, and unpaired *t* tests were performed at each time point with no significant differences found

t test) between splenectomised rodents (1.05 ± 0.13 mm^3) and those with a sham procedure (1.01 ± 0.06 mm^3).

Splenectomy alters the acute effects of early intravenous MSCs infusion following SCI

Prior to in vivo use, HUCMCs (passages 7–8) were validated with positive expression of mesenchymal cell markers (CD73, CD146, CD44, CD13, and PDGFR) at 80–90% confluence (Fig. 5b). Subsequently, as previously described [22], 2.5×10^6 HUCMCs were infused via the tail vein at 1 h following SCI ($n = 4$ per group). The effects of cell infusion on splenic inflammation were evaluated at 1 day following SCI (Fig. 5c), where statistically significant ($p \leq .05$) differences in cytokine expression levels were found for thymus chemokine/CXCL7 and sICAM (multiple *t* tests with Holm-Sidak correction for multiple comparisons). Spinal cord lesion volume and systemic IL-10 expression were also evaluated at 1 day post-SCI and HUCMC infusion (Fig. 6a). Animals

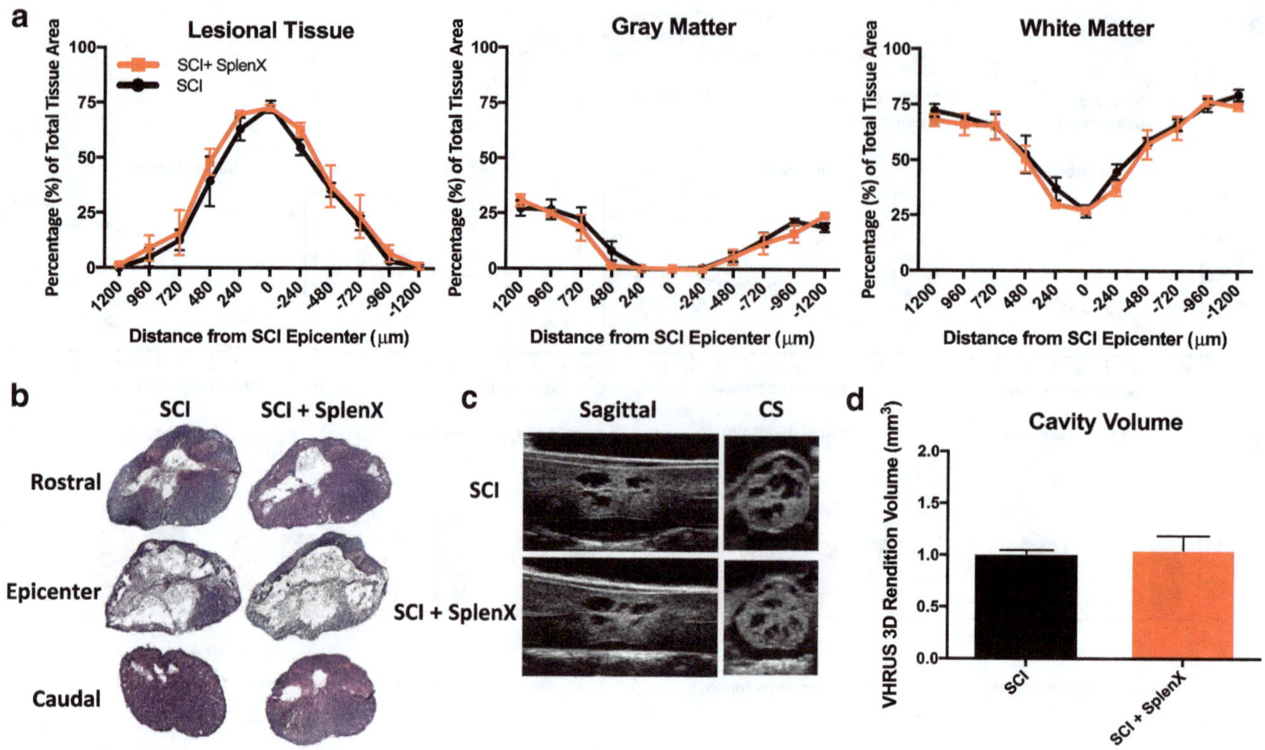

Fig. 4 Tissue preservation and cavitation was unaffected by splenectomy at 8 weeks following SCI. Cross-sectional (30 μm) serial sections ($n = 4$ per group) were stained with Luxol fast blue and H&E and systematically sampled at every 240 μm over a distance of 2400 μm, and unbiased measurements were made with a Cavalieri probe by using Stereo Investigator. Percent area of lesional tissue, gray matter, and white matter are shown (**a**). Data are expressed as percent mean ± SEM. Two-way analysis of variance (ANOVA) with Tukey's multiple comparison was performed, and no significant difference was found between groups. Representative images are shown rostral and caudal to the injury site, as well as at the lesion epicenter (**b**). In vivo very high-resolution ultrasound (VHRUS) imaging ($n = 8$ per group) in B mode was also used to quantify the cavity volume (**c**). Data are expressed as percent mean ± SEM, and unpaired *t* test was performed with no significant difference between groups. Representative sagittal and cross-sectional (CS) VHRUS images are shown (**d**)

that received HUCMCs had a significantly ($p = 0.03$, unpaired *t* test) reduced lesion volume (7.96 ± 0.93 mm^3) compared to that of vehicle controls (11.89 ± 0.60 mm^3). The concentration of plasma ($p = 0.009$, unpaired *t* test) and splenic IL-10 ($p = 0.03$, unpaired *t* test) was also higher in HUCMC-treated animals. Interestingly, when cells were infused to splenectomised animals, some of the effects were lost (Fig. 6b). Specifically, the HUCMC-mediated reduction in VHRUS lesion volume was absent in splenectomized animals ($p = 0.18$, unpaired *t* test), despite a trend ($p = 0.052$, unpaired *t* test) in those with a sham procedure. Similarly, while there was less parenchymal hemorrhage with cells ($p = 0.016$, unpaired *t* test) in shams, this effect was lost in the splenectomy group ($p = 0.93$, unpaired *t* test). The rise in plasma IL-10 levels was missing in both groups ($p = 0.14$ for sham and $p = 0.44$ for splenectomy, unpaired *t* tests).

Discussion

Traumatic SCI drives local as well as systemic inflammation. Although the resulting peripheral pathology is known to contribute to multi-organ dysfunction, post-injury complications, and greater secondary damage to the spinal cord [30], the role of peripheral immune organs is poorly understood. For this reason, the therapeutic potential of lymphoid tissue targets in SCI remains largely unexplored. Here, we characterize the splenic inflammatory cytokine response to injury, demonstrating an early rise in TNFα levels that is followed by a significant influx of pro-inflammatory signaling (with increased expression of IL-17, IL-13, IL-1 β, and CXCL1). Despite previous reports [31], there was no significant difference in spleen weight or length in this injury model (Additional file 1: Figure S1). Relatedly, we further assessed the splenic involvement in secondary damage via splenectomy experiments. There was no significant difference in acute or long-term tissue damage, as well as functional recovery post-SCI, between splenectomised and sham surgery rodents. However, interestingly, when human umbilical cord matrix-derived MSCs (known as HUCMCs) were intravenously infused into splenectomised rodents, the previously reported protective effects [22] were lost. The splenic

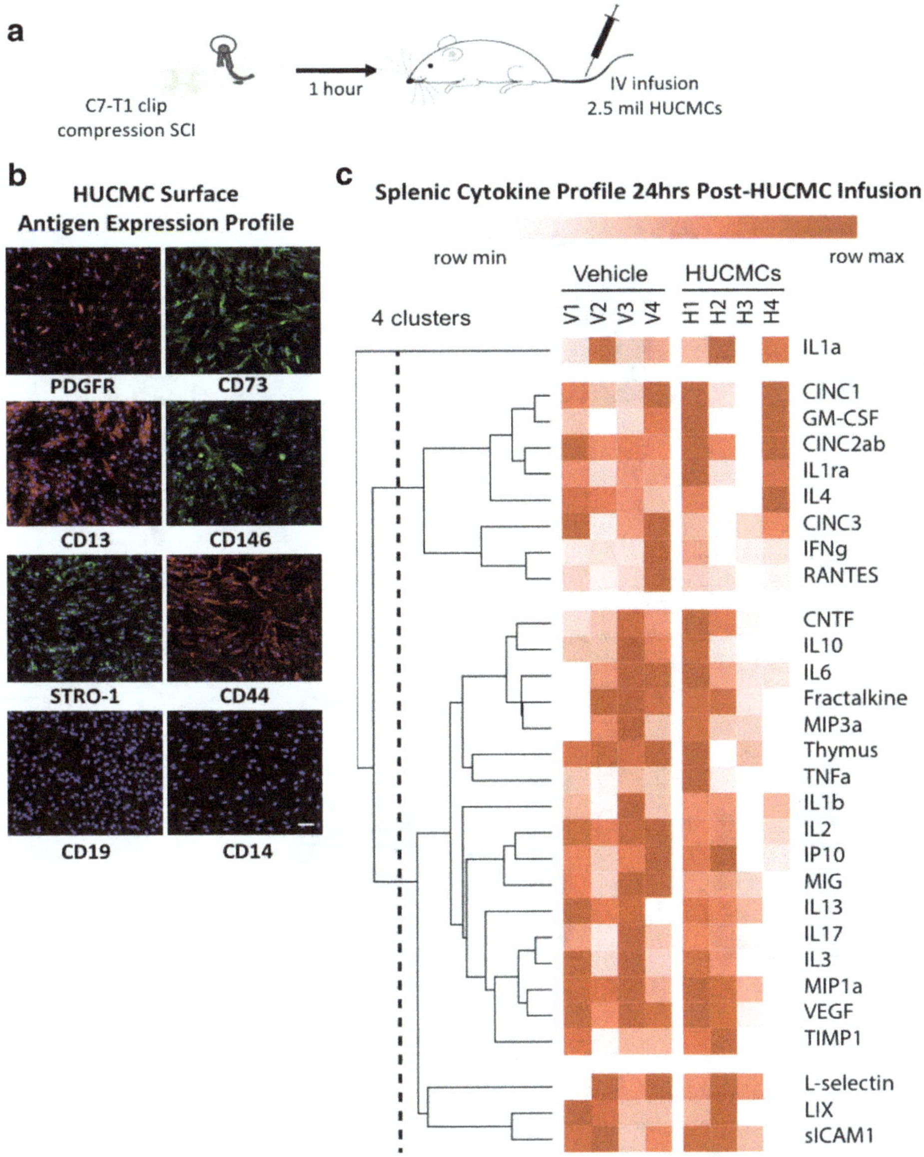

Fig. 5 Early intravenous MSCs infusion alters splenic cytokine expression following SCI. Adult female Wistar rats (~ 250 g) received a C7 35-g clip-compression injury and 2.5×10^6 human umbilical cord matrix cells (HUCMCs) were infused 1 h following SCI (**a**). The surface antigen expression profile of MSC markers was assessed with immunocytochemistry in HUCMCs at passage 7. Representative images were taken at × 20 with the Nikon C2+ microscope (**b**). Scale bar = 10 µm. Splenic cytokines were assessed using the rat cytokine R&D ELISA Proteome Profiler array (ARY008) between vehicle and HUCMC-treated animals. A representative heat map, showing the four replicates (mean gray values), was generated using the BROAD Institute's R implementation of Morpheus and one minus Pearson's correlation hierarchical clustering (**c**). Statistically significant ($p \leq .05$) differences were found for thymus chemokine/CXCL7 and sICAM (multiple *t* tests with Holm-Sidak correction for multiple comparisons)

target of intravenous HUCMC infusion was further validated by demonstrating a significant reduction in inflammatory cytokines, thymus chemokine/CXCL7 and sICAM. Together, this work demonstrates that, while the inflammatory response function of the spleen can be replaced by other immune organs, it may be an important and clinically relevant therapeutic target for acute SCI pathology.

The rapid production of TNFα in the spleen post-trauma is consistent with reports in other models of injury [9], likely triggered by a combination of neural [32] as well as non-neural signaling [33], including angiotensin II. Considering TNFα's role as a mediator of inflammation [34], the subsequent rise in splenic pro-inflammatory molecules, albeit never previously reported, was expected. These results have further implications in the context of cell therapy, where TNFα has been reported to trigger MSC immunomodulatory effects [35–37], specifically through the production of TNFα-stimulated gene-6 (TSG6). It is

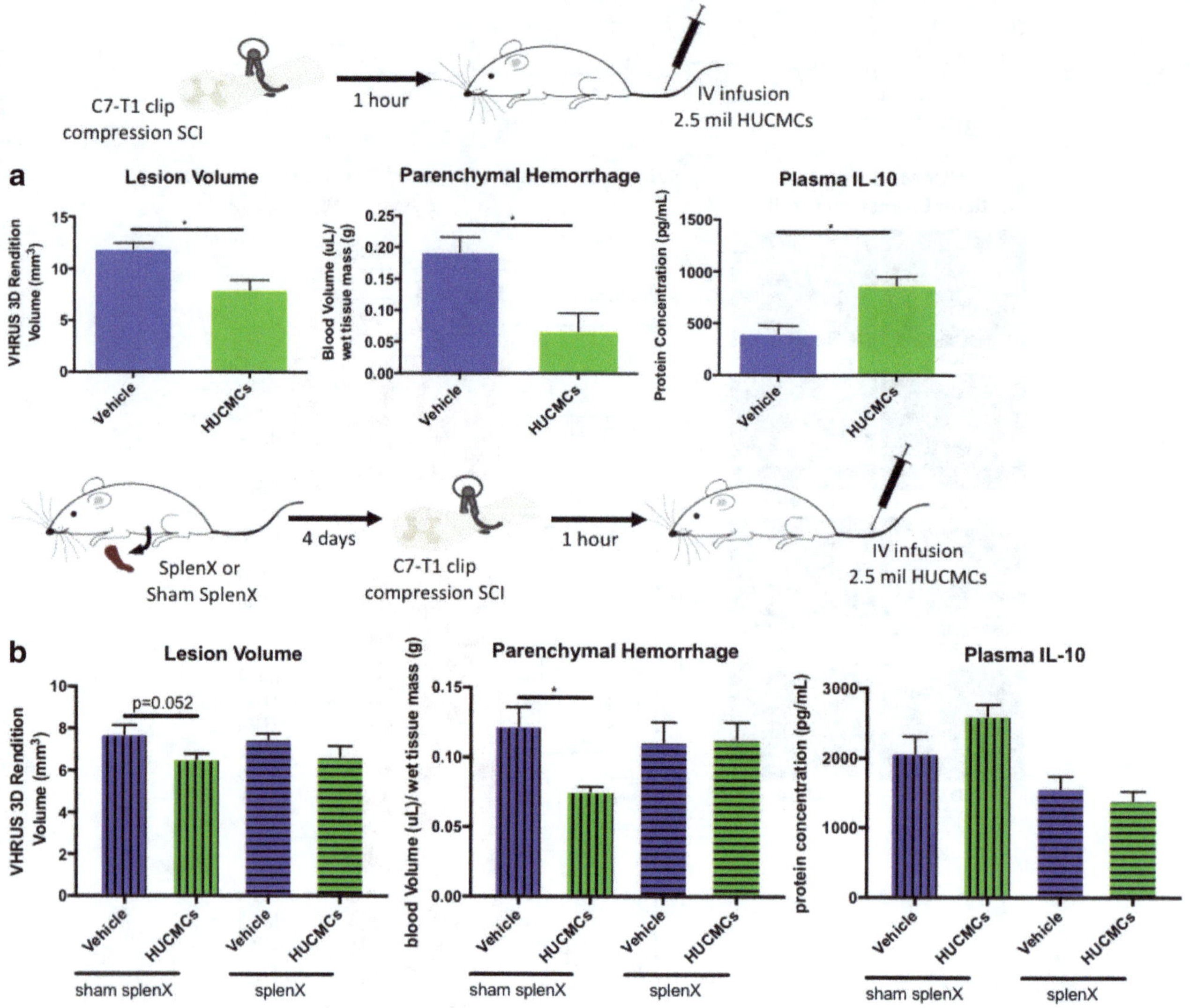

Fig. 6 Splenectomy alters the acute effects of early intravenous MSCs infusion following SCI. When HUCMCs were intravenously infused (via tail vein) at 1 h post-SCI, there was a significant reduction in lesion volume, parenchymal hemorrhage, and plasma IL-10 at 1 day following cell transplant compared to the vehicle control (**a**). Data are expressed as percent mean ± SEM ($n = 4$ per group), unpaired t test, $*p \leq .05$. When the experiment was repeated in the absence of a spleen (splenectomy), some of HUCMC-mediated effects at 1 day post-SCI were lost (**b**). Data are expressed as percent mean ± SEM ($n = 4$–5 per group), and unpaired t test performed (between HUCMCs and vehicle controls), $*p \leq .05$

interesting to note that neonatal MSCs, specifically cells from the human umbilical cord, have been reported to exhibit enhanced and more rapid TSG6 expression with TNFα stimulation [38]. In turn, TSG6 has been shown to drive Mφ polarization to a more anti-inflammatory M2 state [39–41] and these cells are thought to contribute to recovery post-SCI [42, 43]. Other strategies reported to reprogram Mφs towards a more anti-inflammatory phenotype, such as peroxisome proliferator-activated receptor-γ (PPAR-γ) [44], have also shown promise in SCI [45].

It is increasingly recognized that MSCs rarely localize to the site of injury and often mediate effects through short-lived engraftment in peripheral tissue [23]. Aside from the spleen [21], as described in our previous study [22], the lungs have also been widely reported as the tissue source of MSC-mediated effects post-SCI [46] in addition to other disease models [35]. Therefore, in the absence of a spleen, one would expect the lungs to play a central role in immunomodulation with MSCs. Yet, interestingly, reduced secondary pathology (as assessed by lesion volume and parenchymal hemorrhage) as well as the systemic rise in IL-10 following MSC infusion was lost in the splenectomy animals at acute time-points. If, as suggested by the profiling data, splenic TNFα production has an important role in activating transplanted MSCs, the absence may account for the changed outcomes. However, it is important to note that other MSC effects may endure and longer time-points are needed to further understand this relationship. Relatedly, previous work with human multipotent adult stem cells derived from bone marrow, known as multipotent adult progenitor cells (MAPC), demonstrated in stroke that intravenous cell effects on long-term functional recovery were lost with splenectomy [18]. However, there was also evidence of other MAPC targets, as the effects on lesion size were preserved without the spleen.

In contrast to the aforementioned studies, the bone marrow has been traditionally recognized as the primary source of circulating Mφs [47]. While precursors are found in the spleen [48], irradiation and splenectomy studies have demonstrated that the bone marrow alone can replenish circulating populations [47]. Therefore, with bone marrow able to replace some splenic function, the unchanged acute pathology and long-term recovery in splenectomised rodents can be explained by this compensation. Nevertheless, these results differ from the work of Blomster et al., who found that splenectomy improved outcomes in mouse SCI and identified the spleen as a key reservoir of Mφs responsible for exacerbating injury [14]. These differences may stem from species variation [49] as well as timing of splenectomy relative to trauma. Future work should aim to characterize the relationship between systemic, splenic, and bone marrow immune cell population as well as phenotype changes following trauma and MSC infusion.

With considerable blood influx and a large population of immune precursor cells, targeting the spleen for therapeutic purposes has numerous advantages. In one example, systemic delivery of nanoparticles encapsulating short interfering RNA (siRNA) against CCR2 allowed for silencing expression of this chemokine in splenic populations of inflammatory Mφs, thereby attenuating their recruitment and tissue damage in various models of disease [50, 51]. Another study was also able to target the splenic Mφ progenitor recruitment by blocking angiotensin II, leading to improved outcomes in lung adenocarcinoma [52]. Together, these studies highlight the therapeutic potential of peripheral immune organ targets in neurotrauma, with the spleen as an exciting avenue for further exploration.

Herein, this work aimed to characterize a single mechanism of MSC-mediated action in the context of SCI. Although our assessment focused on the spleen, there are likely multiple mechanisms involved in the neuroprotective effects reported. For example, MSCs have been shown to coordinate the production of both matrix metalloproteinases and tissue inhibitors of matrix metalloproteinases (TIMPs) in order to mediate the structure of the vascular basement membrane and thereby vascular integrity [53]. The secretion of TIMPs (such as TIMP-3) by MSCs has been the suggested mechanism of intravenous cell delivery in a model of traumatic brain injury [19]. Other potential mechanisms include modulation of the VE-cadherin/β-catenin signaling pathway [54] and secretion of Wnt3a [55] as well as prostaglandin E2 (PGE2) [56]. Moreover, this study has been largely limited to cytokine profiling, which only provides partial insight into physiological changes. Long-term assessment and further characterization of immune cell populations is warranted.

Conclusions

Overall, our study shows that the spleen, through amplification of inflammatory signaling, is involved in SCI secondary pathophysiology. Further, the spleen plays an important role in MSC-mediated immunomodulation, highlighting that peripheral immune tissues can be a therapeutic target for SCI. This finding can help us tailor cell therapy, as well as all systemic interventions, to maximize efficacy.

Abbreviations

ANOVA: Analysis of variance; BBB: Basso, Beattie, and Bresnahan; ELISA: Enzyme-linked immunosorbent assay; H&E: Hematoxylin-eosin; LFB: Luxol fast blue; MAPC: Multipotent adult progenitor cells; MSCs: Mesenchymal stromal cells; Mφ: Monocytes/macrophages; PPAR-γ: Peroxisome proliferator-activated receptor-γ; RIPA: Radioimmunoprecipitation assay; SCI: Spinal cord injury; SEM: Standard error of the mean; siRNA: Short interfering RNA; TNFα: Tumor necrotic factor-α; VHRUS: Very high-resolution ultrasound

Acknowledgements

The authors would like to acknowledge the Canadian Institutes of Health Research, the Government of Ontario, James F. Crothers Family, the Halbert Foundation, the Krembil Foundation, and the DeZwirek Family Foundation.

Funding

This work was supported by funds from the Canadian Institutes of Health Research Training Program in Regenerative Medicine (A.B.), the Ontario Graduate Scholarship (A.B.), and the James F. Crothers Family Fellowship in Peripheral Nerve Damage (A.B.). M.F. was supported by the Halbert Chair in Neural Repair and Regeneration, Krembil Foundation, and DeZwirek Family Foundation.

Authors' contributions

AB made substantial contributions to the conception and design and acquisition, analysis, and interpretation of the data; was involved in drafting the manuscript and revising it critically for important intellectual content; gave the final approval of the version to be published; and agreed to be accountable for all aspects of the work in ensuring that questions related to the accuracy or integrity of any part of the work are appropriately investigated and resolved. JH made substantial contributions to the acquisition of the data and analysis, gave the final approval of the version to be published, and agreed to be accountable for all aspects of the work in ensuring that questions related to the accuracy or integrity of any part of the work are appropriately investigated and resolved. JH made substantial contributions to the acquisition of the data and analysis, gave the final approval of the version to be published, and agreed to be accountable for all aspects of the work in ensuring that questions related to the accuracy or integrity of any part of the work are appropriately investigated and resolved. MM made substantial contributions to the acquisition of the data and analysis, gave the final approval of the version to be published, and agreed to be accountable for all aspects of the work in ensuring that questions related to the accuracy or integrity of any part of the work are appropriately investigated and resolved. RV made substantial contributions to the acquisition of the data and analysis, gave the final approval of the version to be published, and agreed to be accountable for all aspects of the work in ensuring that questions related to the accuracy or integrity of any part of the work are appropriately investigated and resolved. MGF made substantial contributions to the conception and design, was involved in drafting the manuscript or revising it critically for important intellectual content, gave the final approval of the version to be published, and agreed to be accountable for all aspects of the work in ensuring that questions related to the accuracy or integrity of any part of the work are appropriately investigated and resolved.

Consent for publication
Not applicable.

Competing interests
The authors declare that they have no competing interests.

Author details
[1]Division of Genetics and Development, Krembil Research Institute, University Health Network, 60 Leonard Ave, Toronto, Ontario M5T 2S8, Canada. [2]Institute of Medical Science, University of Toronto, 1 King's College Circle, Toronto, Ontario M5S 1A8, Canada. [3]Division of Neurosurgery, Toronto Western Hospital, 399 Bathurst St. Suite 4WW-449, Toronto, Ontario M5T 2S8, Canada.

References
1. Ulndreaj A, Badner A, Fehlings MG. Promising neuroprotective strategies for traumatic spinal cord injury with a focus on the differential effects among anatomical levels of injury. F1000Res. 2017;6:1907.
2. Tator CH, Fehlings MG. Review of the secondary injury theory of acute spinal cord trauma with emphasis on vascular mechanisms. J Neurosurg. 1991;75:15–26.
3. Anthony DC, Couch Y. The systemic response to CNS injury. Exp Neurol. 2014;258:105–11.
4. Jung W-C, Levesque J-P, Ruitenberg MJ. It takes nerve to fight back: the significance of neural innervation of the bone marrow and spleen for immune function. Semin Cell Dev Biol. 2016.
5. Lucin KM, Sanders VM, Jones TB, Malarkey WB, Popovich PG. Impaired antibody synthesis after spinal cord injury is level dependent and is due to sympathetic nervous system dysregulation. Exp Neurol. 2007;207:75–84.
6. Brommer B, Engel O, Kopp MA, Watzlawick R, Müller S, Prüss H, et al. Spinal cord injury-induced immune deficiency syndrome enhances infection susceptibility dependent on lesion level. Brain J Neurol. 2016;139:692–707.
7. Ueno M, Ueno-Nakamura Y, Niehaus J, Popovich PG, Yoshida Y. Silencing spinal interneurons inhibits immune suppressive autonomic reflexes caused by spinal cord injury. Nat Neurosci. 2016;19:784–7.
8. Ulndreaj A, Tzekou A, Mothe AJ, Siddiqui AM, Dragas R, Tator CH, et al. Characterization of the antibody response after cervical spinal cord injury. J Neurotrauma. 2017;34:1209–26.
9. Swirski FK, Nahrendorf M, Etzrodt M, Wildgruber M, Cortez-Retamozo V, Panizzi P, et al. Identification of splenic reservoir monocytes and their deployment to inflammatory sites. Science. 2009;325:612–6.
10. Ajmo CT, Vernon DOL, Collier L, Hall AA, Garbuzova-Davis S, Willing A, et al. The spleen contributes to stroke-induced neurodegeneration. J Neurosci Res. 2008;86:2227–34.
11. Bao Y, Kim E, Bhosle S, Mehta H, Cho S. A role for spleen monocytes in post-ischemic brain inflammation and injury. J Neuroinflammation. 2010;7:92.
12. Seifert HA, Hall AA, Chapman CB, Collier LA, Willing AE, Pennypacker KR. A transient decrease in spleen size following stroke corresponds to splenocyte release into systemic circulation. J Neuroimmune Pharmacol Off J Soc NeuroImmune Pharmacol. 2012;7:1017–24.
13. Zhang Y, Guan Z, Reader B, Shawler T, Mandrekar-Colucci S, Huang K, et al. Autonomic dysreflexia causes chronic immune suppression after spinal cord injury. J Neurosci. 2013;33:12970–81.
14. Blomster LV, Brennan FH, Lao HW, Harle DW, Harvey AR, Ruitenberg MJ. Mobilisation of the splenic monocyte reservoir and peripheral CX_3 CR1 deficiency adversely affects recovery from spinal cord injury. Exp Neurol. 2013;247:226–40.
15. Kim E, Yang J, Beltran CD, Cho S. Role of spleen-derived monocytes/macrophages in acute ischemic brain injury. J Cereb Blood Flow Metab Off J Int Soc Cereb Blood Flow Metab. 2014;34:1411–9.
16. Zierath D, Shen A, Stults A, Olmstead T, Becker KJ. Splenectomy does not improve long-term outcome after stroke. Stroke. 2017;48:497–500.
17. Acosta SA, Tajiri N, Hoover J, Kaneko Y, Borlongan CV. Intravenous bone marrow stem cell grafts preferentially migrate to spleen and abrogate chronic inflammation in stroke. Stroke. 2015;46:2616–27.
18. Yang B, Hamilton JA, Valenzuela KS, Bogaerts A, Aronowski J, Mays RW, et al. Multipotent adult progenitor cells enhance recovery after stroke by modulating the immune response from the spleen. Stem Cells Dayt Ohio. 2017;35:1290–302.
19. Menge T, Zhao Y, Zhao J, Wataha K, Gerber M, Zhang J, et al. Mesenchymal stem cells regulate blood-brain barrier integrity through TIMP3 release after traumatic brain injury. Sci Transl Med. 2012;4:161ra150.
20. Walker PA, Shah SK, Jimenez F, Gerber MH, Xue H, Cutrone R, et al. Intravenous multipotent adult progenitor cell therapy for traumatic brain injury: preserving the blood brain barrier via an interaction with splenocytes. Exp Neurol. 2010;225:341–52.
21. DePaul MA, Palmer M, Lang BT, Cutrone R, Tran AP, Madalena KM, et al. Intravenous multipotent adult progenitor cell treatment decreases inflammation leading to functional recovery following spinal cord injury. Sci Rep. 2015;5:16795.
22. Badner A, Vawda R, Laliberte A, Hong J, Mikhail M, Jose A, et al. Early intravenous delivery of human brain stromal cells modulates systemic inflammation and leads to vasoprotection in traumatic spinal cord injury. Stem Cells Transl Med. 2016;5:991–1003.
23. Fabian C, Naaldijk Y, Leovsky C, Johnson AA, Rudolph L, Jaeger C, et al. Distribution pattern following systemic mesenchymal stem cell injection depends on the age of the recipient and neuronal health. Stem Cell Res Ther. 2017;8:85.
24. Soubeyrand M, Badner A, Vawda R, Chung YS, Fehlings MG. Very high resolution ultrasound imaging for real-time quantitative visualization of vascular disruption after spinal cord injury. J Neurotrauma. 2014;31:1767–75.
25. Choudhri TF, Hoh BL, Solomon RA, Connolly ES, Pinsky DJ. Use of a spectrophotometric hemoglobin assay to objectively quantify intracerebral hemorrhage in mice. Stroke. 1997;28:2296–302.
26. Forgione N, Karadimas SK, Foltz WD, Satkunendrarajah K, Lip A, Fehlings MG. Bilateral contusion-compression model of incomplete traumatic cervical spinal cord injury. J Neurotrauma. 2014;31:1776–88.
27. Rivlin AS, Tator CH. Objective clinical assessment of motor function after experimental spinal cord injury in the rat. J Neurosurg. 1977;47:577–81.
28. Basso DM, Beattie MS, Bresnahan JC. A sensitive and reliable locomotor rating scale for open field testing in rats. J Neurotrauma. 1995;12:1–21.
29. Nguyen DH, Cho N, Satkunendrarajah K, Austin JW, Wang J, Fehlings MG. Immunoglobulin G (IgG) attenuates neuroinflammation and improves neurobehavioral recovery after cervical spinal cord injury. J Neuroinflammation. 2012;9:224.
30. Sun X, Jones ZB, Chen X-M, Zhou L, So K-F, Ren Y. Multiple organ dysfunction and systemic inflammation after spinal cord injury: a complex relationship. J Neuroinflammation. 2016;13:260.
31. Lankford KL, Arroyo EJ, Nazimek K, Bryniarski K, Askenase PW, Kocsis JD. Intravenously delivered mesenchymal stem cell-derived exosomes target M2-type macrophages in the injured spinal cord. PLoS One. 2018;13:e0190358.
32. Seeley EJ, Barry SS, Narala S, Matthay MA, Wolters PJ. Noradrenergic neurons regulate monocyte trafficking and mortality during gram-negative peritonitis in mice. J Immunol Baltim Md 1950. 2013;190:4717–24.
33. Cortez-Retamozo V, Etzrodt M, Newton A, Rauch PJ, Chudnovskiy A, Berger C, et al. Origins of tumor-associated macrophages and neutrophils. Proc Natl Acad Sci U S A. 2012;109:2491–6.
34. Baud V, Karin M. Signal transduction by tumor necrosis factor and its relatives. Trends Cell Biol. 2001;11:372–7.
35. Lee RH, Pulin AA, Seo MJ, Kota DJ, Ylostalo J, Larson BL, et al. Intravenous hMSCs improve myocardial infarction in mice because cells embolized in lung are activated to secrete the anti-inflammatory protein TSG-6. Cell Stem Cell. 2009;5:54–63.
36. Choi H, Lee RH, Bazhanov N, Oh JY, Prockop DJ. Anti-inflammatory protein TSG-6 secreted by activated MSCs attenuates zymosan-induced mouse

peritonitis by decreasing TLR2/NF-κB signaling in resident macrophages. Blood. 2011;118:330–8.
37. Lee RH, Yu JM, Foskett AM, Peltier G, Reneau JC, Bazhanov N, et al. TSG-6 as a biomarker to predict efficacy of human mesenchymal stem/progenitor cells (hMSCs) in modulating sterile inflammation in vivo. Proc Natl Acad Sci U S A. 2014;111:16766–71.
38. Hamidian Jahromi S, Li Y, Davies JE. Effect of Tumor Necrosis Factor Alpha Dose and Exposure Time on Tumor Necrosis Factor-Induced Gene-6 Activation by Neonatal and Adult Mesenchymal Stromal Cells. Stem Cells Dev. 2018;27(1):44-54. https://doi.org/10.1089/scd.2017.0179.
39. Song W-J, Li Q, Ryu M-O, Ahn J-O, Ha Bhang D, Chan Jung Y, et al. TSG-6 secreted by human adipose tissue-derived mesenchymal stem cells ameliorates DSS-induced colitis by inducing M2 macrophage polarization in mice. Sci Rep. 2017;7:5187.
40. Mittal M, Tiruppathi C, Nepal S, Zhao Y-Y, Grzych D, Soni D, et al. TNFα-stimulated gene-6 (TSG6) activates macrophage phenotype transition to prevent inflammatory lung injury. Proc Natl Acad Sci U S A. 2016;113: E8151–8.
41. Martinez FO, Gordon S. The M1 and M2 paradigm of macrophage activation: time for reassessment. F1000prime Rep. 2014;6:13.
42. Shechter R, London A, Varol C, Raposo C, Cusimano M, Yovel G, et al. Infiltrating blood-derived macrophages are vital cells playing an anti-inflammatory role in recovery from spinal cord injury in mice. PLoS Med. 2009;6:e1000113.
43. Kigerl KA, Gensel JC, Ankeny DP, Alexander JK, Donnelly DJ, Popovich PG. Identification of two distinct macrophage subsets with divergent effects causing either neurotoxicity or regeneration in the injured mouse spinal cord. J Neurosci. 2009;29:13435–44.
44. Ren Y, Young W. Managing inflammation after spinal cord injury through manipulation of macrophage function. Neural Plast. 2013; 2013:945034.
45. McTigue DM, Tripathi R, Wei P, Lash AT. The PPAR gamma agonist Pioglitazone improves anatomical and locomotor recovery after rodent spinal cord injury. Exp Neurol. 2007;205:396–406.
46. White SV, Czisch CE, Han MH, Plant CD, Harvey AR, Plant GW. Intravenous transplantation of mesenchymal progenitors distribute solely to the lungs and improve outcomes in cervical spinal cord injury. Stem Cells Dayt Ohio. 2016;34:1812–25.
47. van Furth R, Cohn ZA. The origin and kinetics of mononuclear phagocytes. J Exp Med. 1968;128:415–35.
48. Geissmann F, Manz MG, Jung S, Sieweke MH, Merad M, Ley K. Development of monocytes, macrophages, and dendritic cells. Science. 2010;327:656–61.
49. Bronte V, Pittet MJ. The spleen in local and systemic regulation of immunity. Immunity. 2013;39:806–18.
50. Leuschner F, Dutta P, Gorbatov R, Novobrantseva TI, Donahoe JS, Courties G, et al. Therapeutic siRNA silencing in inflammatory monocytes in mice. Nat Biotechnol. 2011;29:1005–10.
51. Leavy O. Immunotherapy: stopping monocytes in their tracks. Nat Rev Immunol. 2011;11:715.
52. Cortez-Retamozo V, Etzrodt M, Newton A, Ryan R, Pucci F, Sio SW, et al. Angiotensin II drives the production of tumor-promoting macrophages. Immunity. 2013;38:296–308.
53. Lozito TP, Kuo CK, Taboas JM, Tuan RS. Human mesenchymal stem cells express vascular cell phenotypes upon interaction with endothelial cell matrix. J Cell Biochem. 2009;107:714–22.
54. Menge T, Gerber M, Wataha K, Reid W, Guha S, Cox CS, et al. Human mesenchymal stem cells inhibit endothelial proliferation and angiogenesis via cell-cell contact through modulation of the VE-cadherin/β-catenin signaling pathway. Stem Cells Dev. 2013;22: 148–57.
55. Zhao Y, Gibb SL, Zhao J, Moore AN, Hylin MJ, Menge T, et al. Wnt3a, a protein secreted by mesenchymal stem cells is neuroprotective and promotes neurocognitive recovery following traumatic brain injury. Stem Cells Dayt Ohio. 2016;34:1263–72.
56. Vasandan AB, Jahnavi S, Shashank C, Prasad P, Kumar A, Prasanna SJ. Human mesenchymal stem cells program macrophage plasticity by altering their metabolic status via a PGE2-dependent mechanism. Sci Rep. 2016;6:38308.

9

Environmental enrichment reduces adolescent anxiety- and depression-like behaviors of rats subjected to infant nerve injury

Xingrui Gong[1,2,3], Yongmei Chen[4], Jing Chang[1], Yue Huang[1], Meihau Cai[1] and Mazhong Zhang[1*]

Abstract

Background: Infant nerve injury causes delayed adolescent neuropathic pain, but whether it also leads to psychiatric illness is unknown. Environmental enrichment (EE) increases social communication and activity. Thus, our goal was to test anxiety- and depression-like behaviors after infant peripheral nerve injury and evaluate the effect of environmental enrichment on these models of affective disorders.

Methods: Open field, elevated plus maze, sucrose preference, and pain behaviors (paw withdrawal threshold, spontaneous guarding score, and cold response to acetone) were measured in rats that received infant spared nerve injury (SNI). Enzyme-linked immune absorbent assay of cytokines was performed to evaluate the inflammatory response in the brain. Then, the ability of intracerebroventricular (ICV) injection of a microglia inhibitor, minocycline (MIN), and EE (a free-running wheel, a staircase, a plastic tunnel, a raised platform, and various colored balls) to reverse the infant SNI effects on behaviors and cytokines was examined.

Results: Infant nerve injury resulted in adolescent anxiety- and depression-like behaviors. The medial prefrontal cortex, basolateral amygdala, and ventral hippocampus were skewed to a pro-inflammatory profile. ICV injection of MIN reduced anxiety- and depression-like behaviors without affecting pain behaviors. In addition, ICV MIN skewed the brain towards an anti-inflammatory profile. Finally, environmental enrichment improved anxiety- and depression-like behaviors, as well as pain behaviors. EE increased brain IL-10 and decreased IL-1β and TNF-α.

Conclusions: Infant nerve injury induces adolescent anxiety- and depression-like behaviors and central nervous inflammation. Environmental enrichment reduces these behaviors by normalizing the inflammation balance in the brain.

Keywords: Environmental enrichment, Anxiety, Depression, Inflammation

Background

Anxiety and depression are frequent comorbidities of chronic pain. About 40–60% of patients with chronic pain report anxiety and depression [1], and the prevalence of a lifetime history of psychiatric disorders is higher in chronic pain patients [2]. Both depression and chronic pain are debilitating and have a negative effect on quality of life [3], and both involve neuroinflammation. The causes of psychiatric disorders include monoamine dysfunction, hypothalamic-pituitary-adrenal axis dysfunction, deficiencies in neurogenesis, and neuroimmune activation [4]. Recently, these psychiatric disorders have been increasingly recognized as neuroinflammatory conditions because of the causes as described above and because they respond to anti-inflammatory treatment [5]. Microglia are the primary resident immune cells in the central nervous system. They are sentinels and patrol their surroundings constantly. After an insult, they change their morphology and release inflammatory cytokines [6, 7]. These

* Correspondence: zhangmazhong@scmc.com.cn
[1]Department of Anesthesiology and Pediatric Clinical Pharmacology Laboratory, Shanghai Children's Medical Center, Shanghai Jiao Tong University School of Medicine, 1678 Dongfang Road, 200127 Shanghai, China
Full list of author information is available at the end of the article

inflammatory mediators affect neuron-neuron and neuron-glia communication and lead to affective disorders [5]. This opens up the possibility of treating these affective disorders by targeting microglia-related inflammation.

Neuroinflammation is also critical for the development of chronic pain including neuropathic pain conditions [8]. However, neuropathic pain is absent in infants. Peripheral nerve injury early in life often results in delayed onset of neuropathic pain behaviors starting from adolescence onward. For example, newborns with brachial plexus injury rarely develop chronic pain [9]; phantom pain happens long after congenital limb deficiency or early-life surgical amputation [10]. Population-based studies show that complex regional pain syndrome never occurs before adolescence [11]. Development of neuropathic pain is age-dependent, and chronic pain was rarely prevalent before adolescence [12]. In animal studies [13, 14], rats that received spared nerve injury (SNI) surgery did not develop neuropathic pain until 4 weeks after the injury, which was attributed to suppression of spinal inflammation in the early life. Considering that chronic pain is an important cause of psychiatric disorders [15] and that few clinical studies have focused on affective disorders induced by infant nerve injury, we evaluated anxiety- and depression-like behaviors after infant peripheral nerve injury in rats.

Anxiety and depression can have high morbidity and are often relapsing. Despite considerable effort dedicated to searching for efficacious treatment for these diseases, they are still refractory to treatment. Treating these conditions with psychiatric medications often brings an economic burden to families in addition to some severe side effects to patients. Environmental enrichment (EE) increases social communication and exploration [16], and a voluntary wheel running inhibits anxiety [17] and pain [18]. EE which includes a free-running wheel may be a useful approach to model this effect in preclinical studies. Thus, we tested the effect of EE on behaviors related to psychiatric disorders. Considering previous studies showing that anxiety and depression are inflammatory diseases [5, 6], we also measured the critical inflammatory cytokines IL-10, IL-1β, and TNF-α, after infant spared nerve injury (SNI), and measured changes in these cytokines in the central nervous system after EE treatment to explore potential mechanisms of EE effects.

Methods

The study was approved by the institutional experimental animal use and care committee, Shanghai Children's Medical Center, an affiliate of Shanghai Jiao Tong University School of Medicine, and was conducted under the guidelines of the National Institute of Health. All animals were kept in a controlled environment (25 °C, lights on from 8 AM to 8 PM) with free access to food and water.

Male Sprague-Dawley rat pups aged 1 week with their mothers and prior to weaning were purchased from the Shanghai Experimental Animal Center. The rat pups were numbered by their weight, then every two consecutive rats in weight order were randomly divided into sham or SNI groups by a computer-generated random number "1" or "2," which indicated "sham" or "SNI" group, respectively. Each group was distributed across multiple litters (two to three animals) to allow for possible litter variability. Pups assigned into different groups remained with their single dam mothers until weaning. After weaning, only littermates were housed together in the same cage to avoid unnecessary stress. The surgery was performed as previously described [19]. On postnatal day (P) 10, the rat's skin was prepared under isoflurane anesthesia on the right lateral thigh followed by a small incision to expose the sciatic nerve under a dissecting surgical microscope (Leica M205FA, Germany). The tibia and common peroneal branches were ligated and transected leaving the sural nerve intact. The skin was closed in layers and the rats were returned to their mother cages for recovery in the lab after the surgery, which typically lasted no more than 20–30 min. The cages were returned to the original animal facility on the same day. Rat pups were weaned at P21 and were housed two to three littermates per cage. Behavior tests, drug injections, and ELISA assays were done in a blinded fashion to avoid bias. The study consisted of three experiments as shown in Fig. 1.

In experiment 1, rat pups received sham or SNI surgery at P10, and in adolescence, rats received behavior tests on postoperative days (POD) 20, 40, and 70 ($n = 8$ rats in each group) or were sacrificed on POD 45 for cytokine assays of medial prefrontal cortex (mPFC), basolateral amygdala (BA), and ventral hippocampus (VH) ($n = 6$ rats in each group).

In experiment 2, rat pups received sham or SNI surgery at P10 and then received ICV injection of vehicle or minocycline (MIN) daily from POD 34 to POD 39; behavior tests were performed on POD 20 and POD 40. After the last behavior test on POD 45, all of the rats were decapitated and mPFC, BA, and VH were collected for cytokine assay ($n = 10$ rats per group).

In experiment 3, rat pups received sham or SNI surgery at P10, and EE (or conventional standard housing as a control) was employed starting from POD 11 to the end of the experiment. In four groups of animals, behavior tests were done on POD 20, 40, and 70 ($n = 9$ rats in each group). In another four groups of animals, rats were sacrificed for cytokine assays on POD 45 ($n = 6$ rats in each group). The EE consisted of a free-running wheel and any two of the following toys: a staircase, a plastic

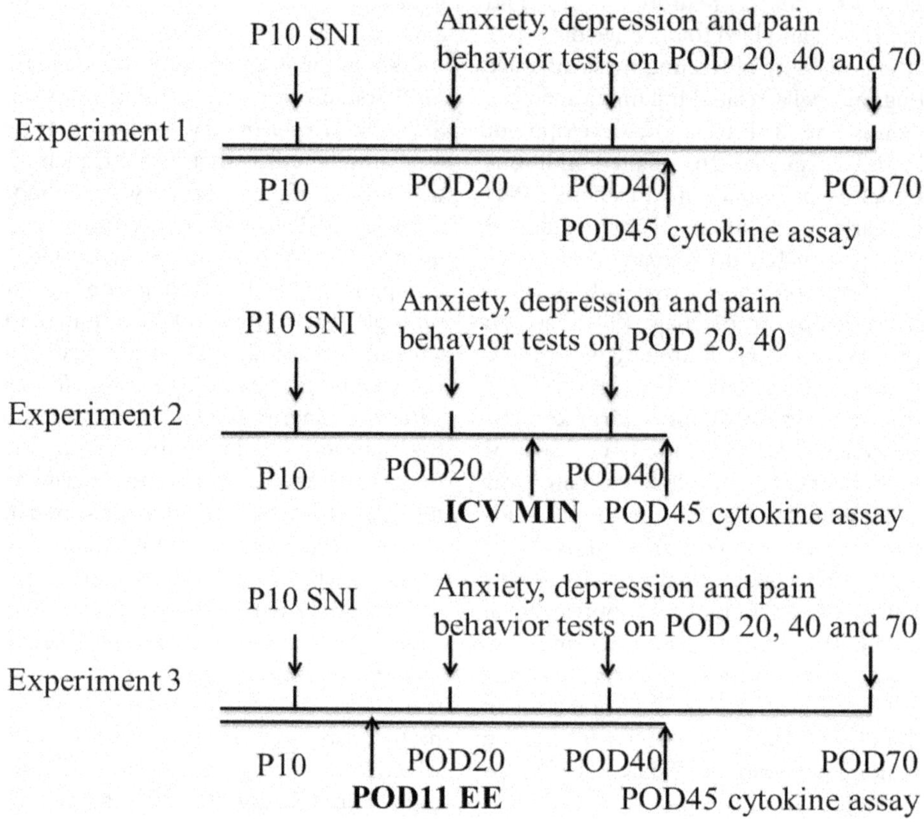

Fig. 1 Experimental procedures and timeline. SNI surgery was performed by ligation and transection of the tibia and common peroneal branches, leaving the sural nerve intact. Experiment 1: Behavior tests and ELISA to measure the anxiety- and depression-like behaviors and inflammatory profile. Experiment 2: ICV MIN to evaluate the effect of a microglia inhibitor on the anxiety- and depression-like behaviors and inflammatory profile. Experiment 3: Test the effects of EE on anxiety- and depression-like behaviors and inflammatory profile of rats subjected to infant SNI. SNI spared nerve injury, ELISA enzyme-linked immune-absorbent assay, ICV intracerebroventricular, MIN minocycline, EE environmental enrichment, P postnatal days, POD postoperative days

tunnel, a raised platform, and various colored balls. The two toys were changed every 3 to 5 days. The rats in the control groups were not exposed to the running wheel and toys.

Pain behavior tests

Spontaneous guarding scores were measured as in a previous study [20]. Briefly, scores were 0 (paw flat on the floor with equal weight on both paws), 1 (mild shift of weight away from ipsilateral paw), 2 (unequal weight bearing and part of the paw lifted), or 3 (foot totally raised and not bearing any weight). Paw withdrawal threshold to mechanical stimulation was measured on POD 11,20, 40, and 70 in accordance with a previous study [18]. In the morning, the rats were placed in a Plexiglas box with a mesh floor 50 cm above the table. After 15 min of acclimation, the ipsilateral paw withdrawal thresholds were measured by an electric apparatus (IITC Life Science, USA). An increasing force was used to stimulate the ipsilateral hind paw, and when the paw withdrawal was observed, the value was recorded. Three repeated measures were averaged to get a mean value. Cold test response rate to acetone was done according to a previous study [20]; the score was recorded as withdrawal or licking or shaking of the hind paw to a drop of acetone applied to the ventral surface of the paw. The guarding behaviors were measured before the paw withdrawal threshold test and acetone test.

Anxiety- and depression-like behavior tests

The open field test was performed on POD 20, 40, and 70 and followed the procedures described previously [21]. The rat was placed in a square arena (50 × 50 × 50 cm). The square was divided into two areas: a peripheral area and a central (17 × 17 cm) square area. The center distance and center duration were recorded as measures of anxiety-like behavior, and total running distance was recorded as a measure of general motor behavior. The running track was recorded for 5 min by a camera 2 m above the box. The field was cleaned with 75% ethanol after each test.

The elevated plus maze test was performed the day after the open field test to assess anxiety-like behavior as described previously [22]. The apparatus was comprised of two open arms and two closed arms (60 × 30 × 20 cm) emerging from a center platform (20 × 20 cm). The maze was covered with PVC material. After preparation, a rat was placed in the center of the platform area, and then, the track was videotaped for 5 min by a camera 1.5 m above the plus maze. The open arm entries and open arm duration were recorded for analysis. After each test, the rat was returned to its cage and the maze was cleaned with 75% ethanol. The videos of open field and elevated plus maze tests were analyzed by tracking software Noldus Ethovision XT (Noldus Information Technology, Leesburg, VA).

After the open field and elevated plus maze tests, the sucrose preference test was performed to assess depression-like behavior. The experiment followed a previous study with minor modifications [21]. Briefly, all of the rats were habituated with 1% sucrose for 48 h before experiments. On POD 25, 45, and 75, each rat received an 8-h fluid and food deprivation and then was exposed for 1 h to two bottles, one filled with 1%sucrose and the other tap water. The water and sucrose intakes were recorded to calculate the sucrose intake percentage (sucrose/(sucrose + water)) × 100%.

Intracerebroventricular catheter placement and injection

Intracerebroventricular (ICV) catheter placement and injection followed the procedures used in a previous study [23]. Briefly, on POD 30, rats were anesthetized with pentobarbital sodium (50 mg/kg). After anesthesia, the rat was fixed on a stereotaxic apparatus. Then, the surgery was performed and a catheter was placed with stereotaxic coordinates: 0.8 mm posterior, 1.5 mm left lateral, and 4.5 mm ventral from the bregma. The guide cannula was fixed with dental cement and the rat was returned to its cage for recovery. The ICV cannulation was verified by injection of methylene blue through the cannula. The environmental enrichment toys were provided as before. Minocycline hydrochloride (purchased from Sigma-Aldrich Corp, St Louis, USA) was dissolved in normal saline. For each daily injection, rats were anesthetized with isoflurane as above; rats received bilateral microinjection of minocycline (160 μg/side) or saline (control) into the cerebral ventricle. A total volume of 4.0 μl was infused into each side over 10 min, and the injection syringe was left in place for an additional 5 min to allow for diffusion [23]. The microinjections were performed daily from POD34 to POD39. The behavior tests resumed on POD 40.

Inflammatory mediators measurement by enzyme-linked immune-absorbent assay

On POD45, rats were deeply anesthetized with pentobarbital sodium (100 mg/kg) followed by decapitation. Tissues were collected for ELISA as previously described [24]. Briefly, the brains were placed in a chilled matrix and microdissected on a chilled glass plate. The mPFC was obtained from a 2-mm-thick slice ranging from approximately 5 to 3 mm anterior of Bregma. The VH was isolated from a 4-mm-thick section ranging from approximately 3.2 to 7.2 mm posterior of Bregma and was separated from cortex and underlying brain structures. The BA was dissected out ranging from approximately 1.2 to 3.2 mm posterior of Bregma just lateral to the optic tracks. After the samples were collected, these tissues were homogenized with normal saline and centrifuged at 2000 rpm, 4 °C for 10 min. The supernatants were used for IL-10, IL-1β, and TNF-α assay with ELISA kits (Nanjingjiancheng Biocompany, Nanjing, China) following the manufacturer's instructions.

Statistical analysis

The data are shown as mean ± SEM and were analyzed with one-way or two-way analysis of variance (ANOVA) with repeated measures. If a statistically significant difference was found, Bonferroni post hoc analysis was conducted. Nonparametric Wilcoxon or unpaired "*t*" test was used for comparison of variables without repeated measure. $P < 0.05$ was considered statistically significant. The statistical analysis was performed using GraphPad Prism software (GraphPad Prism 5.0, version 2.0; GraphPad Software Inc., San Diego, CA, USA).

Results

Infant SNI surgery induced adolescent anxiety- and depression-like behaviors

From adolescence onward, anxiety- and depression-like behaviors were measured. The open field test showed that infant SNI surgery decreased the center duration (group $F_{1,14} = 13.2$, $P = 0.003$; time $F_{2,28} = 1.16$, $P = 0.329$; interaction $F_{2,28} = 1.29$, $P = 0.243$) and center distance (group $F_{1,14} = 11.4$, $P = 0.005$; time $F_{2,28} = 1.06$, $P = 0.359$; interaction $F_{2,28} = 1.07$, $P = 0.355$) compared to the sham surgery group from POD 20 to POD 40 (Fig. 2a, b respectively). The total running distance in the open field was not different between the sham and SNI groups (Fig. 2c) (group $F_{1,14} = 1.09$, $P = 0.315$; time $F_{2,28} = 0.326$, $P = 0.724$; interaction $F_{2,28} = 0.047$, $P = 0.955$). SNI surgery decreased the center distance/total distance ratio (Fig. 2j) (group $F_{1,14} = 7.7$, $P = 0.015$; time $F_{2,28} = 0.745$, $P = 0.484$; interaction $F_{2,28} = 0.737$, $P = 0.487$), a measure which minimizes any small changes in total locomotion

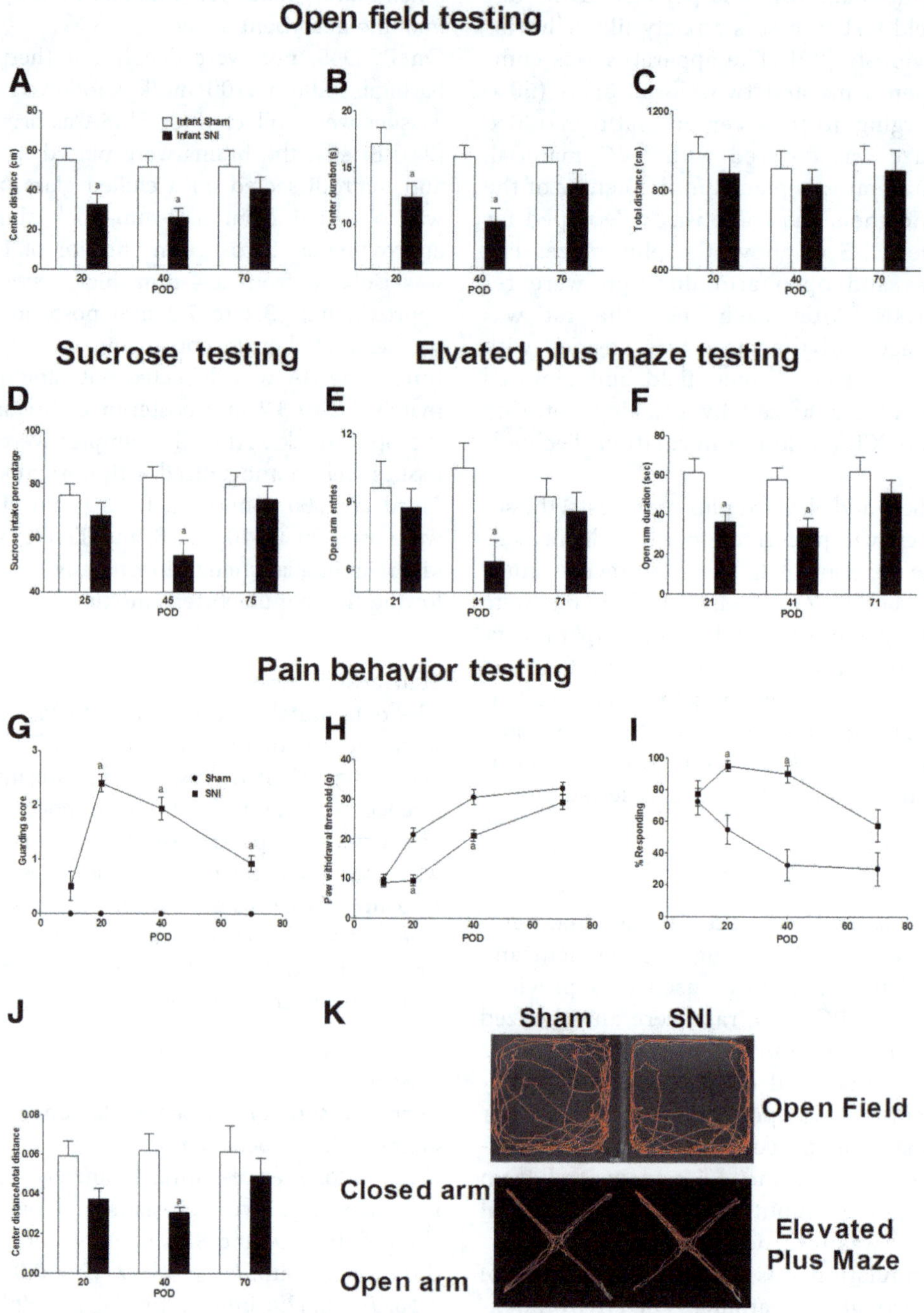

Fig. 2 Infant SNI resulted in adolescent anxiety- and depression-like behaviors. Infant rats that received SNI on P10 showed decreased (**a**) center distance and (**b**) center duration compared to the sham group from POD 20 to POD 40. **c** The total distance traveled in the open field did not differ from the sham group. **d** Infant SNI surgery decreased sucrose intake percentage compared to the sham group on POD 45. In the elevated plus maze test, infant SNI surgery decreased (**f**) open arm duration compared to the sham group from POD 21 to POD 41 and (**e**) open arm entries on POD 41. In addition, infant SNI resulted in decreased (**g**) paw withdrawal threshold from POD 20 to POD 40, increased (**h**) guarding score from POD 20 to POD 70, and increased (**i**) cold sensitivity to acetone from POD 20 to POD 40. **j** SNI decreased the center distance/total distance calculated from the open field test on POD 40. Representative open field and elevated plus maze photos (**k**). $n = 8$. "a" denotes the statistically significant difference compared to the sham group

on the results. Representative open field and elevated plus maze photos are shown in Fig. 2k.

The elevated plus maze test showed that infant SNI surgery decreased open arm duration compared to the sham group from POD 21 to POD 41 (Fig. 2f) (group $F_{1,14} = 8.38$, $P = 0.012$; time $F_{2,28} = 0.270$, $P = 0.766$; interaction $F_{2,28} = 1.763$, $P = 0.190$). The number of open arm entries was decreased on POD 41 compared to the sham group (Fig. 2e) (group $F_{1,14} = 11.6$, $P = 0.004$; time $F_{2,28} = 2.00$, $P = 0.154$; interaction $F_{2,28} = 1.08$, $P = 0.352$). The sucrose preference test showed that the infant SNI surgery decreased the sucrose intake percentage on POD 45 compared to the sham group (Fig. 2d) (group $F_{1,14} = 28.75$, $P = 0.000$; time $F_{2,28} = 1.55$, $P = 0.231$; interaction $F_{2,28} = 3.01$, $P = 0.653$).

The paw withdrawal threshold (Fig. 2g) (group $F_{1,14} = 42.6$, $P = 0.000$; time $F_{3,42} = 75.9$, $P = 0.000$; interaction $F_{3,42} = 4.97$, $P = 0.005$) of rats subjected to infant SNI was decreased on POD 20 and POD 40, spontaneous guarding behavior (Fig. 2h) (group $F_{1,14} = 404$, $P = 0.000$; time $F_{3,42} = 16$, $P = 0.000$; interaction $F_{3,42} = 16$, $P = 0.000$) was increased on POD 20, POD 40, and POD 70, and the response to acetone (Fig. 2i) (group $F_{1,14} = 53.8$, $P = 0.000$; time $F_{3,42} = 5.31$, $P = 0.003$; interaction $F_{3,42} = 2.94$, $P = 0.044$) was increased on POD 20 and POD 40, as compared to sham rats.

Infant SNI surgery increased mPFC, BA, and VH inflammatory mediators on POD 45

The ELISA results showed that SNI surgery increased IL-1β in the mPFC ($P = 0.003$, unpaired t test), BA ($P = 0.004$, unpaired t test), and VH ($P = 0.001$, unpaired t test) and TNF-α in the mPFC ($P = 0.001$, unpaired t test), BA ($P = 0.003$, unpaired t test), and VH ($P = 0.001$, unpaired t test) compared to the sham group (Fig. 3a–c). In contrast, infant SNI surgery decreased IL-10 in the mPFC compared to the sham group ($P = 0.032$, unpaired t test, Fig. 3a). These results showed that SNI caused the adolescent brain to skew towards a pro-inflammatory profile.

ICV MIN reduced adolescent anxiety- and depression-like behaviors

In experiment 2, four rats did not complete the experiment and were excluded, including one in sham + MIN, one in SNI + MIN, and two in SNI + vehicle group. Two rats in the SNI + vehicle group died due to respiratory depression possibly caused by pentobarbital overdose. One rat in the sham + MIN group and one in the SNI + MIN group were excluded from the study due to failure of proper cannulation. The behavior results showed that ICV MIN for 6 days starting at POD34 did not affect anxiety, depression, and pain behaviors of sham rats (Fig. 4a–f). Consistent with experiment 1, SNI surgery induced adolescent anxiety, depression, and pain behaviors compared to sham rats. ICV MIN starting at POD 34 increased the center distance (group $F_{3,24} = 15.3$, $P = 0.000$; time $F_{1,24} = 2.41$, $P = 0.133$; interaction $F_{3,24} = 2.00$, $P = 0.141$) and center duration (group $F_{3,24} = 8.42$, $P = 0.001$; time $F_{1,24} = 0.146$, $P = 0.706$; interaction $F_{3,24} = 1.867$, $P = 0.162$) on POD 40 in the open field test, open arm duration (group $F_{3,24} = 7.91$, $P = 0.000$; time $F_{1,24} = 0.28$, $P = 0.602$; interaction $F_{3,24} = 1.59$, $P = 0.216$) and a number of open arm entries (group $F_{3,24} = 7.1$, $P = 0.000$; time $F_{1,24} = 0.83$, $P = 0.37$; interaction $F_{3,24} = 2.54$, $P = 0.08$) on POD 41 in the elevated plus maze test, and sucrose intake percentage (group $F_{3,24} = 4.83$, $P = 0.001$; time $F_{1,24} = 0.02$, $P = 0.88$; interaction $F_{3,24} = 1.16$, $P = 0.35$) on POD 45 in the sucrose preference test (Fig. 4a–f). Although SNI decreased the paw withdrawal threshold (group $F_{3,28} = 17.93$, $P = 0.000$; time $F_{1,28} = 51.0$, $P = 0.000$; interaction $F_{3,24} = 0.105$, $P = 0.957$) and increased spontaneous guarding behaviors (group $F_{3,28} = 176.7$, $P = 0.000$; time $F_{1,24} = 3.52$, $P = 0.073$; interaction $F_{3,24} = 3.52$, $P = 0.140$) and response to acetone (group $F_{3,28} = 34.1$, $P = 0.000$; time $F_{1,24} = 1.63$, $P = 0.214$; interaction $F_{3,24} = 0.12$, $P = 0.947$), ICV MIN did not affect those behaviors in the sham or SNI rats (Fig. 4g–i). SNI decreased the center/total distance (Fig. 4j) (group $F_{3,24} = 5.93$, $P = 0.004$; time $F_{1,24} = 0.255$, $P = 0.618$; interaction $F_{3,24} = 1.49$, $P = 0.244$) compared to the sham group, while ICV MIN decreased that effect on POD40.

ICV MIN reduced mPFC, BA, and VH inflammation of rats subjected to infant SNI on POD 45 compared to ICV vehicle group

After the behavior tests on POD 45, rats were decapitated and samples were collected for ELISA tests. The ELISA results showed infant SNI increased IL-1β and

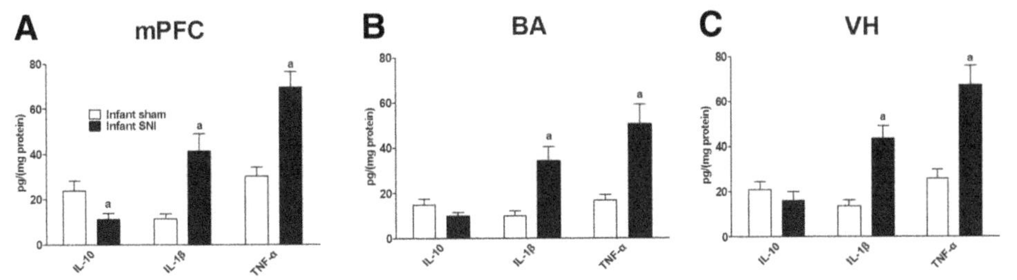

Fig. 3 Infant SNI skewed mPFC, BA, and VH to a pro-inflammatory profile. On POD 45, infant SNI surgery increased **a** mPFC, **b** BA, and **c** VH IL-1β and TNF-α while decreasing mPFC and BA IL-10 expression compared to the sham group. $n = 6$. "a" denotes the statistically significant difference compared to the sham group

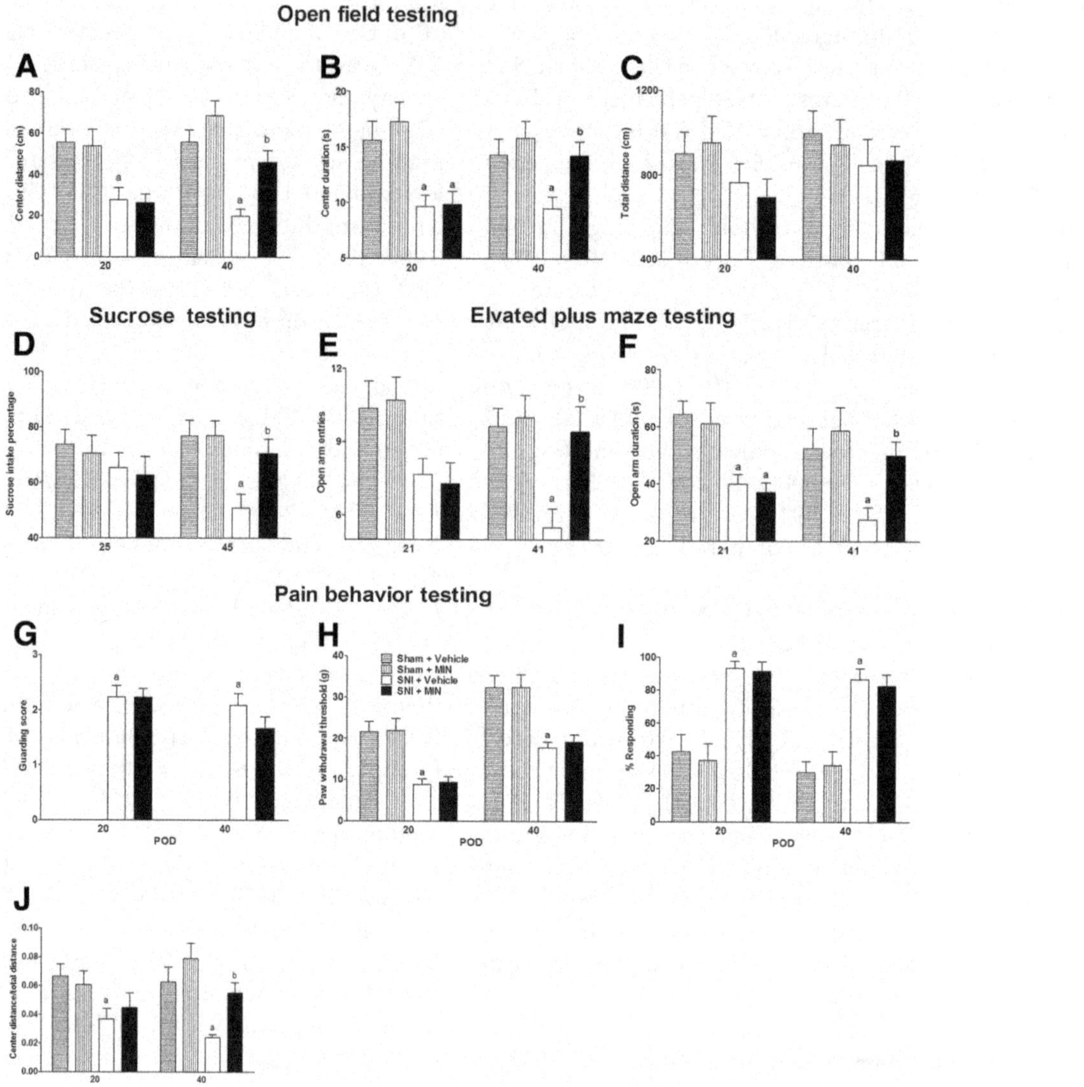

Fig. 4 ICV MIN decreased infant SNI-induced anxiety- and depression-like behaviors. Infant SNI decreased **a** center duration and **b** distance from POD 20 to POD 40 in the open field test, **f** open arm duration from POD 20 to POD 40, **e** open arm entrances on POD 40 in the elevated plus maze test, and **d** sucrose intake percentage on POD 45. ICV MIN increased center duration and distance in the open field test, open duration and open entrance on POD 40 in the elevated plus maze test, and sucrose intake percentage on POD 45. ICV MIN did not affect the total distance traveled in the open field test (no difference between the four groups) and did not affect any behaviors of the sham rats. Infant SNI decreased **g** paw withdrawal threshold and **h** increased guarding score (guarding scores in the two sham groups were zero) and **i** response to acetone from POD 20 to POD 40, while ICV MIN did not affect these values in sham or SNI rats. **k** SNI decreased center/total distance compared to the sham group, while ICV MIN decreased that effect on POD40. $n = 6–8$. "a" denotes the statistically significant difference compared to the sham plus vehicle group. "b" denotes the statistically significant difference compared to the SNI plus vehicle group

TNF-α in mPFC (Fig. 5a–c), BA (Fig. 5d–f), and VH (Fig. 5g–i), while ICV MIN increased IL-10 in mPFC ($F_{3,24} = 4.47$, $P = 0.013$), BA ($F_{3,24} = 4.14$, $P = 0.017$), and VH ($F_{3,24} = 16.23$, $P = 0.000$) and decreased IL-1β in mPFC ($F_{3,24} = 34.85$, $P = 0.000$), BA ($F_{3,24} = 24.87$, $P = 0.000$), and VH ($F_{3,24} = 25.52$, $P = 0.000$) and TNF-α in mPFC ($F_{3,24} = 17.41$, $P = 0.000$), BA ($F_{3,24} = 31.2$, $P = 0.000$), and VH ($F_{3,24} = 39.6$, $P = 0.000$). The increased IL-10 and decreased IL-1β and TNF-α in mPFC, BA, and VH suggested that ICV MIN skewed the SNI-induced pro-inflammatory profile towards an anti-inflammatory profile in those regions.

EE inhibited infant SNI-induced adolescent pain and anxiety- and depression-like behaviors

In the EE intervention experiment, one rat in the sham group was excluded because of incision infection. After EE starting from POD 11, the center duration (group $F_{3,31} = 16.2$, $P = 0.000$; time $F_{2,62} = 0.285$, $P = 0.824$; interaction $F_{6,62} = 0.913$, $P = 0.491$) and center distance

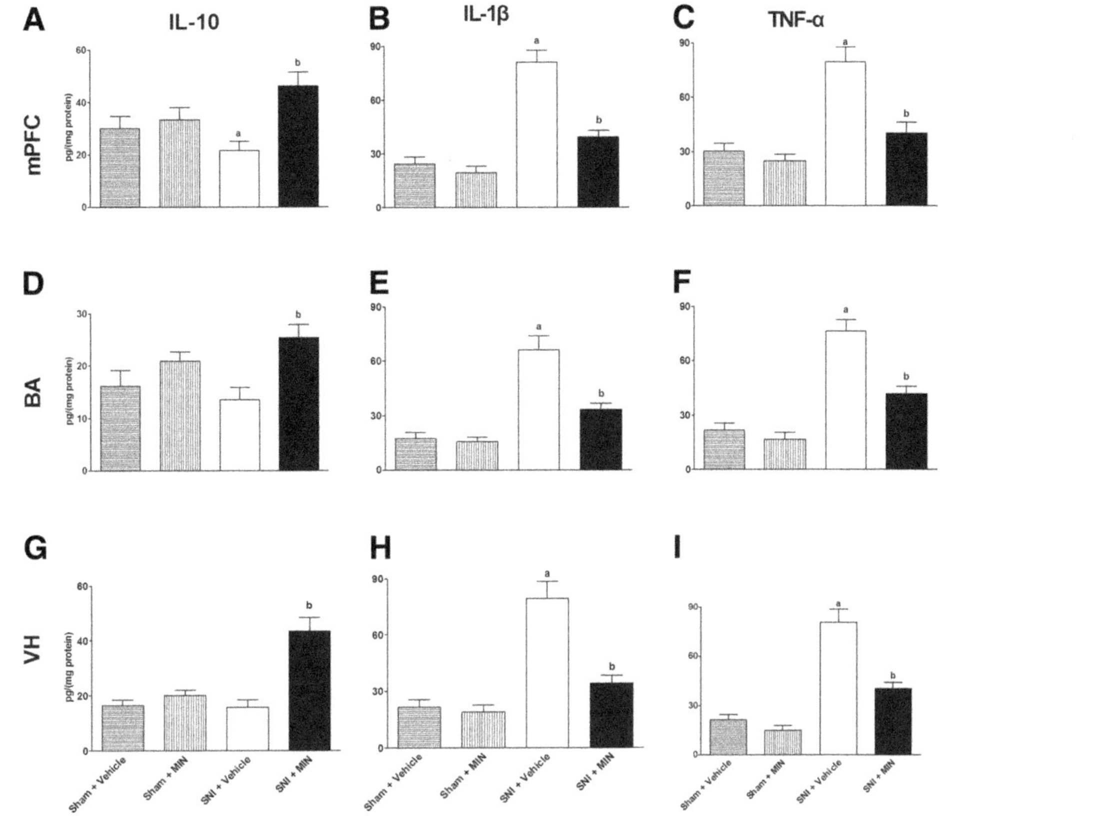

Fig. 5 ICV MIN changed the mPFC, BA, and VH inflammatory profile. Infant SNI decreased IL-10 in mPFC, and ICV MIN increased IL-10 in the **a** mPFC, **d** BA, and **g** VH. Infant SNI increased IL-1β and TNF-α in mPFC, BA, and VH, and ICV MIN decreased IL-1β and TNF-α in the **b, c** mPFC, **e, f** BA, and **g, h** VH. *n* = 6–8. "a" denotes the statistically significant difference compared to the sham plus vehicle group. "b" denotes the statistically significant difference compared to the SNI plus vehicle group

(group $F_{3,31}$ = 9.67, P = 0.000; time $F_{2,62}$ = 0.285, P = 0.753; interaction $F_{6,62}$ = 0.454, P = 0.968) on POD 40 were greatly increased compared to the group without EE in the open field test of rats that received SNI on POD 10 (Fig. 6a, b). The total running distance in the open field was not different between the four groups (Fig. 6c) (group $F_{3,31}$ = 0.593, P = 0.624; time $F_{2,62}$ = 2.38, P = 0.101; interaction $F_{6,62}$ = 0.111, P = 0.995). EE increased open arm duration (group $F_{3,31}$ = 5.79, P = 0.003; time $F_{2,62}$ = 0.744, P = 0.480; interaction $F_{6,62}$ = 0.566, P = 0.756) compared to the group without EE on POD 41 in the elevated plus maze test of rats that received SNI on P10 (Fig. 6f). The sucrose preference test showed that EE increased sucrose intake percentage on POD 25 and POD 45, compared to the group without EE of rats that received SNI on P10 (Fig. 6d) (group $F_{3,31}$ = 12.49, P = 0.000; time $F_{2,62}$ = 1.305, P = 0.278; interaction $F_{6,62}$ = 0.762, P = 0.603). EE did not affect behavior results of sham rats in the open field, elevated plus maze, and sucrose preference tests. SNI decreased center/total distance compared to the sham group, while EE decreased that effect on POD40 in the open field test (Fig. 6k) (group $F_{3,31}$ = 3.33, P = 0.042; time $F_{2,62}$ = 2.12, P = 0.118; interaction $F_{6,62}$ = 0.967, P = 0.455).

In addition, EE increased the paw withdrawal threshold (Fig. 6g) (group $F_{3,31}$ = 12.49, P = 0.000; time $F_{3,93}$ = 185.4, P = 0.000; interaction $F_{9,93}$ = 2.97, P = 0.004) and decreased the spontaneous guarding score (Fig. 6h) (group $F_{3,31}$ = 160.1, P = 0.000; time $F_{3,93}$ = 26.32, P = 0.000; interaction $F_{9,93}$ = 9.67, P = 0.000) on POD 40 compared to the group without EE of rats that received infant SNI. Although SNI increased the response to acetone (Fig. 6i) (group $F_{3,31}$ = 6.81, P = 0.001; time $F_{3,93}$ = 16.1, P = 0.000; interaction $F_{9,93}$ = 0.019, P = 2.36), EE did not affect the response to acetone of sham rats or rats that received SNI.

EE skewed mPFC, BA, and VH to an anti-inflammatory profile on POD 45

After EE intervention from POD21 to POD45, the rats were killed and decapitated on POD45, and samples were obtained from three brain regions and prepared for ELISA assays. The ELISA results showed that EE increased IL-10 in mPFC ($F_{3,20}$ = 8.80, P = 0.001), BA ($F_{3,20}$ = 7.99, P = 0.001), and VH ($F_{3,20}$ = 5.78, P = 0.001) and decreased IL-1β in mPFC ($F_{3,20}$ = 14.5, P = 0.000) and VH ($F_{3,20}$ = 17.1, P = 0.000) and TNF-α in mPFC ($F_{3,20}$ = 9.85, P = 0.001), BA ($F_{3,20}$ = 18.2, P = 0.000), and

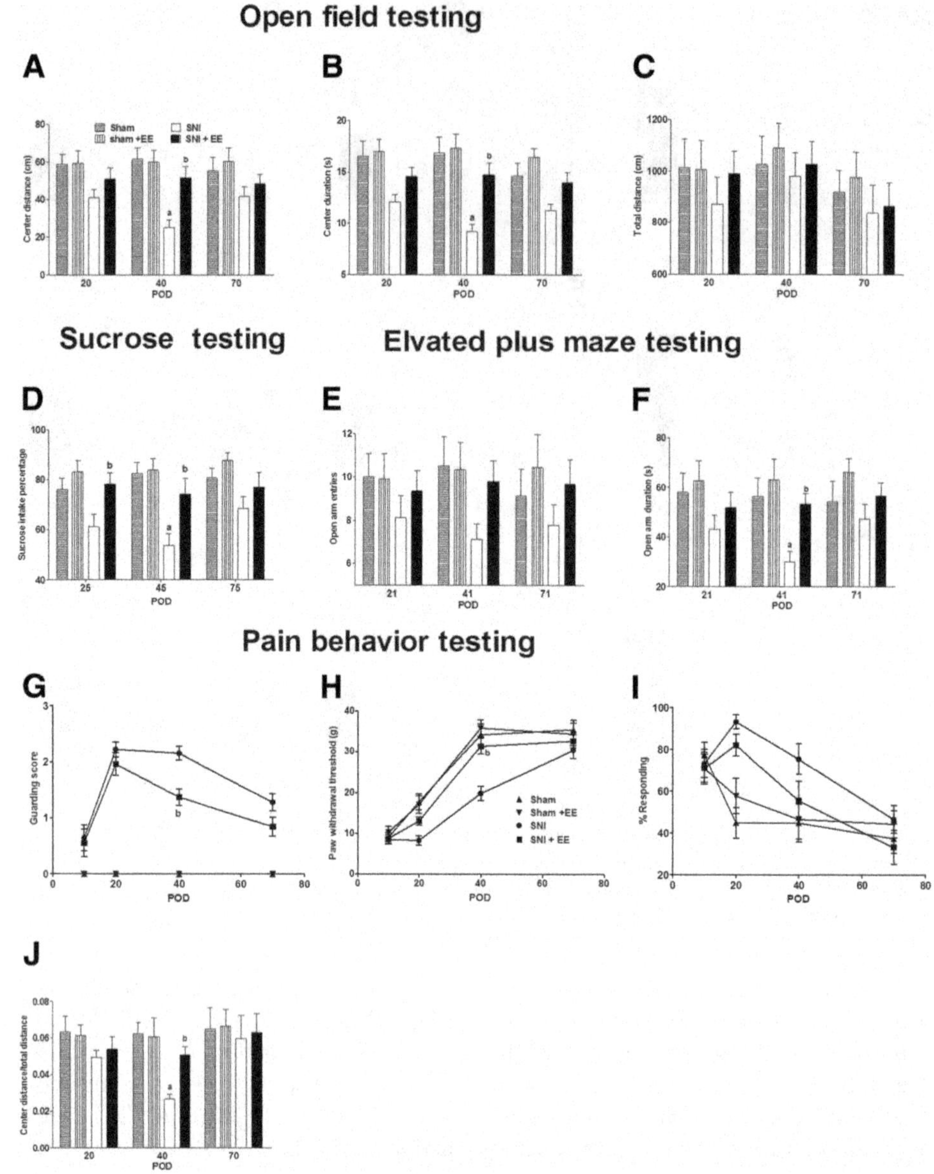

Fig. 6 Environmental enrichment (EE) reduced infant SNI-induced anxiety- and depression-like behavior. After EE intervention starting from POD11, **a** the center distance and **b** duration were greatly increased on POD 40 in the open field test compared to the group without EE. **c** The total distance was not different between the four groups. **d** EE increased sucrose intake percentage compared to the group without EE from POD 25 to POD 45. **f** Open arm duration was increased on POD 41 after EE when compared to the group without EE. After EE, **h** the guarding score was decreased and **g** the paw withdrawal threshold was increased on POD 40 as compared to the SNI group. **i** EE did not decrease the response to acetone of rats subjected to infant SNI. **k** SNI decreased center/total distance compared to the sham group, while ICV MIN decreased that effect on POD40. $n = 8–9$. "a" and "b" denote the statistically significant difference compared to the sham and SNI group, respectively

VH ($F_{3,20} = 19.0$, $P = 0.000$) of rats that received infant SNI (Fig. 7a–c). EE did not affect IL-10, IL-1β, and TNF-α in the mPFC, BA, and VH of sham rats.

Discussion

Our study showed that the infant nerve injury resulted in anxiety- and depression-like behaviors in adolescence, while EE reduced adolescent anxiety- and depression-like behaviors and suppressed central nervous inflammation.

In the study, we found that infant rats with peripheral nerve injury exhibited anxiety- and depression-like behaviors. Anxiety-like behaviors, including open field test and elevated plus maze test measures, peaked on POD 40 and disappeared on POD 70. Sucrose intake percentage, a measure of depression-like behavior, was decreased on POD 45. The total distance traveled was

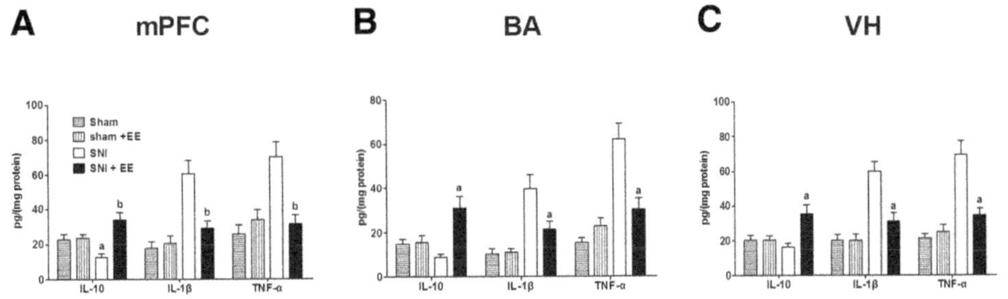

Fig. 7 EE skewed the brain to an anti-inflammatory profile. On POD 45, EE increased IL-10 expression and decreased IL-1β and TNF-α expression in **a** mPFC, **b** BA, and **c** VH compared to without EE. $n = 6$. "a" and "b" denote the statistically significant difference compared to the sham and SNI group, respectively

not different between groups in the open field test, which excluded the possibility that anxiety- and depression-like results were caused by motor impairment. In addition, IL-10 decreased in mPFC and BA, while IL-1β and TNF-α protein expression increased in mPFC, BA, and VH on POD 45, which indicated a CNS shift to pro-inflammatory profile at the time when anxiety- and depression-related behaviors were observed. In addition, our results showed neuropathic pain generally coincided with these behaviors. Since neuropathic pain causes psychiatric disorders [25], it is reasonable to deduce, at least in part, that the delayed neuropathic pain contributed to the anxiety- and depression-like behaviors.

Previous studies have demonstrated substantive links between neuroinflammation and psychological disorders [26]. Microglia are a major source of inflammation in the central nervous system [27], and the application of MIN, a microglia inhibitor, abolished anxiety- and depression-like behavior in a previous study [28]. Thus, we tested injection of MIN to treat anxiety- and depression-like behaviors in rats subjected to infant peripheral nerve injury. Our results showed that ICV MIN reduced adolescent anxiety- and depression-like behaviors induced by infant SNI surgery. This is in agreement with some previous clinical and preclinical studies showing anxiety and depression are associated with microglia activation and are reduced by MIN [6]. In addition, we found that ICV MIN reduced mPFC, BA, and VH inflammation. The inflammatory profile switch was verified by our ELISA results showing that MIN decreased IL-1β and TNF-α protein expression and increased IL-10 expression. These effects on the cytokine profile are similar to those found in a preclinical study of systemic MIN that showed it shifted brain microglia towards an M2 phenotype [29]. However, a limitation of our study is that we did not directly examine brain microglia and cannot exclude other mechanisms such as direct effects on neurons [30]. In contrast, our results showed that ICV MIN did not affect pain behaviors; this may be because the effects of the small dose of MIN were limited to microglial inhibition in the brain only, rather than influencing microglia in the spinal cord, so that MIN did not affect lower extremity reflexes. Another reason may be that MIN is effective for the prevention of neuropathic pain development, but has no effect on established neuropathic pain [31]. Our results showed ICV MIN did not affect delayed adolescent neuropathic pain behaviors induced by infant nerve injury when applied after these behaviors were already established.

After infant nerve injury, EE was employed to counteract the anxiety- and depression-related behaviors. Our results showed that EE is anxiolytic and anti-depressive. On POD 40, the anxiety- and depression-like behaviors were improved. However, on POD 20, the anxiety-like behaviors were not different between groups, possibly because this time point was only 9 days after the start of EE. The ELISA results on POD45 support the behavioral findings and showed decreased proinflammatory cytokines after EE. Previous studies have demonstrated that anxiety and depression are inflammatory diseases and that modulation of inflammation is anxiolytic and anti-depressive [5]. IL-1β and TNF-α are pro-inflammatory cytokines. ICV application of these cytokines provokes anxiety- and depression-like behaviors [32, 33], whereas the ICV application of IL-10, an anti-inflammatory cytokine, abolished these behaviors [34]. This is consistent with our results showing that EE decreased both the anxiety- and depression-like behaviors and inflammation in the brain. Our results indicate EE is anxiolytic and antidepressant and it promotes a switch from a pro-inflammatory to an anti-inflammatory profile in the brain.

Previous studies have demonstrated IL-1β is an important pro-inflammatory cytokine in the formation of psychiatric disorders: blocking IL-1β signaling with an antagonist greatly reduced inflammatory psychiatric disorders, and drugs targeting IL-1β are in phase II clinical trials [33, 35]. TNF-α is another pro-inflammatory cytokine that plays a pivotal role in the development of psychiatric disorders. A single dose of TNF-α by ICV injection induced anxiety- and depression-like behaviors, while antagonizing TNF-α abolished those behaviors [32, 36]. In addition, TNF-α is the main cytokine involved in the genesis of chronic pain. Blocking TNF-α not only reduced psychiatric disorders but also reduced chronic pain at the same time [15]. In contrast, IL-10 is an anti-inflammatory cytokine and is decreased in various affective disorders, whereas central administration of IL-10 antagonized these disorders [34], an effect attributed to the suppression of neuroinflammation. Consistently, $IL\text{-}10^{-}/^{-}$ animals displayed increased depressive-like behavior that was reversed by IL-10. Moreover, mice overexpressing IL-10 showed a decreased depressive-like behavior [37]. Our results showed that EE and ICV MIN switched the brain from a pro-inflammatory towards an anti-inflammatory profile, reversing the increases in IL-1β and TNF-α and decreases in IL-10. Generally, the results confirmed that affective disorders are inflammatory illnesses, and modulation of inflammation is effective for the treatment of affective illnesses [5, 38].

Our results showed that EE also increased the adolescent pain threshold of rats subjected to infant nerve injury. Previous studies demonstrated that environmental enrichment [39] and exercise [40] both relieve neuropathic pain. Thus, the increased pain threshold we observed could be due to the environment and/or voluntary running. Exercise has been known to have mild to moderate anxiolytic and antidepressant effect. Possible mechanisms include changes in monoamine levels, altered levels of stress hormones (e.g., cortisol), and upregulation of neurotrophic factors [41]. A recent meta-analysis study reported that exercise is effective in treating depression in adolescents [42]. Of course, larger trials with clinical samples that adequately minimize the risk of bias are needed to confirm the findings. Exercise is also known to have neuroprotective effects by increasing expression of anti-inflammatory cytokines and decreasing levels of pro-inflammatory cytokines [43]. Since anxiety and depression are increasingly being recognized as inflammatory conditions [26], it is reasonable to believe that exercise-induced inhibition of inflammatory responses contributes to the anxiolytic and antidepressant effects observed in the current study. Since EE is also anti-inflammatory [44] and EE in our protocol includes exercise [22], our study does not distinguish which was the most important in alleviating anxiety and depression behaviors.

Our results showed that infant nerve injury induced adolescent anxiety- and depression-like behaviors. We tested these behaviors beginning at POD20, to avoid possible stress caused by separation from their mothers. In addition, the anxiety- and depression-like behaviors were not permanent and disappeared on POD 70 in untreated rats. This may be due to the following reasons. Chronic pain is an important contributor to anxiety and depression, and with age, chronic pain decreases [14]. Consequently, the rat anxiety- and depression-like behaviors may also improve with age. One of the limitations of the study is that we do not know whether the anxiolytic and anti-depressive effect of EE is due to suppression of brain inflammation, reduced neuropathic pain, or a combination of the two. The relationship between chronic pain and psychiatric illness is rather complex. Chronic pain leads to psychiatric illness, whereas psychiatric illness sensitizes chronic pain. These two disorders often exacerbate each other, leading to a vicious cycle that is refractory to medical treatment [15]. Although it is well recognized that chronic pain and psychiatric illness co-exist, it is not fully explored as to why or how they do so. A better understanding of their relationship may help to resolve both problems. However, our results showed EE reduces adolescent anxiety- and depression-like and neuropathic pain behaviors of rats subject to infant nerve injury.

We targeted mPFC, BA, and VH because many studies have demonstrated that these regions are key sites of inflammation in psychiatric conditions, while suppression of pro-inflammatory cytokines in those sites decreases various affective disorders [15, 45]. mPFC and BA are undergoing continuing development during adolescence [46]. This late development may lead to susceptibilities to psychopathologies that often develop at this time. A previous study [47] has demonstrated that IL-1β is increased in mPFC in chronic stress-treated rats, while decreasing IL-1β in mPFC also decreased anxiety- and depression-like behaviors. Similarly, others report that mice with complete Freund's adjuvant-induced inflammatory pain showed anxiety-like behavior and increased TNF-α in the BA [48]. VH has been reported to participate in psychiatric disorders by sending information to mPFC and BA [49]. Lesions of the ventral hippocampus but not the dorsal hippocampus attenuate anxiety behaviors and prevent the physiological response of increased defecation in response to an anxiogenic environment [50, 51]. Therefore, in our study, those regions were chosen to evaluate the inflammatory conditions.

To avoid estrus cycle effects, only male rats were included in our study. However, recent studies from other groups showed that pain and psychiatric disorders exhibit sex differences. Microglia play a key role in chronic pain initiation and maintenance in males, while in females, adaptive immune cells, likely T lymphocytes, exert a more important role in chronic pain. Estrogen and progesterone suppress innate immunity, and testosterone inhibits adaptive immunity which may contribute to these effects [52]. Similar to pain, anxiety and depression also showed sex differences. Previous studies have demonstrated that females do not show anxiety-like behaviors and had less inflammation [53]. This was attributed to the suppression of neuroinflammation by estradiol [54]. Moreover, large-scale data from the Netherlands Study of Depression and Anxiety reported that inflammation associated with depression is male-specific [55]. Despite sexual dimorphisms in the prevalence of psychiatric illnesses, much current research investigating the neuroimmune impact of stress remains exclusively focused on male subjects. However, in our results, we found that male rat brains skewed to a proinflammatory profile when they presented anxiety- and depression-like behaviors.

Conclusions

In summary, results from our study demonstrate that infant nerve injury induces adolescent anxiety- and depression-like behaviors and that the CNS switches to a proinflammatory profile. Suppression of microglia-related inflammation by MIN counteracts the adolescent anxiety- and depression-like behaviors. EE including exercise, a non-pharmacological method, inhibits adolescent anxiety- and depression-like behaviors and restores the balance of inflammatory mediators.

Abbreviations

ANOVA: Analysis of variance; BA: Basolateral amygdala; EE: Environmental enrichment; ELISA: Enzyme-linked immune-absorbent assay; ICV: Intracerebroventricular; MIN: Minocycline; mPFC: Medial prefrontal cortex; P: Postnatal day; POD: Postoperative day; SNI: Spared nerve injury; VH: Ventral hippocampus

Acknowledgements

We thank Judith A. Strong from the Pain Research Center, Department of Anesthesiology, University of Cincinnati College of Medicine, Cincinnati, Ohio 45267 for her language editing and revision of grammatical errors.

Funding

This research is funded by a grant from the National Natural Science Foundation of China (NSFC, Grant No. 81270414), Shanghai Municipal Commission of Health and Family Planning Founding for Key Developing Disciplines (no. 2015ZB0106), and Shanghai Pudong New Area Science and Technology Development Fund Innovation Capital (no. PKJ2013-Y61).

Authors' contributions

XG and YC did the surgery and behavior tests. JC did the ELISA experiment. YH and MC did the statistical analysis. MZ designed the experiment. All authors read and approved the final manuscript.

Consent for publication

Not applicable

Competing interests

The authors declare that they have no competing interests.

Author details

[1]Department of Anesthesiology and Pediatric Clinical Pharmacology Laboratory, Shanghai Children's Medical Center, Shanghai Jiao Tong University School of Medicine, 1678 Dongfang Road, 200127 Shanghai, China. [2]Department of Anesthesiology, Shiyan Taihe Hospital (Affiliated Hospital of Hubei University of Medicine), Shiyan, Hubei, China. [3]Institute of Anesthesiology, Department of Anesthesiology, Shiyan Taihe Hospital (Affiliated Hospital of Hubei University of Medicine), Shiyan, Hubei, China. [4]Department of Laboratory, Shiyan Taihe Hospital (Affiliated Hospital of Hubei University of Medicine), Shiyan, Hubei, China.

References

1. Bair MJ, Robinson RL, Katon W, Kroenke K. Depression and pain comorbidity: a literature review. Arch Intern Med. 2003;163:2433–45.
2. Epstein SA, Kay G, Clauw D, Heaton R, Klein D, Krupp L, Kuck J, Leslie V, Masur D, Wagner M, Waid R, Zisook S. Psychiatric disorders in patients with fibromyalgia. A multicenter investigation. Psychosomatics. 1999;40:57–63.
3. Argoff CE. The coexistence of neuropathic pain, sleep, and psychiatric disorders: a novel treatment approach. Clin J Pain. 2007;23:15–22.
4. Eyre HA, Papps E, Baune BT. Treating depression and depression-like behavior with physical activity: an immune perspective. Front Psych. 2013;4:3.
5. Wohleb ES, Franklin T, Iwata M, Duman RS. Integrating neuroimmune systems in the neurobiology of depression. Nat Rev Neurosci. 2016;17:497–511.
6. Yirmiya R, Rimmerman N, Reshef R. Depression as a microglial disease. Trends Neurosci. 2015;38:637–58.
7. Wang YL, Han QQ, Gong WQ, Pan DH, Wang LZ, Hu W, Yang M, Li B, Yu J, Liu Q. Microglial activation mediates chronic mild stress-induced depressive- and anxiety-like behavior in adult rats. J Neuroinflammation. 2018;15:21.
8. Vallejo R, Tilley DM, Vogel L, Benyamin R. The role of glia and the immune system in the development and maintenance of neuropathic pain. Pain Pract. 2010;10:167–84.
9. Anand P, Birch R. Restoration of sensory function and lack of long-term chronic pain syndromes after brachial plexus injury in human neonates. Brain. 2002;125:113–22.
10. Melzack R, Israel R, Lacroix R, Schultz G. Phantom limbs in people with congenital limb deficiency or amputation in early childhood. Brain. 1997; 120(Pt 9):1603–20.
11. Sandroni P, Benrud-Larson LM, McClelland RL, Low PA. Complex regional pain syndrome type I: incidence and prevalence in Olmsted county, a population-based study. Pain. 2003;103:199–207.
12. ATHERTON DD, TAHERZADEH O, ELLIOT D, ANAND P. Age-dependent development of chronic neuropathic pain, allodynia and sensory recovery after upper limb nerve injury in children. J Hand Surg Eur Vol. 2008;33:186–91.
13. McKelvey R, Berta T, Old E, Ji RR, Fitzgerald M. Neuropathic pain is constitutively suppressed in early life by anti-inflammatory neuroimmune regulation. J Neurosci. 2015;35:457–66.
14. Gong X, Chen Y, Fu B, Jiang J, Zhang M. Infant nerve injury induces delayed microglial polarization to the M1 phenotype, and exercise reduces delayed neuropathic pain by modulating microglial activity. Neuroscience. 2017;349:76–86.
15. Fasick V, Spengler RN, Samankan S, Nader ND, Ignatowski TA. The hippocampus and TNF: common links between chronic pain and depression. Neurosci Biobehav Rev. 2015;53:139–59.
16. Zhou F, Chen C, Huang Y, Hu H, Li L, Tan Y. The effects of enriched environmental intervention on the parturition outcome and filial health of pregnant mice with chronic pain. Biol Res Nurs. 2018;20:264–71.
17. Salam JN, Fox JH, Detroy EM, Guignon MH, Wohl DF, Falls WA. Voluntary exercise in C57 mice is anxiolytic across several measures of anxiety. Behav Brain Res. 2009;197:31–40.
18. Gong X, Jiang J, Zhang M. Exercise preconditioning reduces neonatal incision surgery-induced enhanced hyperalgesia via inhibition of P38 mitogen-activated protein kinase and IL-1β, TNF-α release. Int J Dev Neurosci. 2016;52:46–54.
19. Decosterd I, Clifford W. Spared nerve injury: an animal model of persistent peripheral neuropathic pain. Pain. 2000;87:149–58.
20. Xie W, Strong JA, Zhang JM. Active nerve regeneration with failed target reinnervation drives persistent neuropathic pain. eNeuro. 2017;4:e8–17.
21. Zhang JM, Tonelli L, Regenold WT, McCarthy MM. Effects of neonatal flutamide treatment on hippocampal neurogenesis and synaptogenesis correlate with depression-like behaviors in preadolescent male rats. Neuroscience. 2010;169:544–54.
22. Ahmadalipour A, Sadeghzadeh J, Vafaei AA, Bandegi AR, Mohammadkhani R, Rashidy-Pour A. Effects of environmental enrichment on behavioral deficits and alterations in hippocampal BDNF induced by prenatal exposure to morphine in juvenile rats. Neuroscience. 2015;305:372–83.

23. Réus GZ, Abelaira HM, Maciel AL, Dos Santos MAB, Carlessi AS, Steckert AV, Ferreira GK, De Prá SD, Streck EL, Macêdo DS, Quevedo J. Minocycline protects against oxidative damage and alters energy metabolism parameters in the brain of rats subjected to chronic mild stress. Metab Brain Dis. 2015;30:545–53.
24. Porterfield VM, Gabella KM, Simmons MA, Johnson JD. Repeated stressor exposure regionally enhances beta-adrenergic receptor-mediated brain IL-1β production. Brain Behav Immun. 2012;26:1249–55.
25. Gerrits MM, Vogelzangs N, van Oppen P, van Marwijk HW, van der Horst H, Penninx BW. Impact of pain on the course of depressive and anxiety disorders. Pain. 2012;153:429–36.
26. Krishnadas R, Cavanagh J. Depression: an inflammatory illness? J Neurol Neurosurg Psychiatry. 2012;83:495–502.
27. Lehmann ML, Cooper HA, Maric D, Herkenham M. Social defeat induces depressive-like states and microglial activation without involvement of peripheral macrophages. J Neuroinflammation. 2016;13:224.
28. Arakawa S, Shirayama Y, Fujita Y, Ishima T, Horio M, Muneoka K, Iyo M, Hashimoto K. Minocycline produced antidepressant-like effects on the learned helplessness rats with alterations in levels of monoamine in the amygdala and no changes in BDNF levels in the hippocampus at baseline. Pharmacol Biochem Behav. 2012;100:601–6.
29. Yang Y, Salayandia VM, Thompson JF, Yang LY, Estrada EY, Yang Y. Attenuation of acute stroke injury in rat brain by minocycline promotes blood-brain barrier remodeling and alternative microglia/macrophage activation during recovery. J Neuroinflammation. 2015;12:26.
30. Ossola B, Lantto TA, Puttonen KA, Tuominen RK, Raasmaja A, Mannisto PT. Minocycline protects SH-SY5Y cells from 6-hydroxydopamine by inhibiting both caspase-dependent and -independent programmed cell death. J Neurosci Res. 2012;90:682–90.
31. Padi SS, Kulkarni SK. Minocycline prevents the development of neuropathic pain, but not acute pain: possible anti-inflammatory and antioxidant mechanisms. Eur J Pharmacol. 2008;601:79–87.
32. Kaster MP, Gadotti VM, Calixto JB, Santos ARS, Rodrigues ALS. Depressive-like behavior induced by tumor necrosis factor-α in mice. Neuropharmacology. 2012;62:419–26.
33. Pan Y, Chen X, Zhang Q, Kong L. Microglial NLRP3 inflammasome activation mediates IL-1β-related inflammation in prefrontal cortex of depressive rats. Brain Behav Immun. 2014;41:90–100.
34. Pan Y, Lin W, Wang W, Qi X, Wang D, Tang M. The effects of central pro- and anti-inflammatory immune challenges on depressive-like behavior induced by chronic forced swim stress in rats. Behav Brain Res. 2013;247: 232–40.
35. Maes M, Song C, Yirmiya R. Targeting IL-1 in depression. Expert Opin Ther Targets. 2012;16:1097–112.
36. Neis VB, Manosso LM, Moretti M, Freitas AE, Daufenbach J, Rodrigues ALS. Depressive-like behavior induced by tumor necrosis factor-α is abolished by agmatine administration. Behav Brain Res. 2014;261:336–44.
37. Mesquita AR, Correia-Neves M, Roque S, Castro AG, Vieira P, Pedrosa J, Palha JA, Sousa N. IL-10 modulates depressive-like behavior. J Psychiatr Res. 2008; 43:89–97.
38. Blume J, Douglas SD, Evans DL. Immune suppression and immune activation in depression. Brain Behav Immun. 2011;25:221–9.
39. Vachon P, Millecamps M, Low L, Thompsosn SJ, Pailleux F, Beaudry F, Bushnell CM, Stone LS. Alleviation of chronic neuropathic pain by environmental enrichment in mice well after the establishment of chronic pain. Behav Brain Funct. 2013;9:22.
40. Ross JL, Queme LF, Lamb JE, Green KJ, Ford ZK, Jankowski MP. Interleukin 1β inhibition contributes to the antinociceptive effects of voluntary exercise on ischemia/reperfusion-induced hypersensitivity. Pain. 2018;159:380–92.
41. Wegner M, Helmich I, Machado S, Nardi AE, Arias-Carrion O, Budde H. Effects of exercise on anxiety and depression disorders: review of meta-analyses and neurobiological mechanisms. CNS Neurol Disord Drug Targets. 2014;13:1002–14.
42. Carter T, Morres ID, Meade O, Callaghan P. The effect of exercise on depressive symptoms in adolescents: a systematic review and meta-analysis. J Am Acad Child Adolesc Psychiatry. 2016;55:580–90.
43. Svensson M, Lexell J, Deierborg T. Effects of physical exercise on neuroinflammation, neuroplasticity, neurodegeneration, and behavior: what we can learn from animal models in clinical settings. Neurorehabil Neural Repair. 2015;29:577–89.
44. Jurgens HA, Johnson RW. Environmental enrichment attenuates hippocampal neuroinflammation and improves cognitive function during influenza infection. Brain Behav Immun. 2012;26:1006–16.
45. Dantzer R, O'Connor JC, Freund GG, Johnson RW, Kelley KW. From inflammation to sickness and depression: when the immune system subjugates the brain. Nat Rev Neurosci. 2008;9:46–56.
46. Koss WA, Belden CE, Hristov AD, Juraska JM. Dendritic remodeling in the adolescent medial prefrontal cortex and the basolateral amygdala of male and female rats. Synapse. 2014;68:61–72.
47. Vialou V, Bagot RC, Cahill ME, Ferguson D, Robison AJ, Dietz DM, Fallon B, Mazei-Robison M, Ku SM, Harrigan E, Winstanley CA, Joshi T, Feng J, Berton O, Nestler EJ. Prefrontal cortical circuit for depression- and anxiety-related behaviors mediated by cholecystokinin: role of DeltaFosB. J Neurosci. 2014; 34:3878–87.
48. Chen J, Song Y, Yang J, Zhang Y, Zhao P, Zhu XJ, Su HC. The contribution of TNF-alpha in the amygdala to anxiety in mice with persistent inflammatory pain. Neurosci Lett. 2013;541:275–80.
49. O'Leary OF, Cryan JF. A ventral view on antidepressant action: roles for adult hippocampal neurogenesis along the dorsoventral axis. Trends Pharmacol Sci. 2014;35:675–87.
50. Pentkowski NS, Blanchard DC, Lever C, Litvin Y, Blanchard RJ. Effects of lesions to the dorsal and ventral hippocampus on defensive behaviors in rats. Eur J Neurosci. 2006;23:2185–96.
51. Kjelstrup KG, Tuvnes FA, Steffenach HA, Murison R, Moser EI, Moser MB. Reduced fear expression after lesions of the ventral hippocampus. Proc Natl Acad Sci U S A. 2002;99:10825–30.
52. Sorge RE, Mapplebeck JCS, Rosen S, Beggs S, Taves S, Alexander JK, Martin LJ, Austin J, Sotocinal SG, Chen D, Yang M, Shi XQ, Huang H, Pillon NJ, Bilan PJ, Tu Y, Klip A, Ji R, Zhang J, Salter MW, Mogil JS. Different immune cells mediate mechanical pain hypersensitivity in male and female mice. Nat Neurosci. 2015;18:1081–3.
53. Nemeth CL, Reddy R, Bekhbat M, Bailey J, Neigh GN. Microglial activation occurs in the absence of anxiety-like behavior following microembolic stroke in female, but not male, rats. J Neuroinflammation. 2014;11:174.
54. Pyter LM, Kelly SD, Harrell CS, Neigh GN. Sex differences in the effects of adolescent stress on adult brain inflammatory markers in rats. Brain Behav Immun. 2013;30:88–94.
55. Ramsey JM, Cooper JD, Bot M, Guest PC, Lamers F, Weickert CS, Penninx BW, Bahn S. Sex differences in serum markers of major depressive disorder in the Netherlands study of depression and anxiety (NESDA). PLoS One. 2016;11:e156624.

Temporal changes in macrophage phenotype after peripheral nerve injury

Joy E. Tomlinson[1], Emilija Žygelytė[1], Jennifer K. Grenier[1], Michael G. Edwards[2] and Jonathan Cheetham[1*]

Abstract

Background: Macrophages play a key role in peripheral nerve repair and demonstrate complex phenotypes that are highly dependent on microenvironmental cues.

Methods: We determined temporal changes in macrophage gene expression over time using RNA sequencing after fluorescence-activated cell sorting (FACS) macrophage populations from injured peripheral nerve. We identified key upstream regulators and dominant pathways using ingenuity pathway analysis and confirmed these changes with NanoString technology. We then investigate the effects of extreme polarizers of macrophage phenotype (IL4 and IFNγ) on nerve regeneration. We determined macrophage gene expression in vivo at the site of peripheral nerve injury with NanoString technology, and assessed recovery from sciatic nerve injury by cranial tibial muscle weights and retrograde labeling motor neurons in mice with deletion of IL4 or IFNγ receptors.

Results: We demonstrate that IL4R and IFNγR deletions provide complementary responses to polarization, and alter expression of genes associated with angiogenesis and axonal extension, but do not influence recovery from peripheral nerve transection at 8 weeks after repair.

Conclusions: Overall, this study provides a framework to evaluate the phenotype of macrophages over time, and provides a broader and more precise assessment of gene expression changes than has previously been commonly used. This data suggests ways in which polarization may be modulated to improve repair.

Keywords: Macrophage, Gene expression, Nerve injury, Regeneration

Background

Macrophages play a wide range of roles during adaptive and innate immunity and can be detected in almost all tissues in the body. They are intimately involved in the processes of homeostasis, tissue repair, and regeneration [1]. The macrophage response to tissue injury is highly plastic and heavily dependent on microenvironmental cues which generate a spectrum of heterogeneous macrophage sub-populations, phenotypes, and functions. In the context of peripheral nerve injury, macrophages play a crucial role in the orchestration of series of events which are essential for successful regeneration and functional recovery to occur [2–5].

In the first 3 days after peripheral nerve injury, resident macrophages and Schwann cells (SC) remove fragmented axonal segments and breakdown the nerve–blood barrier [6]. Denervated SC then recruit hematogenous macrophages to the site of repair [7, 8]. Macrophage accumulation peaks 3 to 7 days after injury [9–12], and these infiltrating monocyte-derived cells encourage proliferation of SC [13], which fail to proliferate and transdifferentiate when migrating macrophages are excluded from the site of injury [10, 14]. Macrophages are the major cell type in the first few days after injury and secrete vascular endothelial growth factor (VEGF-A) which promotes development of the polarized microvasculature that directs SC migration within the regenerative bridge [9]. These data suggest that axonal regrowth, and so functional recovery, is heavily dependent upon the host immune response to nerve injury.

Initial classification of macrophage phenotype was based on extreme polarization states induced by in vitro ligands including interferon gamma (IFNɣ, "M1," classical activation) [15, 16], and IL4 [15, 17–19] and IL10 ("M2," alternative activation) [20, 21]. Extension of this

* Correspondence: jc485@cornell.edu
[1]Cornell University College of Veterinary Medicine, Ithaca, NY, USA
Full list of author information is available at the end of the article

system to an in vivo context has been problematic and has allowed overemphasis of a small number of markers to describe a complex spectrum of macrophage activation [15, 22]. Additionally, prior work has predominantly characterized macrophage phenotype in each experimental context using small numbers of markers [23–31]. Because in vivo macrophage phenotype is not dichotomous, conclusions drawn from studies that rely on a few markers of phenotype are likely to be highly dependent on which markers are chosen. Macrophages can have intermediate phenotypes and often show co-expression of classic M1 or M2 markers. For example, tumor-associated macrophages are often described as M2-like but they also have expression of many interferon stimulated genes [15, 32–34]. In peripheral nerve injury, a predominantly anti-inflammatory phenotype has been identified by gene expression of injured nerve stumps [35].

In this study, we characterize the temporal profile of macrophage gene expression during the early, mid, and late phases of macrophage response at the nerve injury site and identify changes in pathways associated with control of macrophage phenotype, angiogenesis, and cell migration.

We then determine differences in the global immune response to inflammation across a range of transgenic mice selected to capture extremes of macrophage polarization and identify changes in genes associated with angiogenesis and axon extension following polarization to these extremes. We then identify alterations in growth factor and neurotrophin expression associated with alterations in macrophage phenotype and evaluate the effects of macrophage polarization in vivo.

Methods

Animals

The following mouse strains were obtained from Jackson Laboratories: C57BL/6J (Jax # 664), BALBc/J (Jax# 651), *Il4ra*$^{-/-}$ (BALB/c-*Il4ra*^{tm1Sz}/J, Jax# 3514), *Ifngr1*$^{-/-}$ (B6.129S7-*Ifngr1*^{tm1Agt}/J, Jax# 3288), and *Il10rb*$^{-/-}$ (B6.129S2-*Il10rb*^{tm1Agt}/J, Jax# 5027). Mice with myeloid-specific deletion of Interferon gamma receptor 1 (IFNγR1) were generated by crossing mice with a conditional deletion for IFNγR1 (C57BL/6N-Ifngr1$^{tm1.1Rds}$/J, Jax #015859) with myeloid-specific cre transgenic mice (Lys2cre, B6.129P2-*Lyz2*$^{tm1(cre)Ifo}$/J, Jax #004781) and then backcrossing to produce mice homozygous for the floxed IFNγR1 and cre-positive in myeloid cells. The efficacy of the myeloid-specific Cre mice (Lys2cre, Jax #004781) was verified using R26r LacZ reporter mice (B6.129S4Gt(ROSA)26Sortm1Sor/J, Jax #3474). When crossed with the Lys2cre mouse, the STOP codon was excised in macrophages and lacZ was expressed. This was detected via a colorimetric assay resulting in blue coloration in the presence of β-galactosidase. LacZ localization was compared to CD68 (macrophage marker) by immunohistochemistry and expression in bone marrow-derived macrophages (BMDM), and macrophages in the intestine, dermis, and spleen was confirmed. Mice were bred in house in stable colonies, and genotypes were confirmed by PCR (Transnetyx, Cordova, TN).

Animals were allowed to acclimatize for 3 days after being brought into the research unit prior to any procedure. Rodent cages were replaced weekly. Animals were on a 12/12-h light-dark cycle and allowed food and water ad libitum. Group housing of 2–5 mice provided socialization. Daily record logs of medical procedures were maintained.

This study was performed in accordance with the Public Health Service Policy on Humane Care and Use of Laboratory Animals, the NIH guide for Care and Use of Laboratory Animals, federal and state regulations, and was approved by the Cornell University Institutional Animal Care and Use Committee.

Sepsis model

LPS injection

Mice (n = 10–17/strain; mean age 12 weeks, range 8–18 weeks; mean weight 23 g, range 15–27 g; both sexes) were administered 50 mg/kg LPS (*Escherichia coli* O111:B4, Santa Cruz Biotechnology, Dallas, TX) diluted in 300 μl sterile saline via i.p. injection between 1 and 2 am. Animals were maintained under their normal housing conditions and were observed hourly for 48 h. Observers were blinded to mouse strain. Mice were euthanized at a humane endpoint of loss of self-righting reflex [36]. Time of death or euthanasia was recorded for each animal. Survival analysis (Gehan–Breslow--Wilcoxon) was performed using GraphPad Prism (GraphPad Software, v6).

Bone marrow-derived macrophage (BMDM) culture

Culture

Culture was performed in two groups temporally: *Ifngr1*$^{-/-}$, *Il10rb*$^{-/-}$, and C57BL/6J; and *Il4ra*$^{-/-}$ and BALB/cJ. Animals (n = 5/strain; mean age 6 weeks, range 5–8 weeks; female) were euthanized by CO_2 asphyxiation, and bone marrow was harvested from the left tibia and femur. For each mouse, 5×10^5 cells were seeded onto 100-mm sterile non-tissue culture-treated polystyrene petri dishes (Falcon) with 12 mL R10 cell culture medium [RPMI 1640 (Corning) with 10% FBS (ThermoFisher), 1% penicillin/streptomycin (ThermoFisher), and 1% HEPES (Sigma Aldrich)]. Cells were stimulated to differentiate into macrophages with 10 ng/mL M-CSF (eBioscience). Cells were cultured at 37°C and 5% CO_2 for 6 days and were fed every third day. On days 6 and 7 of culture, R10+M-CSF media was refreshed for all samples. M(IFNγ+LPS) cells were stimulated with 50 ng/ml IFNγ (eBioscience) on day 6 and with 50 ng/ml IFNγ +

100 ng/ml LPS (Sigma-Aldrich) on day 7. M(IL4) macrophages were stimulated with 50 ng/ml IL-4 (BD Biosciences) on day 7. Cells were harvested on day 8.

Cultured macrophage harvest

Culture media was replaced with 10 ml PBS and plates incubated at 37 °C for 30 min. PBS was triturated vigorously and collected into a 50-mL conical for a total of three washes of 10 ml each. Cells were centrifuged for 10 min at 300 g and resuspended in 200 μl of 0.1% BSA in PBS. Cells were counted on a hemacytometer. 1.5 × 10^6 cells from each sample were transferred to a v-bottom, 96-well plate (ThermoFisher Scientific) for flow cytometric labeling and analysis.

Flow cytometric analysis

Cultured cells were first labeled with Zombie Aqua fixable viability marker for 15 min at room temperature. Washing steps were performed with 150 μl PBS. Cells were incubated with surface markers for 45 min at 4 °C; washing steps were performed with 0.1% BSA in PBS. Dilutions were determined by titration. Cultured BMDM were labeled with anti-CD11b and CD16/32 antibodies to confirm successful differentiation to macrophages (Table 1). Cells were then fixed and permeabilized with Cytofix/Cytoperm (BD Biosciences) for 20 min at 4 °C. Once fixed, cells were incubated with antibodies to the intracellular markers arginase (Arg1) and nitric oxide synthase (Nos2) for 60 min at 4 °C (Table 1). The remaining wash steps were performed with 1× Perm/Wash (BD Biosciences) in DI water. After staining, cells were resuspended in 0.1% BSA in PBS for analysis.

The stained cells were analyzed by FACSAriaIII (BD Biosciences) using FACSDiva software (BD Biosciences), and final analysis was performed with FlowJo software (Tree Star, v10). The fluorochromes were excited with the instrument's 405, 488, 532, and 633 nm lasers. The appropriate detection filters were used (Additional file 1: Table S1). Compensation beads (OneComp, eBioscience) were used to set the compensation matrix. Fluorescence was determined by gating against appropriate controls (unstained, fluorescence minus one) on samples prepared in parallel. Gates were set such that less than 1% positive events were recorded when acquiring the corresponding negative control. Cells were gated on forward and side scatter area for general cell size, forward scatter height and width to exclude doublets, and side scatter and Zombie Aqua to exclude dead cells. Cultured macrophages were defined as all viable single cells that were $CD11b^+CD16/32^+$ (Additional file 2: Figure S1b).

Nerve injury model

Nerve injury

To identify changes in macrophage gene expression over time, the left sciatic nerves of BALB/cJ mice were transected proximal to the bifurcation and immediately repaired. Mice were anesthetized with 3% isoflurane and maintained under anesthesia with 2% isoflurane and oxygen. Analgesia was provided by subcutaneous meloxicam (4 mg/kg) injection pre-operatively and 24 h after surgery. The sciatic nerve was exposed and transected.

Table 1 Antibodies used for flow cytometric analysis of cultured bone marrow-derived macrophages and for sorting macrophages from injured sciatic nerve

Antibody/probe	Clone	Fluorophore	Distributor/Cat No.	Specificity
CD16/32	2.4G2	BV-605	BD Biosciences/563006	Pan macrophage
F4/80	BM8	PE-Cy7	eBioscience/25-4801	Pan macrophage
CD11b	M1/70	Pacific Blue	BioLegend/101224	Pan macrophage
CD14	Sa2-8	PE	eBioscience/12-0141	Pan macrophage
Arg1		PE	R&D Systems/IC5868P	M2
Nos2	CXNFT	APC	eBioscience/17-5920	M1
Thy1.2	53-2.1	APC	eBioscience/17-0902	Fibroblast
CD19	ID3	APC	eBioscience/17-0193	Pan B cell
Ly6G	1A8-Ly6g	APC	eBioscience/17-9668	Granulocyte
Siglec F	ES22-10D8	APC	Miltenyi Biotec/130-102-241	Eosinophil
Ter119	Ter119	APC	eBioscience/17-5921	RBC
CD31	MEC 13.3	APC	BD Biosciences/551262	Endothelial cell
CD3e	17A2	APC	eBioscience/17-0032	T cell
Propidium iodide		na	eBioscience/00-6990	Dead cell/DNA
Zombie Aqua		na	BioLegend/423101	Fixable viability marker

na not available

Proximal and distal nerve stumps were aligned and sutured 1 mm into 5 mm nerve conduits with 10–0 suture (Ethilon) to create a non-critical defect (3 mm). For retrograde labeling of *Ifngr1* $^{fl/fl,\ cre/-}$ and control mice, the sciatic nerve was repaired by direct coaptation with two epineurial sutures.

Macrophage isolation from regenerative bridges and RNA extraction

Mice were euthanized at 3, 5, 14, or 28 days after repair to describe the early, mid, and late immune responses to nerve injury. The regenerative bridge was harvested within the conduit by transecting the proximal and distal sciatic nerve stumps 1 mm from the end of the 5 mm conduit. The epineurial sutures were cut and the regenerative bridge was removed from the conduit and placed in a petri dish with 1 mL RPMI-1640 (Corning) and was cut into 1 mm pieces. The tissues were then transferred to a 50-mL conical with 10 mL of digestion buffer. Digestion buffer comprised of 3 mg/mL collagenase type I (Sigma), 1 mg/mL hyaluronidase (Sigma), and 0.5 mL of 1 mM HEPES in RPMI-1640. After 1 h digestion in a 37 °C water bath, tissues were strained through a 70-µm mesh strainer (BD Biosciences) to obtain a single-cell suspension. Cells were centrifuged at 300 g for 10 min and resuspended in 1 mL red blood cell lysis buffer (eBioscience) for 10 min on ice then quenched with 5 mL DPBS and centrifuged again at 300 g for 10 min. The cell pellet was resuspended in 0.5% BSA (Sigma) in PBS, and cells were plated on a v-bottom 96-well plate (Nunc, Thermo Scientific) for FACS. Cells were labeled for FACS for 45 min at 4 °C using species-specific antibodies to label macrophages and other immune cells. Exclusion markers included Ly6G (granulocytes), Siglec F (eosinophils), CD19 (B lymphocytes), CD3e (T lymphocytes), Ter119 (RBC), and Thy1.2 (fibroblasts). Positive selection markers for macrophages included CD16/32, CD11b, CD14, and F4/80. Antibody details are provided in Table 1. All wash steps were performed with 0.5% BSA in PBS. Following sorting, aliquots of up to 2.0×10^5 cells were placed into RNase/DNase-free 1.5-ml tubes (Eppendorf). RNA was purified according to the manufacturer's instructions using the Quick-RNA MicroPrep kit (Zymo Research).

RNA sequencing

RNA sample quality was confirmed by spectrophotometry (Nanodrop) to determine concentration and chemical purity (A260/230 and A260/280 ratios) and with a Fragment Analyzer (Advanced Analytical) to determine RNA integrity. PolyA+RNA were isolated with the NEBNext Poly(A) mRNA Magnetic Isolation Module (New England Biolabs). TruSeq-barcoded RNA sequencing (RNASeq) libraries were generated with the NEBNext Ultra RNA Library Prep Kit (New England Biolabs). Each library was quantified with a Qubit 2.0 (dsDNA HS kit; Thermo Fisher) and the size distribution determined with a Fragment Analyzer (Advanced Analytical) prior to pooling. Libraries were sequenced on an Illumina NextSeq500. At least 20 M single-end 75+bp reads were generated per library. Reads were trimmed for low quality and adaptor sequences with cutadapt v1.8. parameters: -m 20 -q 20 –a AGATCGGAAGAGCACACGTCTGAACTCCAG –match-read-wildcards. Reads were mapped to the reference genome/transcriptome (Mouse: UCSC mm10) using tophat v2.0 with the following parameters: –no-novel--juncs -G <ref_genes.gtf>. Cufflinks v2.2 was used to generate FPKM values and statistical analysis of differential gene expression. In addition to statistical significance as determined by cuffdiff, the set of stringent-differentially expressed (stringent-DE) genes also had minimum two-fold expression change and minimum average FPKM 5 in at least one condition. Hierarchical clustering was performed using JMP Pro 11 software (SAS Institute Inc., Cary, NC) on log2-fold change values.

Gene expression analysis with NanoString

Extracted RNA was incubated with a custom panel of 90 (for in vivo samples) or 114 (for in vitro samples) bar-coded probes (NanoString Technologies, Seattle, WA; Additional file 3: Table S2) specific for genes associated with macrophage phenotype and function with an emphasis on the context of peripheral nerve repair [1, 17, 37–42]. Four to five biological replicates per condition were evaluated (Molecular Biology Core Facility at Geisel School of Medicine at Dartmouth, Hanover, NH). RNA quality was evaluated with a fragment analyzer and degraded samples were replaced with an alternative sample if available. Standard NanoString protocols were followed [43, 44]. Reporter probes, hybridization solution, sample, and capture probes were mixed together and hybridized overnight at 65 °C. Following hybridization, samples were transferred and processed in the NanoString nCounter Prep Station. The Prep Station washed away excess probes and purified the target/probe complexes using magnetic beads. The purified target/probe complexes were deposited in a cartridge, laid flat, and immobilized for data collection. Data collection was carried out in the NanoString nCounter Digital Analyzer. Images were processed, and the barcodes were tabulated.

Effects of Il4ra and Ifngr1 deletion on macrophage gene expression and nerve regeneration

Sciatic nerve transection and repair was performed in *Il4ra*$^{-/-}$, *Ifngr1*$^{-/-}$, *Ifngr1*$^{fl/fl\ cre/-}$, and control mice as described above. Macrophages were isolated from *Il4ra*$^{-/-}$

and *Ifngr1*$^{-/-}$ by FACS 3, 5 and 14 days after injury. Gene expression was determined using the custom NanoString panel. To determine the quality of repair, retrograde labeling was performed in a separate cohort of *Il4ra*$^{-/-}$ and *Ifngr1*$^{fl/fl\ cre/-}$ mice and their controls at 8 weeks after injury as previously described [45]. Briefly, mice were anesthetized and the sciatic nerve was transected 5 mm distal to the repair site. The nerve stump was soaked in 10% FluoroRuby in 2% DMSO for 1 h, rinsed, and replaced under the biceps femoris muscle. Mice were sacrificed 5 days later, perfused with chilled saline followed by 4% paraformaldehyde, and the spinal cord was harvested 5 mm cranial and 5 mm caudal to the L4-S3 region, which encompassed all retrograde labeled motor neurons. Explanted cords were fixed in 4% paraformaldehyde overnight and optically cleared with increasing concentrations of tetrahydrofuran followed by dichloromethane, and finally dibenzyl ether. [45] Spinal cords were imaged at 10× magnification with 6.4 μm z-stacks using a confocal microscope (Zeiss 510, Thornwood, NY; 561 nm). The entire motor neuron pool of all labeled cells was counted by a single-blinded observer using a customized automated cell counting program in Matlab (Release 2015a, The MathWorks, inc., Natick, MA) based on 3D Laplacian Gaussian object detection. Cranial tibial muscle weights were performed on the cohort of *Il4ra*$^{-/-}$ and *Ifngr1*$^{fl/fl\ cre/-}$ mice that underwent retrograde tracing 8 weeks after injury and repair as previously described. The cranial tibial muscles were removed prior to perfusion and weighed immediately. Cranial tibial muscle weights of the injured limb were standardized to the contralateral limb.

Statistical analysis

Median fluorescent intensity (MFI)

MFI of each marker in the macrophage gate for each mouse was obtained from FlowJo (Tree star, v10). For cell culture, 4 markers (Nos2, Arg1, CD16/32, and CD11b) and 3 stimulation conditions [M(–), M(IL4), M(IFNγ+LPS)] were examined. The MFI of each marker was analyzed by linear mixed effect model on rank transformed data with mouse as a random effect and an interaction term (strain*stimulation) to determine which markers showed significant variation. Rank transformation was used due to non-homogeneity of variance and the presence of a few negative MFI values, which prevented use of log transformation. Tukey post hoc pairwise comparisons were applied.

Gene expression with NanoString

NanoString nSolver 2.6 Analysis Software (NanoString Technologies) was used to process raw data. Background was calculated from the raw data for each group (strain and stimulation) as the average mRNA count across all negative controls plus twice the standard deviation of the negative controls. Genes with average expression in all groups below background expression were removed from analysis. Eight potential housekeeping genes were included on the panel. Data was normalized using the housekeeping genes Actb, ANKRD27, GAPDH, TBP, and RICTOR, which were expressed in all samples and had < 60% CV. Normalized data were analyzed. Statistical analysis was performed separately by culture group, as described above, to allow for potential differences in cytokine and serum lots.

Hierarchical clustering was performed using JMP Pro 12 software (SAS Institute Inc., Cary, NC) on log transformed data to visualize gene expression patterns by strain and stimulation. ANOVA of a linear mixed effect model with mouse as a random effect and an interaction term of strain*stimulation, followed by Benjamini and Hochberg false discovery rate (FDR) correction was performed using R (R 3.2.3, RStudio Team (2015). RStudio: Integrated Development for R. RStudio, Inc., Boston, MA URL http://www.rstudio.com/) to determine which genes showed significant variation. For genes that passed FDR screening on the interaction term (FDR p value < 0.05), Tukey post hoc pairwise comparison was performed to examine expression differences in individual genes among the strains and stimulations. Log transformation was used to meet the assumptions of the test. Significance was set as $p < 0.05$ throughout.

Bioinformatics analysis

DE transcripts between time points were analyzed for over-representation of biological functions, pathways, and networks using the bioinformatics software ingenuity pathways analysis (IPA) (www.ingenuity.com) [46, 47]. IPA uses a Fisher's exact test to identify over-represented connected biological units in a defined set of genes, which can include pathways, cellular functions, or known targets of regulatory genes. In some cases a confidence score, or z score, can be made on the activation state of the pathway, process, or upstream regulator based on the expression pattern of the associated genes [46]. The more positive or negative the z score, the more confidence the platform has that the pathway, biological process, or upstream regulator is activated or inhibited respectively.

Results

Temporal analysis of macrophage gene expression at the site of nerve injury in wild-type mice demonstrates complex phenotypes

To investigate the range of macrophage phenotypes expressed at the site of nerve injury, we first analyzed temporal changes in macrophage gene expression after sciatic nerve injury in wild-type mice. Macrophages were isolated from the regenerative bridge within the conduit by flow cytometry ($Lin^{-}F4/80^{+}CD14^{+}CD11b^{+}CD16/32^{+}$, Additional file 2: Figure S1) 5, 14, and 28 days after sciatic transection and repair.

Gene expression was quantified with RNASeq and compared pairwise between the time points, and 382 genes met the stringent DE cutoff in at least one time point comparison. Unsupervised hierarchical clustering on differential gene expression and Panther gene ontogeny database (overrepresentation test, release 20160321) identified six clusters associated with common biological functions including macrophage activation, coagulation, immune response, cell communication, cell proliferation and cytokine receptor binding (Fig. 1a). Retnla was in cluster 1 and increased over time from day 5 to day 14, whereas other markers of alternative activation, such as Argl and Chi3l3, were in cluster 4 and decreased in this time period. This emphasizes the complexity of macrophage phenotype and need to include a variety of markers to accurately describe macrophage phenotype and function. DE genes between time points (d5 vs 14; d14 vs 28) were then analyzed for over-representation of biological functions, pathways, and networks using Downstream Effects Analysis through IPA to identify those biological processes and functions that are likely to be causally affected by up- and downregulated genes [46, 47]. IPA identified LPS, IFNɣ, TNF, STAT3, and IL4 as key upstream regulators of changes in macrophage polarization over time, and identified key pathways including granulocyte and agranulocyte adhesion and diapedesis, angiogenesis and dendritic cell maturation (Fig. 1b, c).

RNASeq and NanoString data demonstrate mixed temporal expression of pro- and anti-inflammatory genes and are in agreement

We designed a custom NanoString gene expression panel, including a subset of 90 genes that were highly differentially expressed in the RNASeq data, to confirm these RNASeq findings. The NanoString platform has high reproducibility, sensitivity, and is associated with a low background signal [43, 44]. Genes were selected that describe macrophage phenotype, function, and signaling,

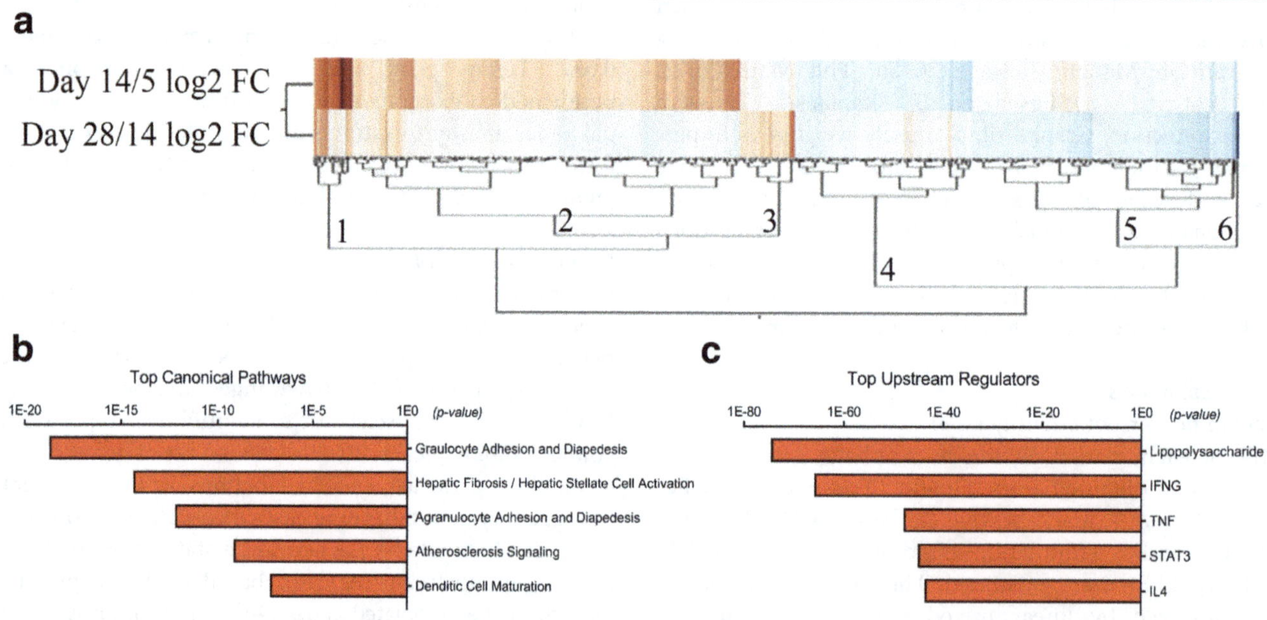

Fig. 1 IFNɣ and IL4 are key upstream regulators of macrophage gene expression in injured nerve. **a** Unsupervised hierarchical clustering on differential gene expression over time identified six clusters of genes. The PANTHER GO database overrepresentation test was performed. Cluster 1 was unclassified, but contained the macrophage alternative activation marker Retnla, which increased from days 5 to 14 (red). Cluster 2 was enriched for the common biological functions of coagulation, immune response, and cell communication and included genes Alox15, Jun, and Egr1. Cluster 3 was unclassified and included genes such as Nes and Clu. Cluster 4 was dominated by cell proliferation and cytokine receptor binding, and included Chi3l3, Arg1, Ccl2, Ccl7, and Il1a, which decreased from days 5 to 14 (blue). Cluster 5 was enriched for genes related to macrophage activation and response to IFNɣ, and included Nos2. This pro-inflammatory signature declined over time. The sixth cluster contained only Sct. Red— increased with time; blue—decreased with time. **b** Ingenuity pathway analysis identified key pathways including granulocyte and agranulocyte adhesion and diapedesis, angiogenesis, and dendritic cell maturation. **c** LPS, IFNγ, STAT3, and IL4 were identified as key upstream regulators of changes in macrophage gene expression. Gene expression was compared pairwise between three time points and 382 genes met the stringent differential expression (DE) cutoff in at least one time point comparison. Stringent cutoffs of FPKM > 5 and fold change > 2 were used. RNASeq was performed on sorted macrophages from BALB/cJ mice 5, 14, and 28 days after sciatic nerve transection and repair ($n = 3$/group). Further analysis of differentially expressed (DE) transcripts between time points (days 5 vs 14; days 14 vs 28) were analyzed for over-representation of biological functions, pathways, and networks using Downstream Effects Analysis to identify those biological processes and functions that are likely to be causally affected by up- and downregulated genes, using the bioinformatics software ingenuity pathways analysis (IPA)

with a preference for including pathways where multiple genes were differentially expressed in the RNASeq data. Cell lineage markers for macrophages and other cell types found in injured peripheral nerve were also included to confirm accuracy of cell sorting. Because the initial time course RNASeq data showed greater differences between days 14 and 5 than between 28 and 14, for this experiment we compared early time points of days 3, 5, and 14.

NanoString data demonstrated a high level of agreement with RNASeq data ($R^2 = 0.67$, $p < 0.001$, Fig. 2a). Greater differences were observed between macrophage gene expression at day 14 and day 5 than between day 5 and day 3 (Fig. 2b, c). Macrophage expression of the major monocyte chemokine, monocyte chemoattractant protein (CCL2), was identified early in the repair process (Fig. 2b) [48]. CX3CR1 ligand (fractalkine), which can also recruit monocytes through the CX3CR1 receptor, was identified later [49]. A variety of collagens (1a1, 1a2, and 3a1) were all elevated at day 14 compared to day 5.

While Ydens et al. [30] found no expression of the classical macrophage markers Nos2 and IL-12p40 in whole nerve lysates of the distal nerve stump up to 14 days after axotomy, we found that some IFNγ-regulated (M1) genes, such as Nos2, were initially highly expressed in macrophages isolated from the regenerative bridge and then declined from 5 to 28 days. Retnla expression increased throughout the time course, whereas Chi3l3 and Arg1 decreased from days 5 to 14 and then partially rebounded by day 28.

Ifngr1 or Il4ra deletion profoundly alter survival after endotoxin challenge

Our RNASeq/IPA data identified IFNɣ and IL4 as key regulators of macrophage phenotype in injured peripheral nerve. To further investigate this finding, we selected three mouse strains with global deletions for receptors of cytokines that control macrophage phenotype, namely *Ifngr1*$^{-/-}$, *Il4ra*$^{-/-}$, and *Il10rb*$^{-/-}$, and first characterized their global inflammatory response and macrophage phenotypes. We first used a model of endotoxemia by intraperitoneal LPS injection. Mice with a less pro-inflammatory (Th1/M1) immune response are expected to have longer survival in this model. *Ifngr1* knockout reduces the ability of immune cells to respond one of the major pro-inflammatory cytokines, IFNγ, and therefore was expected to confer resistance to endotoxin. In contrast, mice with a stronger pro-inflammatory response or less ability to modulate that response should succumb more quickly. IL4 and IL10 are essential to regulate inflammation, and their knockout strains were, therefore, expected to be more susceptible to endotoxin. The strains performed as expected, with *Ifngr1*$^{-/-}$ mice demonstrating longer survival ($p = 0.046$) and *Il10rb*$^{-/-}$ ($p < 0.0001$) and *Il4ra*$^{-/-}$ ($p = 0.014$) having shorter survival than their background strains (Fig. 3, Additional file 4: Table S3). Additionally, BALB/cJ are known to have a more Th2 biased immune response than C57BL/6J [15, 50–52], so these mice were expected to have better survival than C57BL/6J. The difference in immune phenotype between BALB/cJ and C57BL/6J was expected to be less than that between the three knockout strains and their controls; however, it was enough to detect a difference in survival in this model, with BALB/cJ surviving longer ($p = 0.031$), as anticipated. No differences between sexes were observed.

Ifngr1 and Il4ra deletions provide complementary alterations in macrophage phenotype in response to in vitro polarization

The majority of macrophages involved in peripheral nerve repair are monocyte-derived (circulating)

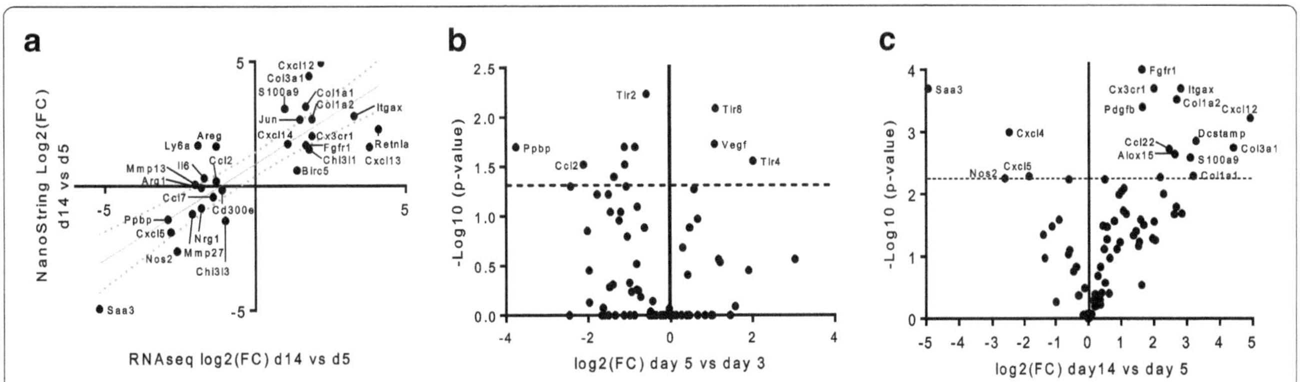

Fig. 2 RNASeq and NanoString data demonstrate mixed expression of pro-inflammatory and anti-inflammatory genes over time. **a** Scatter plot of log2 fold changes between day 5 and 14 in macrophage gene expression detected by RNASeq (FPKM > 5) and NanoString panel. Linear regression and 95% CI are shown. **b**, **c** Differences in gene expression on NanoString panel between days 3 and 5, and 5 and 14 expressed as volcano plots. *P* values for NanoString data for 90 genes were obtained from nSolver software, with the false discovery rate (FDR) corrected level of significance (dotted line). Significance set at $p < 0.05$. Macrophages were sorted from sciatic nerves of BALB/cJ mice that were transected and repaired with an empty conduit 3, 5, or 14 days before harvest. Different mice were used for RNASeq and NanoString ($n = 3$ and 5 per time point)

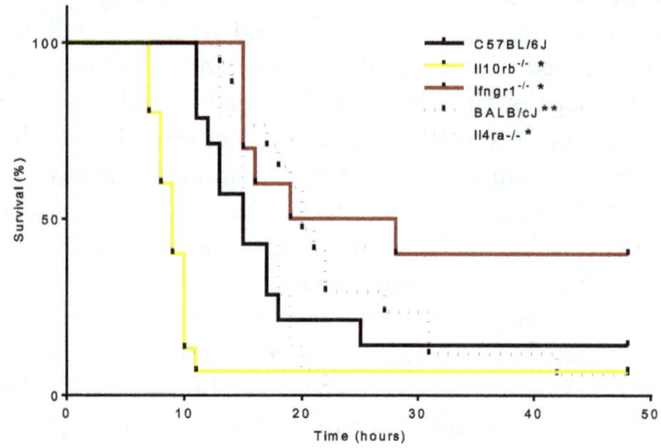

Fig. 3 Global deletion of receptors controlling macrophage phenotype profoundly alters survival after endotoxin challenge. Gehan–Breslow–Wilcoxon survival analysis of mice administered 50 mg/kg LPS i.p. and euthanized at the humane endpoint of loss of self-righting reflex or censored at 48 h if still alive. *Ifngr1*$^{-/-}$ mice demonstrate longer survival ($p = 0.046$) and *Il10rb*$^{-/-}$ ($p < 0.0001$) and *Il4ra*$^{-/-}$ ($p = 0.014$) have a shorter survival than corresponding WT. BALB/cJ survived slightly longer than C57BL/6J ($p = 0.031$). *Il10rb*$^{-/-}$, and *Ifngr1*$^{-/-}$ mice were on a C57BL/6J background; and *Il4ra*$^{-/-}$ on a BALB/cJ background. $N = 10–17$/strain. *Significantly different survival from WT; **significantly different survival between WT strains ($p < 0.05$)

macrophages from the myeloid lineage [53, 54] and the distinct resident population is small [6] and less important [55]. To evaluate the effect of in vitro polarization on myeloid-derived macrophages from *Ifngr1*$^{-/-}$, *Il4ra*$^{-/-}$, and *Il10rb*$^{-/-}$ mice, we polarized BMDM with either IFNγ+LPS or IL4. To evaluate plasticity in macrophage phenotype, we also exposed BMDM to each stimulus sequentially. We use the recently recommended nomenclature for describing in vitro macrophage polarization which is "M(stimulating ligand)." For example, cells polarized with IL4 are identified as M(IL4) instead of M2a. Polarization was confirmed using flow cytometric analysis of the commonly used macrophage phenotype markers, Nos2 (upregulated by IFNγ+LPS) and Arg1 (upregulated by IL4). As expected, expression of Nos2 and Arg1 was reduced in the absence of the receptors for a given ligand (Additional file 5: Figure S2). While CD16/32 has been frequently used as a marker of classical activation [56–59], here, we find that it was more robustly stimulated by M(IL4) than M(IFNγ+LPS) ($p < 0.0001$, Additional file 5: Figure S2). However, *Ifngr1*$^{-/-}$ BMDM showed the most dramatic increase in CD16/32 MFI, suggesting that IFNγ signaling may modulate the effect of LPS on CD16/32 expression. The myeloid lineage marker, CD11b, showed no clear pattern of response to stimulation, with minimal differences between strains.

We then used NanoString gene expression analysis [43, 44] to expand the phenotypic description of these macrophages, because single activation markers provide an incomplete description of macrophage phenotype and because some markers can be expressed in multiple phenotypes. For example, Arg1 is expressed in some M(IFNγ+LPS) cells (Additional file 5: Figure S2a). The panel was designed to include macrophage activation markers across multiple phenotypes.

Low or absent expression of non-macrophage cell lineage markers, including Cd3e (T cells), S100b and Gfap (Schwann cells), Cd19 (B cells), and Thy1.2 (fibroblasts), confirmed the specificity of the sort. Because the panel was designed to focus on markers of activation, M(−) cells were characterized by low expression of the majority of genes in the panel. The following genes were not expressed above background in the *Ifngr1*$^{-/-}$, *Il10rb*$^{-/-}$, and C57BL/6J group: Alox15, Cd19, Ccl1, Ccl11, Ccl17, Ccl20, Egf, Fgf1, Fgf2, Gfap, Il5, Il10, Il23p19, Ly6g, Rtn4r, Ntf3, Ntf5, S100b, Thy1.2, Lama5, and Ngfr. The following genes were not expressed above background in the *Il4ra*$^{-/-}$ and BALBc/J group: Alox15, Bdnf, Cd19, Ccl1, Ccl11, Ccl20, Egf, Fgf2, Gfap, Il5, Il10, Il23p19, Ly6g, Rtn4r, Ntf3, Ntf5, S100b, Thy1.2, Lama5, and Ngfr.

Clustering analysis was performed on the NanoString data by both gene and strain-stimulation (Fig. 4). Specific genes in each cluster are reported in Additional file 6: Table S4. Clustering by strain-stimulation showed that M(−) and M(IL4) gene expression profiles tended to cluster together (row cluster S1, Fig. 4a, b), while M(IFNγ+LPS) formed a distinct cluster (row cluster S2, Fig. 4a, b). For the *Ifngr1*$^{-/-}$, *Il10rb*$^{-/-}$, and C57BL/6J group (Fig. 4a), column clusters 1a–3a represent genes that are highly expressed in M(IL4). Cluster 1a genes, including Cxcl13, Itgam, and Il17a, were also upregulated in *Ifngr1*$^{-/-}$ M(IFNγ + LPS), suggesting they can be upregulated by LPS in the absence of IFNγ signaling. Cluster 2a genes were also highly expressed in M(−) macrophages and included many genes that are commonly associated with a pro-regenerative/M2 phenotype such as Cd163, Mrc1 (a.k.a CD206), and Tgfb (cluster 2a, Fig. 4a). This is consistent with prior reports that macrophages in an adherent culture with M-CSF develop a somewhat M2-like phenotype [60, 61]. Cluster 3a genes were only expressed highly in the M(IL4) group and included M2 phenotype markers such as Chil3 and Retnla. In contrast, clusters 4a and 5a represent genes that were highly expressed in M(IFNγ + LPS). Cluster 4a genes were also upregulated in *Ifngr1*$^{-/-}$ M(IFNγ + LPS) compared to M(−), suggesting LPS alone was adequate to stimulate their expression to some degree. These included Stat1, Il1a, Tnf, Ccr7, Cxcl9, Il12b, Il6, and Nos2. While Ccr7, Cxcl9, Il12b, Il6, and Nos2 were upregulated in *Ifngr1*$^{-/-}$ M(IFNγ + LPS) compared to M(−), it was to a significantly lesser degree than in C57BL/6J and *Il10rb*$^{-/-}$ M(IFNγ + LPS). Cluster 5a genes were not

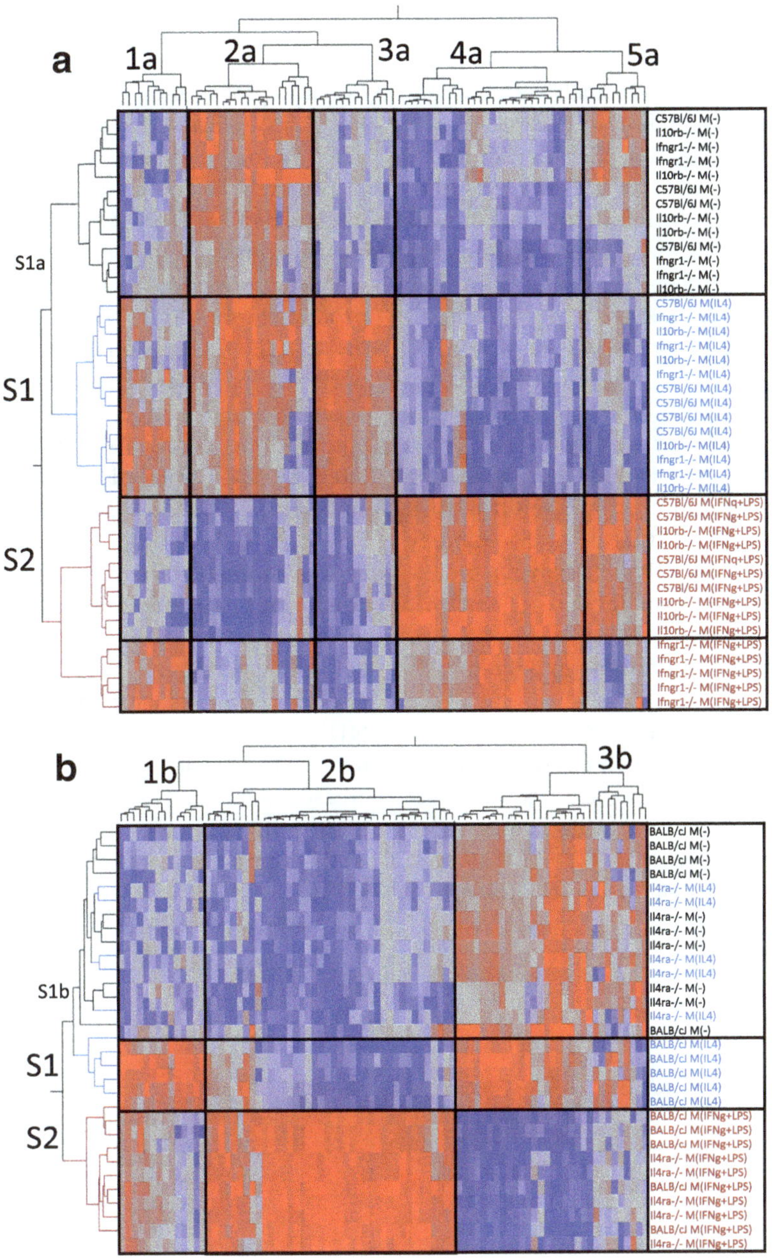

Fig. 4 M(–) BMDM show moderate to high expression of genes that are commonly associated with a pro-regenerative/M2 phenotype. Cluster analysis of log transformed gene expression data from BMDM that were stimulated in vitro with polarizing ligands IL4 or IFNγ+LPS. Three transgenic mouse strains and their background WT strains were compared. Clustering was performed separately by background strain. In both groups, M(–) BMDM expressed many genes that are classically considered pro-regenerative or M2 (**a**, cluster 2; **b**, cluster 3). **a** *Ifngr1*$^{-/-}$ showed a distinct pattern of gene expression after IFNγ+LPS stimulation, but *Il10rb*$^{-/-}$ showed no difference from WT. **b** *Il4ra*$^{-/-}$ did not respond to IL4 stimulation and *Il4ra*$^{-/-}$ M(IL4) clustered with WT M(–). $n = 4$–5/group

upregulated in *Ifngr1*$^{-/-}$ M(IFNγ + LPS), suggesting IFNγ signaling is required for their upregulation. These included Cd86, Stat3, Vegfa, and Cd80. Overall, *Il10rb*$^{-/-}$ showed no difference from wild-type in any polarization condition (Fig. 4a), and *Ifngr1*$^{-/-}$ mice demonstrated reduced expression of pro-inflammatory genes that are stimulated by IFNγ, such as Nos2, Ccr7, Cxcl9, Il12, and Il6, compared to WT after stimulation with IFNγ+LPS, but demonstrated minimal alteration in response to IL4 stimulation compared to WT (Fig. 4a).

For the *Il4ra*$^{-/-}$ and BALB/cJ group (Fig. 4b), cluster 1b represented genes that were highly expressed in WT M(IL4) and expressed to a variable degree in

M(IFNγ+LPS), which largely corresponds to cluster 3a in the *Ifngr1*$^{-/-}$ group (Fig. 4a). Cluster 1b genes included M2 markers such as Arg1, Chil3, and Retnla. Cluster 2b (Fig. 4b) represented genes that were upregulated in M(IFNγ+LPS), corresponding to clusters 4a and 5a in the *Ifngr1*$^{-/-}$ group (Fig. 4a). Cluster 3b represented genes that were expressed in M(−) were either up- or downregulated in WT M(IL4), and were downregulated in M(IFNγ+LPS) (Fig. 4b). These corresponded largely to cluster 2a in the *Ifngr1*$^{-/-}$ group (Fig. 4a). *Il4ra*$^{-/-}$ mice showed no response to IL4 stimulation and *Il4ra*$^{-/-}$ M(IL4) clustered with WT and *Il4ra*$^{-/-}$ M(−) in row cluster S1b (Fig. 4b). *Il4ra*$^{-/-}$ mice had minimal to no alteration in response to IFNγ+LPS stimulation compared to WT (row cluster S2, Fig. 4b).

In summary, mice with Ifngr1 and Il4ra deletions showed orthogonal alterations in macrophage phenotype in response to in vitro polarization (Fig. 5), thereby representing possibly useful models for studying the effects of macrophage polarization on nerve regeneration.

Increased expression of growth factors is not limited to the M(IL4) phenotype

M2-like macrophages are often referred to as pro-regenerative and are associated with improved wound healing and tissue regeneration [1]. This is frequently attributed to increased production of growth factors, especially those regulating angiogenesis [1, 62–67]; however, this is controversial. There is increasing evidence that pro-inflammatory macrophages, which often predominate in early stages of tissue injury and repair [64, 65, 68, 69], are essential for the initiation of angiogenesis and attraction and proliferation of precursor cells required for repair [68–71]. We investigated expression of growth and angiogenic factors known to be important in nerve repair. Approximately half were upregulated by IL4 and half were upregulated by IFNγ+LPS (Fig. 6). We found increased Vegfa expression in M(IFNγ+LPS) which is consistent with many reports that pro-inflammatory macrophages produce more VEGF [69, 70, 72–74]. Reports surrounding PDGFb expression have been conflicting, with reports of both increased expression with alternative activation [69], and, conversely, with pro-inflammatory stimulation [75, 76]. We found PDGFb was downregulated by IL4 stimulation. Major neurotrophic factors, such as IGF1, IGF2, NGF, BDNF, NT-3, and NT-4/5 can be produced by macrophages [77–79] and are greatly upregulated in peripheral nerve injury, often concurrent with the influx of macrophages [80, 81]. We included these factors in our gene expression panel to determine whether IL4 or IFNɣ+LPS stimulation could directly induce macrophages to express neurotrophins. Igf1 was markedly downregulated by IFNɣ+LPS polarization, and Igf2 expression was markedly increased with IL4 stimulation (Fig. 6). Brain-derived neurotrophic factor (BDNF) was increased by IFNɣ+LPS stimulation; whereas hepatocyte growth factor (HGF) was reduced. NGF and CNTF expression was not affected. GDNF, NT3, and NT5 were not

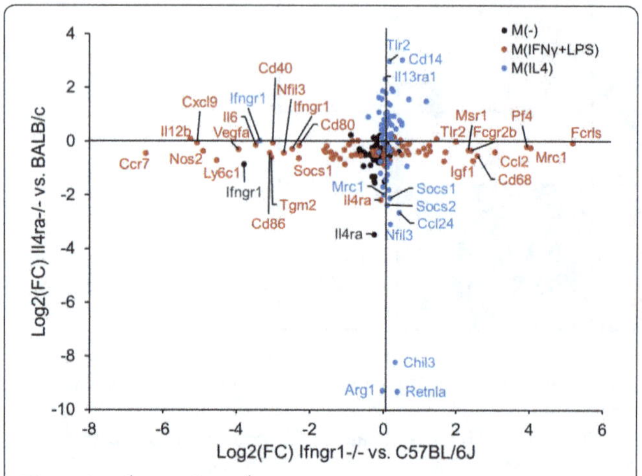

Fig. 5 *Il4ra*$^{-/-}$ and *Ifngr1*$^{-/-}$ provide orthogonal alterations in macrophage phenotype in response to in vitro polarization. Gene expression Log2(fold change) over the control strain for *Il4ra*$^{-/-}$ and *Ifngr1*$^{-/-}$ BMDM under 3 polarization conditions: M(−), M(IL4), and M(IFNγ+LPS). *Ifngr1*$^{-/-}$ macrophages demonstrate reduced expression of pro-inflammatory, or M1, markers compared to wild-type after stimulation with IFNγ+LPS, but have minimal to no alteration in response to IL4 stimulation. *Il4ra*$^{-/-}$ mice have marked reduction in the classical M2 markers Arg1, Chil3, and Retnla after IL4 stimulation, with no difference in response to IFNγ+LPS stimulation. $n = 4–5$/group

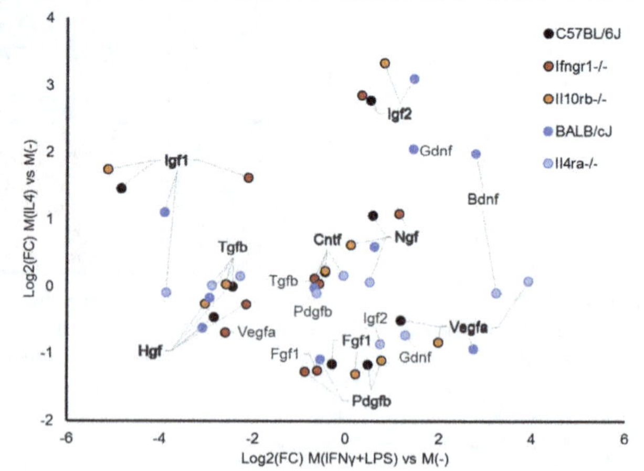

Fig. 6 Macrophage phenotype influences gene expression of neurotrophic and growth factors relevant to peripheral nerve repair. Pro-inflammatory macrophages have higher expression of pro-angiogenic growth factors: Vegfa is consistently upregulated by IFNγ+LPS stimulation, while Pdgfb is downregulated by IL4 stimulation. Insulin-like growth factors, Igf1 and Igf2 are upregulated by IL4. Plot of gene expression Log2(fold change) over the unstimulated M(−) condition for BMDM of 5 strains of mice exposed to IL4 or IFNγ+LPS stimulation. $n = 4–5$/group

consistently expressed above the detection limit of the assay and, when expressed, did not show consistent response to stimulation between the control strains. It is possible that local environmental factors, such as exposure to myelin or oxidized galectin-1, are required to drive more robust expression of some neurotrophic factors [79, 82].

Effect of Il4ra and Ifngr1 deletion on macrophage gene expression and neural regeneration after sciatic nerve transection

Based on the above data, *Ifngr1* and *Il4ra* deleted mouse strains were selected to investigate the effects of macrophage polarization on sciatic nerve regeneration. Sciatic nerves were transected and repaired as before, and macrophages were isolated from the regenerative bridge within the conduit by FACS. Macrophages from $Il4ra^{-/-}$ mice had significantly higher expression of Pak1, part of the VEGF/angiogenesis pathway, at all time points (days 3, 5, and 14) compared to WT controls (Fig. 7a). Effects were more pronounced at earlier time points. Mice with global $Ifngr1^{-/-}$ deletion had significantly lower expression of Col1a2, Cx3cr1, and Pdgfb which are all known to be important in peripheral nerve repair [66, 83, 84]. Effects were more pronounced at day 3 compared with day 5 (Fig. 7b). Overall, the effect of genotype on macrophage gene expression at the site of peripheral nerve injury in vivo was reduced compared to the effect seen in vitro.

The effect of these genotypes on regeneration was examined through retrograde labeling of motor neurons, and through cranial tibial muscle weight at 8 weeks after injury. For this purpose, a myeloid-specific $Ifngr1^{Lys2Cre}$ $_{fl/fl,\ cre/-}$ mouse had been developed and was used. No myeloid specific Il4ra knockout was available at the time and the global knockout was used. Although, some changes in macrophage gene expression had been identified with the global knockouts, myeloid-specific deletion of Ifngr1 and global deletion of Il4ra did not produce significant differences in standardized cranial tibial muscle weights or the number of retrograde-labeled motor neurons 8 weeks after injury (Fig. 8). Myeloid-specific $Ifngr1^{\ fl/fl,\ cre/-}$ were compared to litter-matched $Ifngr1^{fl/fl,-/-}$ controls. No effect of sex was detected.

Discussion

We developed an approach to isolate macrophages from peripheral nerve and characterize temporal changes in gene expression using RNA sequencing confirmed by a digital bar coded panel of 90 genes that are differentially expressed during peripheral nerve repair. We provide the first description of macrophage gene expression over time after nerve injury. RNASeq data and NanoString data showed that IL4 and IFNγ signaling pathways play pivotal roles in macrophage phenotype 5–28 days after nerve injury and that there is an early pro-inflammatory response that declines over time.

The application of causal network analysis (IPA) to RNASeq data from macrophages isolated from injured peripheral nerve allowed identification of changes in key upstream regulators of macrophage phenotype over time including IL4, IFNγ, TNF, and STAT3 [15, 17]. It also identified changes in key pathways over time including granulocyte and agranulocyte adhesion and diapedesis, angiogenesis and dendritic cell maturation. Traditionally, interpretation of high-throughput gene-expression data has been performed using statistical gene-set-enrichment methods where differentially expressed genes are intersected with sets of genes

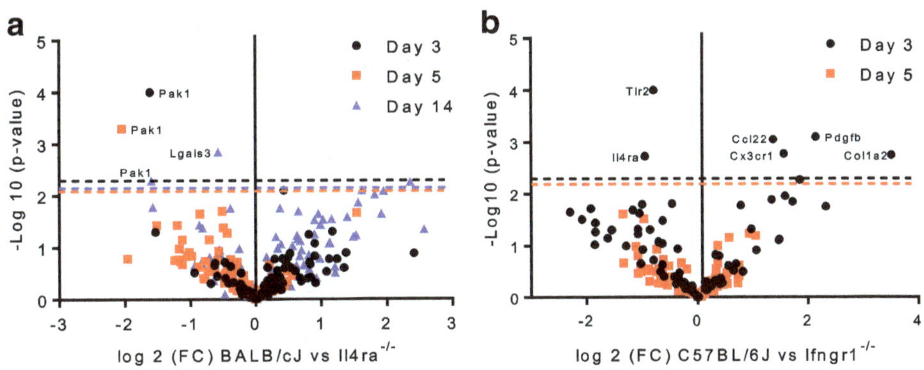

Fig. 7 $Il4ra^{-/-}$ and $Ifngr1^{-/-}$ produce minimal changes in macrophage gene expression in injured nerve. **a** Macrophages from $Il4ra^{-/-}$ mice had significantly higher expression of Pak1, part of the VEGF/angiogenesis pathway, at all time points (days 3, 5, and 14) compared to WT controls. **b** $Ifngr1^{-/-}$ causes reduced expression of Col1a2, Pdgfb and Cx3cr1 (the receptor for fractaline), which are all known to be important in peripheral nerve repair. Volcano plot of NanoString data comparing the fold difference in macrophage gene expression between $Il4ra^{-/-}$ mice and $Ifngr1^{-/-}$ with WT at key time points after sciatic nerve repair. *P* values were obtained from nSolver software, with the false discovery rate corrected level of significance indicated by the horizontal dotted line. Significance set at $p < 0.05$

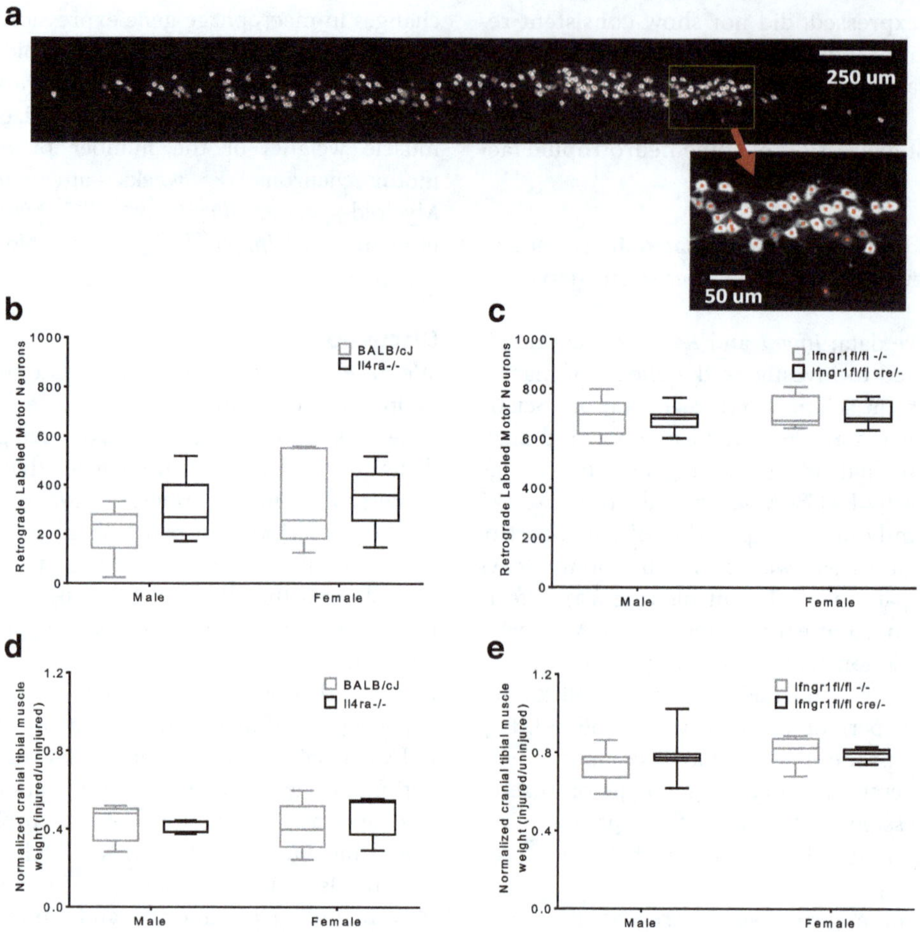

Fig. 8 Deletion of Il4ra or Ifngr1 does not alter the quality of reinnervation. A representative image of a retrograde labeled spinal cord in shown (**a**) with red dots denoting counted cells. The total number of retrograde labeled motor neurons per mouse 8 weeks after sciatic nerve transection and repair are shown (**b**, **c**). Il4ra$^{-/-}$ and control BALB/cJ mice underwent sciatic transection and empty conduit repair with a 3 mm gap (**b**). Ifngr1$^{fl/fl\ cre/-}$ and control mice underwent sciatic transection and direct coaptation (**c**). The cranial tibial muscle weights of the injured limb normalized to the contralateral limb 8 weeks after sciatic nerve transection and repair are shown (**d**, **e**). No differences were detected between strains or sexes. $n = 6$/sex/strain, except male Ifngr1$^{fl/fl\ cre/-}$ and control ($n = 18$ each). ANOVA ($p > 0.05$)

that are associated with a particular biological function or pathway [85]. A more recent approach involves the application of causal networks that integrate previously observed cause–effect relationships reported in the literature. While still depending on statistics, this is more powerful than gene-set enrichment as it leverages knowledge about the direction of effects rather than mere associations [46, 86, 87]. This causal network analysis is based on a large structured collection of observations in various experimental contexts with nearly five million findings manually curated from the biomedical literature or integrated from third-party databases. The network contains ~ 40,000 nodes that represent mammalian genes and their products, chemical compounds, microRNA molecules and biological functions. Nodes are connected by ~ 1,480,000 edges representing experimentally observed cause–effect relationships that relate to expression, transcription, activation, molecular modification, and transport as well as binding events. Network edges are also associated with a direction of the causal effect, i.e., either activating or inhibiting [46].

This study also provides a standardized description of the effects of endotoxin exposure in vivo and macrophage stimulation in vitro across a range of mouse strains commonly used to manipulate macrophage phenotype. This is the first report directly comparing the response of these mouse strains to lethal endotoxin injection. Reported survival times and lethal doses of i.p. endotoxin vary widely [88–97], preventing useful comparison between strains that are not examined concurrently. The reported variability may be partly related to endotoxin preparation and handling, as LPS rapidly binds plastics and the actual dose administered can be less than calculated. All mice used in this experiment were injected with the same batch of endotoxin, prepared simultaneously, and administered in a block randomized pattern, to minimize any variability in endotoxin concentration. This allows accurate comparison of the strains and description of their susceptibility to endotoxemia. In the LPS model of sepsis, there was markedly reduced survival in the *Il10rb*$^{-/-}$ mice, which is consistent with findings in IL10 deficient mice [88], but which has not been previously reported.

Ifngr1$^{-/-}$ and *Il4ra*$^{-/-}$ mice provide complementary alterations in macrophage phenotype that could be useful in studying the effect of macrophages on various pathologic and regenerative processes. As expected, *Ifngr1*$^{-/-}$ mice showed reduced polarization toward an M1-like phenotype when stimulated with IFNγ+LPS. Because this stimulation condition included LPS, the phenotype achieved in these cells was distinct from M(−) as well as from M(IFNγ+LPS) in wild-type mice. These two strains of mice provide non-overlapping alterations in macrophage phenotype that could be useful in studying the biological influence of macrophage phenotype or response to treatment with either cytokine.

In this study, we demonstrate the effect of macrophage polarization on expression of several growth factors known to be important in nerve injury, and show that pro-inflammatory as well as alternatively activated macrophages express these factors. Macrophage depletion has been shown to cause reduced angiogenesis, while exogenous addition of macrophages promotes angiogenesis [66, 98–100]. We show that pro-inflammatory stimulation of macrophages could enhance this effect because Vegfa was consistently increased by IFNγ+LPS stimulation; while Pdgfb was consistently downregulated by IL4 stimulation. Neurotrophins are also crucial to the process of axonal regrowth and have been investigated as therapeutic targets [101–104]. M(IFNγ+LPS) macrophages showed higher expression of Bdnf, while M(IL4) macrophages showed higher expression of Igf1, Igf2, and Hgf than M(IFNγ+LPS) macrophages. Together these data suggest that alteration of macrophage phenotype may offer a therapeutic target mediated by altered angiogenesis or neurotrophin expression.

Despite the promising findings regarding the role of IFNγ and IL4 signaling in peripheral nerve regeneration, we did not find a difference in quality of final regenerative outcome of mice with deletion in receptors for either cytokine. The number of motor neurons that regenerate axons across an injury site is one measure of the quality of regeneration, with greater numbers of regenerated neurons corresponding to improved fine motor control. Cranial tibial muscle weight was used as a proxy for functional recovery, with weights closer to the contralateral limb indicating greater recovery from denervation atrophy. In this study, we evaluated outcome at 8 weeks after injury, at which point mice are often maximally repaired, and we found no difference between the groups. It is possible that differences in rate of regeneration could be observed at earlier time points, or that supraphysiologic addition of exogenous cytokines could have greater effect than receptor deletion models. These are areas for future investigation.

Conclusions

Overall, this study provides a framework to evaluate gene expression in macrophages over time at the site of peripheral nerve injury and defines the effects of specific deletions for genes that control macrophage phenotype in the context of peripheral nerve repair. This methodology provides a broader and more precise assessment of changes in macrophage gene expression at the site of nerve injury than has been previously commonly used. We also specifically assess gene expression in isolated macrophage populations rather than whole nerve lysates. Prior approaches emphasizing a small number of markers to describe a complex spectrum of macrophage activation may lead to differing conclusions dependent on which markers are chosen [15, 22]. For instance, reliance on Retnla vs. Arg1 as single markers would give opposing conclusions regarding the alternative activation status of the macrophages in these in vivo experiments. Assessing changes in macrophage gene expression in an in vivo system is important because manipulations of BMDM in vitro using ligands designed to produce extremes in polarization do not necessarily reflect changes in the context of the extracellular matrix environment and other cell types.

Additional files

Additional file 1: Table S1. Excitation and detection settings for antibodies and conjugates used.

Additional file 2: Figure S1. Sorting strategy for macrophage isolation from injured nerve (a) or cell culture (b). Cells were isolated from regenerative bridges and identified as F4/80+, CD14+, CD16/32+ and CD11b+. Gates for activation markers were set by the fluorescence minus one controls such that < 1% of events were positive.

Additional file 3: Table S2. NanoString gene expression panels for in vitro and in vivo experiments

Additional file 4: Table S3. Survival after intraperitoneal endotoxin injection[1]. 1 Survival times of 5 mouse strains exposed to 50 mg/kg LPS I.P. Gehan–Breslow–Wilcoxon test and Mantel–Haenszel hazard ratios were calculated in GraphPad Prism. *Ifngr1*$^{-/-}$ and *IL10rb*$^{-/-}$ were compared to their background strain C57BL/6J. Il4ra$^{-/-}$ were compared to their background strain, BALB/cJ. C57BL/6J were compared to BALB/cJ.

Additional file 5: Figure S2. In vitro stimulation of BMDM with IFNγ+LPS or IL4 resulted in differentiation into classically activated and alternatively activated macrophage phenotypes, respectively. Cross-polarization, with each stimulus delivered sequentially, resulted in intermediate phenotypes, demonstrating macrophage plasticity.

Representative dot plots of cultured BMDM from (a) an *Ifngr1*$^{-/-}$ mouse (red) compared to a C57BL/6J mouse (black) under M(IFNγ+LPS) stimulation condition and from (b) an*Il4ra*$^{-/-}$ mouse (blue) compared to a BALB/cJ mouse (black) under M(IL4) stimulation condition with an inset histogram of the same data.Nos2 and Arg1 expression of WT strains confirm polarization to M(IFNγ+LPS) and M(IL4). (c) Median fluorescent intensity (MFI) of BMDM macrophages in the CD11b + CD16/32+ macrophage gate when exposed to 5 stimulation conditions. CD16/32 was more robustly stimulated by M(IL4) than M(IFNγ+LPS) ($p < 0.0001$). However, *Ifngr1*$^{-/-}$ BMDM showed the most dramatic increase in CD16/32 MFI, suggesting that IFNγ signaling may modulate the effect of LPS on CD16/32 expression. CD11b showed no clear pattern of response to stimulation, with minimal differences between strains. BALB/cJ and *Il4ra*$^{-/-}$ were analyzed separately, and Tukey groups are indicated by letters/numbers. Groups with the same letter or number are not significantly different. Significance was determined by linear mixed effect model with Tukey post-hoc comparison within stimulation. Significance was set as $p < 0.05$. $n = 5$ mice/strain. nd, no significant difference.

Additional file 6: Table S4a. Gene expression of bone marrow-derived macrophages from 3 mouse strains under 3 in vitro stimulation conditions. Log transformed mRNA transcript count mean +/− standard deviation & Tukey letters from linear mixed effect model with mouse as a random effect and an interaction term of strain* stimulation, followed by Benjamini and Hochberg false discovery rate (FDR) correction. *p* value for the interaction term is displayed. **Table S4b.** Gene expression of bone marrow-derived macrophages from 2 mouse strains under 3 in vitro stimulation conditions. Log transformed mRNA transcript count mean +/−standard deviation & Tukey letters from linear mixed effect model with mouse as a random effect and an interaction term of strain*stimulation, followed by Benjamini and Hochberg false discovery rate (FDR) correction.

Abbreviations

BMDM: Bone marrow-derived macrophages; DE: Differential expression; FACS: Fluorescence activated cell sorting; IPA: Ingenuity pathway analysis; MFI: Median fluorescent intensity; RNASeq: RNA sequencing; SC: Schwann cells; WT: Wild type

Funding

Funding for this work was provided by the National Institute of Health, R03 DC013376 (Cheetham) and the Harry M. Zweig Memorial Fund for Equine Research (Tomlinson).

Authors' contributions

JET and JC conceived and planned the study. JET, EZ, JG, ME, and JC performed the work. JET, JG, ME, and JC wrote the manuscript. ME performed the ingenuity pathway analysis of the RNASeq data. All authors read and approved the final manuscript.

Competing interests

The authors declare that they have are no competing interests.

Author details

[1]Cornell University College of Veterinary Medicine, Ithaca, NY, USA. [2]Bioinfo Solutions LLC, Parker, CO, USA.

References

1. Wynn TA, Vannella KM. Macrophages in tissue repair, regeneration, and fibrosis. Immunity. 2016;44:450–62.
2. Gaudet AD, Popovich PG, Ramer MS. Wallerian degeneration: gaining perspective on inflammatory events after peripheral nerve injury. J Neuroinflammation. 2011;8:110. Available from: http://www.jneuroinflammation.com/content/8/1/110
3. Corfas G, Velardez MO, Ko C-P, Ratner N, Peles E. Mechanisms and roles of axon-Schwann cell interactions. J Neurosci. 2004;24:9250–60.
4. Fu SY, Gordon T. The cellular and molecular basis of peripheral nerve regeneration. Mol Neurobiol. 1997;14:67–116. Available from: http://www.scopus.com/inward/record.url?eid=2-s2.0-0031063473&partnerID=tZOtx3y1
5. Waller A. Experiments on the section of the glossopharyngeal and hypoglossal nerves of the frog, and observations of the alterations produced thereby in the structure of their primitive fibres. Philos Trans R Soc Lond. 1850;140:423–9. Available from: http://www.jstor.org/stable/108444
6. Müller M, Leonhard C, Krauthausen M, Wacker K, Kiefer R. On the longevity of resident endoneurial macrophages in the peripheral nervous system: a study of physiological macrophage turnover in bone marrow chimeric mice. J Peripher Nerv Syst. 2010;15:357–65.
7. Martini R, Fischer S, López-Vales R, David S. Interactions between schwann cells and macrophages in injury and inherited demyelinating disease. Glia. 2008;56:1566–77. Available from: http://doi.wiley.com/10.1002/glia.20766
8. Tofaris GK, Patterson PH, Jessen KR, Mirsky R. Denervated Schwann cells attract macrophages by secretion of leukemia inhibitory factor (LIF) and monocyte chemoattractant protein-1 in a process regulated by interleukin-6 and LIF. J Neurosci. 2002;22:6696–703.
9. Cattin A-L, Burden JJ, Van Emmenis L, Mackenzie FE, Hoving JJA, Garcia Calavia N, et al. Macrophage-induced blood vessels guide Schwann cell-mediated regeneration of peripheral nerves. Cell. 2015;162:1127–39. Available from: http://www.pubmedcentral.nih.gov/articlerender.fcgi?artid=4553238&tool=pmcentrez&rendertype=abstract. [cited 2016 May 23]
10. Chen P, Piao X, Bonaldo P. Role of macrophages in Wallerian degeneration and axonal regeneration after peripheral nerve injury. Acta Neuropathol. 2015;130(5):605–18. Available from: http://link.springer.com/10.1007/s00401-015-1482-4
11. Mueller M, Leonhard C, Wacker K, Ringelstein EB, Okabe M, Hickey WF, et al. Macrophage response to peripheral nerve injury: the quantitative contribution of resident and hematogenous macrophages. Lab Invest. 2003; 83:175–85. Available from:http://www.nature.com/doifinder/10.1097/01.LAB.0000056993.28149.BF.
12. Taskinen HS, Röyttä M. The dynamics of macrophage recruitment after nerve transection. Acta Neuropathol. 1997;93:252–9. Available from: http://www.ncbi.nlm.nih.gov/pubmed/9083556
13. Baichwal RR, Bigbee JW, DeVries GH. Macrophage-mediated myelin-related mitogenic factor for cultured Schwann cells. Proc Natl Acad Sci U S A. 1988; 85:1701–5. Available from: https://www.pubmedcentral.nih.gov/articlerender.fcgiartid=279842&tool=pmcentrez&rendertype=abstract.
14. Dahlin LB. Prevention of macrophage invasion impairs regeneration in nerve grafts. Brain Res. 1995;679:274–80. Available from: http://www.ncbi.nlm.nih.gov/pubmed/7633888
15. Martinez FO, Gordon S. The M1 and M2 paradigm of macrophage activation: time for reassessment. F1000Prime Rep. 2014;6:1–13. Available from: http://www.f1000.com/prime/reports/b/6/13
16. Hu X, Ivashkiv LB. Cross-regulation of signaling pathways by interferon-gamma: implications for immune responses and autoimmune diseases. Immunity. 2009;31:539–50. Available from: http://www.ncbi.nlm.nih.gov/pubmed/19833085
17. Murray PJ, Allen JE, Biswas SK, Fisher EA, Gilroy DW, Goerdt S, et al. Macrophage activation and polarization: nomenclature and experimental guidelines. Immunity. 2014;41:14–20. Available from: https://doi.org/10.1016/j.immuni.2014.06.008
18. Novak ML, Koh TJ. Macrophage phenotypes during tissue repair. J Leukoc Biol. 2013;93:875–81. Available from: http://www.jleukbio.org/cgi/doi/10.1189/jlb.1012512
19. Gordon S. Alternative activation of macrophages. Nat Rev Immunol. 2003;3: 23–35. Available from: http://www.ncbi.nlm.nih.gov/pubmed/12511873. [cited 2013 Aug 1]
20. Fiorentino DF, Bond MW, Mosmann TR. Two types of mouse T helper cell. IV. Th2 clones secrete a factor that inhibits cytokine production by Th1 clones. J Exp Med. 1989;170:2081–95. Available from: http://www.ncbi.nlm.nih.gov/pubmed/2531194
21. Park-Min KH, Antoniv TT, Ivashkiv LB. Regulation of macrophage phenotype by long-term exposure to IL-10. Immunobiology. 2005;210:77–86.
22. Xue J, Schmidt SV, Sander J, Draffehn A, Krebs W, Quester I, et al. Transcriptome-based network analysis reveals a spectrum model of human

macrophage activation. Immunity. 2014;40:274–88. Available from: https://doi.org/10.1016/j.immuni.2014.01.006
23. Bitsaktsis C, Huntington J, Winslow G. Production of IFN-gamma by CD4 T cells is essential for resolving Ehrlichia infection. J Immunol. 2004;172:6894–901.
24. Carow B, qun YX, Gavier-Widén D, Bhuju S, Oehlmann W, Singh M, et al. Silencing suppressor of cytokine signaling-1 (SOCS1) in macrophages improves Mycobacterium tuberculosis control in an interferon-gamma (IFN-gamma)-dependent manner. J Biol Chem. 2011;286:26873–87.
25. Dai WJ, Bartens W, Köhler G, Hufnagel M, Kopf M, Brombacher F, et al. Impaired macrophage listericidal and cytokine activities are responsible for the rapid death of Listeria monocytogenes-infected IFN-gamma receptor-deficient mice. J Immunol. 1997;158:5297–304.
26. Car BD, Eng VM, Schnyder B, Ozmen L, Huang S, Gallay P, et al. Interferon gamma receptor deficient mice are resistant to endotoxic shock. J Exp Med. 1994;179:1437–44.
27. Krause P, Morris V, Greenbaum JA, Park Y, Bjoerheden U, Mikulski Z, et al. IL-10-producing intestinal macrophages prevent excessive antibacterial innate immunity by limiting IL-23 synthesis. Nat Commun. 2015;6:7055.
28. Atochina O, Da'dara AA, Walker M, Harn DA. The immunomodulatory glycan LNFPIII initiates alternative activation of murine macrophages in vivo. Immunology. 2008;125:111–21.
29. Daley JM, Brancato SK, Thomay AA, Reichner JS, Albina JE. The phenotype of murine wound macrophages. J Leukoc Biol. 2010;87:59–67.
30. Egawa M, Mukai K, Yoshikawa S, Iki M, Mukaida N, Kawano Y, et al. Inflammatory monocytes recruited to allergic skin acquire an anti-inflammatory M2 phenotype via basophil-derived interleukin-4. Immunity. 2013;38:570–80.
31. Brombacher F, Arendse B, Peterson R, Hölscher A, Hölscher C. Analyzing classical and alternative macrophage activation in macrophage/neutrophil-specific IL-4 receptor-alpha-deficient mice. Methods Mol Biol. 2009;531:225-52.
32. Sindrilaru A, Peters T, Wieschalka S, Baican C, Baican A, Peter H, et al. An unrestrained proinflammatory M1 macrophage population induced by iron impairs wound healing in humans and mice. J Clin Invest. 2011;121:985–97.
33. Biswas SK, Gangi L, Paul S, Schioppa T, Saccani A, Sironi M, et al. A distinct and unique transcriptional program expressed by tumor-associated macrophages (defective NF- B and enhanced IRF-3/STAT1 activation). Blood. 2006;107:2112–22.
34. Lawrence T, Natoli G. Transcriptional regulation of macrophage polarization: enabling diversity with identity. Nat Rev Immunol. 2011;11:750–61. Available from: https://doi.org/10.1038/nri3088
35. Ydens E, Cauwels A, Asselbergh B, Goethals S, Peeraer L, Lornet G, et al. Acute injury in the peripheral nervous system triggers an alternative macrophage response. J Neuroinflammation. 2012;9:176.
36. Nemzek JA, Xiao HY, Minard AE, Bolgos GL, Remick DG. Humane endpoints in shock research. Shock. 2004;22:17–25.
37. Liu G, Yang H. Modulation of macrophage activation and programming in immunity. J Cell Physiol. 2013;228:502–12.
38. Mantovani A, Sica A, Sozzani S, Allavena P, Vecchi A, Locati M. The chemokine system in diverse forms of macrophage activation and polarization. Trends Immunol. 2004;25:677–86.
39. Dougherty KD, Dreyfus CF, Black IB. Brain-derived neurotrophic factor in astrocytes, oligodendrocytes, and microglia/macrophages after spinal cord injury. Neurobiol Dis. 2000;7:574–85.
40. Gautier EL, Shay T, Miller J, Greter M, Jakubzick C, Ivanov S, et al. Gene-expression profiles and transcriptional regulatory pathways that underlie the identity and diversity of mouse tissue macrophages. Nat Immunol. 2012;13: 1118–28.
41. Gordon S, Martinez FO. Alternative activation of macrophages: mechanism and functions. Immunity. 2010;32:593–604.
42. Mosser DM, Edwards JP. Exploring the full spectrum of macrophage activation. Nat Rev Immunol. 2008;8:958–69. Available from: http://www.pubmedcentral.nih.gov/articlerender.fcgi?artid=2724991&tool=pmcentrez&rendertype=abstract. [cited 2013 Aug 1]
43. Guerrero AD, Dong MB, Zhao Y, Lau-Kilby A, Tarbell KV. IL-2-mediated inhibition of DC development correlates with decreased flt3 expression and increased monocyte-macrophage precursors. Immunology. 2014;143(4):640–50. Available from: http://www.ncbi.nlm.nih.gov/pubmed/24954893.
44. Geiss GK, Bumgarner RE, Birditt B, Dahl T, Dowidar N, Dunaway DL, et al. Direct multiplexed measurement of gene expression with color-coded probe pairs. Nat Biotechnol. 2008;143(4):640–50. Available from: http://www.nature.com/doifinder/10.1038/nbt1385.
45. Žygelytė E, Bernard ME, Tomlinson JE, Martin MJ, Terhorst A, Bradford HE, et al. RetroDISCO: clearing technique to improve quantification of retrograde labeled motor neurons of intact mouse spinal cords. J Neurosci Methods. 2016;271:34–42. Available from: http://linkinghub.elsevier.com/retrieve/pii/S0165027016301194.[cited 2017 Sep 25]
46. Krämer A, Green J, Pollard J, Tugendreich S. Causal analysis approaches in ingenuity pathway analysis. Bioinformatics. 2014;30:523–30.
47. Hoffman O, Burns N, Vadász I, Eltzschig HK, Edwards MG, Vohwinkel CU. Detrimental ELAVL-1/HuR-dependent GSK3β mRNA stabilization impairs resolution in acute respiratory distress syndrome. PLoS One. 2017;12:1–15.
48. Perrin FE, Lacroix S, Avilés-Trigueros M, David S. Involvement of monocyte chemoattractant protein-1, macrophage inflammatory protein-1alpha and interleukin-1beta in Wallerian degeneration. Brain. 2005;128:854–66. Available from: http://www.ncbi.nlm.nih.gov/pubmed/15689362. [cited 2013 Aug 4]
49. Chapman GA, Moores KE, Gohil J, Berkhout TA, Patel L, Green P, et al. The role of fractalkine in the recruitment of monocytes to the endothelium. Eur Aust J Pharm. 2000;392:189–95. Available from: http://www.ncbi.nlm.nih.gov/pubmed/10762673. [cited 2017 Jul 7]
50. Mills CD. Macrophage arginine metabolism to ornithine/urea or nitric oxide/citrulline: a life or death issue. Crit Rev Immunol. 2001;21:28. Available from: http://www.dl.begellhouse.com/journals/2ff21abf44b198 38,5ce6ad235835b45a,53c29c740807e053.html
51. Mills CD, Kincaid K, Alt JM, Heilman MJ, Hill AM. M-1/M-2 macrophages and the Th1/Th2 paradigm. J Immunol. 2000;164:6166–73. Available from: http://www.jimmunol.org/cgi/doi/10.4049/jimmunol.164.12.6166
52. Ebrahimpoor S, Pakzad S, Ajdary S. IgG1 and IgG2a profile of serum antibodies to Leishmania major amastigote in BALB/c and C57BL/6 mice. Iran J Allergy Asthma Immunol. 2013;12:361–7.
53. Davies LC, Jenkins SJ, Allen JE, Taylor PR. Tissue-resident macrophages. Nat Immunol. 2013;14:986–95. Available from: http://www.pubmedcentral.nih.gov/articlerender.fcgi?artid=4045180&tool=pmcentrez&rendertype=abstract.
54. Hashimoto D, Chow A, Noizat C, Teo P, Beasley MB, Leboeuf M, et al. Tissue-resident macrophages self-maintain locally throughout adult life with minimal contribution from circulating monocytes. Immunity. 2013;38:792–804. Available from: http://www.ncbi.nlm.nih.gov/pubmed/23601688
55. Shen ZL, Lassner F, Bader A, Becker M, Walter GF, Berger A. Cellular activity of resident macrophages during Wallerian degeneration. Microsurgery. 2000;20: 255–61. Available from: http://www.ncbi.nlm.nih.gov/pubmed/11015722
56. Li K, Xu W, Guo Q, Jiang Z, Wang P, Yue Y, et al. Differential macrophage polarization in male and female BALB/c mice infected with coxsackievirus B3 defines susceptibility to viral myocarditis. Circ Res. 2009;105:353–64.
57. Hirai T, Uchida K, Nakajima H, Guerrero AR, Takeura N, Watanabe S, et al. The prevalence and phenotype of activated microglia/macrophages within the spinal cord of the hyperostotic mouse (twy/twy) changes in response to chronic progressive spinal cord compression: implications for human cervical compressive myelopathy. PLoS One. 2013;8:e64528.
58. Kigerl KA, Gensel JC, Ankeny DP, Alexander JK, Donnelly DJ, Popovich PG. Identification of two distinct macrophage subsets with divergent effects causing either neurotoxicity or regeneration in the injured mouse spinal cord. J Neurosci. 2009;29:13435–44. Available from: http://www.pubmedcentral.nih.gov/articlerender.fcgi?artid=2788152&tool=pmcentrez&rendertype=abstract
59. Liu C, Li Y, Yu J, Feng L, Hou S, Liu Y, et al. Targeting the shift from M1 to M2 macrophages in experimental autoimmune encephalomyelitis mice treated with fasudil. PLoS One. 2013;8(2):e54841. Available from: http://journals.plos.org/plosone/article?id=10.1371/journal.pone.0054841.
60. Grotenhuis N, Vd Toom HFE, Kops N, Bayon Y, Deerenberg EB, Mulder IM, et al. In vitro model to study the biomaterial-dependent reaction of macrophages in an inflammatory environment. Br J Surg. 2014;101: 983–92.
61. Lacey DC, Achuthan a F a J, Dinh H, Roiniotis J, Scholz GM, et al. Defining GM-CSF- and macrophage-CSF-dependent macrophage responses by in vitro models. J Immunol. 2012;8(2):e54841. https://doi.org/10.1371/journal.pone.0054841.
62. Zajac E, Schweighofer B, T a K, Juncker-Jensen A, Minder P, Quigley JP, et al. Angiogenic capacity of M1- and M2-polarized macrophages is determined by the levels of TIMP-1 complexed with their secreted proMMP-9. Blood. 2013;122:4054–67.
63. Takeda Y, Costa S, Delamarre E, Roncal C, Leite de Oliveira R, Squadrito

ML, et al. Macrophage skewing by Phd2 haplodeficiency prevents ischaemia by inducing arteriogenesis. Nature. 2011;479:122–6.
64. Nahrendorf M, Swirski FK, Aikawa E, Stangenberg L, Wurdinger T, J-LJ-L F, et al. The healing myocardium sequentially mobilizes two monocyte subsets with divergent and complementary functions. J Exp Med. 2007; 204:3037–47.
65. Deng B, Wehling-Henricks M, Villalta SA, Wang Y, Tidball JG. IL-10 triggers changes in macrophage phenotype that promote muscle growth and regeneration. J Immunol. 2012;189:3669–80.
66. Jetten N, Verbruggen S, Gijbels MJ, Post MJ, De Winther MPJ, Donners MMPC. Anti-inflammatory M2, but not pro-inflammatory M1 macrophages promote angiogenesis in vivo. Angiogenesis. 2014;17:109–18.
67. Lucas T, Waisman A, Ranjan R, Roes J, Krieg T, Muller W, et al. Differential roles of macrophages in diverse phases of skin repair. J Immunol. 2010;184: 3964–77.
68. Spiller KL, Nassiri S, Witherel CE, Anfang RR, Ng J, Nakazawa KR, et al. Sequential delivery of immunomodulatory cytokines to facilitate the M1-to-M2 transition of macrophages and enhance vascularization of bone scaffolds. Biomaterials. 2015;37:194–207. Available from: http://linkinghub.elsevier.com/retrieve/pii/S0142961214010643
69. Spiller KL, Anfang RR, Spiller KJ, Ng J, Nakazawa KR, Daulton JW, et al. The role of macrophage phenotype in vascularization of tissue engineering scaffolds. Biomaterials. 2014;35:4477–88. Available from: https://doi.org/10.1016/j.biomaterials.2014.02.012
70. Lolmede K, Campana L, Vezzoli M, Bosurgi L, Tonlorenzi R, Clementi E, et al. Inflammatory and alternatively activated human macrophages attract vessel-associated stem cells, relying on separate HMGB1- and MMP-9-dependent pathways. J Leukoc Biol. 2009;85:779–87.
71. Saclier M, Yacoub-Youssef H, Mackey AL, Arnold L, Ardjoune H, Magnan M, et al. Differentially activated macrophages orchestrate myogenic precursor cell fate during human skeletal muscle regeneration. Stem Cells. 2013;31:384–96.
72. Berse B, Brown LLFLF, Van De Water L, Dvorak HFHF, Senger DRDR. Vascular permeability factor (vascular endothelial growth factor) gene is expressed differentially in normal tissues, macrophages, and tumors. Mol Biol Cell. 1992;3:211–20.
73. Kiriakidis S, Andreakos E, Monaco C, Foxwell B, Feldmann M, Paleolog E. VEGF expression in human macrophages is NF-κB-dependent: studies using adenoviruses expressing the endogenous NF-κB inhibitor IκBα and a kinase-defective form of the IκB kinase 2. J Cell Sci. 2003;116:665–74.
74. Willenborg S, Lucas T, Van Loo G, Knipper JA, Krieg T, Haase I, et al. CCR2 recruits an inflammatory macrophage subpopulation critical for angiogenesis in tissue repair. Blood. 2012;120:613–25.
75. Rappolee DA, Mark D, Banda MJ, Werb Z. Wound macrophages express TGF-alpha and other growth factors in vivo: analysis by mRNA phenotyping. Science. 1988;241:708–12.
76. Shimokado K, Raines EW, Madtes DK, Barrett TB, Benditt EP, Ross R. A significant part of macrophage-derived growth factor consists of at least two forms of PDGF. Cell. 1985;43:277–86.
77. Elkabes S, DiCicco-Bloom EM, Black IB. Brain microglia/macrophages express neurotrophins that selectively regulate microglial proliferation and function. J Neurosci. 1996;16:2508–21.
78. Ricci A, Greco S, Mariotta S, Felici L, Amenta F, Bronzetti E. Neurotrophin and neurotrophin receptor expression in alveolar macrophages: an immunocytochemical study. Growth Factors. 2000;18:193–202.
79. Horie H, Kadoya T, Hikawa N, Sango K, Inoue H, Takeshita K, et al. Oxidized galectin-1 stimulates macrophages to promote axonal regeneration in peripheral nerves after axotomy. J Neurosci. 2004;24:1873–80.
80. Raivich G, Makwana M. The making of successful axonal regeneration: genes, molecules and signal transduction pathways. Brain Res Rev. 2007;53: 287–311.
81. Boyd JG, Gordon T. Neurotrophic factors and their receptors in axonal regeneration and functional recovery after peripheral nerve injury. Mol Neurobiol. 2003;27:277–324. Available from: http://www.ncbi.nlm.nih.gov/pubmed/12845152
82. Hikawa N, Takenaka T. Myelin-stimulated macrophages release neurotrophic factors for adult dorsal root ganglion neurons in culture. Cell Mol Neurobiol. 1996;16:517–28. Available from: http://www.ncbi.nlm.nih.gov/pubmed/8879753
83. Mokarram N, Dymanus K, Srinivasan A, Lyon JG, Tipton J, Chu J, et al. Immunoengineering nerve repair. Proc Natl Acad Sci U S A. 2017;114: E5077–84. Available from: http://eutils.ncbi.nlm.nih.gov/entrez/eutils/elink.fcgi?dbfrom=pubmed&id=28611218&retmode=ref&cmd=prlinks%5Cnpapers3://publication/doi/10.1073/pnas.1705757114
84. Hermanson M, Olsson T, Westermark B, Funa K. PDGF and its receptors following facial nerve axotomy in rats: expression in neurons and surrounding glia. Exp Brain Res. 1995;102:415–22.
85. Abatangelo L, Maglietta R, Distaso A, D'Addabbo A, Creanza TM, Mukherjee S, et al. Comparative study of gene set enrichment methods. BMC Bioinformatics. 2009;10:275. Available from: http://www.ncbi.nlm.nih.gov/pubmed/19725948%5Cnhttp://www.pubmedcentral.nih.gov/articlerender.fcgi?artid=PMC2746222
86. Martin F, Thomson TM, Sewer A, D a D, Mathis C, Weisensee D, et al. Assessment of network perturbation amplitudes by applying high-throughput data to causal biological networks. BMC Syst Biol. 2012;6:54. Available from: http://www.pubmedcentral.nih.gov/articlerender.fcgi?artid=3433335&tool=pmcentrez&rendertype=abstract
87. Chindelevitch L, Ziemek D, Enayetallah A, Randhawa R, Sidders B, Brockel C, et al. Causal reasoning on biological networks: interpreting transcriptional changes. Bioinformatics. 2012;28:1114–21.
88. Berg DJ, Kuhn R, Rajewsky K, Muller W, Menon S, Davidson N, et al. Interleukin-10 is a central regulator of the response to LPS in murine models of endotoxic shock and the Shwartzman reaction but not endotoxin tolerance. J Clin Invest. 1995;96:2339–47.
89. Car BBD, Eng VM, Schnyder B, Ozmen L, Huang S, Gallay P, et al. From the *Institute of Toxicology of the Swiss Federal Institute of Technology and University of Ziirich, 8063 Schwerzenbach; CPharmaceutical Research, Hoffmann-La Roche, 4002 Basel; SMolecular Biology, University of Ziirich, HSnggerber~ 8093 Ziirich; and. 1994;179.
90. Howard BM, Muchamuel T, Andrade S. Interleukin 10 protects mice from lethal endotoxemia. J Exp Med. 1993;177:1205–8.
91. Leon LR, Kozak W, Kluger MJ. Role of IL-10 in Inflammation. Studies using cytokine knockout mice. Ann N Y Acad Sci. 1998;856:69–75.
92. Milano S, Arcoleo F, Agostino PD, Cillari E. Intraperitoneal injection of tetracyclines protects mice from lethal endotoxemia downregulating inducible nitric oxide synthase in various organs and cytokine and nitrate secretion in blood. Antimicrob Agents Chemother. 1997;41(1):117–21.
93. Mohler KM, Torrance DS, Smith CA, Goodwin RG, Stremler KE, Fung VP, et al. Soluble tumor necrosis factor (TNF) receptors are effective therapeutic agents in lethal endotoxemia and function simultaneously as both TNF carriers and TNF antagonists. J Immunol. 1993;151:1548–61.
94. Netea MG, Fantuzzi G, Kullberg BJ, Stuyt JL, Pulido EJ, Mcintyre RC, et al. Neutralization of IL-18 reduces neutrophil tissue accumulation and protects mice against lethal Escherichia coli and Salmonella typhimurium endotoxemia. J Immunol. 2000;164(5):2644–9
95. Remick D, Newcomb DE, Bolgos GL, Call DR. Comparison of the mortality and inflammatory response of two models of sepsis: lipopolysaccharide vs. cecal ligation and puncture. Shock. 2000;13(2):110–6.
96. Ulloa L, Ochani M, Yang H, Tanovic M, Halperin D, Yang R, et al. Ethyl pyruvate prevents lethality in mice with established lethal sepsis and systemic inflammation. Proc Natl Acad Sci U S A. 2002;99(19):12351–6.
97. Victor VM, Rocha M, Fuente MDELA. N-acetylcysteine protects mice from lethal endotoxemia by regulating the redox state of immune cells. Free Radic Res. 2003;37:919–29.
98. Sakurai E, Anand A, Ambati BK, Van Rooijen N, Ambati J. Macrophage depletion inhibits experimental choroidal neovascularization. Invest Ophthalmol Vis Sci. 2003;44:3578–85.
99. Fantin A, Vieira JM, Gestri G, Denti L, Schwarz Q, Prykhozhij S, et al. Tissue macrophages act as cellular chaperones for vascular anastomosis downstream of VEGF-mediated endothelial tip cell induction. Blood. 2010;116:829–40.
100. Rivera LB, Bergers G. Intertwined regulation of angiogenesis and immunity by myeloid cells. Trends Immunol. 2015;36:240–9. Available from: https://doi.org/10.1016/j.it.2015.02.005
101. Kanje M, Skottner A, Sjöberg J, Lundborg G. Insulin-like growth factor I (IGF-I) stimulates regeneration of the rat sciatic nerve. Brain Res. 1989;486:396–8. Available from: http://www.ncbi.nlm.nih.gov/pubmed/2731041
102. Kemp SWP, Webb AA, Dhaliwal S, Syed S, Walsh SK, Midha R. Dose and duration of nerve growth factor (NGF) administration determine the extent of behavioral recovery following peripheral nerve injury in the rat. Exp Neurol. 2011;229:460–70. Available from: http://www.ncbi.nlm.nih.gov/pubmed/21458449. [cited 2013 Nov 4]

11

Macrophage depletion reduced brain injury following middle cerebral artery occlusion in mice

Yuanyuan Ma[1], Yaning Li[2], Lu Jiang[2], Liping Wang[1], Zhen Jiang[1], Yongting Wang[2], Zhijun Zhang[2*] and Guo-Yuan Yang[1,2*]

Abstract

Background: Macrophages are involved in demyelination in many brain diseases. However, the role of macrophages in the recovery phase of the ischemic brain is unknown. The present study aims to explore the role of macrophages in the ischemic brain injury and tissue repair following a 90-min transient middle cerebral artery occlusion in mice.

Methods: Clodronate liposomes were injected into mice to deplete periphery macrophages. These mice subsequently underwent middle cerebral artery occlusion. F4/80$^+$ and CD68$^+$ cells were examined in the mouse spleen and brain to confirm macrophage depletion at 14 days after middle cerebral artery occlusion. Modified neurological severity scores were used to evaluate the behavioral function between 1 and 14 days after middle cerebral artery occlusion. MBP, Iba1, and CD31 immunostaining were performed to determine myelin lesion, microglia activation, and microvessel density.

Results: Clodronate liposomes depleted 80 % of the macrophages in the mouse spleen and reduced macrophage infiltration in the mouse brain. Macrophage depletion reduced the myelin damage in the ipsilateral striatum and microglia activation in both the ipsilateral cortex and striatum, enhanced the microvessel density in the peri-infarct region, attenuated brain atrophy, and promoted neurological recovery following middle cerebral artery occlusion.

Conclusions: Our results suggested that macrophage depletion is a potential intervention that can promote tissue repair and remodeling after brain ischemia, reduce demyelination and microglia activation, and enhance focal microvessel density.

Keywords: Brain, Ischemia, Macrophage, Microglia, Myelin

Background

Ischemic stroke is the second leading cause of death and the most common cause of disability worldwide [1, 2]. There still lacks effective therapy except for timely endovascular treatment and thrombolysis of ischemic stroke onset [3, 4]. However, only 4–7 % of patients with acute ischemic stroke are eligible for thrombolytic treatment due to the narrow therapeutic time window and the risk of hemorrhagic transformation [5]. It remains critical to develop new strategies to reduce brain injury and promote neurological function recovery after ischemic stroke [6].

* Correspondence: zhangzhij@gmail.com; gyyang0626@163.com
[2]Neuroscience and Neuroengineering Research Center, Med-X Research Institute and School of Biomedical Engineering, Shanghai Jiao Tong University, 1954 Hua Shan Road, Shanghai 200030, China
[1]Department of Neurology, Ruijin Hospital, School of Medicine, Shanghai Jiao Tong University, Shanghai 200025, China

Ischemic stroke is caused by severe stenosis or occlusion of a cerebral artery. It can subsequently lead to evere neural injury, neuronal necrosis, and apoptosis. Necrotic or apoptotic tissues release a variety of pro-inflammatory cytokines and damage-associated molecular patterns (DAMPs), which activate brain resident microglia and recruit peripheral immune cells into the brain. Macrophages and neutrophils are the key players in ischemia-induced inflammatory response [7]. However, there are different infusion patterns among macrophages, neutrophils, and other immune cells in mice following middle cerebral artery occlusion (MCAO). Periphery macrophages infiltrate into the brain as early as 12 h and recruit more neutrophils into the ischemic brain by releasing pro-inflammatory cytokines and up-regulating adhesion molecules in endothelial cells [8, 9]. The infiltration of neutrophils and lymphocytes is mostly limited at the early stage of ischemic stroke while the infiltration of periphery macrophages persists through the recovery phase of ischemic stroke [10]. The role of periphery macrophages during ischemic stroke is under debate. On the one hand, macrophage infiltration was thought to exacerbate focal inflammatory response and further damage the brain [11–13]. Macrophages can specifically bind with myelin oligodendrocyte glycoprotein (MOG) and infiltrate into the ischemic brain, increase brain infarct volume, and exacerbate neurological deficit after 4 days of transient MCAO in mice [14]. On the other hand, macrophages also participate in phagocytosis of necrotic debris at 3 and 6 days after transient MCAO [15]. Macrophage infiltration at the early stage of tissue injury is critical for tissue repair and remodeling but is not as important during the late phase of tissue recovery [16, 17]. In a mouse model of spinal cord injury, periphery macrophages contributed to fibrotic scar formation and inhibited axonal growth at the recovery phase of spinal cord injury [18]. Based on these reported observations, we hypothesized that the infiltration of periphery macrophages possibly is detrimental for tissue repair at the recovery phase of ischemic stroke.

To directly explore the role of periphery macrophages during the recovery phase of ischemic stroke, we depleted the periphery macrophages by intraperitoneally injecting clodronate liposomes into mice at 1 day before and 4 and 9 days after transient MCAO. This strategy ensures persistent macrophage depletion during the whole period of ischemic brain injury [17–19]. We aim to explore (1) whether macrophage depletion facilitates the neurological functional recovery during the recovery phase after ischemic stroke, (2) whether macrophage depletion reduces myelin lesion, (3) whether macrophage depletion affects brain resident microglia response, and (4) whether macrophage depletion enhances the microvessel density.

Methods

Transient MCAO in mice

All animal procedures were carried out in accordance with the guideline of the Institutional Animal Care and Use Committee (IACUC) of Shanghai Jiao Tong University, Shanghai, China. The experimental protocol is illustrated in Fig. 1. Forty-four adult male Institute of Cancer Research (ICR) mice (Sippr-BK, Shanghai, China) weighing 25–30 g were used in the study. Transient MCAO surgery was performed as described previously [20]. Briefly, mice were anesthetized with ketamine/xylazine (100 mg/10 mg/kg, Sigma, St. Louis, MO). After making an incision at the midline of the neck, the left common carotid artery, external carotid artery, and internal carotid artery were isolated. A 6-0 silica-coated nylon suture was gently inserted through the external carotid artery and advanced along the internal carotid artery and stopped at the origin of middle cerebral artery. After 90 min of ischemia, the suture was withdrawn and reperfusion was achieved. The successful ischemia and reperfusion were validated by monitoring the changes of cerebral blood flow using a laser Doppler flowmetry (Moor Instruments, Axminster, Devon, UK). Animals were included into further characterizations when the brain blood flow decreased for at least 80 % compared to the baseline and returned to 80 % of the baseline after suture withdrawal (Fig. 2). The mortality rates of animals following MCAO for the control liposome (Vehicle), phosphate-buffered saline (PBS), and clodronate liposome (CLP) groups were 21.4, 14.3, and 18.8 %, respectively. There was no significant difference of the mortality among the groups.

Neurobehavioral examination

Neurobehavioral tests were carried out by two investigators who were blinded to the experimental groups using a modified neurological severity score (mNSS) system. mNSS ranges from 0 to 14, in which 0 represents normal and 14 represents the highest degree of neurological deficiency [21]. mNSS is a comprehensive assessment of neurological function including motor, sensory, balance, and reflex tests. For the motor test, the bend and torsion of limbs were observed by holding up the tail of the mouse (0–3). The posture of walking on the floor was also assessed (0–3). For the balance test, the mice were placed on a beam. The neurological deficiency was assessed according to whether the mouse could keep balance on the beam, limbs fall off the beam, and walk through the beam (0–6). For the sensory and reflex tests, pinna and corneal reflex were examined, respectively (0–2). The higher the scores, the more severe is the injury.

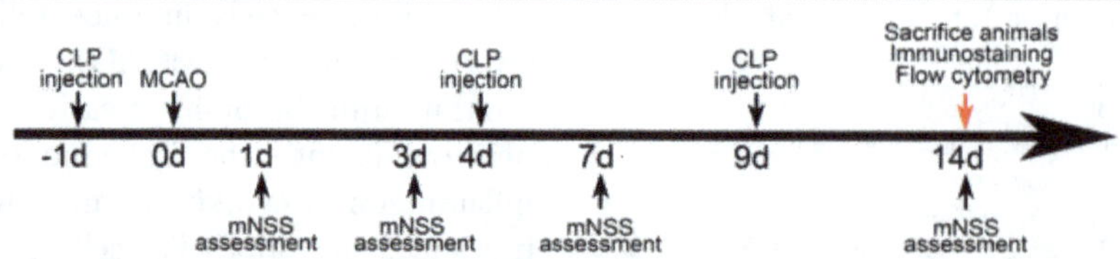

Fig. 1 A diagram of the experimental design. Mice were treated with clodronate liposomes 1 day before transient MCAO. Neurological functions were assessed using modified neurological severity scores following 1, 3, 7, and 14 days after transient MCAO. The mouse brain was collected for the immunohistochemistry, and the spleens were obtained for flow cytometry at 14 days after MCAO

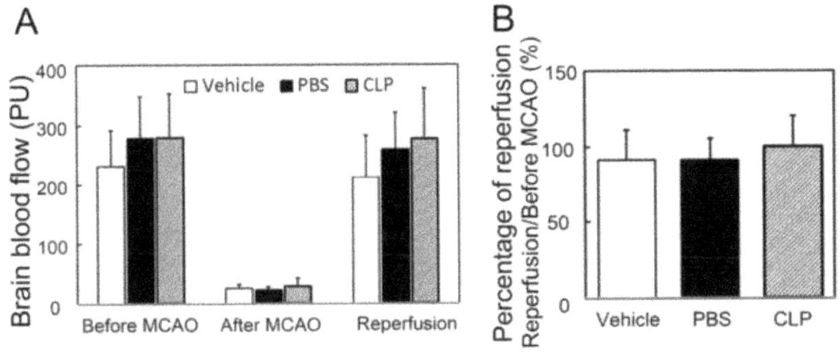

Fig. 2 Brain blood flow in mice during MCAO. **a** Representation of brain blood flow before MCAO (as a baseline), after MCAO (when the cerebral artery was occluded), and reperfusion (when the suture was withdrawn from the cerebral artery). **b** Percentage of brain blood flow reperfusion (reperfusion/before MCAO) among groups. There was no significance on the percentage of brain blood flow reperfusion among groups. $n = 11–13$ per group

The measurement of brain atrophy volume

The mice were sacrificed following 14 days of transient MCAO and perfused with 0.9 % saline followed by 4 % paraformaldehyde. The brain samples were removed and post-fixed in 4 % paraformaldehyde for 6 h and dehydrated in 30 % sucrose until the brain sank into the bottom of a 15-ml tube. Then the brains were frozen in −80 °C for 2 days and cut into 20-μm sections from the anterior commissure to the hippocampus. A total of 20 coronal sections were mounted on the slide and used for cresyl violet staining. The distance between adjacent sections was 200 μm. The other sections used for immunohistochemistry were collected in the anti-freezing solution and stored at −20 °C until use. The atrophy area was measured using the ImageJ software (National Institutes of Health, Bethesda, MD). The atrophy volume was calculated with the formula $V = \sum_1^n \left[\left(S_n + \sqrt{S_n * S_{n+1}} + S_{n+1} \right) * \frac{h}{3} \right]$, in which h was the distance between two adjacent sections and S_n and S_{n+1} were the atrophy areas of two adjacent sections [22, 23].

Macrophage depletion and clodronate liposome administration

Clodronate liposomes were widely used to deplete peripheral macrophages [24, 25]. Clodronate was encapsulated in liposomes with a concentration of 7 mg clodronate per milliliter, a concentration that can ensure the depletion of 90 % of macrophages within 24 to 36 h after systemic administration [26]. Clodronate liposomes (F70101C-A, FormuMax Scientific, Inc., Palo Alto, CA) were intraperitoneally injected at 1 day before and 4 and 9 days after transient MCAO. Control liposomes (F70101C-A, FormuMax Scientific, Inc., Palo Alto, CA) and PBS were used as the controls. The dose of clodronate liposomes was adjusted according to the manufacturer's instructions (0.2 ml/20–25 g). The efficiency of macrophage depletion was verified at 14 days after MCAO by examining the number of F4/80$^+$ macrophages in the spleen and CD68$^+$ macrophages in the brain by flow cytometry and immunostaining.

Spleen cell isolation and flow cytometry

Flow cytometry was performed on the spleen samples collected on day 14 after MCAO. The mice were deeply anesthetized and the spleens were removed and collected in a 1.5-ml tube. To obtain single cell suspension, the spleens were grinded in PBS using a mechanical trituration method through a 100-μm cell strainer (Corning, New York, NY). The cell suspension was centrifuged for 5 min at 1000 rpm at 25 °C, and the supernatant was discarded. Red blood cells were removed by re-suspending the cells in red blood cell lysis buffer (NH4Cl 8.29 g, KHCO3 1 g, EDTA-2Na 37.2 mg, diluted in distilled water, at pH = 7.4) for 30 s. Then the cell suspension was centrifuged for 5 min at 1000 rpm at 25 °C again and the supernatant was discarded. After washing in PBS, the cells were re-suspended in 1 ml PBS. Single cell suspension of 200 μl was incubated with fluorescence-conjugated rat–anti-mouse F4/80-FITC (1:200, BioLegend, San Diego, CA) for 30 min at 4 °C. Then the cells were centrifuged for 5 min at 2500 rpm at 25 °C. After discarding the supernatant, the cells were washed once with PBS. Then the cells were re-suspended in 300 μl PBS and analyzed by a flow cytometry (BD Biosciences, San Jose, CA). A minimum of 10,000 events were acquired for each sample.

Western blot

The ischemic striatum was collected and sonicated in the protein lysis buffer (RIPA with protease cocktail inhibitor, phosphatase inhibitor). The brain homogenate was centrifuged at 12,000 rpm and the supernatant was collected. Protein concentrations were determined with a BCA kit (Thermo Scientific, Waltham, UK). Equal amounts of protein were loaded onto 15 % resolving gel

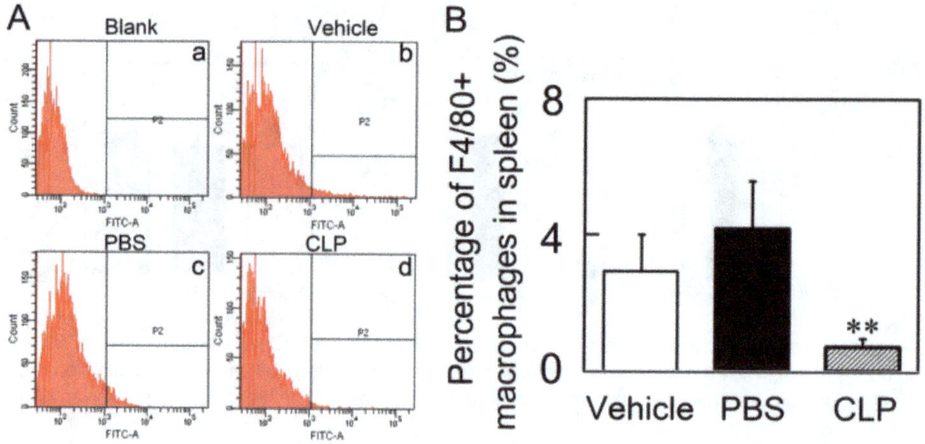

Fig. 3 Clodronate liposome treatment depleted macrophages in the spleen. **a** Flow cytometry analysis shows the percentage of F4/80$^+$ macrophages in the spleen of Vehicle (**b**), PBS (**c**), and CLP (**d**) groups at14 days after MCAO. **b** Bar graph shows quantification of the percentage of F4/80$^+$ macrophages in the spleen of Vehicle, PBS, and CLP groups. Data are mean ± SD, $n = 5–8$ per group. **$p < 0.01$, CLP vs. Vehicle or PBS. CLP = clodronate liposomes, PBS = phosphate-buffered saline, Vehicle = control liposomes

for electrophoresis. The proteins were transferred onto a nitrocellulose membrane (Whatman Inc., Florham Park, NJ) and incubated with the primary antibodies of MBP (1:1000 dilution, Abcam, Cambridge, MA) and β-actin (1:1000 dilution, Abcam, Cambridge, MA) at 4 °C overnight. After washing three times using a TBST buffer, the membrane was incubated with horseradish peroxidase (HRP)-conjugated anti-rat or anti-mouse immunoglobulin G for 1 h at room temperature, washed, and then reacted with an enhanced chemiluminescence substrate (Pierce, Rockford, IL). The result of chemiluminescence was semi-quantified using the ImageJ software (National Institutes of Health, Bethesda, MD).

Immunohistochemistry

Myelin basic protein (MBP) immunostaining was performed following DAB immunostaining protocol (Vector Labs, Burlingame, CA) as previously described with minor modifications [20]. Briefly, the brain sections were incubated with 0.3 % H_2O_2 for 30 min at room temperature. After rinsing with PBS, 0.3 % Triton X-100 was added for 10 min, then the coronal sections were incubated with

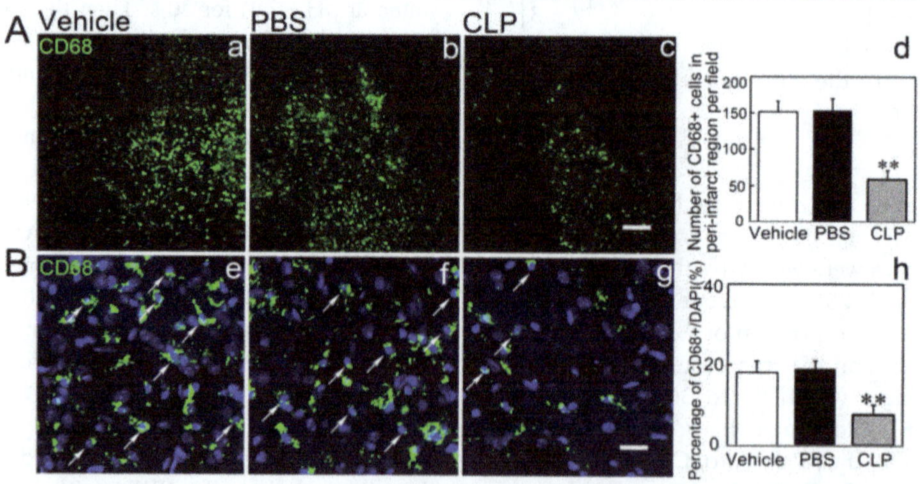

Fig. 4 Clodronate liposome treatment reduced macrophage infiltration in the brain after MCAO. **a** Representative images of CD68$^+$ macrophages (*green*) of the ipsilateral striatum in Vehicle (*a*), PBS (*b*), and CLP (*c*) groups at 14 days after MCAO. *Scale bar* = 100 μm. Quantification of the number of CD68$^+$ macrophages in the peri-infarct region of the ipsilateral striatum (*d*). **b** Representative images of CD68$^+$ macrophages (*green*) and DAPI-stained cells (*blue*) of the ipsilateral striatum in Vehicle (*e*), PBS (*f*), and CLP (*g*) groups at 14 days after MCAO. *Scale bar* = 20 μm. Quantification of the percentage of CD68$^+$/DAPI cells in the peri-infarct region of the ipsilateral striatum (*h*). Data are mean ± SD, $n = 4$ per group. **$p < 0.01$, CLP vs. Vehicle or PBS. CLP = clodronate liposomes, PBS = phosphate-buffered saline, Vehicle = control liposomes

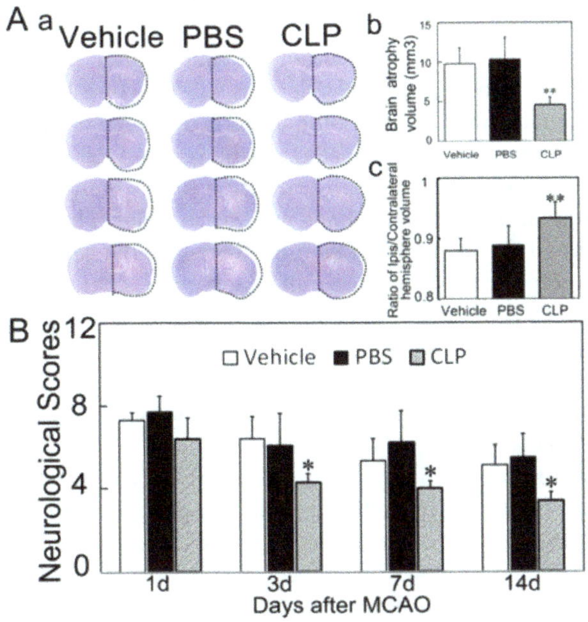

Fig. 5 Macrophage depletion improved neurological outcomes in mice following transient MCAO. **a** A series of cresyl violet stained coronal sections represented the brain atrophy in CLP, PBS, and Vehicle groups at 14 days after MCAO (**a**). Quantification of the brain atrophy volume is presented by the brain volume of contralateral subtracted ipsilateral hemisphere at 14 days after MCAO (*b*). Quantification of brain volume presented by ratio of ipsilateral/contralateral hemisphere brain volume at 14 days after MCAO (*c*). Data are mean ± SD, $n = 7–8$ per group. $^{**}p < 0.01$, CLP vs. Vehicle or PBS. **b** Bar graph shows the mNSS assessment in CLP, PBS, and Vehicle groups at 1, 3, 7, and 14 days after MCAO. Data are mean ± SD, $n = 5–8$ per group. $^{*}p < 0.05$, CLP vs. Vehicle or PBS. mNSS = modified neurological severity scores

horse serum for 1 h at room temperature. The brain sections were then incubated in a primary antibody of MBP (1:500, Abcam, Cambridge, MA) at 4 °C overnight. After rinsing with PBS for three times, the brain sections were incubated with a biotinylated secondary antibody and Vectastain ABC solution (Vector Labs, Burlingame, CA) for 1 h. The brain sections were then examined under an optical microscope. Three fields in the peri-infarct region of the ipsilateral striatum and the corresponding contralateral striatum were imaged in each section. A total of five sections (taking every other section spaced 200 μm apart) were evaluated for each mouse. The mean integrated optical density (IOD) was measured by the ImageJ Pro Plus 6.0 software (Media Cybernetics, Bethesda, MO). The ratio of mean IOD between the ipsilateral and contralateral was used for further analysis.

For macrophage, microglia, and microvessel immunostaining, the brain sections were incubated in the primary antibodies of CD68 (1:200, AbD Serotec, Kidlington, UK), Ibal (1:200, WAKO, Osaka, Japan), and CD31 (1:150, R&D, Minneapolis, MN) at 4 °C overnight. After rinsing with PBS for three times, the brain sections were incubated with the secondary antibodies: Alexa Fluor 488-conjugated donkey anti-rat, Alexa Fluor 488-conjugated donkey anti-rabbit, or Alexa Fluor 594-conjugated donkey anti-goat (1:500, Invitrogen, Carlsbad, CA) for 1 h at room temperature. Then the brain sections were rinsed with PBS for three times and incubated with 4′, 6-diamidino-2-phenylindole (DAPI, Life Technologies, Mulgrave, VIC, Australia) for 5 min at room temperature. After rinsing with PBS, the brain sections were covered and sealed with mounting medium (Vector Labs, Burlingame, CA) for further study. Negative controls (without primary antibodies) were included in each immunohistochemistry experiment. Additional figures show this in more detail (see Additional file 1).

Cell and vessel counting

The brain tissues were visualized using a confocal microscope (Leica, Solms, Germany). For $Ibal^+$ microglia counting, the field in the peri-infarct region of the cortex and striatum was imaged per section. For $CD68^+$ macrophages and $CD31^+$ microvessels, three fields in the peri-infarct region of the striatum were imaged per section. A total of five sections with a 200-μm interval were selected per mouse. The number of positive cells was counted by the investigators who were blinded to the experimental groups. DAPI-stained nuclei were counted by the ImageJ Pro Plus 6.0 software (Media Cybernetics, Bethesda, MO). The average number of positive cells per section and the percentage of the positive cells to total cells stained by DAPI were used for data analysis [27].

Statistical analysis

Data were presented as mean ± SD. Statistical significance among groups were evaluated by one-way ANOVA followed by the Bonferroni (homogeneity of variance) or the Tamhane test (heterogeneity of variance) using the SPSS 18.0 software (SPSS Inc., Chicago, IL). For nonparametric analysis, the Kruskal–Wallis test and Mann–Whitney *U* test were applied. A value of $p < 0.05$ was considered significant.

Results

Macrophages were successfully depleted by clodronate liposome treatment

To deplete periphery macrophages during transient MCAO, the mice were subjected to clodronate liposome injection. At 14 days after injection, 80 % of $F4/80^+$ macrophages were depleted in the spleen in the clodronate liposome-treated mice compared to the control mice (Fig. 3, $p < 0.05$), this result suggested the success of macrophage depletion. Animals that received clodronate liposomes showed no visible disorders such as infection, reduced appetite, or inhibition of motor activity.

Macrophage infiltration was reduced in the brain of MCAO after clodronate liposome injection

To further clarify whether periphery macrophage depletion could reduce macrophage infiltration in the brain, we examined the number of $CD68^+$ macrophages in the peri-infarct region of the ipsilateral striatum. We found that macrophages were reduced in the clodronate liposome-treated mice compared to the control mice (Fig. 4, $p < 0.05$); this result indicated that periphery macrophage depletion could reduce macrophage infiltration in the brain after ischemia.

Macrophage depletion reduced the brain atrophy volume and neurological deficits in MCAO mice

To analyze the influence of macrophage depletion on tissue repair, we measured the brain atrophy volume at 14 days after MCAO. The result showed that the brain atrophy volume was much smaller in the clodronate liposome-treated mice than that in the control mice (Fig. 5a, $p < 0.05$). To examine the role of macrophage depletion on neurological outcomes, we assessed the neurological deficits using the mNSS system at 1, 3, 7, and 14 days after MCAO. The results showed that neurological scores were lower at 3 days and maintained at low level for 14 days after MCAO in the clodronate liposome-treated mice compared to the control mice (Fig. 5b, $p < 0.05$).

Macrophage depletion reduced myelin lesion in ischemic mice

Myelin, a major component of the white matter, is vulnerable to ischemia, and the loss of myelin contributes to impaired neurological outcomes. To understand why macrophage depletion facilitated the recovery of ischemic stroke, we examined MBP expression to assess the myelin lesion using immunostaining and western blot. The results showed that MBP expression was higher in the clodronate liposome-treated mice compared to the control mice (Fig. 6, $p < 0.05$), suggesting that macrophage depletion reduced myelin lesion.

Macrophage depletion reduced microglia activation both in the cortex and striatum

Brain resident microglia activation participates in myelin lesion induced by ischemia, and periphery macrophage infiltration might contribute to microglia activation [10]. To further explore the effect of macrophage depletion on microglia activation, we examined microglia activation by Iba1 immunostaining. We found that microglia displayed a classical ramified shape, with long and thin processes in the cortex and striatum in the macrophage depletion group (Fig. 7a). Microglia displayed distinct cell morphology with a larger cell body and more processes in the control groups compared to the macrophage depletion group. Furthermore, we found that macrophage depletion significantly reduced the number

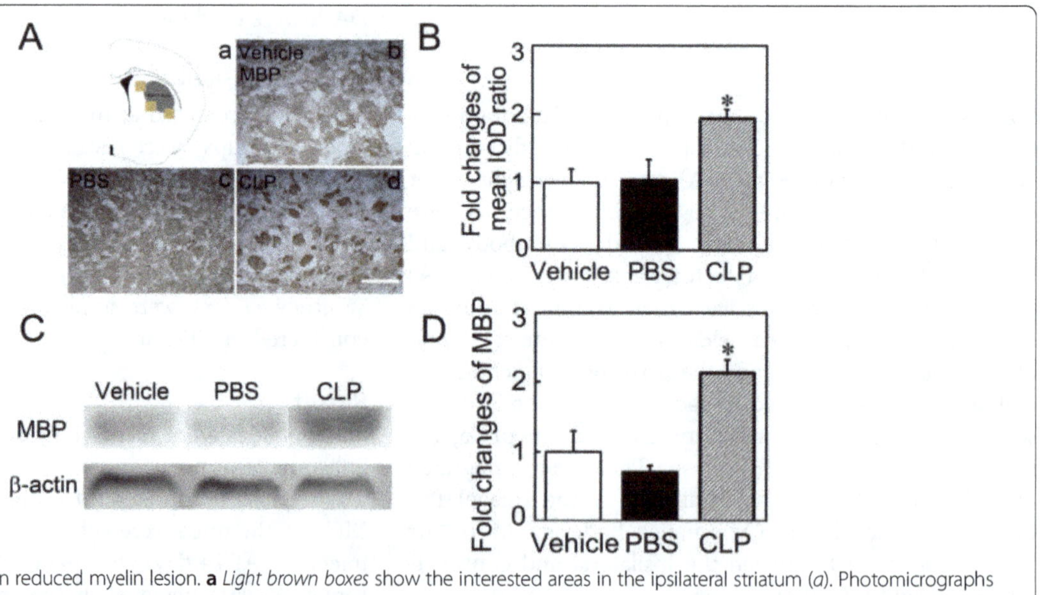

Fig. 6 Macrophage depletion reduced myelin lesion. **a** *Light brown boxes* show the interested areas in the ipsilateral striatum (*a*). Photomicrographs show MBP-stained myelin in the peri-infarct region of the ischemic striatum in Vehicle (*b*), PBS (*c*), and CLP (*d*) groups at 14 days after MCAO. *Scale bar* = 100 μm. **b** Bar graph represents quantification of fold changes of mean IOD ratio (ipsilateral/contralateral hemisphere) in the CLP group compared to the PBS or Vehicle group. Data are mean ± SD, $n = 4$ per group. *$p < 0.05$, CLP vs. Vehicle or PBS. IOD = integrated optical density. **c** MBP expression in the ischemic striatum was determined by western blot. **d** Quantification of MBP expression by normalizing to the β-actin level in each group and set the Vehicle treated group as 1. Data are mean ± SD, $n = 3$ per group. *$p < 0.05$, CLP vs. Vehicle or PBS

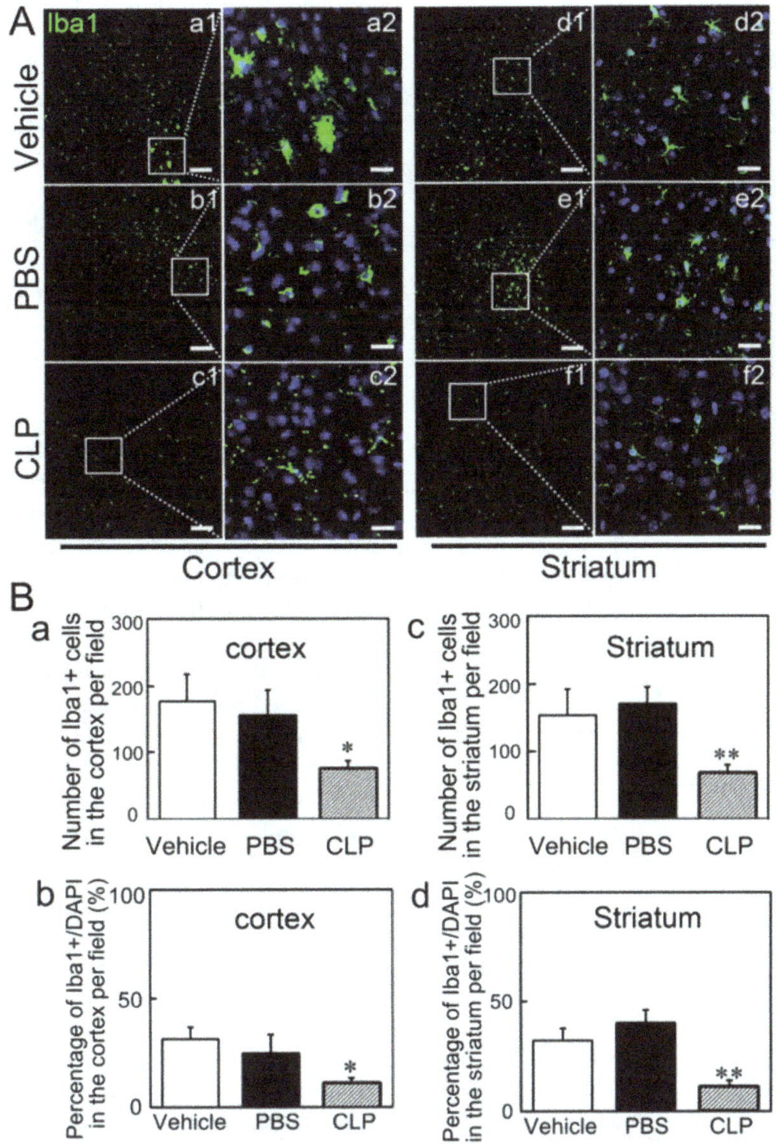

Fig. 7 Macrophage depletion reduced microglia activation. **a** Photomicrographs represented Iba1 (*green*)-stained microglia in the cortex and striatum in CLP, PBS, and Vehicle groups at 14 days after MCAO. *Right panels* at each column (*a2 to f2*) presented a higher magnification of the images of *left panels* labeled by the *boxes* (*a1 to f1*). *Scale bar* = 100 μm in *a1* to *f1* and 20 μm in *a2* to *f2*. **b** Quantification of the number of $Iba1^+$ microglia located in the cortex (**a**) and striatum (**c**) and the percentage of $Iba1^+$ /DAPI cells located in the cortex (*b*) and striatum (*d*) at 14 days after MCAO. Data are mean ± SD, $n = 4$ per group. $^*p < 0.05$, $^{**}p < 0.01$, CLP vs. Vehicle or PBS

of microglia both in the ipsilateral cortex and striatum (Fig. 7b, $p < 0.05$). These data suggested that macrophage depletion reduced microglia activation at least at 14 days after MCAO.

Macrophage depletion enhanced the microvessel density in MCAO mice

Macrophages were reported to reduce the microvessel density in diabetic mice, while the microvessel density in the peri-infarct region contributed to recovery after brain injury [22, 23]. Therefore, we explored whether macrophage depletion affected the microvessel density during MCAO. We counted $CD31^+$ microvessels in the peri-infarct region of the ipsilateral striatum (Fig. 8a–c). The number of $CD31^+$ microvessels increased by 40 % in the macrophage depletion mice compared to the control mice (Fig. 8d, $p < 0.05$). The result suggested that macrophage depletion could increase the microvessel density in the peri-infarct region of the lesion striatum.

Discussion

In this study, we found that macrophage depletion improved neurological outcomes and promoted tissue repair for 14 days after MCAO. The beneficial outcomes

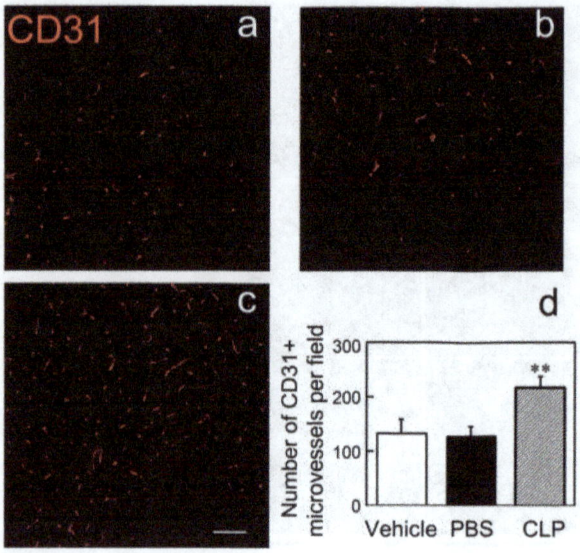

Fig. 8 Macrophage depletion enhanced the microvessel density in the peri-infarct region of mice brain after MCAO. Photomicrographs show that CD31$^+$ microvessels in the peri-infarct region of the ipsilateral striatum in Vehicle (**a**), PBS (**b**), and CLP (**c**) groups at 14 days after MCAO. *Scale bar* = 100 μm. Bar graph shows the quantification of the number of CD31$^+$ cells in the peri-infarct region of the ipsilateral striatum (**d**). Data are mean ± SD, $n = 4$ per group. $^{**}p < 0.01$, CLP vs. Vehicle or PBS

of macrophage depletion correlate with the decrease of myelin loss and microglia activation and the increase of focal microvessel density.

We aimed to explore whether macrophage depletion affects the neurological function recovery at the recovery phase of MCAO. To achieve the maximum efficiency of macrophage depletion, mice were subjected to clodronate liposome injection at 1 day prior to transient MCAO. We gave two additional injections of clodronate liposomes at a 4-day interval until 14 days after transient MCAO [19]. The success of macrophage depletion was verified by quantifying F4/80$^+$ macrophages in the spleen at 14 days after MCAO, which showed a reduction of 80 % F4/80$^+$ macrophages in the clodronate liposome-treated mice compared to the control mice. Macrophage infiltration was also reduced in the brain after ischemia, which was validated by immunostaining of CD68$^+$ macrophages in the brain. Our results showed that persistent macrophage depletion reduced the brain atrophy volume and improved the neurological outcomes at 14 days after MCAO, which suggested that macrophages could impede the neurological function recovery after ischemic stroke.

Both peripheral infiltrated macrophages and brain resident microglia activation were implicated in demyelination-associated diseases such as globoid cell leukodystrophy, multiple sclerosis, spinal cord injury, and traumatic brain injury [28–31]. LPS injection-induced brain inflammation resulted in myelin lesion, which was accompanied by enhanced microglia activation and morphological transition [32]. The number of periphery macrophages correlated with the severity of tissue damage [33]. Macrophage infiltration and brain resident microglia activation contributed to myelin damage via producing pro-inflammatory cytokines, chemokines, reactive oxygen species, and glutamate [34]. Iba1$^+$ and CD68$^+$ cells infiltrated around the damaged myelin after MCAO, the result suggested that these cells were implicated in ischemia-induced myelin lesion [35]. However, these past studies could not elucidate the specific contribution of brain resident microglia activation and infiltrated macrophages to myelin lesion, because Iba1 and CD68 are markers for both brain resident microglia and peripheral infiltrated macrophages [36, 37]. In our study, we specifically depleted the peripheral macrophages by intraperitoneal injection of clodronate liposomes; thus, the Iba1$^+$ cells in the cortex and striatum were dominated by brain resident microglia. There were less Iba1$^+$ microglia accumulated in the peri-infarct region of the ipsilateral cortex and striatum in the macrophage depletion mice compared to the control. In addition, macrophage depletion also caused microglia morphological changes in the ipsilateral cortex and striatum in MCAO mice. Microglia displayed a large cell body and thick and short processes in the control brain while displaying small round cell body and ramified morphology in the clodronate liposome-treated mice. These results suggested that peripheral macrophages participated in re-populating microglia in the peri-infarct region after MCAO and contributed to exacerbating myelin damage. The peripheral macrophages could be a potential target for the development of intervention strategies to treat ischemic myelin damage.

Macrophages are critical in promoting angiogenesis by releasing pro-angiogenic factors or supporting the process of microvessel sprouting in tumor [38]. Infiltration of macrophages within 24 h after limb amputation is essential for limb regeneration and tissue recovery via enhancing the microvessel density in the salamanders [25]. To explore whether macrophage depletion affected angiogenesis after ischemic stroke, we examined CD31$^+$ microvessels in the peri-infarct region of the striatum at 14 days after ischemia. We found that the number of CD31$^+$ cells increased in the peri-infarct region of the ischemic striatum in the macrophage depletion mice compared to the control. This result suggested that macrophage depletion enhanced the microvessel density. Studies demonstrated that macrophage depletion attenuated kidney injury by up-regulating stromal cell-derived factor-1 (SDF-1) expression [39]. SDF-1 could enhance pro-angiogenic factors such as CCL and vascular endothelial growth factor (VEGF) expression and promote angiogenesis under different pathological conditions [22, 40]. Therefore, one possible explanation for the macrophage depletion to enhance the microvessel density is possibly the up-regulation of pro-angiogenic factors such as VEGF or chemokines such as SDF-1 in the brain. Furthermore, macrophage depletion may improve neurological function via promoting bone marrow stem cell mobilization to the ischemic brain [41]. The relationship of macrophages and the mobilization of bone marrow stem cells during ischemic stroke awaits further investigation.

Conclusions

Although macrophage depletion prior to ischemic stroke onset is inappropriate for clinical application, it is conducted to explore the role of macrophages during ischemic stroke. Our results showed that macrophage depletion is beneficial for reducing brain injury and promoting tissue recovery following 14 days of ischemic stroke. However, the mechanism by which macrophage depletion improved recovery after ischemia needs to be further investigated. In conclusion, we explored the role of macrophages at the recovery phase of ischemic stroke via peripheral macrophage depletion induced by clodronate liposomes. Our results showed that macrophage depletion reduced the brain atrophy volume and improved neurological outcomes after MCAO. Alleviation of ischemic brain injury induced by macrophage depletion may be due to the reduced myelin lesion and microglia activation and the enhanced microvessel density. Our study suggested that temporary inhibition of peripheral macrophages could be a promising intervention strategy for the ischemic stroke therapy.

Abbreviations

CLP: clodronate liposomes; DAMPs: damage-associated molecular patterns; DAPI: 4′, 6-diamidino-2-phenylindole; HRP: horseradish peroxidase; IACUC: institutional animal care and use committee; ICR: institute of cancer research; IOD: integrated optical density; MBP: myelin basic protein; MCAO: middle cerebral artery occlusion; mNSS: modified neurological severity scores; MOG: myelin oligodendrocyte glycoprotein; PBS: phosphate-buffered saline; SDF-1: stromal cell-derived factor-1; Vehicle: control liposomes.

Competing interests

The authors declare that they have no competing interests.

Authors' contributions

YYM designed the study, performed the animal experiments, and drafted the manuscript. YNL participated in the design of the study. JL and LPW carried out the assessment of neurological deficiency. JZ helped establish the ischemic models. ZJZ and YTW participated in the design of the study and instructed the experiments. GYY conceived of the study and participated in its design and coordination and helped to draft the manuscript. All authors read and approved the final manuscript.

Acknowledgements

This work was supported by the National Natural Science Foundation of China (81471178 and U1232205, GYY; 81522015, YTW), K. C. Wong Education Foundation (GYY), and the Science and Technology Commission of Shanghai Municipality (13ZR1422600, ZJZ).

References

1. Lozano R, Naghavi M, Foreman K, Lim S, Shibuya K, Aboyans V, et al. Global and regional mortality from 235 causes of death for 20 age groups in 1990 and 2010: a systematic analysis for the Global Burden of Disease Study 2010. Lancet. 2012;380:2095–128.
2. Go AS, Mozaffarian D, Roger VL, Benjamin EJ, Berry JD, Blaha MJ, et al. Heart disease and stroke statistics—2014 update: a report from the American Heart Association. Circulation. 2014;129:e28–292.
3. Albers GW, Goyal M, Jahan R, Bonafe A, Diener HC, Levy EI, et al. Relationships between imaging assessments and outcomes in solitaire with the intention for thrombectomy as primary endovascular treatment for acute ischemic stroke. Stroke. 2015;46:2786–94.
4. Jauch EC, Saver JL, Adams Jr HP, Bruno A, Connors JJ, Demaerschalk BM, et al. Guidelines for the early management of patients with acute ischemic stroke: a guideline for healthcare professionals from the American Heart Association/American Stroke Association. Stroke. 2013;44:870–947.
5. Schwamm LH, Ali SF, Reeves MJ, Smith EE, Saver JL, Messe S, et al. Temporal trends in patient characteristics and treatment with intravenous thrombolysis among acute ischemic stroke patients at Get With The Guidelines-Stroke hospitals. Circ Cardiovasc Qual Outcomes. 2013;6:543–9.
6. Prabhakaran S, Ruff I, Bernstein RA. Acute stroke intervention: a systematic review. JAMA. 2015;313:1451–62.
7. Shichita T, Sakaguchi R, Suzuki M, Yoshimura A. Post-ischemic inflammation in the brain. Front Immunol. 2012;3:132.
8. Gelderblom M, Leypoldt F, Steinbach K, Behrens D, Choe CU, Siler DA, et al. Temporal and spatial dynamics of cerebral immune cell accumulation in stroke. Stroke. 2009;40:1849–57.
9. Huang J, Upadhyay UM, Tamargo RJ. Inflammation in stroke and focal cerebral ischemia. Surg Neurol. 2006;66:232–45.
10. Tanaka R, Komine-Kobayashi M, Mochizuki H, Yamada M, Furuya T, Migita M, et al. Migration of enhanced green fluorescent protein expressing bone marrow-derived microglia/macrophage into the mouse brain following permanent focal ischemia. Neurosci. 2003;117:531–9.
11. Lo EH. Degeneration and repair in central nervous system disease. Nat Med. 2010;16:1205–9.
12. Moskowitz MA, Lo EH, Iadecola C. The science of stroke: mechanisms in search of treatments. Neuron. 2010;67:181–98.
13. Barrett JP, Costello DA, O'Sullivan J, Cowley TR, Lynch MA. Bone marrow-derived macrophages from aged rats are more responsive to inflammatory stimuli. J Neuroinflammation. 2015;12:67.
14. Ren X, Akiyoshi K, Grafe MR, Vandenbark AA, Hurn PD, Herson PS, et al. Myelin specific cells infiltrate MCAO lesions and exacerbate stroke severity. Metab Brain Dis. 2012;27:7–15.
15. Schroeter M, Jander S, Huitinga I, Witte OW, Stoll G. Phagocytic response in photochemically induced infarction of rat cerebral cortex. The role of resident microglia. Stroke. 1997;28:382–6.
16. Lucas T, Waisman A, Ranjan R, Roes J, Krieg T, Muller W. Differential roles of macrophages in diverse phases of skin repair. J Immunol. 2010;184:3964–77.
17. Kotter MR, Setzu A, Sim FJ, Van Rooijen N, Franklin RJ. Macrophage depletion impairs oligodendrocyte remyelination following lysolecithin-induced demyelination. Glia. 2001;35:204–12.
18. Zhu Y, Soderblom C, Krishnan V, Ashbaugh J, Bethea JR, Lee JK. Hematogenous macrophage depletion reduces the fibrotic scar and increases axonal growth after spinal cord injury. Neurobiol Dis. 2015;74:114–25.
19. Zattoni M, Mura ML, Deprez F, Schwendener RA, Engelhardt B, Frei K, et al. Brain infiltration of leukocytes contributes to the pathophysiology of temporal lobe epilepsy. J Neurosci. 2011;31:4037–50.
20. Huang J, Li Y, Tang Y, Tang G, Yang GY, Wang Y. CXCR4 antagonist AMD3100 protects blood-brain barrier integrity and reduces inflammatory response after focal ischemia in mice. Stroke. 2013;44:190–7.
21. Li Y, Chopp M, Chen J, Wang L, Gautam SC, Xu YX, et al. Intrastriatal transplantation of bone marrow nonhematopoietic cells improves functional recovery after stroke in adult mice. J Cereb Blood Flow Metab. 2000;20:1311–9.
22. Li Y, Huang J, He X, Tang G, Tang YH, Liu Y, et al. Postacute stromal cell-derived factor-1alpha expression promotes neurovascular recovery in ischemic mice. Stroke. 2014;45:1822–9.

23. Chen C, Lin X, Wang J, Tang G, Mu Z, Chen X, et al. Effect of HMGB1 on the paracrine action of EPC promotes post-ischemic neovascularization in mice. Stem Cells. 2014;32:2679–89.
24. Gliem M, Mausberg AK, Lee JI, Simiantonakis I, van Rooijen N, Hartung HP, et al. Macrophages prevent hemorrhagic infarct transformation in murine stroke models. Ann Neurol. 2012;71:743–52.
25. Godwin JW, Pinto AR, Rosenthal NA. Macrophages are required for adult salamander limb regeneration. Proc Natl Acad Sci U S A. 2013;110:9415–20.
26. Seiler P, Aichele P, Odermatt B, Hengartner H, Zinkernagel RM, Schwendener RA. Crucial role of marginal zone macrophages and marginal zone metallophils in the clearance of lymphocytic choriomeningitis virus infection. Eur J Immunol. 1997;27:2626–33.
27. Pires PW, Girgla SS, Moreno G, McClain JL, Dorrance AM. Tumor necrosis factor-alpha inhibition attenuates middle cerebral artery remodeling but increases cerebral ischemic damage in hypertensive rats. Am J Physiol Heart Circ Physiol. 2014;307:H658–69.
28. Matthes F, Andersson C, Stein A, Eistrup C, Fogh J, Gieselmann V, et al. Enzyme replacement therapy of a novel humanized mouse model of globoid cell leukodystrophy. Exp Neurol. 2015;271:36–45.
29. Choi BY, Kim JH, Kho AR, Kim IY, Lee SH, Lee BE, et al. Inhibition of NADPH oxidase activation reduces EAE-induced white matter damage in mice. J Neuroinflammation. 2015;12:104.
30. Haan N, Zhu B, Wang J, Wei X, Song B. Crosstalk between macrophages and astrocytes affects proliferation, reactive phenotype and inflammatory response, suggesting a role during reactive gliosis following spinal cord injury. J Neuroinflammation. 2015;12:109.
31. Morganti JM, Jopson TD, Liu S, Riparip LK, Guandique CK, Gupta N. CCR2 antagonism alters brain macrophage polarization and ameliorates cognitive dysfunction induced by traumatic brain injury. J Neurosci. 2015;35:748–60.
32. Cardoso FL, Herz J, Fernandes A, Rocha J, Sepodes B, Brito MA, et al. Systemic inflammation in early neonatal mice induces transient and lasting neurodegenerative effects. J Neuroinflammation. 2015;12:82.
33. Ajami B, Bennett JL, Krieger C, McNagny KM, Rossi FM. Infiltrating monocytes trigger EAE progression, but do not contribute to the resident microglia pool. Nat Neurosci. 2011;14:1142–9.
34. Cao L, He C. Polarization of macrophages and microglia in inflammatory demyelination. Neurosci Bull. 2013;29:189–98.
35. Moxon-Emre I, Schlichter LC. Evolution of inflammation and white matter injury in a model of transient focal ischemia. J Neuropathol Exp Neurol. 2010;69:1–15.
36. Simard AR, Rivest S. Bone marrow stem cells have the ability to populate the entire central nervous system into fully differentiated parenchymal microglia. FASEB J. 2004;18:998–1000.
37. Varvel NH, Grathwohl SA, Baumann F, Liebig C, Bosch A, Brawek B, et al. Microglial repopulation model reveals a robust homeostatic process for replacing CNS myeloid cells. Proc Natl Acad Sci U S A. 2012;109:18150–5.
38. Murdoch C, Muthana M, Coffelt SB, Lewis CE. The role of myeloid cells in the promotion of tumour angiogenesis. Nat Rev Cancer. 2008;8:618–31.
39. Wan X, Xia W, Gendoo Y, Chen W, Sun W, Sun D, et al. Upregulation of stromal cell-derived factor 1 (SDF-1) is associated with macrophage infiltration in renal ischemia-reperfusion injury. PLoS One. 2014;9:e114564.
40. Amantea D, Nappi G, Bernardi G, Bagetta G, Corasaniti MT. Post-ischemic brain damage: pathophysiology and role of inflammatory mediators. FEBS J. 2009;276:13–26.
41. Albiero M, Poncina N, Ciciliot S, Cappellari R, Menegazzo L, Ferraro F, et al. Bone marrow macrophages contribute to diabetic stem cell mobilopathy by producing oncostatin M. Diabetes. 2015;64:2957–68.

Fluoxetine attenuates neuroinflammation in early brain injury after subarachnoid hemorrhage: a possible role for the regulation of TLR4/MyD88/NF-κB signaling pathway

Fu-yi Liu, Jing Cai, Chun Wang, Wu Ruan, Guo-ping Guan, Hai-zhou Pan, Jian-ru Li, Cong Qian, Jing-sen Chen, Lin Wang and Gao Chen*

Abstract

Background: Neuroinflammation is closely associated with functional outcome in subarachnoid hemorrhage (SAH) patients. Our recent study demonstrated that fluoxetine inhibited NLRP3 inflammasome activation and attenuated necrotic cell death in early brain injury after SAH, while the effects and potential mechanisms of fluoxetine on neuroinflammation after SAH have not been well-studied yet.

Methods: One hundred and fifty-three male SD rats were subjected to the endovascular perforation model of SAH. Fluoxetine (10 mg/kg) was administered intravenously at 6 h after SAH induction. TAK-242 (1.5 mg/kg), an exogenous TLR4 antagonist, was injected intraperitoneally 1 h after SAH. SAH grade, neurological scores, brain water content, Evans blue extravasation, immunofluorescence/TUNEL staining, quantitative real-time polymerase chain reaction (qRT-PCR), and western blot were performed.

Results: Fluoxetine administration attenuated BBB disruption, brain edema, and improved neurological function after SAH. In addition, fluoxetine alleviated the number of Iba-1-positive microglia/macrophages, neutrophil infiltration, and cell death. Moreover, fluoxetine reduced the levels of pro-inflammatory cytokines, downregulated the expression of TLR4 and MyD88, and promoted the nuclear translocation of NF-κB p65, which *were* also found in rats with TAK-242 administration. Combined administration of fluoxetine and TAK-242 did not enhance the neuroprotective effects of fluoxetine.

Conclusion: Fluoxetine attenuated neuroinflammation and improved neurological function in SAH rats. The potential mechanisms involved, at least in part, TLR4/MyD88/NF-κB signaling pathway.

Keywords: Subarachnoid hemorrhage, Early brain injury, Neuroinflammation, Fluoxetine

* Correspondence: d-chengao@zju.edu.cn
Department of Neurosurgery, The Second Affiliated Hospital of Zhejiang University School of Medicine, Hangzhou, China

Background

Subarachnoid hemorrhage (SAH) is a severe subtype of stroke with high mortality and morbidity; 25% of SAH patients died within 2 days, and cognitive and functional deficits present in about 20% of SAH survivors [1, 2]. In recent years, the importance of early brain injury has been concerned by researchers. Initial clinical severity after SAH has been shown to be the most important predictor for clinical outcomes in patients [3]. In addition, alleviating early brain injury has been reported to exert neuroprotective effects in SAH model [4–6].

Neuroinflammation is a well-recognized consequence of SAH and considered as an important contributor for early brain injury, cerebral vasospasm, and delayed brain injury after SAH [7, 8]. In addition, neuroinflammation is closely associated with functional outcome in SAH patients [9, 10]. Toll-like receptors (TLRs) belong to a large family of pattern recognition receptors that play a key role in inflammatory responses [11]. Of all the TLR family members, TLR4 is widely expressed in the central nervous system, including microglia, neurons, astrocytes, endothelial cells [12]. After stimulation of TLR4 with ligands, the MyD88-dependent pathway activates NF-κB, which produces pro-inflammatory cytokines mediators such as tumor necrosis factor (TNF-α) [13]. Thus, therapies target TLR4 signaling pathway, and subsequent neuroinflammation may offer potential treatment to protect against neuroinflammation after SAH.

Fluoxetine is one of the serotonin selective reuptake inhibitors. Since the least toxicity and side effects, fluoxetine has been widely prescribed depression and anxiety disorders [14]. Neuroprotective effects of fluoxetine have been demonstrated in different neurological diseases [15–18]. Fluoxetine has been shown to exert a capacity to regulate neuroinflammation [19, 20]. Our recent study also demonstrated that fluoxetine inhibited NLRP3 inflammasome activation and subsequent necrotic cell death in early brain injury after SAH [18]. Importantly, recent studies also demonstrated that fluoxetine inhibits TLR4 activation and subsequent NF-κB signaling pathway in vivo and in vitro [21–24]. In the present study, we investigated the effects of fluoxetine in neuroinflammation and the potential TLR4/MyD88/NF-κB signaling pathway in early brain injury after SAH.

Methods

Study design

Experiment 1

Male SD rats were randomly divided into four groups: sham, sham+fluoxetine, SAH+vehicle, and SAH+fluoxetine group. Fluoxetine was purchased from Selleck and dissolved in sterile 0.9% NaCl. Fluoxetine (10 mg/kg) or vehicle was injected intravenously at 6 h after SAH induction as previously described [18]. SAH grade and neurological scores were measured in all groups. Brain edema ($n = 6$/group), Evans blue extravasation ($n = 6$/group), immunofluorescence/TUNEL staining ($n = 5$/group), quantitative real-time polymerase chain reaction (qRT-PCR) ($n = 5$/group), and western blot ($n = 6$/group) were performed.

Experiment 2

Male SD rats were randomly divided into four groups: SAH+vehicle, SAH+TAK-242, and SAH+fluoxetine, SAH+fluoxetine+TAK-242 group. TAK-242 (1.5 mg/kg), an exogenous TLR4 antagonist, was injected intraperitoneally 1 h after SAH as previously described [25]. Neurological scores, Evans blue extravasation ($n = 6$/group), qRT-PCR ($n = 5$/group), and western blot ($n = 6$/group) were performed.

SAH model

Male Sprague-Dawley (SD) rats were purchased from SLAC Laboratory Animal Company (Shanghai, China) and housed in a controlled humidity and temperature conditions. The endovascular perforation model was performed to induce rat SAH as previously described [26]. Briefly, we isolated the left carotid artery and its branches under anesthesia of pentobarbital (50 mg/kg). Then, we divided the external carotid artery (ECA) and advanced a 4-0 monofilament suture until resistance was felt. Subsequently, we punctured the vessel and induced SAH. The sham rats underwent the same procedure without puncturing.

SAH grade and neurological scores

SAH grade and neurological scores were blindly assessed at 24 h after SAH as previously described [27]. Briefly, the basal cistern was divided into six segments. Each part was blindly obtained a grade from 0 to 3 judging by the amount of the blood clot in subarachnoid space. Then, the rats have received a total score ranging from 0 to 18. Neurological scores were blindly evaluated with a modification of the Garcia scoring system [28]. This scoring system has six parts as follow: spontaneous activity, spontaneous movements of all limbs, movement of forelimbs, climbing wall of the wire cage, reaction to touch on both side of trunk, and response to vibrissae touch. Then, the rats have received a total score ranging from 3 to 18. In this study, rats with SAH grade < 9 were excluded.

Brain edema and blood-brain barrier disruption

Brain edema and blood-brain barrier (BBB) disruption were evaluated at 24 h after SAH as previously described

[29]. Brain water content and Evans blue leakage were used to assessing brain edema and BBB disruption. Briefly, under deep anesthesia, rats were sacrificed. Then, brains were removed and divided into the left hemisphere, right hemisphere, cerebellum, and brainstem. The left hemispheres were weighed immediately to get the wet weight and dried at 105 °C for 3 days to obtain dry weight. Brain water content was calculated as [(wet weight-dry weight)/wet weight] × 100%. Evans blue dye (2%, 5 ml/kg) was administrated via the left femoral vein and circulated for 1 h. Under deep anesthesia, rats were sacrificed by cardiac perfusion. Then, we removed and separated the brain to get the left hemispheres immediately. Subsequently, we weighted the brain samples and homogenized with 3 ml of 50% trichloroacetic acid, then centrifuged at 15000 g for 30 min. The supernatant was mixed with an equal volume of trichloroacetic acid with ethanol. After overnight incubation (4 °C), the samples were centrifuged again (15,000*g*, 30 min) and measured by spectrofluorophotometer (excitation wavelength 620 nm and emission wavelength 680 nm).

Quantitative real-time polymerase chain reaction

The left basal cortical specimen (about 50–100 mg) in the face of the blood clot was collected for PCR detection at 24 h after SAH (as shown in Additional file 1: Figure S1). The total mRNA was then extracted using TRIzolTM Plus RNA Purification Kit (#12183-555, Invitrogen, China). Then, we determined the quantity of the purified RNA using UV absorbance at 260 nm. Subsequently, 1 μg of purified RNA from each sample was reverse-transcribed to cDNA. Superscript™ III First-Stand Synthesis SuperMix for qRT-PCR (#11752-050) was used to synthesize cDNA. The specific sequence of primers used was described as follows: TNF-α: sense primer 5′-GGT CCC AAC AAG GAG GAG AAG TTC-3′, antisense primer 5′-CCG CTT GGT GGT TTG CTA CGA C-3′; IL-1β: sense primer 5′-CGT GGG ATG ATG ACG ACC TGC-3′, antisense primer 5′-GGA GAA TAC CAC TTG TTG GCT TAT-3′; IL-6: sense primer 5′-GAC AGC CAC TGC CTT CCC TAC TT-3′, antisense primer 5′-CAG AAT TGC CAT TGC ACA ACT CT-3′; CD86: sense primer 5′-CAT CTA AGC AAG GAT ACC CGA AAC-3′, and antisense primer 5′-GAG ATA GGC TGA TGG AGA CAC TGA A-3′. PCR amplification was performed with a program of 95 °C for 1 min, followed by 40 cycles of 95 °C for 15 s, and 63 °C for 25 s. The relative mRNA level of each target gene was calculated using the $2^{-\nabla\nabla CT}$ methods as previously described [30].

Immunofluorescence staining

Immunofluorescence staining was performed at 24 h after SAH as previously described [29]. Briefly, rats were deeply euthanized and perfused with 4% paraformaldehyde in 0.1-mM phosphate-buffered saline (PBS, PH7.4). Brain samples were immersed in 30% sucrose until sinking to the bottom; 18 um-thick slices were cut with a cryostat. The primary antibodies were polyclonal goat anti-Iba-1(1:500, ab5076, Abcam), monoclonal mouse anti-NeuN (1:500, ab104224, Abcam), and polyclonal rabbit anti-MPO (1:300, ab65871, Abcam). Alexa Fluor 594 donkey anti-goat IgG (1:500, Invitrogen) and donkey anti-mouse (1:500, Invitrogen) were used as secondary antibody. Terminal deoxynucleotide transferase-deoxyuridine triphosphate (dUTP) nick end labeling (TUNEL) was performed following the manufacturer's protocol (Roche, Switzerland). Finally, the slices were covered by DAPI and observed under a fluorescence microscope. All procedures were conducted by two investigators blind to the experimental condition.

To quantify Iba-1-positive, MPO-positive, TUNEL-positive cells, we selected at least three sections per rats with similar areas of ipsilateral cortex (Additional file 1: Figure S1) and three fields with a magnification of × 200 or × 400 per section. For quantification of Iba-1-positive and MPO-positive cells, the numbers from these fields were averaged and expressed as positive cells per square millimeter for each mouse. For quantification of apoptotic neurons, the percentage of TUNEL-positive neurons was calculated as follows: (number of TUNEL-positive neurons/total number of neurons) × 100%. Tissue sections were analyzed by an observer who was blinded to the experimental cohorts.

Western blot

Western blot was performed at 24 h after SAH as previously described [26]. Under deep anesthesia, rats were sacrificed by cardiac perfusion with 0.1 M PBS, then brains were removed and the left basal cortical specimens in the face of the blood clot were obtained. The nuclear proteins were prepared by the NE-PER nuclear extraction reagents (Thermo, Rockford). Briefly, the ipsilateral cortex was homogenized and centrifuged for 10 min (1000*g*, 4 °C). Total protein was determined by BCA Protein Assay Kit (Beyotime, Shanghai, China). An equal amount of protein (60 μg) was suspended in loading buffer (denatured at 95 °C for 5 min) and loaded on an SDS-PAGE and transferred to nitrocellulose membranes. Then, we blocked the membranes with a nonfat dry milk buffer for 2 h, followed by incubation overnight with the following primary antibodies: polyclonal rabbit anti-NF-κB p65 (1:1000, ab16502, Abcam), monoclonal mouse anti-TLR4 (1:200, sc-293,072, Santa Cruz Biotechnology), polyclonal rabbit anti-MyD88 (1:1000, ab2064, Abcam), monoclonal rabbit anti-MMP9 (1:5000, ab137867, Abcam), polyclonal rabbit anti-ZO-1 (1:2000, ab96587, Abcam); polyclonal goat anti-claudin-5 (1:500, sc-17,668, Santa Cruz Biotechnology), monoclonal rabbit anti-occludin (1:50000, ab167161,

Abcam). The membranes were then incubated with horseradish peroxidase-conjugated secondary antibody for 1 h at room temperature. Blot bands were detected by X-ray film and quantified using Image J software (NIH).

Statistical analysis

Data were presented as mean ± SD. For the data satisfying normal distribution, comparisons between groups were performed by one-way ANOVA as appropriate. For the data satisfying non-normal distribution, comparisons between groups were performed by Kruskal-Wallis test or Mann-Whitney test. Differences were considered significant at $p < 0.05$. All statistical analyses were performed using GraphPad Prism and SPSS software.

Results

Physiological parameters, mortality, and SAH grade

During the surgical procedures, no significant difference was observed in all physiological parameters including the mean arterial pressure, arterial PH, PO_2, PCO_2, and

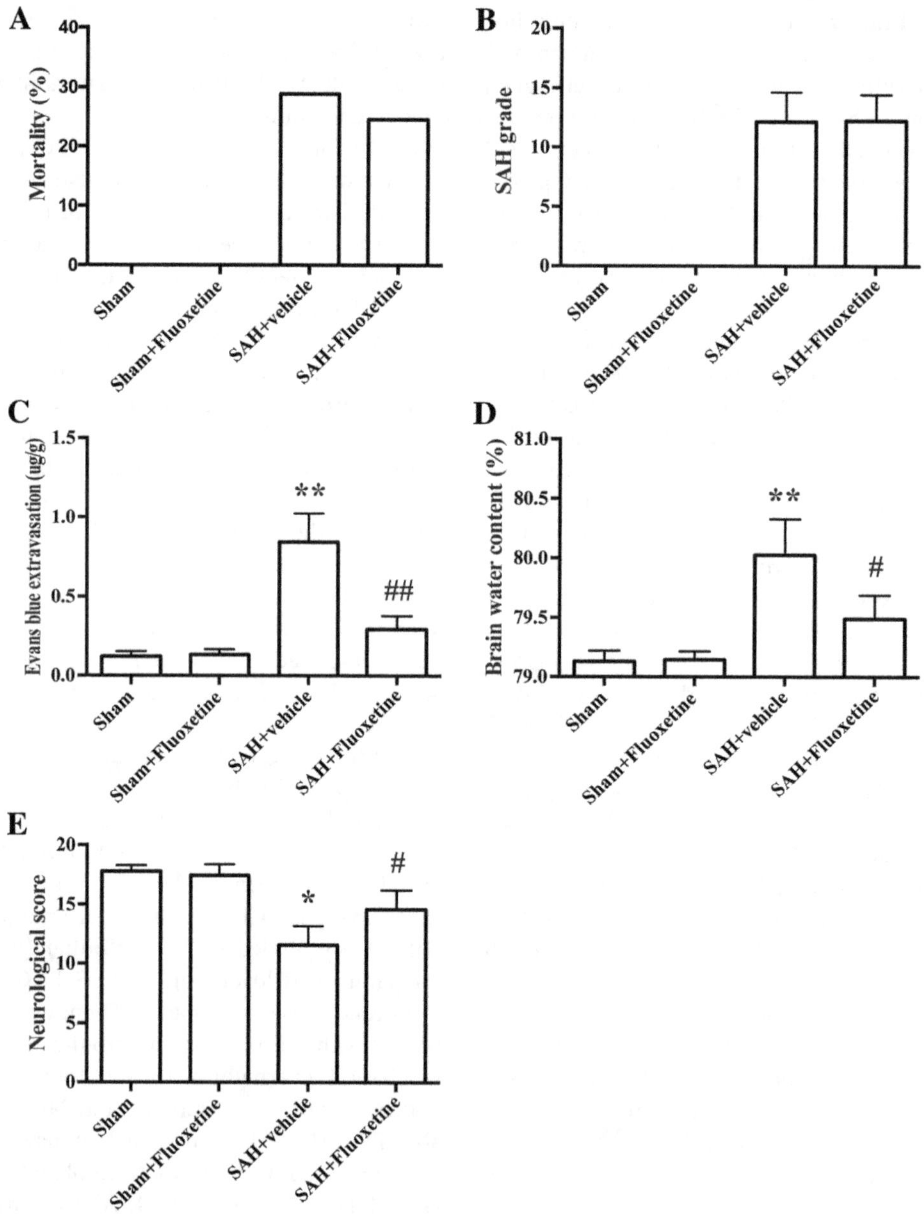

Fig. 1 The effects of fluoxetine on mortality, SAH grade, neurological scores, Evans blue extravasation, and brain edema. **a** The quantification of mortality. **b** The quantification of SAH grade. $n = 28$/group. **c** The quantification of Evans blue extravasation. *$p < 0.05$ vs sham. #$p < 0.05$ vs SAH +vehicle. $n = 6$/group. **d** The quantification of brain water content. **$p < 0.01$ vs sham. #$p < 0.05$ vs SAH+vehicle. $n = 6$/group. **e** The quantification of neurological score. *$p < 0.05$ vs sham. #$p < 0.05$ vs SAH+vehicle. $n = 28$/group

blood glucose levels (data not shown). None of the rats died in the sham and sham+fluoxetine group. In experiment 1, the mortality of SAH+vehicle and SAH+fluoxetine group were 28.2% (11/39, Fig. 1a) and 24.5% (9/37, Fig. 1a), respectively. In experiment 2, the mortality of SAH+vehicle, SAH+TAK-242, SAH+fluoxetine, and SAH +fluoxetine+TAK-242 group were 29.2% (7/24), 22.7% (5/22), 22.7% (5/22), and 19.0% (4/21), respectively. SAH grade was blindly evaluated in our study. However, there is no significant difference between SAH groups ($p > 0.05$, Fig. 1b).

Fluoxetine attenuated BBB disruption, brain edema, and neurological deficits

SAH induction increased the amount of Evans blue extravasation, indicating the disruption of BBB ($p < 0.01$,

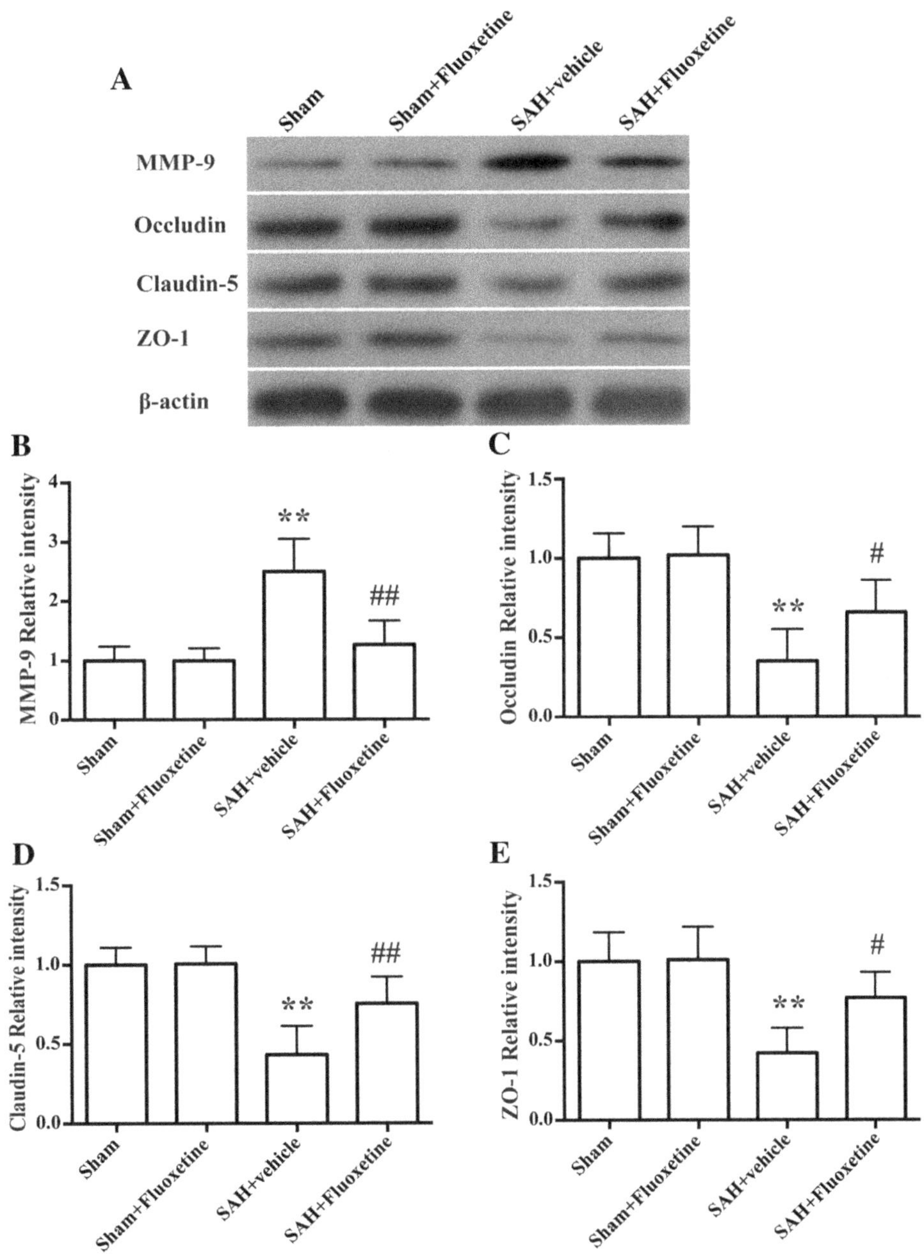

Fig. 2 Fluoxetine downregulated MMP-9 expression and prevented degradation of the tight junction proteins in the ipsilateral cortex at 24 h after SAH. **a** Representative western blot bands of MMP-9, occludin, claudin-5, and ZO-1. **b** Densitometric quantification of MMP-9. $^{**}p < 0.01$ vs sham. $^{\#\#}p < 0.01$ vs SAH+vehicle. $n = 6$/group. **c** Densitometric quantification of occludin. $^{**}p < 0.01$ vs sham. $^{\#}p < 0.05$ vs SAH+vehicle. $n = 6$/group. **d** Densitometric quantification of claudin-5. $^{**}p < 0.01$ vs sham. $^{\#\#}p < 0.01$ vs SAH+vehicle. $n = 6$/group. **e** Densitometric quantification of ZO-1. $^{**}p < 0.01$ vs sham. $^{\#}p < 0.05$ vs SAH+vehicle. $n = 6$/group

Fig. 1c). Similarly, SAH also increased the ratio of brain water content, indicating brain edema ($p < 0.01$, Fig. 1d). In addition, neurological scores were lower in the SAH +vehicle group than in the sham rats, indicating neurological impairments ($p < 0.01$, Fig. 1e). The BBB disruption and brain edema were significantly attenuated by fluoxetine administration ($p < 0.01$, Fig. 1c and $p < 0.05$, Fig. 1d). Fluoxetine treatment also improved neurological function compared with the SAH+vehicle group ($p < 0.05$, Fig. 1e).

Fluoxetine downregulated MMP-9 expression and decreased the degradation of tight junction proteins

Rats in SAH+vehicle group had high levels of MMP-9 than control rats ($p < 0.01$, Fig. 2a, b), and rats post-treated with fluoxetine had a lower MMP-9 expression ($p < 0.01$, Fig. 2a, b). The protein levels of tight junction proteins, including occludin, claudin-5, and ZO-1, were significantly decreased in the SAH+vehicle group when compared with the sham group ($p < 0.01$, Fig. 2 a, c–e), whereas fluoxetine treatment significantly upregulated their protein levels ($p < 0.05$, Fig. 2c, e, and $p < 0.01$, Fig. 2d).

Fluoxetine decreased the expression of pro-inflammatory cytokines

qRT-PCR results showed the mRNA levels of pro-inflammatory cytokines TNF-α, IL-1β, IL-6, and CD86 were significantly increased in the SAH+vehicle group compared with the sham group ($p < 0.01$, Fig. 3a–d), while fluoxetine administration significantly reduced the mRNA levels of TNF-α ($p < 0.01$, Fig. 3a), IL-1β ($p < 0.05$, Fig. 3b), IL-6 ($p < 0.01$, Fig. 3c), and CD86 ($p < 0.01$, Fig. 3d).

Fluoxetine reduced Iba-1-positive microglia/macrophages, neutrophil infiltration, and neuronal apoptosis

A significant increase of Iba-1positive cells was detected in SAH+vehicle group compared with the sham group ($p < 0.01$, Fig. 4a, b), whereas fluoxetine

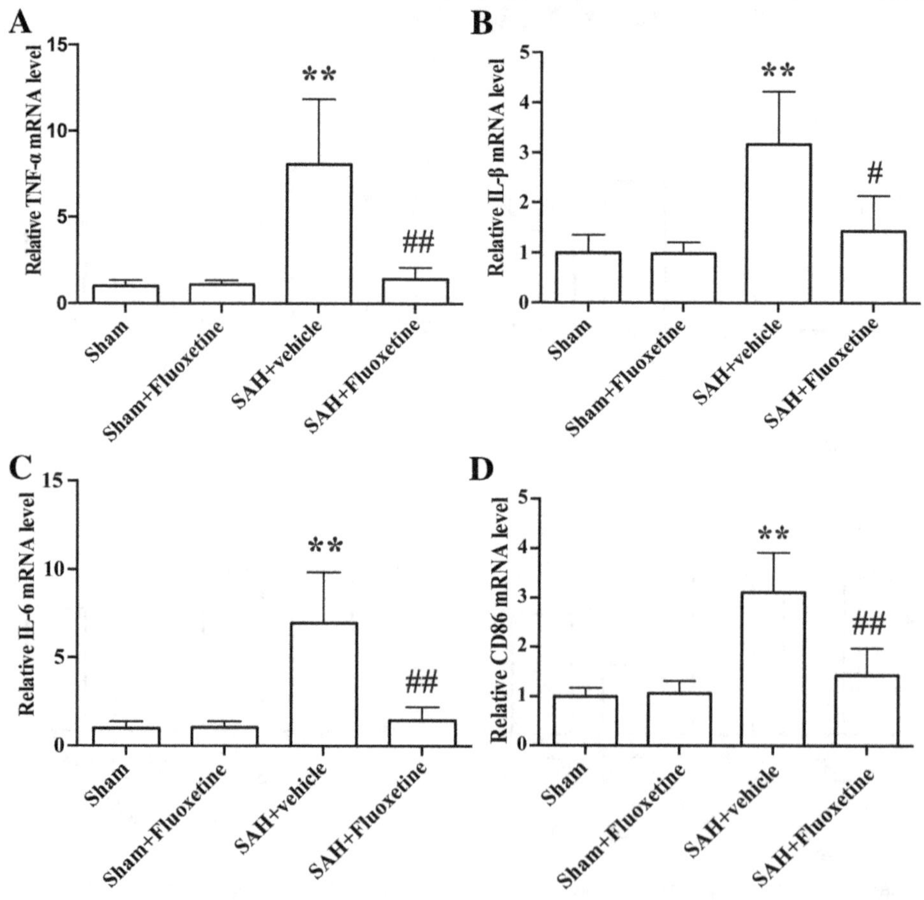

Fig. 3 Fluoxetine decreased the mRNA levels of pro-inflammatory cytokines. **a** The quantification of TNF-α mRNA levels. $^{**}p < 0.01$ vs sham. $^{\#\#}p < 0.01$ vs SAH+vehicle. $n = 5$/group. **b** The quantification of IL-1β mRNA levels. $^{**}p < 0.01$ vs sham. $^{\#}p < 0.05$ vs SAH + vehicle. $n = 5$/group. **c** The quantification of IL-6 mRNA levels. $^{**}p < 0.01$ vs sham. $^{\#\#}p < 0.01$ vs SAH+vehicle. $n = 5$/group. **d** The quantification of CD86 mRNA levels. $^{**}p < 0.01$ vs sham. $^{\#\#}p < 0.01$ vs SAH+vehicle. $n = 5$/group

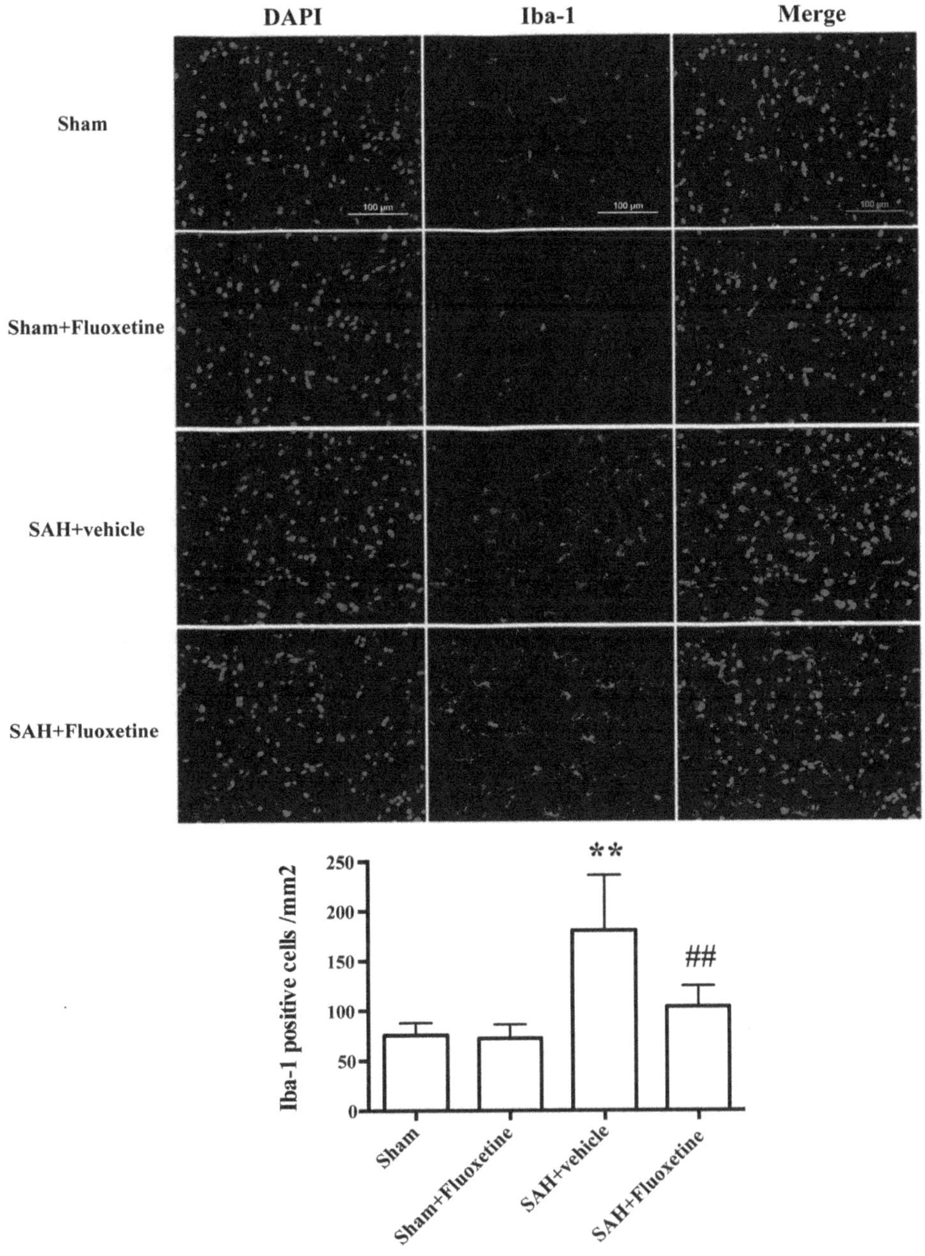

Fig. 4 Fluoxetine decreased the number of Iba-1-positive microglia/macrophages in the ipsilateral cortex at 24 h after SAH. **a** Representative Iba-1 staining. **b** The quantification of Iba-1-positive cells. $^{**}p < 0.01$ vs sham. $^{\#\#}p < 0.01$ vs SAH+vehicle. Scale bar = 100 μm. $n = 5$/group

significantly decreased the number of Iba-1 positive cells ($p < 0.01$, Fig. 4a, b). MPO-positive cells markedly increased in the ipsilateral cortex after SAH when compared with the sham group ($p < 0.01$, Fig. 5a, b), while administration of fluoxetine significantly reduced the number of MPO-positive cells after SAH ($p < 0.01$, Fig. 5a, b). The percentage of TUNEL-positive neurons was significantly higher in the SAH+vehicle group than the control group ($p < 0.01$, Fig. 6a, b), whereas fluoxetine administration significantly decreased the percentage of TUNEL-positive neurons ($p < 0.01$, Fig. 6a, b).

Fluoxetine attenuated TLR4 and MyD88 and reduced the nuclear translocation of NF-κB p65

The protein levels of TLR4 and MyD88 were significantly increased in the cortex in the SAH+vehicle group as compared with the sham group ($p < 0.01$, Fig. 7a–c). The protein levels of TLR4 and MyD88 in SAH+fluoxetine group were significantly lower than those of SAH +vehicle group ($p < 0.01$, Fig. 7a–c). We also examined the nuclear levels of NF-κB p65, an indicator of the activation of the NF-κB signaling pathway. The protein levels of NF-κB p65 were significantly increased in the

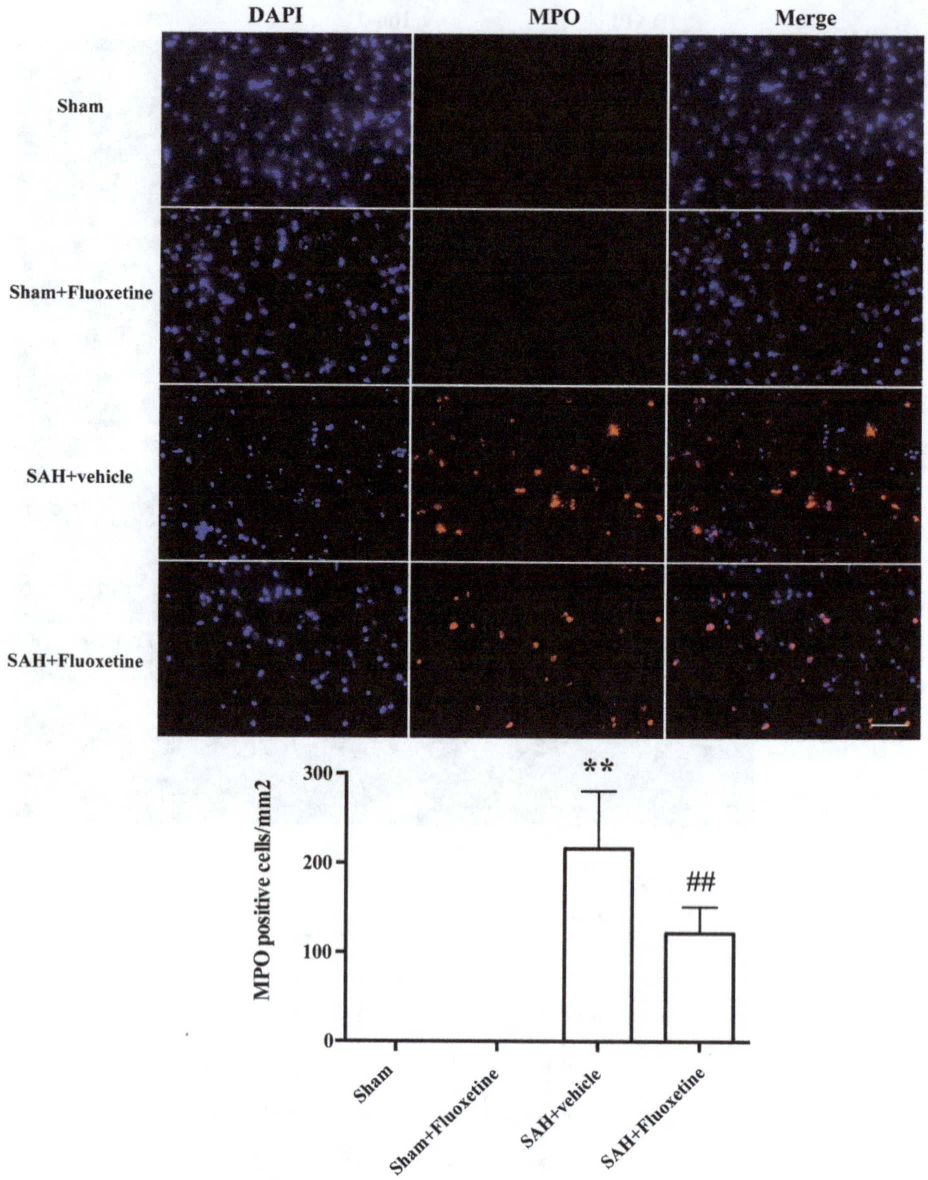

Fig. 5 Fluoxetine inhibited neutrophil infiltration in the ipsilateral cortex at 24 h after SAH. **a** Representative MPO staining. **b** The quantification of MPO-positive cells. $^{**}p < 0.01$ vs sham. $^{\#\#}p < 0.01$ vs SAH+vehicle. Scale bar = 50 μm. $n = 5$/group

SAH+vehicle group as compared with the sham group ($p < 0.01$, Fig. 7a, d). The protein levels of NF-κB p65 in SAH+fluoxetine group were significantly lower than those of SAH+vehicle group ($p < 0.01$, Fig. 7a, d).

Combined administration of fluoxetine and TAK-242 did not enhance the effects of fluoxetine in the expression of TLR4, MyD88, nuclear NF-κB, and pro-inflammatory cytokines, BBB disruption, and neurological function

The protein levels of TLR4, MyD88, and nuclear NF-κB were significantly decreased in the cortex in the SAH +TAK242, SAH+fluoxetine, and SAH+fluoxetine+TAK-242 group as compared with the SAH+vehicle group ($p < 0.01$, Fig. 8a–d). There was no significant difference between SAH+fluoxetine and SAH+fluoxetine +TAK-242 in proteins level of TLR4, MyD88, and nuclear NF-κB ($p > 0.05$, Fig. 8a–d). The mRNA levels of pro-inflammatory cytokines TNF-α, IL-1β, and IL-6 were significantly decreased in the cortex in the SAH +TAK242, SAH+fluoxetine, and SAH+fluoxetine+TAK-242 group as compared with the SAH+vehicle group ($p < 0.01$, Fig. 8e, $p < 0.05$, Fig. 8f, and $p < 0.01$, Fig. 8g). No significant difference was observed in these mRNA levels between SAH+fluoxetine and SAH+fluoxetine+TAK-242 group ($p > 0.05$, Fig. 8e–g). Combined administration of fluoxetine and TAK-242 prevented the

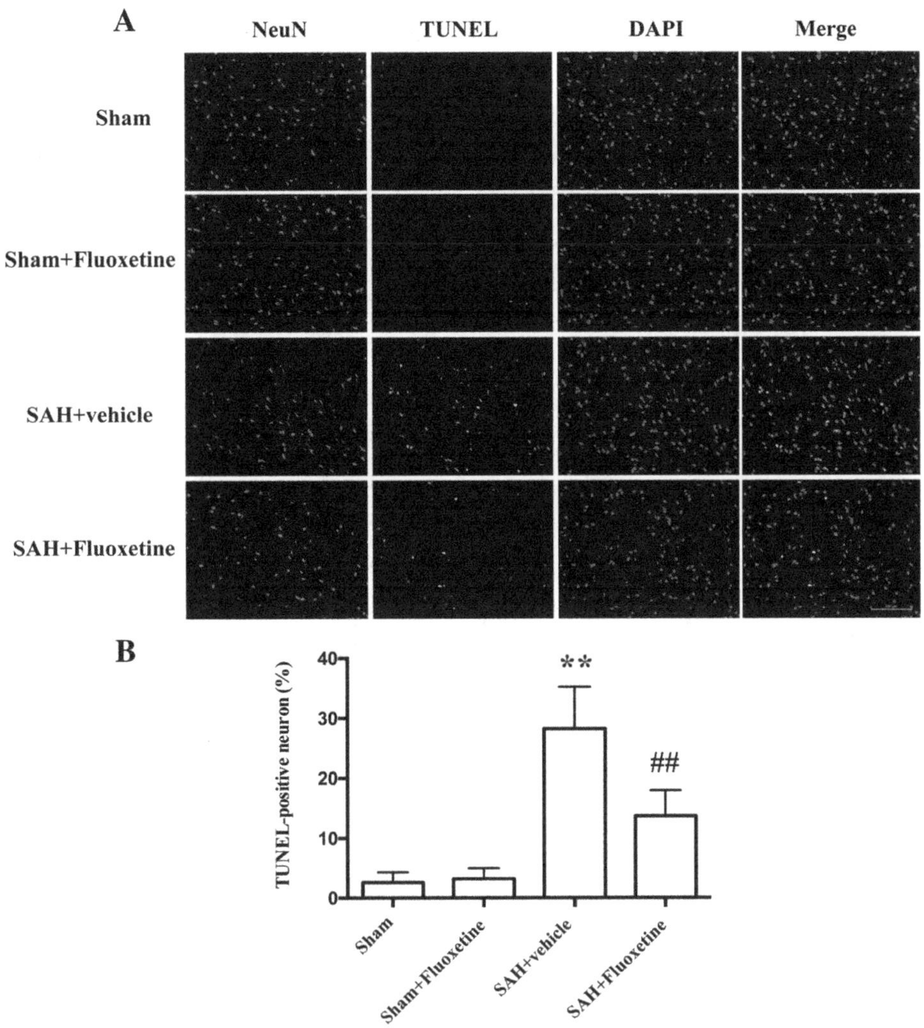

Fig. 6 Fluoxetine attenuated neuronal apoptosis in the ipsilateral cortex at 24 h after SAH. **a** Representative TUNEL staining. **b** The percentage of TUNEL-positive neurons. $^{***}p < 0.01$ vs sham. $^{\#\#}p < 0.01$ vs SAH+vehicle. Scale bar = 100 μm. $n = 5$/group

Evans blue extravasation ($p < 0.01$, Fig. 8h) and improved the neurological function ($p < 0.05$, Fig. 8i), which was similar with fluoxetine treatment ($p > 0.05$, Fig. 8h, i).

Discussion

The current study presented several novel findings:(1) fluoxetine attenuated BBB disruption, brain edema, and improved neurological function after SAH. (2) Fluoxetine alleviated the number of Iba-1-positive microglia/ macrophages, neutrophil infiltration, and cell death. (3) Fluoxetine reduced the levels of pro-inflammatory cytokines, and the underlying mechanisms, at least in part, involved the TLR4/MyD88/NF-κB signaling pathway (Fig. 9).

At present, no therapies are available to cure the neurological deficits in SAH patients [31]; however, an increasing number of studies show that inflammation contributes to early brain injury after SAH and inhibition of inflammation can ameliorate brain injury after SAH [10, 32–34]. One of the most important mediators in inflammation-induced brain injury after SAH is MMP-9. Notably, both clinical and basic studies have reported an elevation of MMP-9 in brain tissue, serum, and cerebrospinal fluid after SAH [35–37]. The MMP-9 elevation is responsible for the degradation of tight junction proteins, which are critical in the maintenance of BBB integrity. In the present study, we observed fluoxetine treatment alleviated MMP-9 expression and degradation of tight junction proteins (ZO-1, occludin, and claudin-5), attenuated BBB disruption and brain edema, and improved neurological function after SAH. The effects of fluoxetine on MMP-9 expression and subsequent BBB disruption were consistent with previous reports about fluoxetine treatment in experimental transient global ischemia and spinal cord injury [38, 39]. BBB disruption facilitates infiltration of peripheral inflammatory cells, including macrophage and

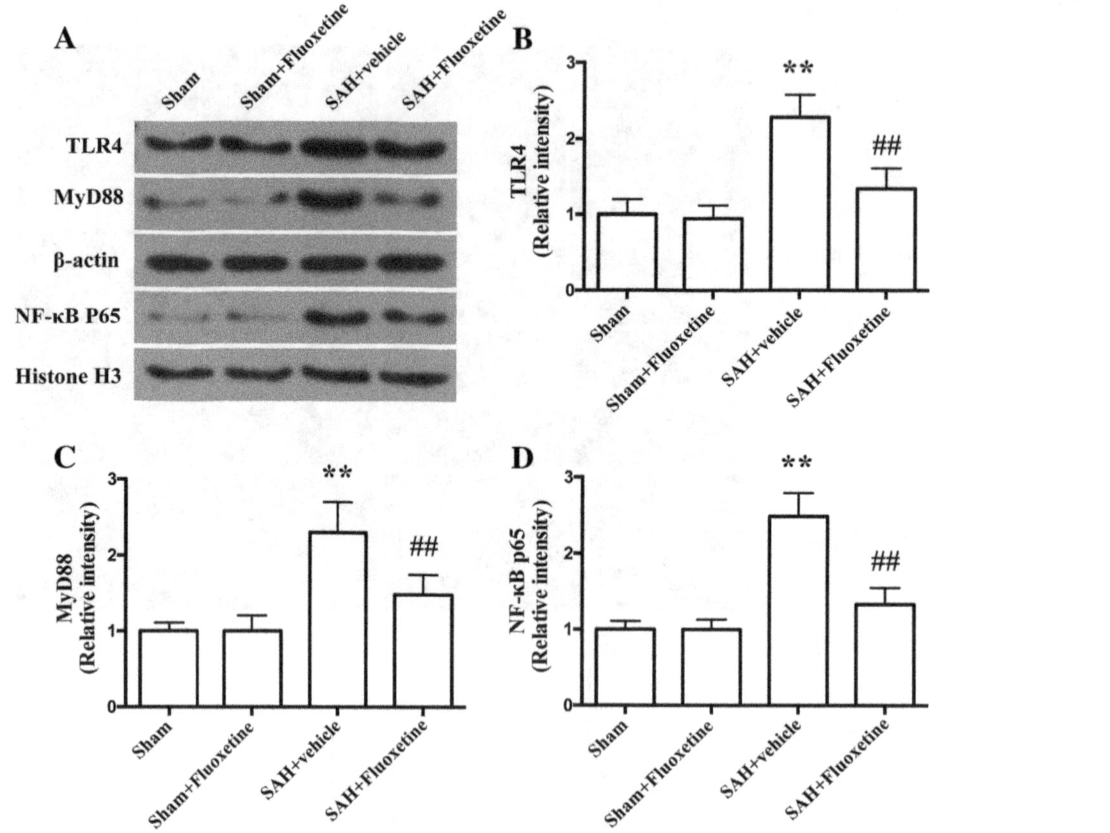

Fig. 7 Fluoxetine downregulated the protein levels of TLR4 and MyD88, but increased the nuclear protein levels of NF-κB p65 in the ipsilateral cortex at 24 h after SAH. **a** Representative western blot bands of TLR4, MyD88, and nuclear NF-κB p65. **b** Densitometric quantification of TLR4. $^{**}p < 0.01$ vs sham. $^{\#\#}p < 0.01$ vs SAH+vehicle. $n = 6$/group. **c** Densitometric quantification of MyD88. $^{**}p < 0.01$ vs sham. $^{\#\#}p < 0.01$ vs SAH+vehicle. $n = 6$/group. **d** Densitometric quantification of nuclear NF-κB p65. $^{**}p < 0.01$ vs sham. $^{\#\#}p < 0.01$ vs SAH+vehicle. $n = 6$/group

neutrophils, which aggravate neuroinflammation by releasing a multitude of inflammatory factors [40]. In addition, BBB disruption also results in neuronal cell death [38]. In the current study, we found that fluoxetine inhibited the neutrophils infiltration and reduced neural cell death in early brain injury after injury.

Inflammatory cytokines are important regulators in MMP-9 activation and subsequent BBB disruption. A previous study demonstrated that the selective inhibitor of IL-1β blocked JNK-mediated MMP-9 activation and improved neurological function in SAH rats [41]. IL-6 induced MMP-9 expression through the JAK-mediated pathway in macrophages [42]. TNF-α was also reported as an upstream regulator for MMP-9 [43]. In our study, we found that fluoxetine downregulated these inflammatory cytokines, which is in accordance with previous studies [44, 45]. TLRs belong to a large family of pattern recognition receptors that play a key role in innate immunity and inflammatory responses. Of the TLR family members, TLR4 was of vital importance in this family. TLR4 is activated by many endogenous ligands such as heme, fibrinogen, heat shock proteins, all of which are produced after SAH [13, 46]. In fact, patients with aneurysmal SAH was reported to have higher TLR4 levels on peripheral blood mononuclear cells, which were associated with more massive SAH, occurrence of cerebral vasospasm, delayed cerebral infarction, and worse functional recovery [47]. TLR4 interacts with two distinct adaptor proteins, MyD88 and Toll-receptor-associated activator of interferon (TRIF), and activates two parallel signaling pathways to initiate activation of transcription factors that regulate expression of proinflammatory cytokines genes [12]. In addition, the TRIF-dependent pathway induces late phase activation of NF-κB, while the faster TLR4 route through MyD88 is the early activation of NF-κB. Many previous studies have demonstrated the anti-inflammatory effects of fluoxetine in other system disorders in vivo and in vitro [20–24, 48]. In these studies, TLR4 and downstream NF-κB were hotspots. However, limited studies focused on the effects of fluoxetine in the TLR4 signaling pathway after SAH. Therefore, we examined the TLR4-mediated MyD88 pathway in the current study. Our results showed that the protein levels of TLR4 and

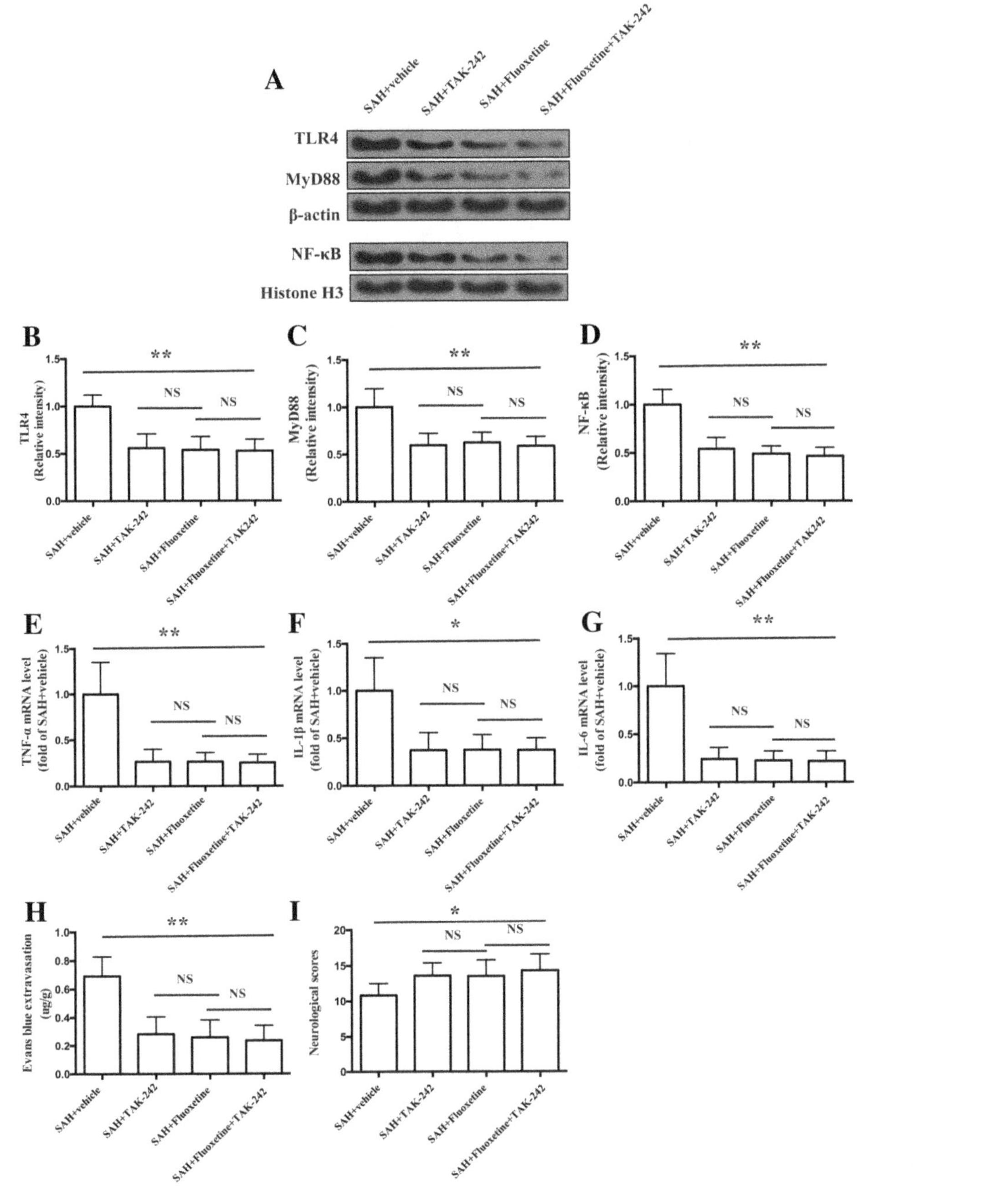

Fig. 8 Combined administration of fluoxetine and TAK-242 did not enhance the effects of fluoxetine in the expression of TLR4, MyD88, nuclear NF-κB, and pro-inflammatory cytokines, BBB disruption, and neurological function. **a** Representative western blot bands of TLR4, MyD88, and nuclear NF-κB p65. **b** Densitometric quantification of TLR4. **$p < 0.01$ vs SAH+vehicle. $n = 6$/group. **c** Densitometric quantification of MyD88. **$p < 0.01$ vs SAH+vehicle. $n = 6$/group. **d** Densitometric quantification of nuclear NF-κB p65. **$p < 0.01$ vs SAH+vehicle. $n = 6$/group. **e** The quantification of TNF-α mRNA levels. **$p < 0.01$ vs SAH+vehicle. $n = 5$/group **f** The quantification of IL-1β mRNA levels. *$p < 0.05$ vs SAH+vehicle. $n = 5$/group. **g** The quantification of IL-6 mRNA levels. **$p < 0.01$ vs SAH+vehicle. $n = 5$/group. **h** The quantification of Evans blue extravasation. **$p < 0.01$vs SAH+vehicle. $n = 6$/group. **i** The quantification of neurological score. *$p < 0.05$ vs sham. #$p < 0.05$ vs SAH + vehicle. $n = 17$/group

MyD88 were significantly increased in early brain injury after SAH and fluoxetine downregulated their expression. In addition, we found that fluoxetine also reduced the nuclear translocation of NF-κB p65, an indicator of NF-κB activation. What is more important is that we also used TAK-242, a small-molecule inhibitor of the TLR4 signaling pathway. We found that the combined administration of fluoxetine and TAK-242 reduced the expression of TLR4, MyD88, and nuclear NF-κB, decreased the mRNA levels of pro-inflammatory cytokines,

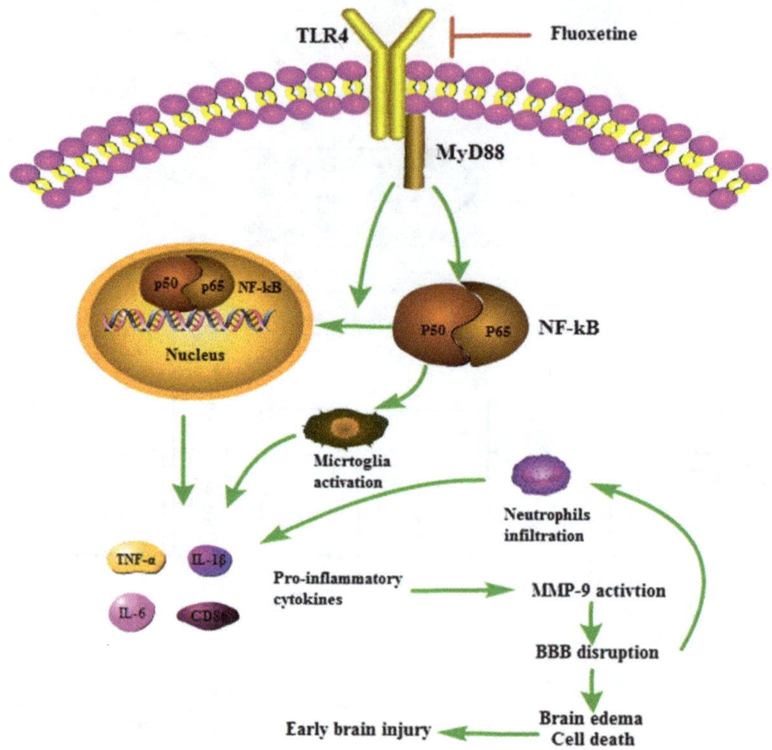

Fig. 9 The potential molecular mechanisms of anti-inflammatory effects of fluoxetine through TLR4/MyD88/NF-κB signaling pathway

prevented BBB disruption, and improved neurological function after SAH. These beneficial effects of combined administration were similar to alone fluoxetine treatment. Taken together, our study indicated that TLR4/MyD88/NF-κB signaling pathway was involved in anti-inflammatory effects of fluoxetine in early brain injury after SAH.

There are some limitations in our study. First, the present study aimed at investigating the effects and potential mechanism of fluoxetine in neuroinflammation in early brain injury after SAH, the long-term study of fluoxetine after SAH is still needed in the future. Second, previous studies showed anti-apoptotic effects of fluoxetine, which did not deeply evaluate in the current study.

Conclusions

The current study has demonstrated that fluoxetine attenuated neuroinflammation and improved neurological function after SAH. The potential mechanisms involved, at least in part, TLR4/MyD88/NF-κB signaling pathway.

Abbreviations

BBB: Blood-brain barrier; ECA: External carotid artery; IL-1β: Interleukin-1β; IL-6: Interleukin-6; MMP-9: Matrix metallopeptidase 9; MPO: Myeloperoxidase; MyD88: Myeloid differentiation primary response 88; NF-κB: Nuclear factor kappa B; qRT-PCR: Quantitative real-time polymerase chain reaction; SAH: Subarachnoid hemorrhage; SD: Sprague-Dawley; TLRs: Toll-like receptors; TNF-α: Tumor necrosis factor-α; TUNEL: Terminal deoxynucleotidyl transferase dUTP nick end labeling

Acknowledgements

Not applicable.

Funding

This work was supported by the National Natural Science Foundation of China (NO.81771246, 81571106, 81701152), Natural Science Foundation of Zhejiang province (LY17H090008, LY17H090007 and Y18H090019).

Authors' contributions

This work includes significant contributions from all authors. GC and FYL conceived the study and contributed to its experimental design. JC, CW, WR, HZP, GPG, and JRL carried out the laboratory experiments, CQ, JSC, GPG, and LW analyzed the data. FYL, JC, and GC wrote the manuscript. CW and GC contributed to the editing of the manuscript. All authors read and approved the final manuscript.

Consent for publication

Not applicable.

Competing interests

The authors declare that they have no competing interests.

References

1. Connolly ES Jr, Rabinstein AA, Carhuapoma JR, Derdeyn CP, Dion J, Higashida RT, Hoh BL, Kirkness CJ, Naidech AM, Ogilvy CS, et al. Guidelines for the management of aneurysmal subarachnoid hemorrhage: a guideline for healthcare professionals from the American Heart Association/American Stroke Association. Stroke. 2012;43:1711–37.
2. Springer MV, Schmidt JM, Wartenberg KE, Frontera JA, Badjatia N, Mayer SA. Predictors of global cognitive impairment 1 year after subarachnoid hemorrhage. Neurosurgery. 2009;65:1043–50 discussion 1050-1041.
3. Mocco J, Ransom ER, Komotar RJ, Schmidt JM, Sciacca RR, Mayer SA, Connolly ES Jr. Preoperative prediction of long-term outcome in poor-grade aneurysmal subarachnoid hemorrhage. Neurosurgery. 2006;59:529–38 discussion 529-538.
4. Zhang X, Wu Q, Zhang Q, Lu Y, Liu J, Li W, Lv S, Zhou M, Zhang X, Hang C. Resveratrol attenuates early brain injury after experimental subarachnoid hemorrhage via inhibition of NLRP3 inflammasome activation. Front Neurosci. 2017;11:611.
5. Fan R, Enkhjargal B, Camara R, Yan F, Gong L, ShengtaoYao TJ, Chen Y, Zhang JH. Critical role of EphA4 in early brain injury after subarachnoid hemorrhage in rat. Exp Neurol. 2017;296:41–8.
6. Liu L, Kawakita F, Fujimoto M, Nakano F, Imanaka-Yoshida K, Yoshida T, Suzuki H. Role of periostin in early brain injury after subarachnoid hemorrhage in mice. Stroke. 2017;48:1108–11.
7. Suzuki H, Kawakita F. Tenascin-C in aneurysmal subarachnoid hemorrhage: deleterious or protective? Neural Regen Res. 2016;11:230–1.
8. Schneider UC, Schiffler J, Hakiy N, Horn P, Vajkoczy P. Functional analysis of pro-inflammatory properties within the cerebrospinal fluid after subarachnoid hemorrhage in vivo and in vitro. J Neuroinflammation. 2012;9:28.
9. Niwa A, Osuka K, Nakura T, Matsuo N, Watabe T, Takayasu M. Interleukin-6, MCP-1, IP-10, and MIG are sequentially expressed in cerebrospinal fluid after subarachnoid hemorrhage. J Neuroinflammation. 2016;13:217.
10. Lucke-Wold BP, Logsdon AF, Manoranjan B, Turner RC, McConnell E, Vates GE, Huber JD, Rosen CL, Simard JM. Aneurysmal subarachnoid hemorrhage and neuroinflammation: a comprehensive review. Int J Mol Sci. 2016;17:497.
11. De Nardo D. Toll-like receptors: activation, signalling and transcriptional modulation. Cytokine. 2015;74:181–9.
12. Buchanan MM, Hutchinson M, Watkins LR, Yin H. Toll-like receptor 4 in CNS pathologies. J Neurochem. 2010;114:13–27.
13. Kawakita F, Fujimoto M, Liu L, Nakano F, Nakatsuka Y, Suzuki H. Effects of toll-like receptor 4 antagonists against cerebral vasospasm after experimental subarachnoid hemorrhage in mice. Mol Neurobiol. 2017;54: 6624–33.
14. Wong DT, Bymaster FP, Engleman EA. Prozac (fluoxetine, Lilly 110140), the first selective serotonin uptake inhibitor and an antidepressant drug: twenty years since its first publication. Life Sci. 1995;57:411–41.
15. Khodanovich M, Kisel A, Kudabaeva M, Chernysheva G, Smolyakova V, Krutenkova E, Wasserlauf I, Plotnikov M, Yarnykh V. Effects of fluoxetine on hippocampal neurogenesis and neuroprotection in the model of global cerebral ischemia in rats. Int J Mol Sci. 2018;19(1):162.
16. Lee JY, Choi HY, Yune TY. Fluoxetine and vitamin C synergistically inhibits blood-spinal cord barrier disruption and improves functional recovery after spinal cord injury. Neuropharmacology. 2016;109:78–87.
17. Lee JY, Kang SR, Yune TY. Fluoxetine prevents oligodendrocyte cell death by inhibiting microglia activation after spinal cord injury. J Neurotrauma. 2015;32:633–44.
18. Li JR, Xu HZ, Nie S, Peng YC, Fan LF, Wang ZJ, Wu C, Yan F, Chen JY, Gu C, et al. Fluoxetine-enhanced autophagy ameliorates early brain injury via inhibition of NLRP3 inflammasome activation following subarachnoid hemorrhage in rats. J Neuroinflammation. 2017;14:186.
19. Alboni S, Poggini S, Garofalo S, Milior G, El Hajj H, Lecours C, Girard I, Gagnon S, Boisjoly-Villeneuve S, Brunello N, et al. Fluoxetine treatment affects the inflammatory response and microglial function according to the quality of the living environment. Brain Behav Immun. 2016;58:261–71.
20. Liechti FD, Grandgirard D, Leib SL. The antidepressant fluoxetine protects the hippocampus from brain damage in experimental pneumococcal meningitis. Neuroscience. 2015;297:89–94.
21. Koh SJ, Kim JM, Kim IK, Kim N, Jung HC, Song IS, Kim JS. Fluoxetine inhibits NF-kappaB signaling in intestinal epithelial cells and ameliorates experimental colitis and colitis-associated colon cancer in mice. Am J Physiol Gastrointest Liver Physiol. 2011;301:G9–19.
22. Zhang F, Zhou H, Wilson BC, Shi JS, Hong JS, Gao HM. Fluoxetine protects neurons against microglial activation-mediated neurotoxicity. Parkinsonism Relat Disord. 2012;18(Suppl 1):S213–7.
23. Ha E, Jung KH, Choe BK, Bae JH, Shin DH, Yim SV, Baik HH. Fluoxetine increases the nitric oxide production via nuclear factor kappa B-mediated pathway in BV2 murine microglial cells. Neurosci Lett. 2006;397:185–9.
24. Waiskopf N, Ofek K, Gilboa-Geffen A, Bekenstein U, Bahat A, Bennett ER, Podoly E, Livnah O, Hartmann G, Soreq H. AChE and RACK1 promote the anti-inflammatory properties of fluoxetine. J Mol Neurosci. 2014;53:306–15.
25. Hua F, Tang H, Wang J, Prunty MC, Hua X, Sayeed I, Stein DG. TAK-242, an antagonist for Toll-like receptor 4, protects against acute cerebral ischemia/reperfusion injury in mice. J Cereb Blood Flow Metab. 2015;35:536–42.
26. Li J, Chen J, Mo H, Chen J, Qian C, Yan F, Gu C, Hu Q, Wang L, Chen G. Minocycline protects against NLRP3 inflammasome-induced inflammation and P53-associated apoptosis in early brain injury after subarachnoid hemorrhage. Mol Neurobiol. 2016;53:2668–78.
27. Ying GY, Jing CH, Li JR, Wu C, Yan F, Chen JY, Wang L, Dixon BJ, Chen G. Neuroprotective effects of valproic acid on blood-brain barrier disruption and apoptosis-related early brain injury in rats subjected to subarachnoid hemorrhage are modulated by heat shock protein 70/matrix metalloproteinases and heat shock protein 70/AKT pathways. Neurosurgery. 2016;79:286–95.
28. Chen J, Wang L, Wu C, Hu Q, Gu C, Yan F, Li J, Yan W, Chen G. Melatonin-enhanced autophagy protects against neural apoptosis via a mitochondrial pathway in early brain injury following a subarachnoid hemorrhage. J Pineal Res. 2014;56:12–9.
29. Xu H, Li J, Wang Z, Feng M, Shen Y, Cao S, Li T, Peng Y, Fan L, Chen J, et al. Methylene blue attenuates neuroinflammation after subarachnoid hemorrhage in rats through the Akt/GSK-3beta/MEF2D signaling pathway. Brain Behav Immun. 2017;65:125–39.
30. Livak KJ, Schmittgen TD. Analysis of relative gene expression data using real-time quantitative PCR and the 2(−Delta Delta C(T)) method. Methods. 2001;25:402–8.
31. Young AM, Karri SK, Helmy A, Budohoski KP, Kirollos RW, Bulters DO, Kirkpatrick PJ, Ogilvy CS, Trivedi RA. Pharmacologic management of subarachnoid hemorrhage. World Neurosurg. 2015;84:28–35.
32. Savarraj JPJ, Parsha K, Hergenroeder GW, Zhu L, Bajgur SS, Ahn S, Lee K, Chang T, Kim DH, Liu Y, Choi HA. Systematic model of peripheral inflammation after subarachnoid hemorrhage. Neurology. 2017;88: 1535–45.
33. Frontera JA, Provencio JJ, Sehba FA, McIntyre TM, Nowacki AS, Gordon E, Weimer JM, Aledort L. The role of platelet activation and inflammation in early brain injury following subarachnoid hemorrhage. Neurocrit Care. 2017; 26:48–57.
34. You W, Wang Z, Li H, Shen H, Xu X, Jia G, Chen G. Inhibition of mammalian target of rapamycin attenuates early brain injury through modulating microglial polarization after experimental subarachnoid hemorrhage in rats. J Neurol Sci. 2016;367:224–31.
35. Feiler S, Plesnila N, Thal SC, Zausinger S, Scholler K. Contribution of matrix metalloproteinase-9 to cerebral edema and functional outcome following experimental subarachnoid hemorrhage. Cerebrovasc Dis. 2011;32:289–95.
36. Fischer M, Dietmann A, Beer R, Broessner G, Helbok R, Pfausler B, Schmutzhard E, Lackner P. Differential regulation of matrix-metalloproteinases and their tissue inhibitors in patients with aneurysmal subarachnoid hemorrhage. PLoS One. 2013;8:e59952.
37. Triglia T, Mezzapesa A, Martin JC, Verdier M, Lagier D, Dufour H, Bruder N, Alessi MC, Velly LJ. Early matrix metalloproteinase-9 concentration in the first 48 h after aneurysmal subarachnoid haemorrhage predicts delayed cerebral ischaemia: an observational study. Eur J Anaesthesiol. 2016;33:662–9.
38. Lee JY, Lee HE, Kang SR, Choi HY, Ryu JH, Yune TY. Fluoxetine inhibits transient global ischemia-induced hippocampal neuronal death and memory impairment by preventing blood-brain barrier disruption. Neuropharmacology. 2014;79:161–71.
39. Lee JY, Kim HS, Choi HY, Oh TH, Yune TY. Fluoxetine inhibits matrix metalloprotease activation and prevents disruption of blood-spinal cord barrier after spinal cord injury. Brain. 2012;135:2375–89.
40. Obermeier B, Daneman R, Ransohoff RM. Development, maintenance and disruption of the blood-brain barrier. Nat Med. 2013;19:1584–96.
41. Sozen T, Tsuchiyama R, Hasegawa Y, Suzuki H, Jadhav V, Nishizawa S, Zhang JH. Role of interleukin-1beta in early brain injury after subarachnoid hemorrhage in mice. Stroke. 2009;40:2519–25.

42. Kothari P, Pestana R, Mesraoua R, Elchaki R, Khan KM, Dannenberg AJ, Falcone DJ. IL-6-mediated induction of matrix metalloproteinase-9 is modulated by JAK-dependent IL-10 expression in macrophages. J Immunol. 2014;192:349–57.
43. Xue H, Sun K, Xie W, Hu G, Kong H, Wang Q, Wang H. Etanercept attenuates short-term cigarette-smoke-exposure-induced pulmonary arterial remodelling in rats by suppressing the activation of TNF-a/NF-kB signal and the activities of MMP-2 and MMP-9. Pulm Pharmacol Ther. 2012;25:208–15.
44. Aksu U, Guner I, Yaman OM, Erman H, Uzun D, Sengezer-Inceli M, Sahin A, Yelmen N, Gelisgen R, Uzun H, Sahin G. Fluoxetine ameliorates imbalance of redox homeostasis and inflammation in an acute kidney injury model. J Physiol Biochem. 2014;70:925–34.
45. Yang JM, Rui BB, Chen C, Chen H, Xu TJ, Xu WP, Wei W. Acetylsalicylic acid enhances the anti-inflammatory effect of fluoxetine through inhibition of NF-kappaB, p38-MAPK and ERK1/2 activation in lipopolysaccharide-induced BV-2 microglia cells. Neuroscience. 2014;275:296–304.
46. Fang H, Wang PF, Zhou Y, Wang YC, Yang QW. Toll-like receptor 4 signaling in intracerebral hemorrhage-induced inflammation and injury. J Neuroinflammation. 2013;10:27.
47. Ma C, Zhou W, Yan Z, Qu M, Bu X. Toll-like receptor 4 (TLR4) is associated with cerebral vasospasm and delayed cerebral ischemia in aneurysmal subarachnoid hemorrhage. Neurol Med Chir (Tokyo). 2015;55:878–84.
48. Habib M, Shaker S, El-Gayar N, Aboul-Fotouh S. The effects of antidepressants "fluoxetine and imipramine" on vascular abnormalities and Toll like receptor-4 expression in diabetic and non-diabetic rats exposed to chronic stress. PLoS One. 2015;10:e0120559.

13

Molecular and cellular identification of the immune response in peripheral ganglia following nerve injury

Jane A. Lindborg[1†], Jon P. Niemi[1†], Madeline A. Howarth[1,2], Kevin W. Liu[1], Christian Z. Moore[1], Deepti Mahajan[1] and Richard E. Zigmond[1,3*]

Abstract

Background: Neuroinflammation accompanies neural trauma and most neurological diseases. Axotomy in the peripheral nervous system (PNS) leads to dramatic changes in the injured neuron: the cell body expresses a distinct set of genes known as regeneration-associated genes, the distal axonal segment degenerates and its debris is cleared, and the axons in the proximal segment form growth cones and extend neurites. These processes are orchestrated in part by immune and other non-neuronal cells. Macrophages in ganglia play an integral role in supporting regeneration. Here, we explore further the molecular and cellular components of the injury-induced immune response within peripheral ganglia.

Methods: Adult male wild-type (WT) and *Ccr2*$^{-/-}$ mice were subjected to a unilateral transection of the sciatic nerve and axotomy of the superior cervical ganglion (SCG). Antibody arrays were used to determine the expression of chemokines and cytokines in the dorsal root ganglion (DRG) and SCG. Flow cytometry and immunohistochemistry were utilized to identify the cellular composition of the injury-induced immune response within ganglia.

Results: Chemokine expression in the ganglia differed 48 h after nerve injury with a large increase in macrophage inflammatory protein-1γ in the SCG but not in the DRG, while C-C class chemokine ligand 2 was highly expressed in both ganglia. Differences between WT and *Ccr2*$^{-/-}$ mice were also observed with increased C-C class chemokine ligand 6/C10 expression in the WT DRG compared to C-C class chemokine receptor 2 (CCR2)$^{-/-}$ DRG and increased CXCL5 expression in CCR2$^{-/-}$ SCG compared to WT. Diminished macrophage accumulation in the DRG and SCG of *Ccr2*$^{-/-}$ mice was found compared to WT ganglia 7 days after nerve injury. Interestingly, neutrophils were found in the SCG but not in the DRG. Cytokine expression, measured 7 days after injury, differed between ganglion type and genotype. Macrophage activation was assayed by colabeling ganglia with the anti-inflammatory marker CD206 and the macrophage marker CD68, and an almost complete colocalization of the two markers was found in both ganglia.

Conclusions: This study demonstrates both molecular and cellular differences in the nerve injury-induced immune response between DRG and SCG and between WT and *Ccr2*$^{-/-}$ mice.

Keywords: Axotomy, Dorsal root ganglion (DRG), Macrophage, Neuroinflammation, Neutrophil, Regeneration, Superior cervical ganglion (SCG)

* Correspondence: rez@case.edu
[†]Jane A. Lindborg and Jon P. Niemi contributed equally to this work.
[1]Department of Neurosciences, School of Medicine, Case Western Reserve University, Cleveland, OH, USA
[3]Present Address: Department Neurosciences, School of Medicine, 10900 Euclid Avenue, Robbins E701, Cleveland, OH 44106-4975, USA
Full list of author information is available at the end of the article

Background

While the inflammatory response to injury in the peripheral nervous system (PNS) is complex and involves a number of immune cells, including dendritic, T, and B cells [1, 2], it is largely dominated by macrophages [3]. Macrophage responses to a peripheral axonal injury occur in two distinct compartments: the nerve distal to the injury site and the axotomized ganglion. The largest contribution to macrophage accumulation within injured PNS tissues come from monocyte-derived macrophages. In the sciatic nerve 7 days after injury, infiltrating macrophages outnumber the resident population 3:1 [4]. Infiltration of the sciatic nerve begins 48 h after injury with peak accumulation occurring between 7 and 14 days [3, 5]. Additionally, macrophage numbers remain elevated in the nerve for at least 30 days after injury [6].

In peripheral ganglia, monocyte infiltration and macrophage accumulation follow a similar timeline to that seen in the sciatic nerve [7–9]. In the superior cervical ganglion (SCG), monocyte-derived macrophages are present at 48 h after injury and remain for at least 2 weeks following transection of the internal and external carotid nerves [9, 10]. Likewise, the lumbar dorsal root ganglion (DRG) shows accumulation beginning 48 to 72 h after sciatic nerve injury with an increased number of monocyte-derived macrophages remaining for at least 28 days [11, 12].

The signal-mediating monocyte/macrophage entry into PNS tissue following injury is thought to be the C-C motif chemokine ligand 2 (CCL2), as a global knockout of its primary receptor C-C class chemokine receptor 2 (CCR2) yields a significant decrease in macrophage accumulation in the sciatic nerve following injury [13, 14]. CCL2, also known as monocyte chemoattractant protein-1 (MCP-1), recruits monocytes to sites of inflammation, infection, and injury. CCL2 also has the ability to act as a chemokine for neutrophils, T cells, and dendritic cells [15, 16].

While the function of macrophages in peripheral ganglia following nerve injury has been unknown until recently, evidence in the DRG and SCG indicates a role in axonal regeneration [11, 14, 17, 18]. Since there is very little cell death and degeneration occurring in peripheral ganglia after injury [19, 20], the stereotypical phagocytic function of macrophages is likely not their main function in the cell body compartment after axonal injury, suggesting an alternate purpose [21, 22]. Recent work by our laboratory has demonstrated that macrophage accumulation near injured neuronal cell bodies is both necessary and sufficient for peripheral axon regeneration [14, 17]. By inhibiting macrophage accumulation within the SCG and DRG following axotomy using a global knockout of the chemokine receptor *Ccr2* (*Ccr2*$^{-/-}$), we showed that in vitro axonal regeneration is significantly reduced when the injury-induced immune response in ganglia is impaired [14].

Numerous studies on peripheral nerve regeneration and the neuronal cell body response to axonal injury exclusively utilize injury to the sciatic nerve and DRG as a model system. However, the DRG is a very unique ganglion in that the sensory neurons lack dendrites and synaptic input within the cell body region, the neurons within the DRG are a heterogeneous population composed of multiple subtypes, and the ganglia lack a blood-ganglion barrier [23]. The differences between the DRG and other peripheral ganglia could allow for unique mechanisms to arise in response to peripheral axonal injury. Thus, a comparison of the injury responses, and more specifically the axotomy-induced immune responses, between the DRG and other peripheral ganglia could identify cellular and molecular mechanisms that are common elements of peripheral injury or unique elements that are specific to the DRG. The SCG, the largest sympathetic ganglia, has many characteristics that directly oppose those of the DRG such as the presence of presynaptic innervation within the ganglia, a more homogeneous neuronal population, and the existence of a blood-ganglion barrier [24–26].

Nevertheless, very little is known about the complete molecular and cellular components of the injury-induced immune response within peripheral ganglia. Here, we utilize unbiased antibody protein arrays, flow cytometry, and immunohistochemistry (IHC) to identify and characterize the molecular and cellular profile of the immune response after nerve injury within the DRG and SCG of wild-type (WT) and *Ccr2*$^{-/-}$ mice.

Methods

Mice

Male (8–12-week-old) WT (C57BL/6J; The Jackson Laboratory, Bar Harbor, ME, USA) and *Ccr2*$^{-/-}$ (B6.129S4-*Ccr2*^{tm1Ifc}/J backcrossed to C57BL/6J; The Jackson Laboratory) mice were used for this study. All mice had ad libitum access to food and water and were housed under a 12-h light/dark cycle.

Injury model

Mice were anesthetized under isoflurane, and the external carotid nerve (ECN) and internal carotid nerve (ICN) of the right SCG were exposed and transected. For axotomy of neurons in the fourth, fifth, and sixth DRG, the right sciatic nerve was exposed and transected at the hip level, and 1 mm of the nerve was removed. The nerves on the left side of the animal were exposed but not transected, and the ganglia served as sham-operated controls. One, two, three, or seven days after injury, mice were killed by CO_2 inhalation, and the SCG and a combination of the L4, L5, and L6 DRG were harvested for analysis. All surgical procedures were approved by the Case Western Reserve University Institutional Animal Care and Use Committee.

Antibody arrays

L4 and L5 DRG and SCG from WT and *Ccr2*$^{-/-}$ mice were collected at 48 h (for chemokine assay) and 7 days (for cytokine assay) after right sciatic nerve transection and right SCG axotomy and flash frozen for chemokine and cytokine determination by Proteome Profiler Array ARY020 and ARY006 (R&D Systems, Minneapolis, MN, USA), respectively. Ganglia from five mice/group were pooled for each sample, and protein was isolated through homogenization in RIPA buffer (Santa Cruz Biotechnology, Dallas, TX, USA). Protein (180 μg per sample) was diluted and mixed with a cocktail of biotinylated detection antibodies and then incubated with mouse chemokine or cytokine array membrane. After washing, streptavidin-horseradish peroxidase and chemiluminescent detection reagents were added. Array images were obtained using a LI-COR Odyssey Fc Imaging System (LI-COR Biosciences, Lincoln, NE, USA) with a 10-min exposure time and analyzed by densitometry for integral optical density using ImageJ software. The optical density of each pair of chemokine or cytokine spots was normalized to the corresponding positive control spots. The data were then represented as a fold increase of the injured chemokine or cytokine expression compared to the WT sham results. Three arrays were run per condition, and the results were averaged. *t* tests were used to evaluate statistical differences between injured and uninjured tissues within a genotype and in the injured tissue between genotypes. The following chemokines were assessed at 48 h post injury in the DRG and SCG: 6Ckine, BLC, C10, C5/C5a, CCL28, chemerin, CTACK, CXCL16, eotaxin, CX_3CL1, interleukin (IL)-16, IP-10, I-TAC, CCL2, CXCL1, LIX, CCL8/MCP-2, MCP-5, MDC, MIG, macrophage inflammatory protein-1 (MIP-1)α/β, macrophage inflammatory protein-1 gamma (MIP-1γ), MIP-2, RANTES, and SDF-1. The following cytokines were assessed at 7 days post injury in the DRG and SCG: CXCL13, C5a, G-CSF, GM-CSF, CCL1, CCL11, soluble intercellular adhesion molecule-1 (sICAM-1), IFN-γ, IL-1α, IL-1β, interleukin-1 receptor antagonist (IL-1ra), IL-2, IL-3, IL-4, IL-5, IL-6, IL-7, IL-10, IL-13, IL-12p70, IL-16, IL-17, IL-23, IL-27, IP-10, CXCL11, KC, M-CSF, CCL2, CCL12, CXCL9, CCL3, CCL4, CXCL2, CCL5, CXCL12, CCL17, tissue inhibitor of metalloproteinase-1 (TIMP-1), tumor necrosis factor alpha (TNF-α), and TREM-1.

Flow cytometry

A pooled sample of L4, L5, and L6 DRG and single SCG was enzymatically digested in 0.125% collagenase for 1 h at 37 °C. Mechanical digestion using a 23-gauge needle attached to a 1-ml syringe produced single cell suspensions which were filtered through a 35-μm cell strainer. Dead cells were labeled using a Live/Dead Fixable Blue Dead Cell Stain kit (Thermo Fisher Scientific, Waltham, MA, USA) for 30 min at 4 °C. Cells were then washed in FACS buffer (PBS, 1% BSA) and blocked with a monoclonal antibody to CD16/CD32 (1:500; Thermo Fisher Scientific) for 10 min at 4 °C. Cells were incubated with fluorophore-conjugated antibodies against F4/80, CD11b, Ly6G (1A8), and p75 ([F4/80] Cat no. 123130; [CD11b] Cat no. 101206; [Ly6G] Cat no. 127610; [p75] Cat no. 113405) for 1 h at 4 °C. Cells were washed and resuspended in FACS buffer and then run on a BD FACSAria (BD Biosciences, San Jose, CA, USA) and analyzed using FlowJo (BD Biosciences). CD45 was not used to gate leukocyte populations, and therefore, non-leukocyte populations may be included in the analysis [27]. All events were gated based on viable single cells. Compensation and gating were performed using negative, single-stained, and isotype controls. Cell populations were gated as follows: F4/80$^+$CD11b$^+$ (macrophages), CD11b$^+$Ly6G$^-$ (monocytes/macrophages), CD11b$^+$Ly6G$^+$ (neutrophils), and p75$^+$ (Schwann cells).

IHC

L5 DRG and SCG from WT and *Ccr2*$^{-/-}$ mice were removed 1, 3, or 7 days post injury, and the ganglia were desheathed and fixed by immersion in 4% paraformaldehyde. The tissues were cryoprotected in 30% sucrose and embedded in Tissue-Tek O.C.T. compound (Electron Microscopy Sciences, Hatfield, PA, USA). IHC was performed on 10-μm cryostat sections to double label tissue with a macrophage marker, CD68, and an anti-inflammatory macrophage marker, CD206. A goat polyclonal antibody to CD206 (1:200; R&D Systems) was incubated with tissue sections overnight at 4 °C. After washing, the sections were incubated in Alexa Fluor 488 secondary antibody (1:400; Thermo Fisher Scientific) for 1 h and washed in PBS. Next, a rat monoclonal antibody against CD68 (1:200; AbD Serotec, Oxford, UK) was incubated with tissue sections overnight at 4 °C. After additional washes, the sections were incubated with a Cy3 secondary antibody (1:200; Jackson ImmunoResearch Laboratories, Inc., West Grove, PA, USA) for 1 h. The sections were then stained with DAPI (1:1000; Thermo Fisher Scientific). IHC was also performed to label neutrophils in the ganglia using a rabbit polyclonal antibody to myeloperoxidase (MPO; 1:100; Abcam, Cambridge, UK) overnight at 4 °C and a Cy3 donkey anti-rabbit secondary antibody (1:400; Jackson ImmunoResearch Laboratories, Inc.). Additionally, IHC was performed on L3, L4, L5, and L6 DRG and SCG to identify the percentage of injured neurons after axotomy using a mouse monoclonal anti-HuC/D (1:100; Thermo Fisher Scientific) and a rabbit polyclonal anti-activating transcription factor 3 (ATF3) antibody (1:100; Sigma-Aldrich, St. Louis, MO, USA) by incubating sections overnight at 4 °C. Prior to the addition of primary ATF3 and HuC/D antibodies, the tissue underwent citrate buffer antigen retrieval and an endogenous mouse antibody blocking step by incubating the tissue with a donkey anti-mouse-unconjugated IgG (1:400; Jackson ImmunoResearch Laboratories, Inc., West Grove, PA, USA). ATF3 and HuC/D were visualized by incubation with goat anti-rabbit Alexa Fluor 594 (1:400; Jackson ImmunoResearch Laboratories, Inc.) and goat anti-mouse IgG2a Alexa Fluor 488 (1:400; Thermo Fisher Scientific). In all experiments, sections not exposed to the primary antibody were included for each experimental group. Images were captured at × 10 or × 25 magnification using HCImage software (Hamamatsu Corporation, Bridgewater, NJ, USA), and then cell counts were performed using ImageJ software. Cell counts were performed to quantify the number of CD68$^+$, CD206$^+$, CD68$^+$CD206$^+$, HuC/D$^+$, ATF3$^+$, and HuC/D$^+$ATF3$^+$ cells. Data are represented as the sum of the cells counted from three distinct images per ganglion per animal. Five samples were included for each group.

Statistical analysis

Data in graphs are presented as mean ± SEM. For experiments involving multiple genotypes, treatments, and time points, a two-way ANOVA was performed, followed by a Tukey's post hoc test. For independent two-group experiments, an unpaired Student's t test (two-tailed) was used to determine statistical significance. Statistical analyses were performed using SigmaPlot, version 12.3 (Systat Software, Inc., San Jose, CA, USA). Values were considered statistically significant at $p < 0.05$. The number of experimental replicates (n), the designation of n belonging to the number of animals, and experiment repetition are indicated in the figure legends. Data from all experiments were included in the analysis. IHC experiments were performed with the experimenter blinded to genotype.

Results

SCG axotomy and sciatic nerve transection injury paradigms

Complete or partial injury to the sciatic nerve is one of the most widely used models to study peripheral nerve regeneration, degeneration, and neuropathic pain [28]. The sciatic nerve is a mixed nerve containing sensory, motor, and sympathetic axons. Sensory axons from the DRG at lumbar levels L4, L5, and L6 project into the sciatic nerve [29, 30]. To examine the injury-induced neuroimmune response within the lumbar DRG, we employed a sciatic nerve transection to injure neuronal cell bodies of L4, L5, and L6 DRG (Fig. 1a). ATF3 is a transcription factor that is highly upregulated in injured DRG and SCG neurons [31, 32]. To determine the extent of injury in the DRG at different lumbar levels, L3, L4, L5, and L6 DRG were collected 7 days after a sciatic nerve transection or sham operation and colabeled with ATF3 and the neuronal marker HuC/D [33]. L4, L5, and L6 DRG all showed significant increases in ATF3 with 26.9, 41.3, and 22.1% of HuC/D$^+$ neurons expressing the injury marker, respectively (Fig. 1b–j). The L3 DRG did not exhibit ATF3 upregulation after sciatic nerve transection (Fig. 1b, c, g).

To study the injury-induced cellular and molecular neuroimmune changes in the SCG, the ECN and ICN, the two major postganglionic nerves of the ganglia, were transected (Fig. 1k). A previous study utilizing retrogradely transported horseradish peroxidase to identify the localization of SCG neurons that project into the ICN and ECN found that when both nerves were cut, approximately 80% of the SCG neurons were injured [34]. SCG were harvested 7 days after axotomy or a sham surgery and colabeled with HuC/D and ATF3. In the SCG, 67.5% of HuC/D$^+$ sympathetic neurons expressed ATF3 7 days after injury (Fig. 1l–n).

Chemokine expression in the axotomized ganglia

To begin to assess the inflammatory response that occurs near injured neuronal cell bodies following peripheral nerve injury, we first measured the expression of chemokines, the proteins which play a critical role in immune cell recruitment to tissues [35]. Macrophages, the major immune cell type studied in peripheral nerve injury, have been shown to accumulate in the DRG and SCG within 48 to 72 h after nerve injury [9, 12]. Therefore, we assessed the expression of chemokines in ganglia using antibody arrays in WT and *Ccr2*$^{-/-}$ mice 48 h after axotomy. In the DRG, WT mice displayed significant injury-induced expression of multiple chemokines and immune-related factors including a 3.0-fold increase in CCL6/C10, a 2.2-fold increase in complement cascade component C5/C5a, a 1.8-fold increase in CXCL5, a 1.9-fold increase in CCL8/MCP-2, and a 3.9-fold increase in CCL2 compared to WT sham DRG (Fig. 2a, b, e). Axotomized *Ccr2*$^{-/-}$ mice exhibited a significant 2.1-fold increase in CCL6/C10, a 2.3-fold increase in CXCL5, a 1.7-fold increase in CCL8/MCP-2, and a 3.5-fold increase in CCL2 compared to *Ccr2*$^{-/-}$ sham DRG (Fig. 2a', b', e). Comparison of the DRG chemokine expression profiles between genotypes found that CCL6/C10 and C5/C5a were more highly expressed in the axotomized WT DRG compared to *Ccr2*$^{-/-}$ DRG (Fig. 2e).

In the SCG, WT mice displayed significant injury-induced expression of multiple chemokines and immune-related factors including a 3.9-fold increase in CCL6/C10, a 1.5-fold increase in CXCL5, a 2.1-fold

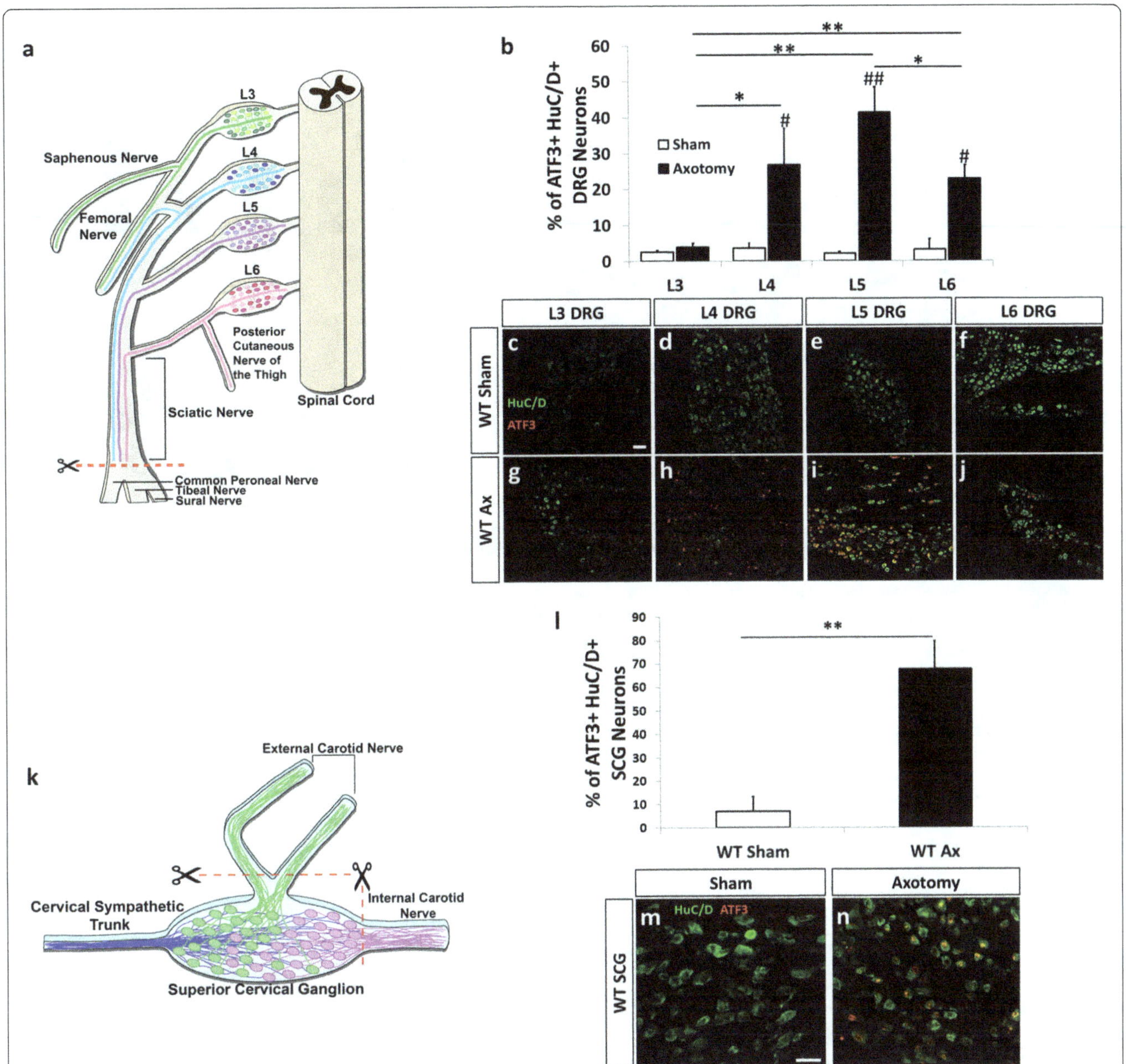

Fig. 1 The axonal injury-induced marker ATF3 is highly upregulated in L4, L5, and L6 DRG and in the SCG 7 days after axotomy. A diagram illustrating the sciatic nerve transection injury and the relative innervation of the sciatic nerve by the individual lumbar DRG (**a**). WT mice underwent a unilateral transection of the right sciatic nerve and lumbar DRG were removed and stained for the injury marker ATF3 and the neuronal marker HuC/D. The percentage of ATF3$^+$HuC/D$^+$ neurons were quantified 7 days after injury (**b**). Representative images of sham-operated (**c**–**f**) and axotomized (**g**–**j**) DRG for L3 (**c**, **g**), L4 (**d**, **h**), L5 (**e**, **i**), and L6 (**f**, **j**) DRG are shown. A diagram illustrating the SCG axotomy and the relative innervation of the external and internal carotid nerves (**k**). In the SCG diagram, blue represents the preganglionic fibers, the green cell bodies are neurons that project into the ECN, and the purple cell bodies project into the ICN. Mice underwent a unilateral transection of the ECN and ICN of the right SCG. SCG were removed 7 days post injury and stained with ATF3 and HuC/D. The percentage of ATF3$^+$ HuC/D$^+$ SCG neurons were quantified (**l**). Representative images of sham-operated (**m**) and axotomized (**n**) SCG are shown. The data are presented as the mean ± SEM. DRG images were taken at × 10 magnification. SCG images were taken at × 25 magnification. Scale bar = 50 μm. $n = 5$ per group. $^*p < 0.05$. $^{**}p < 0.001$ between groups. $^{\#}p < 0.05$. $^{\#\#}p < 0.001$ between sham and axotomy within groups

increase in CCL8/MCP-2, a 5.1-fold increase in MIP-1γ, and a 1.9-fold increase in CCL2 compared to WT sham SCG (Fig. 2c, d, f). Axotomized *Ccr2*$^{-/-}$ mice exhibited a significant 4.1-fold increase in CCL6/C10, a 2.2-fold increase in CXCL5, a 1.9-fold increase in CCL8/MCP-2, a 5.9-fold increase in MIP-1γ, and a 2.1-fold increase in CCL2 compared to *Ccr2*$^{-/-}$ sham DRG (Fig. 2c′, d′, f). A comparison of the SCG injury-induced chemokine

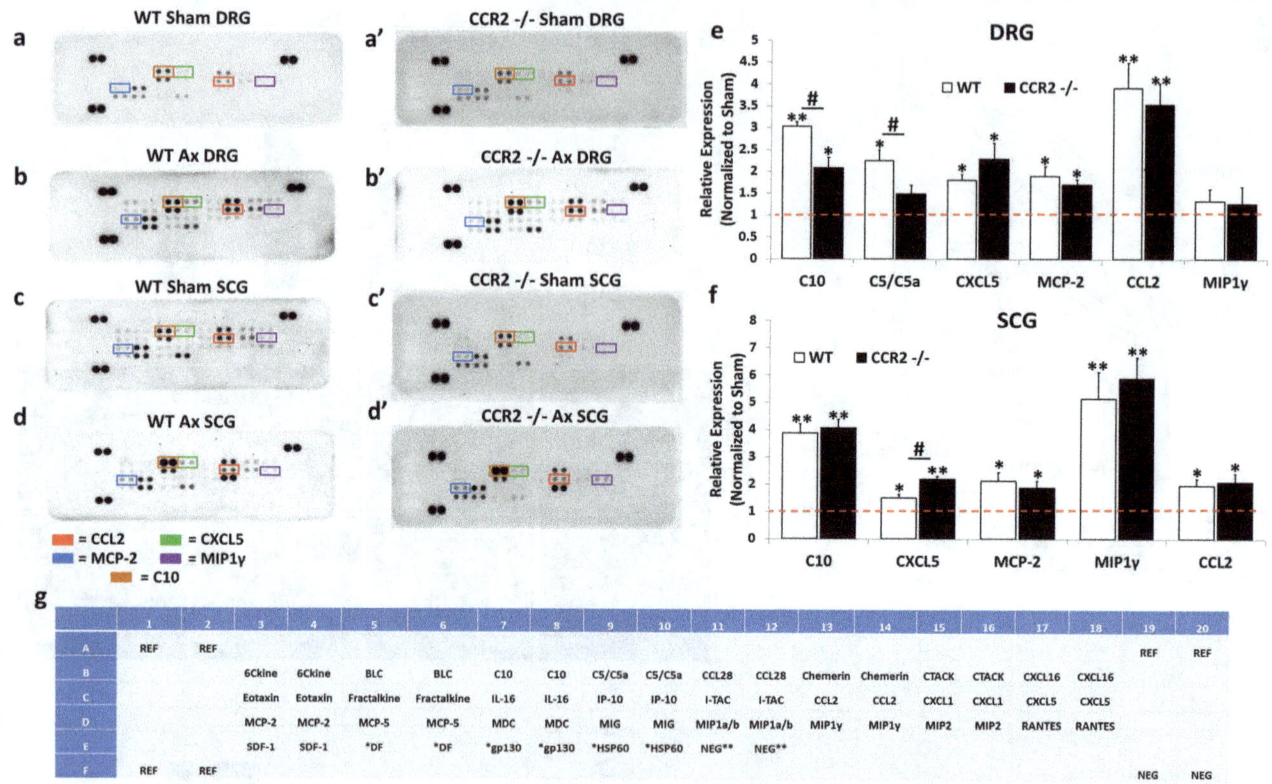

Fig. 2 Chemokines are differentially expressed in the DRG and SCG 48 h after axotomy. Mice underwent a unilateral transection of the right sciatic nerve and the right ICN and ECN of the SCG. Forty-eight hours after axotomy, the injured and contralateral sham-operated L4/L5 DRG and SCG were collected and flash frozen. Protein was isolated from sham and injured ganglia pooled from five mice and used for measurement of chemokines using a Proteome Profiler Mouse Array kit (**g**). Representative arrays for WT [85] and *Ccr2*$^{-/-}$ (**a'**–**d'**) mice for DRG (**a**, **a'**, **b**, **b'**) and SCG (**c**, **c'**, **d**, **d'**) are shown. Array images were analyzed by densitometry for integral optical density using ImageJ. The optical density for each cytokine was then normalized to the internal control for each blot. The data are represented as the fold increase in the expression of the injured condition compared to the sham for each genotype for DRG (**e**) and SCG (**f**). The spots corresponding to the cytokines CCL2, CXCL5, CCL8/MCP-2, MIP-1γ, and CCL6/C10 are highlighted in the representative arrays based on the template indicating the location of controls and various chemokine capture antibodies (**g**). *N* = 3 arrays per group. The data are presented as mean ± SEM. *$p < 0.05$. **$p < 0.001$ represents significance of expression relative to sham within genotype. $^{\#}p < 0.05$. $^{\#\#}p < 0.001$ represents significance between genotypes

expression profiles between genotypes found that CXCL5 was more highly expressed in the *Ccr2*$^{-/-}$ SCG compared to the WT SCG 48 h after injury (Fig. 2f). The most prominent differences in expression patterns between DRG and SCG are in C5/C5a and MIP-1γ. C5/C5a is significantly increased in the WT DRG but is not upregulated in WT or Ccr2$^{-/-}$ SCG 48 h after injury (Fig. 2e, f). Alternately, MIP-1γ shows a greater than fivefold upregulation in the injured WT and *Ccr2*$^{-/-}$ SCG but is not increased in the DRG after injury (Fig. 2e, f).

Cellular analysis of non-neuronal populations in the injured ganglia

Since analysis of chemokine protein expression between axotomized WT and *Ccr2*$^{-/-}$ ganglia revealed differences in the relative expression of macrophage and neutrophil chemoattractants, we used flow cytometry to determine whether these differences translate into differential cellular accumulations within the ganglia after injury. We observed an increase in CCL2 expression 2 days after injury in both WT and *Ccr2*$^{-/-}$ DRG (Fig. 2e); however, significant increases in macrophage accumulation (CD11b$^+$F4/80$^+$ and CD11b$^+$Ly6G$^-$) were not yet seen for either genotype 3 days after injury (Fig. 3a–c). At 7 days after injury and in line with previous findings that used immunohistochemical analysis to identify macrophage populations in the axotomized DRG [14], flow cytometry confirmed a robust increase in macrophages in the injured WT DRG over its sham-operated control (80.0 ± 1.7% for CD11b$^+$F4/80$^+$ macrophages). While macrophage accumulation was also significantly enhanced in the axotomized *Ccr2*$^{-/-}$ DRG over its sham-operated control (55.9 ± 1.9%), the injured WT DRG displayed a more robust increase in CD11b$^+$F4/80$^+$ macrophages compared to injured *Ccr2*$^{-/-}$ DRG (55.5 ± 0.4%, Fig. 3d).

Neutrophil accumulation (CD11b$^+$Ly6G$^+$) in the DRG was negligible for both genotypes at either time point

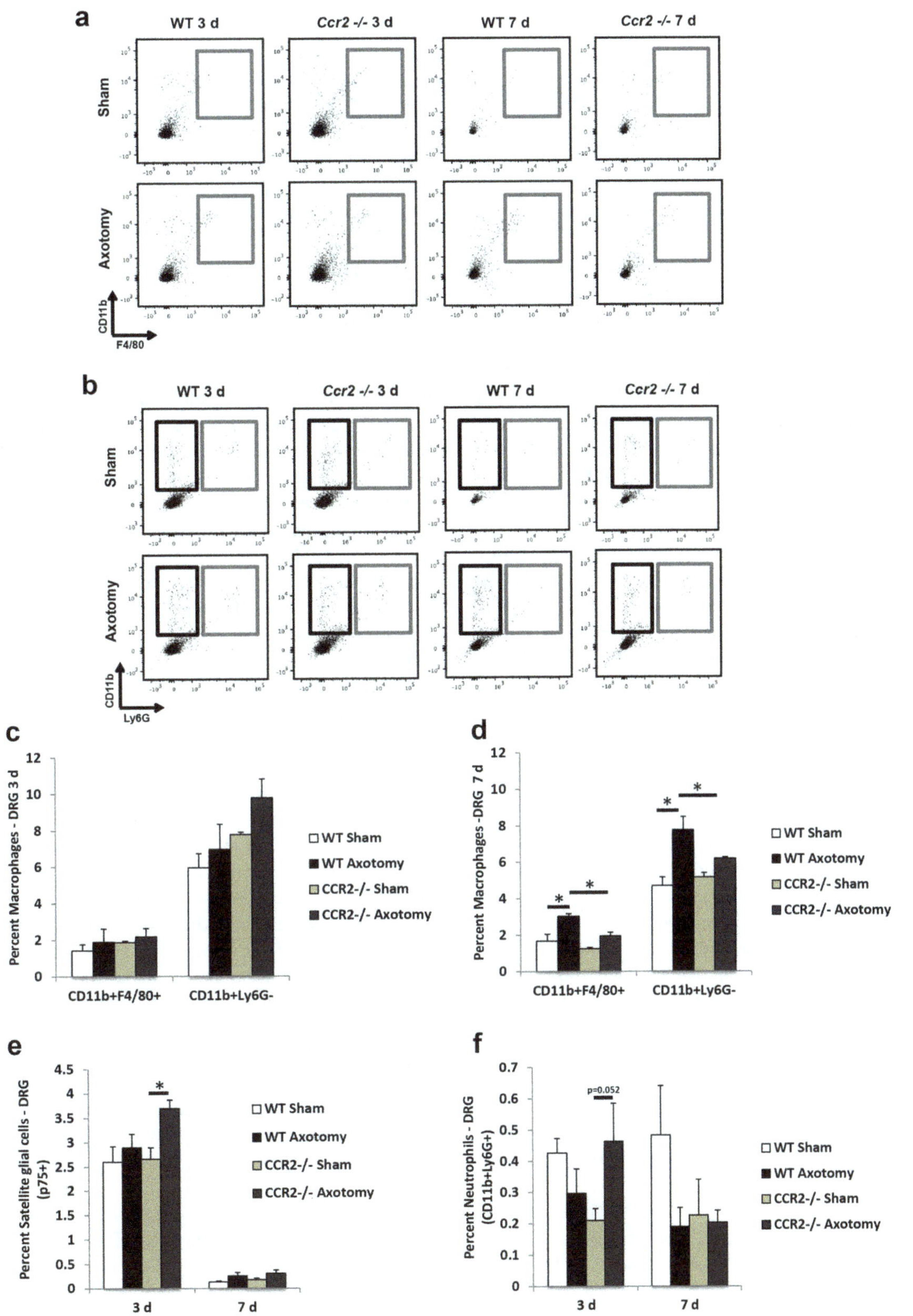

Fig. 3 (See legend on next page.)

(See figure on previous page.)

Fig. 3 Macrophage accumulation is significantly diminished in the axotomized DRG of *Ccr2*$^{-/-}$ mice compared to WT mice, while satellite glial cells and neutrophils are comparable between genotypes. Three and seven days after sciatic nerve transection, L4, L5 and L6 DRG were dissected and examined using flow cytometry. Both sham and axotomized nerves were analyzed. Gray boxes in **a** indicate CD11b$^+$F4/80$^+$ cells. In **b**, black boxes indicate CD11b$^+$Ly6G$^-$ cells and gray boxes indicate CD11b$^+$Ly6G$^+$ cells. Flow cytometric analysis of macrophage populations in the injured DRG (**a**, **b**) shows similar percentages of CD11b$^+$F4/80$^+$ and CD11b$^+$Ly6G$^-$ cells between genotypes at 3 days (**c**) and significant attenuation in *Ccr2*$^{-/-}$ mice compared to WT mice at 7 days (**d**) post injury. A significant increase in the percentage of satellite glial cells after axotomy was seen in 3 days in *Ccr2*$^{-/-}$ DRG alone, with a trend towards a significant increase over injured WT DRG (**e**). No differences were observed for CD11b$^+$Ly6G$^+$ neutrophils after injury in WT mice, while a trend towards a significant increase was observed 3 days after injury in *Ccr2*$^{-/-}$ mice (**f**). Mean ± SEM, two-way ANOVA, Tukey's post hoc test corrected (within individual time points). $^*p < 0.05$. $^{**}p < 0.001$. $n = 3$ mice per genotype per time point

(Fig. 3b, f). In addition to macrophages, satellite glial cells are another population of non-neuronal cells that are abundant in sensory and sympathetic ganglia [36–38]. Satellite glial cells localize to and surround neurons, and it has been suggested that these cells regulate neuronal function by releasing trophic factors, bradykinin, and other proteins [38–40]. p75 is a neurotrophin receptor that is downregulated by neurons after injury and conversely upregulated by satellite glial cells that surround the neurons [37, 41]. Increased p75 expression in satellite glial cells has been observed in both the ipsilateral and contralateral ganglia after injury [42]. Here, the percent of p75$^+$ satellite glial cells in the DRG were comparable between genotypes at both time points, and axotomy induced an increase in p75$^+$ cells after 3 days in *Ccr2*$^{-/-}$ DRG alone (Fig. 3e). p75$^+$ cells were absent in all DRG 7 days after injury, indicating reduced expression in neuronal and glial populations.

Evaluating the macrophage response in the injured SCG indicated an increase in CD11b$^+$F4/80$^+$ cells in the axotomized WT ganglia compared to sham 3 days post injury, and a larger increase in CD11b$^+$Ly6G$^-$ cells in the injured WT SCG relative to injured *Ccr2*$^{-/-}$ SCG (Fig. 4a–c). Similar to prior studies using CD11b$^+$ immunostaining [14], flow cytometry revealed a macrophage response to injury in the axotomized *Ccr2*$^{-/-}$ SCG compared to its sham control 7 days post injury (Fig. 4d). But while CD11b$^+$Ly6G$^-$ and CD11b$^+$F4/80$^+$ macrophage accumulation was significantly increased 7 days after injury in the *Ccr2*$^{-/-}$ SCG, the axotomized WT SCG displayed a substantial increase in CD11b$^+$Ly6G$^-$ macrophages compared to the mutant (15.5 ± 1.4% for WT SCG and 11.9 ± 0.3% for *Ccr2*$^{-/-}$ SCG, Fig. 4d). Furthermore, uninjured WT SCG boast a significantly higher population of CD11b$^+$Ly6G$^-$ resident macrophages compared to uninjured *Ccr2*$^{-/-}$ SCG (6.3 ± 0.2% for WT SCG and 3.0 ± 0.5% for *Ccr2*$^{-/-}$ SCG, Fig. 4d). Injury produced no change in the expression of p75$^+$ satellite glial cells for either genotype at either time point (Fig. 4e).

Unlike with the DRG, axotomy induced an increase in neutrophils in the SCG for both genotypes 3 days after injury (Fig. 4b, f). Interestingly, a significantly larger influx of neutrophils in the *Ccr2*$^{-/-}$ SCG was observed at 3 days post injury compared to the WT SCG. To visualize the localization of neutrophils in the ganglia, immunohistochemical analyses of these polymorphonuclear cells were performed using MPO, which is a common neutrophil marker [43, 44]. While no MPO$^+$ neutrophils were identified in the DRG (data not shown), significant increases in MPO$^+$ neutrophil accumulation were observed in the axotomized SCG in both WT and *Ccr2*$^{-/-}$ mice compared to their respective sham-operated controls (Fig. 5a–g). However, in contrast to flow cytometry data that used Ly6G and CD11b to label neutrophils (Fig. 4f), the percent of MPO$^+$ neutrophils in *Ccr2*$^{-/-}$ ganglia at 3 days post injury were comparable to WT ganglia (Fig. 5a, d, e). No differences in fluorescent staining were observed 1 day post injury between genotypes (Fig. 5a–c). Unexpectedly, an increase in MPO$^+$ cells was observed in the WT SCG 7 days after axotomy, while expression was significantly decreased in the *Ccr2*$^{-/-}$ SCG (Fig. 5a, f, g).

Cytokine expression in the axotomized ganglia

The cellular immune response in ganglia following axotomy defined by flow cytometry (Figs. 3 and 4) displayed differences in the myeloid cell population present in the DRG and SCG between WT and *Ccr2*$^{-/-}$ mice 7 days after axotomy. To assess how the molecular immune response may be impacted by differences in the cellular immune populations with peripheral ganglia, the cytokine expression profile in the DRG and SCG of WT and *Ccr2*$^{-/-}$ mice was assayed 7 days after axotomy. In the DRG, WT mice displayed significant injury-induced expression of multiple cytokines and immune-related factors including a 3.6-fold increase in TIMP-1, a 2.1-fold increase in sICAM-1, a 3.3-fold increase in CCL2, and a 2.8-fold increase in IL-1ra compared to WT sham DRG (Fig. 6a, b, e). In contrast, *Ccr2*$^{-/-}$ mice only exhibited a significant 2.3-fold increase in C5/C5a and a 3.2-fold increase in IL-16 compared to *Ccr2*$^{-/-}$ sham DRG (Fig. 6a', b', e). Furthermore, comparison of the DRG cytokine expression profiles between genotypes found that TIMP-1, CCL2, and IL-1ra were more highly expressed in the axotomized WT DRG compared to *Ccr2*$^{-/-}$ DRG, while C5/C5a and IL-16 were more highly expressed in the *Ccr2*$^{-/-}$ DRG compared to WT 7 days after injury (Fig. 6e).

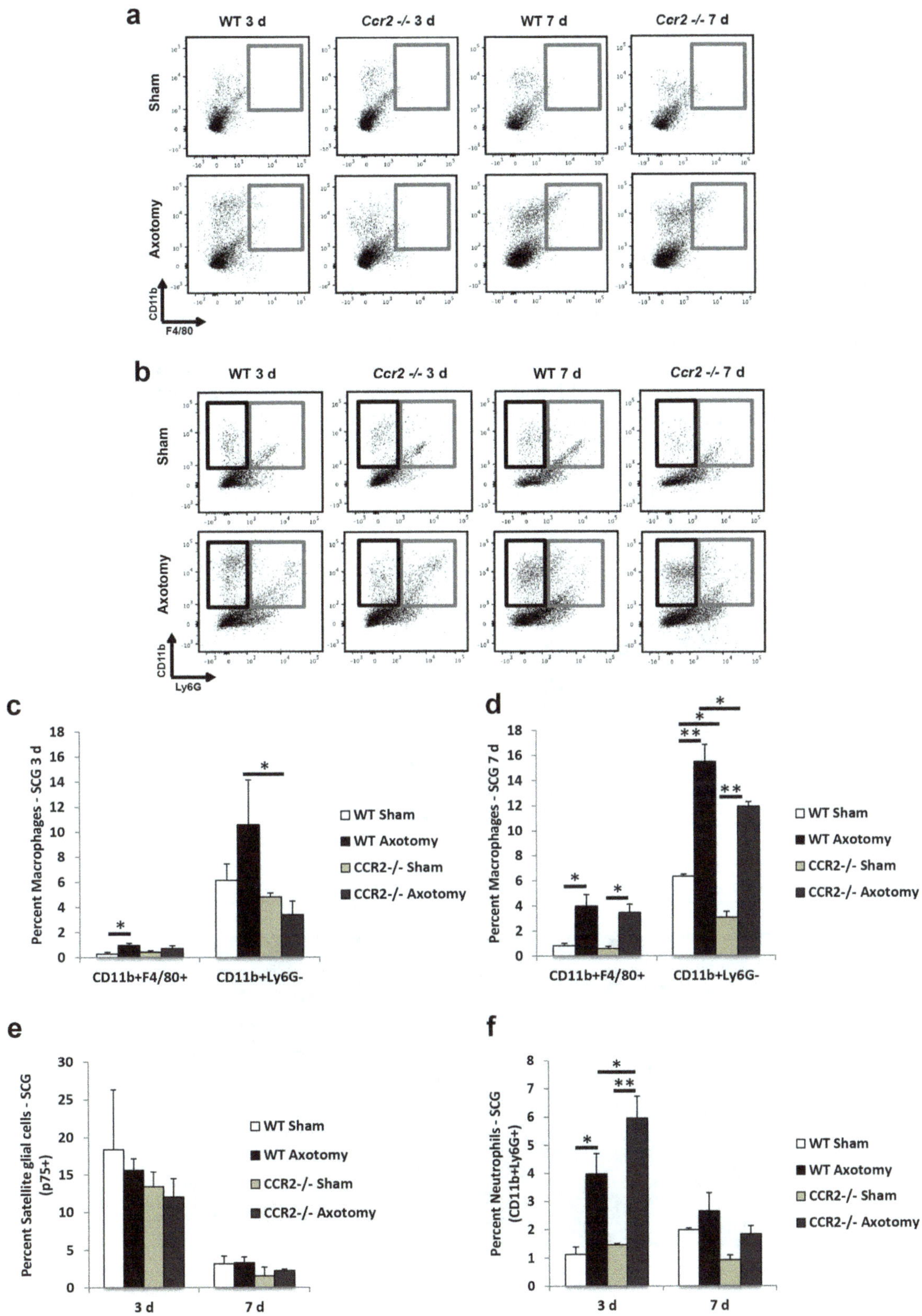

Fig. 4 (See legend on next page.)

(See figure on previous page.)

Fig. 4 Macrophage accumulation is attenuated in the axotomized SCG of *Ccr2*$^{-/-}$ mice compared to WT mice, while *Ccr2*$^{-/-}$ SCG show a larger increase in neutrophil accumulation 3 days after injury, compared to the WT SCG. Three and seven days after axotomy, SCG were dissected and examined using flow cytometry. Both sham and axotomized nerves were analyzed. Gray boxes in **a** indicate CD11b$^+$F4/80$^+$ cells. In **b**, black boxes indicate CD11b$^+$Ly6G$^-$ cells and gray boxes indicate CD11b$^+$Ly6G$^+$ cells. Flow cytometric analysis of macrophage populations in the injured SCG (**a**, **b**) indicates increased percentages of CD11b$^+$F4/80$^+$ cells 3 days after axotomy in WT mice alone and a significant increase in CD11b$^+$Ly6G$^-$ cells in injured WT mice compared to *Ccr2*$^{-/-}$ mice (**c**). Axotomy induced significant increases in macrophages in both genotypes 7 days post injury, with WT mice displaying a larger increase in CD11b$^+$Ly6G$^-$ cells over *Ccr2*$^{-/-}$ mice (**d**). No changes were observed between genotypes in the satellite glial cell population at either time point (**e**). Significant increases in CD11b$^+$Ly6G$^+$ neutrophils were seen in WT and *Ccr2*$^{-/-}$ SCG 3 days post injury (**f**). Neutrophils were more prevalent in the *Ccr2*$^{-/-}$ SCG 3 days after axotomy compared to the WT SCG. Mean ± SEM, two-way ANOVA, Tukey's post hoc test corrected (within individual time points). *$p < 0.05$. **$p < 0.001$. $n = 3$ mice per genotype per time point

In the SCG, WT mice displayed significant injury-induced expression of multiple cytokines and immune-related factors including a 2.6-fold increase in C5/C5a, a 4.8-fold increase in TIMP-1, a 3.0-fold increase in sICAM-1, a 2.1-fold increase in IL-16, and a 3.2-fold increase in IL-1ra compared to WT sham SCG (Fig. 6c, c, f). Axotomized *Ccr2*$^{-/-}$ mice exhibited a significant 2.2-fold increase in the TIMP-1 and a 1.9-fold increase in M-CSF compared to *Ccr2*$^{-/-}$ sham SCG (Fig. 6c', d', f). A comparison of the SCG cytokine expression profiles between genotypes found that C5/C5a, TIMP-1, IL-16, and sICAM-1 were more highly expressed in the WT SCG compared to *Ccr2*$^{-/-}$ SCG 7 days after injury (Fig. 6f). The most striking differences in injury-induced expression patterns between DRG and SCG are in C5/C5a and IL-16. In the DRG, C5/C5a and IL-16 are more highly expressed in *Ccr2*$^{-/-}$ mice than in WT mice; however, the expression pattern is the exact opposite in the SCG where these

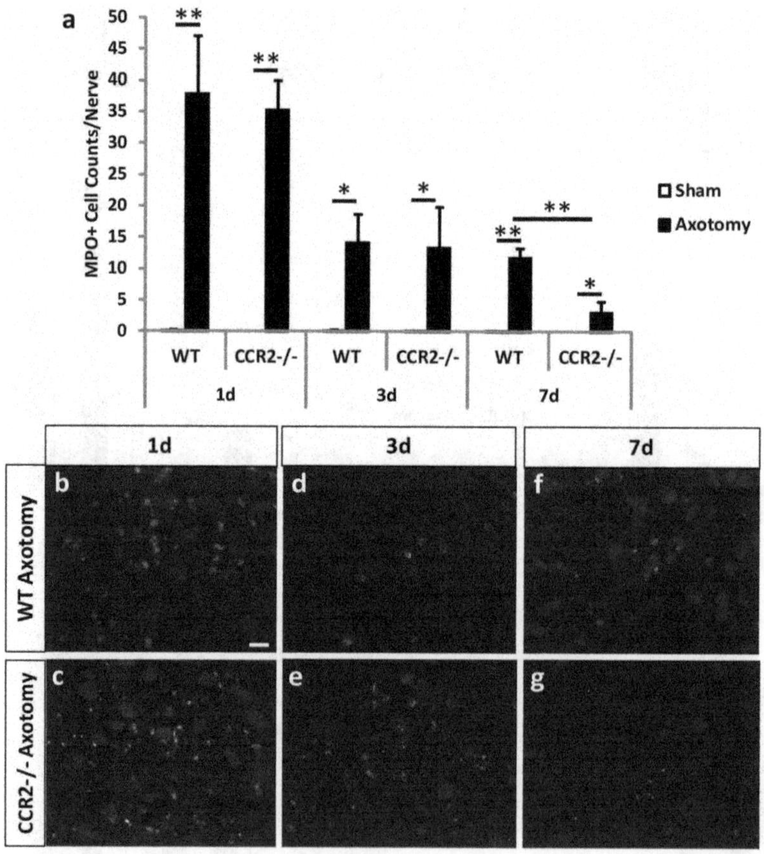

Fig. 5 Myeloperoxidase staining of neutrophils in the axotomized SCG 1, 3, and 7 days after axotomy. Immunohistochemical staining of neutrophils with an antibody against MPO showed comparable neutrophil cell counts between WT and *Ccr2*$^{-/-}$ SCG 1 and 3 days after injury and a significantly higher number of cells in WT ganglia compared to mutants 7 days after injury. Cell counts were performed using ImageJ at 1, 3, and 7 days post injury (**a**). The counts represent the sum of cells from three images per section. Representative images of IHC staining in the SCG at 1, 3, and 7 days post axotomy are shown for WT Ax (**b**, **d**, **f**) and *Ccr2*$^{-/-}$ Ax (**c**, **e**, **g**). All images were taken at × 25 magnification. Scale bar = 20 μm. $n = 5$ per group. *$p < 0.05$. **$p < 0.001$

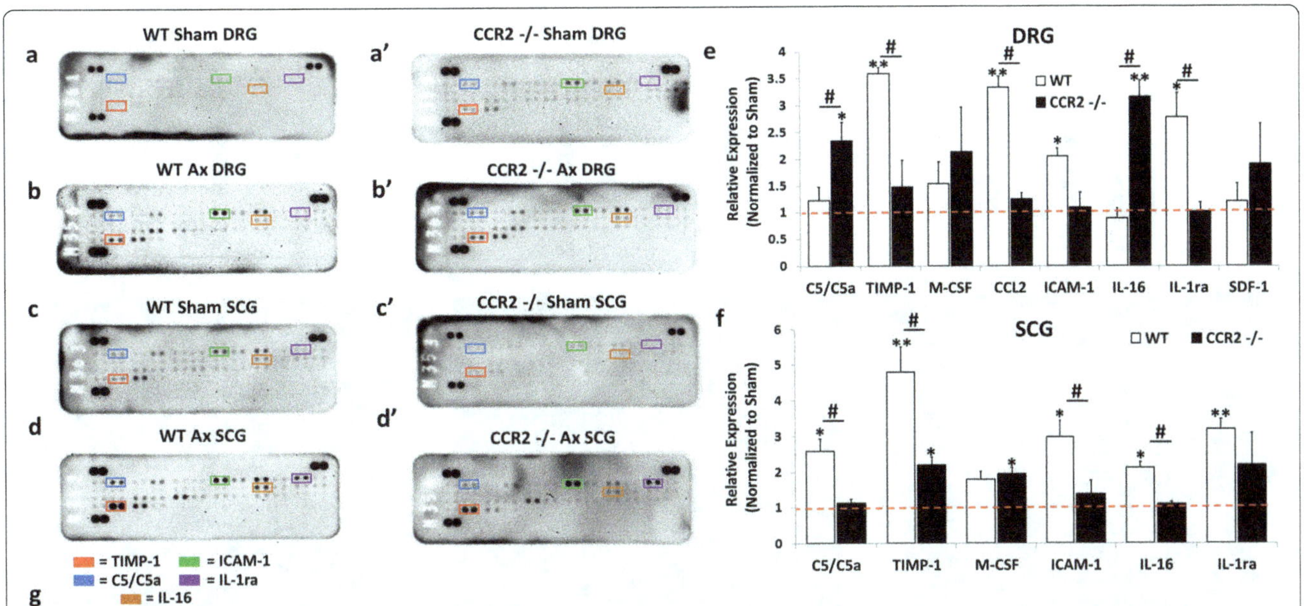

	1	2	3	4	5	6	7	8	9	10	11	12	13	14	15	16	17	18	19	20	21	22	23	24
A	REF	REF																					REF	REF
B	BLC	BLC	C5	C5	G-CSF	G-CSF	GM-CSF	GM-CSF	CCL1	CCL1	Eotaxin	Eotaxin	ICAM-1	ICAM-1	IFN-γ	IFN-γ	IL-1a	IL-1a	IL-1B	IL-1B	IL-1ra	IL-1ra	IL-2	IL-2
C	IL-3	IL-3	IL-4	IL-4	IL-5	IL-5	IL-6	IL-6	IL-7	IL-7	IL-10	IL-10	IL-13	IL-13	IL-12 P70	IL-12 P70	IL-16	IL-16	IL-17	IL-17	IL-23	IL-23	IL-27	IL-27
D	CXCL10	CXCL10	CXCL11	CXCL11	CXCL1	CXCL1	M-CSF	M-CSF	CCL2	CCL2	MCP=5	MCP-5	MIG	MIG	MIP1-A	MIP-1A	MIP-1B	MIP-1B	MIP2	MIP2	RANTES	RENTES	SDF-1	SDF-1
E	CCL17	CCL17	TIMP-1	TIMP-1	TNF-A	TNF-A	TREM-1	TREM-1																
F	REF	REF																					NEG	NEG

Fig. 6 Injury-induced cytokine profiles in the DRG and SCG 7 days after axotomy. Mice underwent a unilateral transection of the right sciatic nerve and the right ICN and ECN of the SCG. Seven days after axotomy, the injured and contralateral sham-operated L4/L5 DRG and SCG were collected and flash frozen. Protein was isolated from sham and injured ganglia pooled from five mice and used for measurement of cytokines using a Proteome Profiler Mouse Array kit (**g**). Representative arrays for WT [85] and *Ccr2*$^{-/-}$ (**a'**–**d'**) mice for DRG (**a**, **a'**, **b**, **b'**) and SCG (**c**, **c'**, **d**, **d'**) are shown. Array images were analyzed by densitometry for integral optical density using ImageJ. The optical density for each cytokine was then normalized to the internal control for each blot. The data are represented as the fold increase in the expression of the injured condition compared to the sham for each genotype for DRG (**e**) and SCG (**f**). The spots corresponding to the cytokines TIMP-1, sICAM-1, C5/C5a, IL-1ra, and IL-16 are highlighted in the representative arrays based on the template indicating the location of controls and various chemokine capture antibodies (**g**). *N* = 3 arrays per group. The data are presented as the mean ± SEM. *$p < 0.05$. **$p < 0.001$ represents significance of expression relative to sham within genotype. $^{\#}p < 0.05$. $^{\#\#}p < 0.001$ represents significance between genotypes

immune-related factors are more highly expressed by WT mice compared to *Ccr2*$^{-/-}$ mice (Fig. 6e, f).

Activation state of macrophages in peripheral ganglia following nerve injury

Macrophages have been shown to increase the regenerative response of DRG neurons through releasable factors [45]; however, this ability was dependent upon the activation state of the macrophages. Conditioned medium derived from macrophages stimulated to an anti-inflammatory state was growth promoting compared to conditioned medium taken from pro-inflammatory macrophages to DRG neurons plated on inhibitory substrates [45, 46]. Given the differences in the molecular and cellular immune response between the SCG and DRG and WT and *Ccr2*$^{-/-}$ mice, we sought to determine if macrophages in our system expressed an activation state which would be expected to support regeneration. Expression of the anti-inflammatory marker CD206 was assessed in the SCG and DRG at 1, 3, and 7 days after axotomy. CD206, a mannose receptor, is a useful marker of anti-inflammatory polarization as pro-inflammatory macrophages do not express this receptor [47–49]. In the DRG, significant accumulation of CD68^{+} macrophages was not seen until 3 days post injury compared to sham-operated controls (Fig. 7f–j). Macrophage accumulation was sustained at 7 days post injury, where 91.3 ± 3.7% of CD68^{+} cells colocalized with CD206 (Fig. 7k–o). *Ccr2*$^{-/-}$ mice displayed a significant reduction in both CD68^{+} cells and CD68^{+}CD206^{+}-colocalized cells 7 days post injury (Fig. 7k). The reduction in colocalized cells in the *Ccr2*$^{-/-}$ DRG does not represent a specific reduction in the expression of CD206 as 85.3 ± 5.5% of CD68^{+} cells present coexpressed CD206.

In the axotomized SCG, significant macrophage accumulation was detected in WT mice as early as 1 day post axotomy (Fig. 8a), an effect that was sustained out to

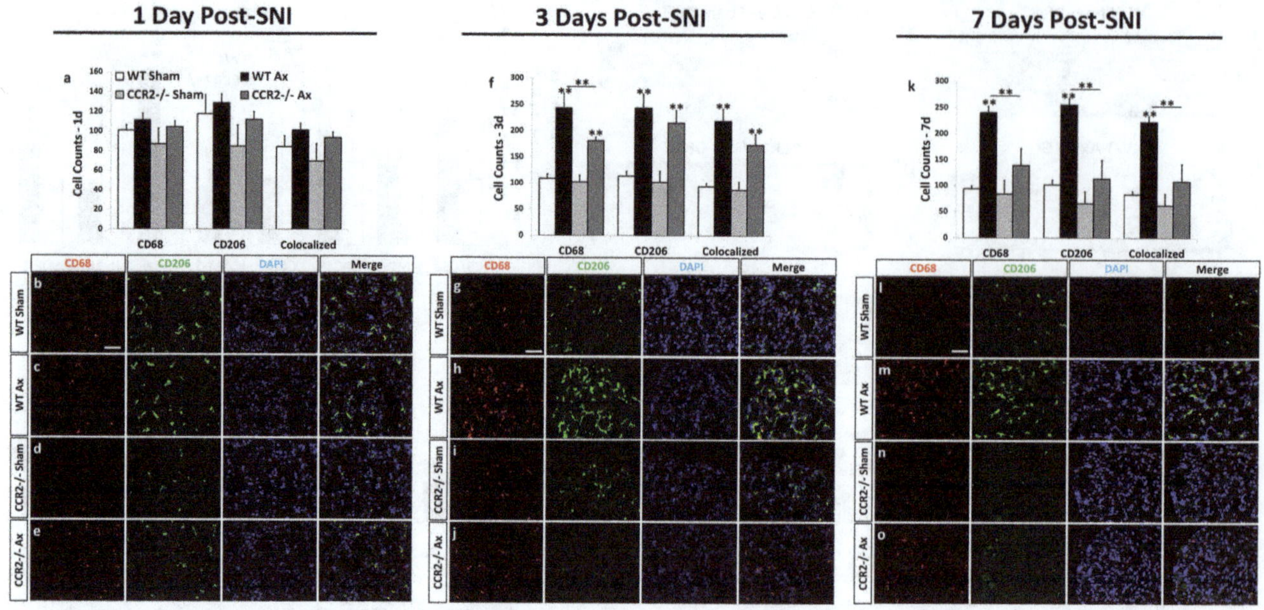

Fig. 7 The anti-inflammatory marker, CD206, is highly expressed in CD68$^+$ macrophages in the WT DRG 3 and 7 days after sciatic nerve transection. Immunohistochemical labeling of DRG sections with antibodies against a macrophage marker, CD68, and an anti-inflammatory marker, CD206, shows that a majority of macrophages in the WT DRG at 7 days post injury express CD206 (**k**). The number of CD68$^+$ and CD206$^+$ cells was significantly diminished in *Ccr2*$^{-/-}$ mice at 3 days (**f**) and 7 days (**k**) post injury. Cell counts were performed using ImageJ at 1, 3, and 7 days post injury for CD68$^+$-, CD206$^+$-, and CD68$^+$CD206$^+$-colocalized cells (**a**, **f**, **k**). The counts represent the sum of cells from three images per section. Representative images of IHC staining in the L5 DRG at 1, 3, and 7 days post axotomy are shown for WT sham (**b**, **g**, **l**), WT Ax (**c**, **h**, **m**), *Ccr2*$^{-/-}$ sham (**d**, **i**, **n**), and *Ccr2*$^{-/-}$ Ax (**e**, **j**, **o**). All images were taken at × 25 magnification. Scale bar = 50 μm. $n = 5$ per group. $^*p < 0.05$. $^{**}p < 0.001$

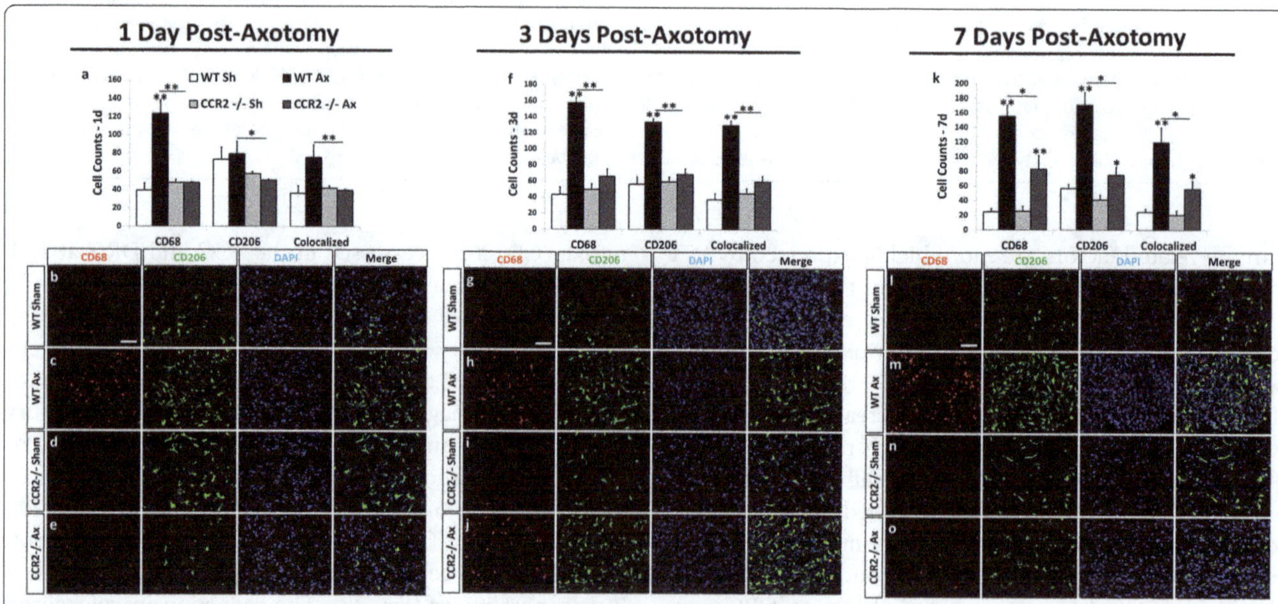

Fig. 8 The anti-inflammatory marker, CD206, is highly expressed in CD68$^+$ macrophages in the WT SCG at 1, 3, and 7 days after axotomy. Immunohistochemical labeling of SCG sections with antibodies against a macrophage marker, CD68, and an anti-inflammatory marker, CD206, shows that a majority of macrophages in the WT SCG at 3 and 7 days post injury express CD206 (**f**, **k**). The number of CD68$^+$ and CD206$^+$ cells was significantly diminished in *Ccr2*$^{-/-}$ mice at 3 and 7 days post injury (**f**, **k**). Cell counts were performed using ImageJ at 1, 3, and 7 days post injury for CD68$^+$-, CD206$^+$-, and CD68$^+$CD206$^+$-colocalized cells (**a**, **f**, **k**). The counts represent the sum of cells from three images per section. Representative images of IHC staining in the SCG at 1, 3, and 7 days post axotomy are shown for WT sham (**b**, **g**, **l**), WT Ax (**c**, **h**, **m**), *Ccr2*$^{-/-}$ sham (**d**, **i**, **n**), and *Ccr2*$^{-/-}$ Ax (**e**, **j**, **o**). All images were taken at × 25 magnification. Scale bar = 50 μm. $n = 5$ per group. $^*p < 0.05$. $^{**}p < 0.001$

7 days post injury (Fig. 8k). A high level of colocalization between CD206 and CD68 is seen in that 77.6 ± 9.5% of $CD68^+$ cells were also labeled with CD206. The *Ccr2*$^{-/-}$ SCG displayed reduced $CD68^+$ macrophage accumulation compared to WT at all time points (Fig. 8a, f, k). These data indicate that macrophages present within peripheral ganglia after nerve injury may be anti-inflammatory in nature.

Discussion

CCL2 overexpression in sensory ganglia has been shown to be sufficient to cause macrophage accumulation in the DRG without a nerve injury [17]. Here, we have shown that CCL2 protein expression is increased in both the WT and *Ccr2*$^{-/-}$ axotomized DRG and SCG early after injury. CCL2 upregulation is associated with a heightened macrophage response in both ganglia, albeit this response is markedly reduced in *Ccr2*$^{-/-}$ mice. Indeed, deletion of the receptor alone showed almost complete blockade of macrophage accumulation in the DRG and a significant but only partial reduction in the SCG after nerve injury [14]. These results suggest that a second chemokine and/or action through a second chemokine receptor is facilitating monocyte-mediated chemotaxis to the injured sympathetic ganglia.

An obvious candidate for this role is MIP-1γ, which we found, using the unbiased chemokine array, to be increased only in the injured SCG of both WT and *Ccr2*$^{-/-}$ mice. MIP-1γ acts through CCR1 expressed on monocytes, neutrophils, dendritic cells, and T cells [50–53]. Some evidence indicates that MIP-1γ may act in an autocrine fashion on macrophages to promote their activation and survival [53], while other studies point to dendritic cells as important producers of this chemokine for extravasation of inflammatory cells from the bloodstream [51]. Regardless of its source, heightened expression of MIP-1γ in the SCG is associated with increased macrophage accumulation. Furthermore, robust expression of both MIP-1γ and CCL2 in the SCG could explain the early and significant accumulation of macrophages that we observed in the axotomized sympathetic ganglia at 1 day post injury, compared to the typical increase in the macrophage response observed in the injured DRG after 3 days [11, 12]. However, we would need to confirm that MIP-1γ is upregulated in the SCG earlier than the 48-h time point that was used in this study.

What are the consequences of inhibiting macrophage accumulation in these ganglia after nerve injury? The most well-described function of macrophages is their role in the distal nerve segment where they promote regeneration of injured neurons through growth factor release and the removal of inhibitory axonal and myelin debris at the distal nerve that would otherwise obstruct the path for regenerating axons [54–57]. Though peripheral nerve degeneration involves the actions of multiple cells, hematogenous macrophages that infiltrate as monocytes from the blood to the injury site have been considered to be necessary for the phagocytosis of myelin and axonal fragments [13, 58–60]. It is believed that while Schwann cells initiate myelin uptake and removal [61, 62], infiltrating macrophages complete the clearance process [60, 63, 64]. However, recent studies have shown that myelin clearance is normal in *Ccr2*$^{-/-}$ sciatic nerves after an injury [14], and that neutrophils play a pivotal role in this clearance [65].

Of late, a new site of macrophage action has been proposed in promoting nerve regeneration. Following injury to the sciatic nerve or ICN and ECN, macrophages accumulate within the DRG and SCG, respectively [14]. Mice lacking CCR2 exhibited diminished macrophage accumulation in the ganglia and a concomitant decrease in axonal regeneration [14], while a similar study that administered the antibiotic minocycline to reduce macrophage numbers in the DRG also observed a reduction in regeneration [11]. Moreover, our lab provided evidence that simply overexpressing CCL2 in sensory ganglia without a nerve injury is sufficient to mount an injury-like macrophage response in the DRG and to prompt robust neurite growth [17].

What remains to be determined is how these macrophages promote regeneration at the level of the neuronal cell bodies. The most likely mechanism of action is through a macrophage-derived releasable factor, such as a cytokine, that stimulates the neuronal expression of regeneration-associated genes [45, 66–68]. Analysis of regeneration-associated genes in the uninjured DRG in which CCL2 was overexpressed highlighted increased expression of leukemia inhibitory factor (*Lif*) mRNA [17], a gene that had been previously described as promoting sensory and sympathetic neuron regeneration [69, 70].

In the cytokine array, we observe differential expression of cytokines between genotypes in the injured DRG 7 days after injury, many of which are downregulated in the *Ccr2*$^{-/-}$ model compared to WT mice. This is not surprising if we consider evidence that the lack of CCR2 and a resulting decrease in macrophage accumulation in the injured ganglia reveal an inhibition of in vitro regeneration of both sensory and sympathetic neurons [14]. TIMP-1, a protein that we find is reduced in the axotomized *Ccr2*$^{-/-}$ DRG and SCG compared to their axotomized WT counterparts, has been shown to be important in supporting regeneration in the central nervous system [71]. TIMP-1 functions to inhibit the activity of metalloproteinases which cleave myelin-associated glycoproteins that accumulate in the central nervous system after nerve injury and obstruct the path of regenerating DRG neurons [72]. Peripheral nerve injury has been shown to induce TIMP-1 expression in the DRG

[73]. Furthermore, a preconditioning injury to the peripheral nerve process of the DRG followed by an injury to the central nerve process results in TIMP-1 upregulation in the DRG and the spinal cord in addition to increased neurite outgrowth into the spinal cord [71].

The specific contribution of macrophage releasable factors to the cytokine microenvironment has been shown to be indicative of the macrophage phenotype, i.e., pro-inflammatory or anti-inflammatory [46]. Pro-inflammatory macrophages are characterized by the increased production of nitric oxide and specifically the enzyme inducible nitric oxide synthase (iNOS) [74, 75], while anti-inflammatory macrophages upregulate expression of the mannose receptor CD206 [76]. These distinctions of macrophage activation states are important because of recent work that has shown that conditioned media taken from anti-inflammatory macrophage cultures was able to stimulate DRG neurite outgrowth on both growth-permissive and growth-inhibiting substrates [45]. We previously reported increased CD206 transcript levels in the uninjured DRG of WT mice where CCL2 was overexpressed, resulting in increased macrophage accumulation and neurite outgrowth [17]. Here, we find that a majority of macrophages in the axotomized WT DRG and SCG at 1, 3, and 7 days post injury express the anti-inflammatory marker CD206, which suggests that these macrophages are of an anti-inflammatory nature. It should be noted that most macrophages in the axotomized *Ccr2*$^{-/-}$ DRG and SCG also express CD206, but the overall accumulation of these myeloid cells is drastically reduced relative to WT mice. Furthermore, the hypothesis that monocyte-derived macrophages that infiltrate the DRG and SCG after injury are of an anti-inflammatory type is evidence of the small number of macrophages that express the pro-inflammatory marker iNOS (data not shown).

In addition to the evaluation of macrophage activation states and the evident differences in macrophage accumulation between genotypes in the axotomized ganglia, we also note a genotype-specific alteration in neutrophil chemotaxis to the SCG. *Ccr2*$^{-/-}$ sympathetic ganglia boast a larger neutrophil population than its WT counterpart 3 days following nerve injury. This increase is associated with heightened expression of CXCL5, a neutrophil chemokine, in the *Ccr2*$^{-/-}$ SCG [77]. Interestingly, upregulation of another neutrophil chemokine MIP-2 (CXCL2) was not observed, though this chemokine most likely plays a role in increased neutrophil accumulation in the injured *Ccr2*$^{-/-}$ sciatic nerve compared to WT nerves [65].

Interestingly, our data suggest that different subpopulations of neutrophils may exist in the SCG after nerve injury. Flow cytometry analysis demonstrated that CD11b^{+}Ly6G^{+} neutrophils were significantly more abundant in the *Ccr2*$^{-/-}$ SCG 3 days following injury compared to the WT SCG; however, IHC data showed comparable MPO^{+} neutrophil accumulation in the sympathetic ganglia between genotypes at this same time point. The idea of neutrophil heterogeneity has gained considerable traction with evidence that has shown that these polymorphonuclear cells develop distinct phenotypes in response to a range of stimuli [78].

Unlike in the SCG, we do not identify a significant population of neutrophils in the DRG after sciatic nerve transection in either genotype. However, the role of neutrophils in the DRG has been extensively characterized in experimental paradigms of neuropathic pain. Neutrophils reportedly infiltrate both the DRG and the sciatic nerve in response to chronic nerve constriction [79] and partial nerve ligation [2]. These types of injuries manifest neuropathic pain due to the sensitization of neurons by exposure to a prolonged inflammatory response [1]. Neutrophils and other immune cells including macrophages and T cells have been shown to contribute to neuropathic pain via the release of TNF-α, IL-1β, and IL-6 through directly engaging cognate receptors on sensory neurons (for a summary, see [80]). Chemotactic disruption of these immune cells using pharmacological or genetic methods has been shown to ameliorate the severity of neuropathic pain [81–83].

Clear differences in chemokine and cytokine expression profiles were observed between DRG and SCG following axotomy. Forty-eight hours after injury, C5/C5a is significantly increased in the WT DRG but is not upregulated in the WT SCG, while MIP-1γ is highly upregulated in the injured WT SCG but is not increased in the DRG after injury. Seven days after injury, IL-1ra is significantly upregulated in the WT SCG but not the WT DRG. The distinct expression of specific immune signaling molecules between ganglia could be a result of the presence of a significant neutrophil population found in the SCG but not the DRG 3 days after injury. However, other ganglion-specific aspects such as the presence of a blood-ganglion barrier in the SCG or the significant heterogeneity of neurons in the DRG could play a contributing factor [24, 84].

Conclusions

Through the characterization of cellular components that populate sensory and sympathetic ganglia in WT and *Ccr2*$^{-/-}$ mice, which, in turn, influence changes in the cytokine microenvironment surrounding the axotomized neurons, we can begin to carve out unexplored territories for future research. Here, we have identified differences in the macrophage response between genotypes after injury in both DRG and SCG, but there remains a similarity of macrophage phenotype (i.e., anti-inflammatory). Additionally, a probable alternative compensatory chemokine network (MIP-1γ) that may facilitate monocyte extravasation to the injured SCG in the absence of CCR2 expression has emerged from this study. CCR2 deletion also induced increased neutrophil accumulation in the injured SCG, but the consequence of this increase is as yet unknown. Taken together, this study has revealed important molecular and cellular differences between WT and $Ccr2^{-/-}$ mice and between axotomized DRG and SCG and has posed interesting new questions for future studies.

Abbreviations

ANOVA: Analysis of variance; ATF3: Activating transcription factor 3; CCL2: C-C class chemokine ligand 2; CCR2: C-C class chemokine receptor 2; DRG: Dorsal root ganglion; ECN: External carotid nerve; ICN: Internal carotid nerve; IHC: Immunohistochemistry; IL: Interleukin; IL-1ra: Interleukin-1 receptor antagonist; iNOS: Inducible nitric oxide synthase; LIF: Leukemia inhibitory factor; MCP-1: Monocyte chemoattractant protein-1; MIP-1γ: Macrophage inflammatory protein-1 gamma; MPO: Myeloperoxidase; PNS: Peripheral nervous system; SCG: Superior cervical ganglion; sICAM-1: Soluble intercellular adhesion molecule-1; TIMP-1: Tissue inhibitor of metalloproteinase-1; TNF-α: Tumor necrosis factor alpha; WT: Wild type

Acknowledgements

Breeding and genotyping of animals were carried out by the Case Western Reserve Visual Sciences Specialized Animal Research and the Molecular Biology and Genotyping Cores (EY11373). The authors thank Mike Sramkoski of the Cytometry and Imaging Microscopy Core at Case Western Reserve University for providing guidance with flow cytometry setup and analysis. The authors also thank Dr. Franklin Echevarria for constructing the diagrams in Fig. 1 and Jeong Seo and Aaron Talsma for their careful review and feedback on the manuscript.

Funding

This work was supported by the National Institutes of Health grants DK097223 and NS095017 to R.E.Z. J.A.L was supported by a training grant NS067431 and an NIH NRSA Award F31NS093694. J.P.N was supported by training grants NS067431 and NS077888.

Authors' contributions

JAL, JPN, and REZ designed the research; JAL, JPN, MEH, CZM, DM, and KWL performed the research; JAL, JPN, and REZ analyzed the data; JAL, JPN, and REZ wrote the paper. All authors read and approved the final manuscript.

Consent for publication

Not applicable.

Competing interests

The authors declare that they have no competing interests.

Author details

[1]Department of Neurosciences, School of Medicine, Case Western Reserve University, Cleveland, OH, USA. [2]Science and Engineering Program, Hathaway Brown School, Shaker Heights, OH, USA. [3]Present Address: Department Neurosciences, School of Medicine, 10900 Euclid Avenue, Robbins E701, Cleveland, OH 44106-4975, USA.

References

1. Austin PJ, Moalem-Taylor G. The neuro-immune balance in neuropathic pain: involvement of inflammatory immune cells, immune-like glial cells and cytokines. J Neuroimmunol. 2010;229:26–50.
2. Kim CF, Moalem-Taylor G. Detailed characterization of neuro-immune responses following neuropathic injury in mice. Brain Res. 2011;1405:95–108.
3. Perry VH, Brown MC, Gordon S. The macrophage response to central and peripheral nerve injury. A possible role for macrophages in regeneration. J Exp Med. 1987;165:1218–23.
4. Mueller M, Leonhard C, Wacker K, Ringelstein EB, Okabe M, Hickey WF, Kiefer R. Macrophage response to peripheral nerve injury: the quantitative contribution of resident and hematogenous macrophages. Lab Investig. 2003;83:175–85.
5. Nadeau S, Filali M, Zhang J, Kerr BJ, Rivest S, Soulet D, Iwakura Y, de Rivero Vaccari JP, Keane RW, Lacroix S. Functional recovery after peripheral nerve injury is dependent on the pro-inflammatory cytokines IL-1beta and TNF: implications for neuropathic pain. J Neurosci. 2011;31:12533–42.
6. Perry VH, Brown MC. Role of macrophages in peripheral nerve degeneration and repair. Bioessays. 1992;14:401–6.
7. Hu P, McLachlan EM. Distinct functional types of macrophage in dorsal root ganglia and spinal nerves proximal to sciatic and spinal nerve transections in the rat. Exp Neurol. 2003;184:590–605.
8. Schmid AB, Coppieters MW, Ruitenberg MJ, McLachlan EM. Local and remote immune-mediated inflammation after mild peripheral nerve compression in rats. J Neuropathol Exp Neurol. 2013;72:662–80.
9. Schreiber RC, Shadiack AM, Bennett TA, Sedwick CE, Zigmond RE. Changes in the macrophage population of the rat superior cervical ganglion after postganglionic nerve injury. J Neurobiol. 1995;27:141–53.
10. Schreiber RC, Vaccariello SA, Boeshore K, Shadiack AM, Zigmond RE. A comparison of the changes in the non-neuronal cell populations of the superior cervical ganglia following decentralization and axotomy. J Neurobiol. 2002;53:68–79.
11. Kwon MJ, Kim J, Shin H, Jeong SR, Kang YM, Choi JY, Hwang DH, Kim BG. Contribution of macrophages to enhanced regenerative capacity of dorsal root ganglia sensory neurons by conditioning injury. J Neurosci. 2013;33:15095–108.
12. Lu X, Richardson PM. Responses of macrophages in rat dorsal root ganglia following peripheral nerve injury. J Neurocytol. 1993;22:334–41.
13. Siebert H, Sachse A, Kuziel WA, Maeda N, Bruck W. The chemokine receptor CCR2 is involved in macrophage recruitment to the injured peripheral nervous system. J Neuroimmunol. 2000;110:177–85.
14. Niemi JP, DeFrancesco-Lisowitz A, Roldan-Hernandez L, Lindborg JA, Mandell D, Zigmond RE. A critical role for macrophages near axotomized neuronal cell bodies in stimulating nerve regeneration. J Neurosci. 2013;33:16236–48.
15. Colonna M, Trinchieri G, Liu Y-J. Plasmacytoid dendritic cells in immunity. Nat Immunol. 2004;5:1219–26.
16. Reichel CA, Rehberg M, Lerchenberger M, Berberich N, Bihari P, Khandoga AG, Zahler S, Krombach F. Ccl2 and Ccl3 mediate neutrophil recruitment via induction of protein synthesis and generation of lipid mediators. Arterioscler Thromb Vasc Biol. 2009;29:1787–93.
17. Niemi JP, DeFrancesco-Lisowitz A, Cregg JM, Howarth M, Zigmond RE. Overexpression of the monocyte chemokine CCL2 in dorsal root ganglion neurons causes a conditioning-like increase in neurite outgrowth and does so via a STAT3 dependent mechanism. Exp Neurol. 2016;275:25–37.
18. Kwon MJ, Shin HY, Cui Y, Kim H, Le Thi AH, Choi JY, Kim EY, Hwang DH, Kim BG. CCL2 mediates neuron–macrophage interactions to drive proregenerative macrophage activation following preconditioning injury. J Neurosci. 2015;35:15934–47.
19. Tandrup T, Woolf CJ, Coggeshall RE. Delayed loss of small dorsal root ganglion cells after transection of the rat sciatic nerve. J Comp Neurol. 2000;422:172–80.
20. Vestergaard S, Tandrup T, Jakobsen J. Effect of permanent axotomy on number and volume of dorsal root ganglion cell bodies. J Comp Neurol. 1997;388:307–12.
21. Himes B, Tessler A. Death of some dorsal root ganglion neurons and plasticity of others following sciatic nerve section in adult and neonatal rats. J Comp Neurol. 1989;284:215–30.

22. Tessler A, Himes B, Krieger N, Murray M, Goldberger M. Sciatic nerve transection produces death of dorsal root ganglion cells and reversible loss of substance P in spinal cord. Brain Res. 1985;332:209–18.
23. Devor M. Unexplained peculiarities of the dorsal root ganglion. Pain. 1999;82(Suppl 6):S27–35.
24. Depace DM. Evidence for a blood-ganglion barrier in the superior cervical ganglion of the rat. Anat Rec. 1982;204:357–63.
25. Andrews TJ, Thrasivoulou C, Nesbit W, Cowen T. Target-specific differences in the dendritic morphology and neuropeptide content of neurons in the rat SCG during development and aging. J Comp Neurol. 1996;368:33–44.
26. Wright LL, Cunningham TJ, Smolen AJ. Developmental neuron death in the rat superior cervical sympathetic ganglion: cell counts and ultrastructure. J Neurocytol. 1983;12:727–38.
27. Schnizlein-Bick CT, Mandy FF, O'Gorman MR, Paxton H, Nicholson JK, Hultin LE, Gelman RS, Wilkening CL, Livnat D. Use of CD45 gating in three and four-color flow cytometric immunophenotyping: guideline from the national institute of allergy and infectious diseases, division of AIDS. Cytometry Part A. 2002;50:46–52.
28. Geuna S. The sciatic nerve injury model in pre-clinical research. J Neurosci Methods. 2015;243:39–46.
29. Jankowski MP, Lawson JJ, McIlwrath SL, Rau KK, Anderson CE, Albers KM, Koerber HR. Sensitization of cutaneous nociceptors after nerve transection and regeneration: possible role of target-derived neurotrophic factor signaling. J Neurosci. 2009;29:1636–47.
30. Decosterd I, Woolf CJ. Spared nerve injury: an animal model of persistent peripheral neuropathic pain. Pain. 2000;87:149–58.
31. Hyatt Sachs H, Schreiber RC, Shoemaker SE, Sabe A, Reed E, Zigmond RE. Activating transcription factor 3 induction in sympathetic neurons after axotomy: response to decreased neurotrophin availability. Neuroscience. 2007;150:887–97.
32. Tsujino H, Kondo E, Fukuoka T, Dai Y, Tokunaga A, Miki K, Yonenobu K, Ochi T, Noguchi K. Activating transcription factor 3 (ATF3) induction by axotomy in sensory and motoneurons: a novel neuronal marker of nerve injury. Mol Cell Neurosci. 2000;15:170–82.
33. Phillips RJ, Hargrave SL, Rhodes BS, Zopf DA, Powley TL. Quantification of neurons in the myenteric plexus: an evaluation of putative pan-neuronal markers. J Neurosci Methods. 2004;133:99–107.
34. Bowers CW, Zigmond RE. Localization of neurons in the rat superior cervical ganglion that project into different postganglionic trunks. J Comp Neurol. 1979;185:381–91.
35. Fernandez EJ, Lolis E. Structure, function, and inhibition of chemokines. Annu Rev Pharmacol Toxicol. 2002;42:469–99.
36. Donegan M, Kernisant M, Cua C, Jasmin L, Ohara PT. Satellite glial cell proliferation in the trigeminal ganglia after chronic constriction injury of the infraorbital nerve. Glia. 2013;61:2000–8.
37. Hall A, Landis S. Division and migration of satellite glia in the embryonic rat superior cervical ganglion. J Neurocytol. 1992;21:635–47.
38. Hanani M. Satellite glial cells in sensory ganglia: from form to function. Brain Res Brain Res Rev. 2005;48:457–76.
39. Shinder V, Govrin-Lippmann R, Cohen S, Belenky M, Ilin P, Fried K, Wilkinson HA, Devor M. Structural basis of sympathetic-sensory coupling in rat and human dorsal root ganglia following peripheral nerve injury. J Neurocytol. 1999;28:743–61.
40. Fenzi F, Benedetti MD, Moretto G, Rizzuto N. Glial cell and macrophage reactions in rat spinal ganglion after peripheral nerve lesions: an immunocytochemical and morphometric study. Arch Ital Biol. 2001;139:357–65.
41. Verge VM, Riopelle RJ, Richardson PM. Nerve growth factor receptors on normal and injured sensory neurons. J Neurosci. 1989;9:914–22.
42. Zhou X-F, Rush RA, McLachlan EM. Differential expression of the p75 nerve growth factor receptor in glia and neurons of the rat dorsal root ganglia after peripheral nerve transection. J Neurosci. 1996;16:2901–11.
43. Haqqani AS, Sandhu JK, Birnboim HC. A myeloperoxidase-specific assay based upon bromide-dependent chemiluminescence of luminol. Anal Biochem. 1999;273:126–32.
44. Amanzada A, Malik IA, Nischwitz M, Sultan S, Naz N, Ramadori G. Myeloperoxidase and elastase are only expressed by neutrophils in normal and in inflammed liver. Histochem Cell Biol. 2011;135:305–15.
45. Kigerl KA, Gensel JC, Ankeny DP, Alexander JK, Donnelly DJ, Popovich PG. Identification of two distinct macrophage subsets with divergent effects causing either neurotoxicity or regeneration in the injured mouse spinal cord. J Neurosci. 2009;29:13435–44.
46. Gordon S, Taylor PR. Monocyte and macrophage heterogeneity. Nat Rev Immun. 2005;5:953–64.
47. Alan R, Ezekowitz B, Gordon S. Alterations of surface properties by macrophage activation: expression of receptors for Fc and mannose-terminal glycoproteins and differentiation antigens. In: Adams DO, editor. Macrophage activation. New York: Springer; 1984. p. 33–56.
48. Murray PJ, Allen JE, Biswas SK, Fisher EA, Gilroy DW, Goerdt S, Gordon S, Hamilton JA, Ivashkiv LB, Lawrence T. Macrophage activation and polarization: nomenclature and experimental guidelines. Immunity. 2014;41:14–20.
49. Porcheray F, Viaud S, Rimaniol AC, Leone C, Samah B, Dereuddre-Bosquet N, Dormont D, Gras G. Macrophage activation switching: an asset for the resolution of inflammation. Clin Exp Immunol. 2005;142:481–9.
50. Poltorak A, Bazzoni F, Smirnova I, Alejos E, Thompson P, Luheshi G, Rothwell N, Beutler B. MIP-1 gamma: molecular cloning, expression, and biological activities of a novel CC chemokine that is constitutively secreted in vivo. J Inflamm. 1995;45:207–19.
51. Mohamadzadeh M, Poltorak AN, Bergstressor P, Beutler B, Takashima A. Dendritic cells produce macrophage inflammatory protein-1 gamma, a new member of the CC chemokine family. J Immunol. 1996;156:3102–6.
52. Lean JM, Murphy C, Fuller K, Chambers TJ. CCL9/MIP-1γ and its receptor CCR1 are the major chemokine ligand/receptor species expressed by osteoclasts. J Cell Biochem. 2002;87:386–93.
53. Okamatsu Y, Kim D, Battaglino R, Sasaki H, Späte U, Stashenko P. MIP-1γ promotes receptor activator of NF-κB ligand-induced osteoclast formation and survival. J Immunol. 2004;173:2084–90.
54. Dailey AT, Avellino AM, Benthem L, Silver J, Kliot M. Complement depletion reduces macrophage infiltration and activation during Wallerian degeneration and axonal regeneration. J Neurosci. 1998;18:6713–22.
55. Barrette B, Hebert MA, Filali M, Lafortune K, Vallieres N, Gowing G, Julien JP, Lacroix S. Requirement of myeloid cells for axon regeneration. J Neurosci. 2008;28:9363–76.
56. Bisby MA, Chen S. Delayed wallerian degeneration in sciatic nerves of C57BL/Ola mice is associated with impaired regeneration of sensory axons. Brain Res. 1990;530:117–20.
57. Perry VH, Brown MC. Macrophages and nerve regeneration. Curr Opin Neurobiol. 1992;2:679–82.
58. Liefner M, Siebert H, Sachse T, Michel U, Kollias G, Bruck W. The role of TNF-alpha during Wallerian degeneration. J Neuroimmunol. 2000;108:147–52.
59. Bruck W. The role of macrophages in Wallerian degeneration. Brain Path. 1997;7:741–52.
60. Beuche W, Friede RL. The role of non-resident cells in Wallerian degeneration. J Neurocytol. 1984;13:767–96.
61. Stoll G, Griffin JW, Li CY, Trapp BD. Wallerian degeneration in the peripheral nervous system: participation of both Schwann cells and macrophages in myelin degradation. J Neurocytol. 1989;18:671–83.
62. Bigbee JW, Yoshino JE, DeVries GH. Morphological and proliferative responses of cultured Schwann cells following rapid phagocytosis of a myelin-enriched fraction. J Neurocytol. 1987;16:487–96.
63. Griffin JW, George R, Lobato C, Tyor WR, Yan LC, Glass JD. Macrophage responses and myelin clearance during Wallerian degeneration: relevance to immune-mediated demyelination. J Neuroimmunol. 1992;40:153–65.
64. Lunn ER, Perry VH, Brown MC, Rosen H, Gordon S. Absence of Wallerian degeneration does not hinder regeneration in peripheral nerve. Eur J Neurosci. 1989;1:27–33.
65. Lindborg JA, Mack M, Zigmond RE. Neutrophils are critical for myelin removal in a peripheral nerve injury model of Wallerian degeneration. J Neurosci. 2017;37:10258–77.
66. Lu X, Richardson PM. Inflammation near the nerve cell body enhances axonal regeneration. J Neurosci. 1991;11:972–8.
67. Lu X, Richardson PM. Changes in neuronal mRNAs induced by a local inflammatory reaction. J Neurosci Res. 1995;41:8–14.
68. Gensel JC, Kigerl KA, Mandrekar-Colucci SS, Gaudet AD, Popovich PG. Achieving CNS axon regeneration by manipulating convergent neuro-immune signaling. Cell Tissue Res. 2012;349:201–13.
69. Cafferty WB, Gardiner NJ, Gavazzi I, Powell J, McMahon SB, Heath JK, Munson J, Cohen J, Thompson SW. Leukemia inhibitory factor determines the growth status of injured adult sensory neurons. J Neurosci. 2001;21:7161–70.
70. Hyatt Sachs H, Rohrer H, Zigmond RE. The conditioning lesion effect on sympathetic neurite outgrowth is dependent on gp130 cytokines. Exp Neurol. 2010;223:516–22.

71. Liu H, Angert M, Nishihara T, Shubayev I, Dolkas J, Shubayev VI. Spinal glia division contributes to conditioning lesion-induced axon regeneration into the injured spinal cord: potential role of cyclic AMP-induced tissue inhibitor of metalloproteinase-1. J Neuropathol Exp Neurol. 2015;74:500–11.
72. Milward E, Kim KJ, Szklarczyk A, Nguyen T, Melli G, Nayak M, Deshpande D, Fitzsimmons C, Hoke A, Kerr D. Cleavage of myelin associated glycoprotein by matrix metalloproteinases. J Neuroimmunol. 2008;193:140–8.
73. Huang B, Zhao X, Zheng L-B, Zhang L, Ni B, Wang Y-W. Different expression of tissue inhibitor of metalloproteinase family members in rat dorsal root ganglia and their changes after peripheral nerve injury. Neuroscience. 2011;193:421–8.
74. Mantovani A, Sica A, Sozzani S, Allavena P, Vecchi A, Locati M. The chemokine system in diverse forms of macrophage activation and polarization. Trends Immunol. 2004;25:677–86.
75. Martinez FO, Gordon S. The M1 and M2 paradigm of macrophage activation: time for reassessment. F1000Prime Rep. 2014;6:13.
76. Gordon S, Martinez FO. Alternative activation of macrophages: mechanism and functions. Immunity. 2010;32:593–604.
77. Koltsova EK, Ley K. The mysterious ways of the chemokine CXCL5. Immunity. 2010;33:7–9.
78. Beyrau M, Bodkin JV, Nourshargh S. Neutrophil heterogeneity in health and disease: a revitalized avenue in inflammation and immunity. Open Biol. 2012;2:120134.
79. Morin N, Owolabi SA, Harty MW, Papa EF, Tracy TF Jr, Shaw SK, Kim M, Saab CY. Neutrophils invade lumbar dorsal root ganglia after chronic constriction injury of the sciatic nerve. J Neuroimmunol. 2007;184:164–71.
80. Sommer C, Kress M. Recent findings on how proinflammatory cytokines cause pain: peripheral mechanisms in inflammatory and neuropathic hyperalgesia. Neurosci Lett. 2004;361:184–7.
81. Perkins NM, Tracey DJ. Hyperalgesia due to nerve injury: role of neutrophils. Neuroscience. 2000;101:745–57.
82. Sommer C, Schafers M. Painful mononeuropathy in C57BL/Wld mice with delayed wallerian degeneration: differential effects of cytokine production and nerve regeneration on thermal and mechanical hypersensitivity. Brain Res. 1998;784:154–62.
83. Costigan M, Scholz J, Woolf CJ. Neuropathic pain: a maladaptive response of the nervous system to damage. Annu Rev Neurosci. 2009;32:1.
84. Li C-L, Li K-C, Wu D, Chen Y, Luo H, Zhao J-R, Wang S-S, Sun M-M, Lu Y-J, Zhong Y-Q. Somatosensory neuron types identified by high-coverage single-cell RNA-sequencing and functional heterogeneity. Cell Res. 2016;26:83.
85. Yin Y, Cui Q, Gilbert HY, Yang Y, Yang Z, Berlinicke C, Li Z, Zaverucha-do-Valle C, He H, Petkova V, et al. Oncomodulin links inflammation to optic nerve regeneration. Proc Natl Acad Sci U S A. 2009;106:19587–92.

14

Interactions between Sirt1 and MAPKs regulate astrocyte activation induced by brain injury in vitro and in vivo

Dan Li[1], Nan Liu[1], Hai-Hua Zhao[1], Xu Zhang[1], Hitoshi Kawano[2], Lu Liu[1], Liang Zhao[1] and Hong-Peng Li[1*]

Abstract

Background: Astrocyte activation is a hallmark of traumatic brain injury resulting in neurological dysfunction or death for an overproduction of inflammatory cytokines and glial scar formation. Both the silent mating type information (Sirt1) expression and mitogen-activated protein kinase (MAPK) signal pathway activation represent a promising therapeutic target for several models of neurodegenerative diseases. We investigated the potential effects of Sirt1 upregulation and MAPK pathway pharmacological inhibition on astrocyte activation in vitro and in vivo. Moreover, we attempted to confirm the underlying interactions between Sirt1 and MAPK pathways in astrocyte activation after brain injury.

Methods: The present study employs an interleukin-1β (IL-1β) stimulated primary cortical astrocyte model in vitro and a nigrostriatal pathway injury model in vivo to mimic the astrocyte activation induced by traumatic brain injury. The activation of GFAP, Sirt1, and MAPK pathways were detected by Western blot; astrocyte morphological hypertrophy was assessed using immunofluorescence staining; in order to explore the neuroprotective effect of regulation Sirt1 expression and MAPK pathway activation, the motor and neurological function tests were assessed after injury.

Results: GFAP level and morphological hypertrophy of astrocytes are elevated after injury in vitro or in vivo. Furthermore, the expressions of phosphorylated extracellular regulated protein kinases (p-ERK), phosphorylated c-Jun N-terminal kinase (p-JNK), and phosphorylated p38 activation (p-p38) are upregulated, but the Sirt1 expression is downregulated. Overexpression of Sirt1 significantly increases the p-ERK expression and reduces the p-JNK and p-p38 expressions. Inhibition of ERK, JNK, or p38 activation respectively with their inhibitors significantly elevated the Sirt1 expression and attenuated the astrocyte activation. Both the overproduction of Sirt1 and inhibition of ERK, JNK, or p38 activation can alleviate the astrocyte activation, thereby improving the neurobehavioral function according to the modified neurological severity scores (mNSS) and balance latency test.

Conclusions: Thus, Sirt1 plays a protective role against astrocyte activation, which may be associated with the regulation of the MAPK pathway activation induced by brain injury in vitro and in vivo.

Keywords: Brain injury, Sirt1, ERK pathway, JNK pathway, p38MAPK pathway, Astrocyte activation

* Correspondence: hpli@cmu.edu.cn
[1]Department of Human Anatomy, College of Basic Medical Sciences, China Medical University, Shenyang, China
Full list of author information is available at the end of the article

Background

Traumatic brain injury can be a serious insult caused by a wide variety of stimuli, enclosing a large range of severities [1]. These severities not only induce direct and immediate neuronal injury but also have the potential for long-term and gradually evolving sequelae, such as overactivation of glial cells and secretion of circulating leucocytes around the lesion site, contributing to the failure of functional recovery. Astrocytes tile the brain and localize to all cellular environments, which are the key players in response to injury [2, 3]. In an environment encompassing a wide range of neuroinflammatory factors such as IL-1β induced by central nervous system (CNS) injury, the astrocytes are transformed as "activated" [4]. The activated astrocytes produce multiple molecular and morphological features that have been considered as hallmarks of astrocyte activation in response to CNS injury by histopathologists and researchers [5–9]. The most prominent of these hallmarks are hypertrophy of astrocyte cellular processes and upregulation of the glial fibrillary acidic protein (GFAP), which is the main constituent of the intermediate filament system of adult astrocytes [10]. Several studies have shown that GFAP upregulation accompanied hypertrophy and migration of astrocytes after a traumatic brain injury [11, 12]. Our previous study also confirmed that the downregulation of GFAP expression could attenuate the astrocyte activation after brain injury [13], suggesting that its upregulation is crucial for astrocyte activation.

Sirtuins are mammalian homologs of the *Saccharomyces cerevisiae* silent mating type information 2 (Sirt2), which are members of the class III histone/lysine deacetylase family. The Sirts use NAD^+ as an obligatory co-substrate to remove an acetyl group from the epsilon amine of lysine [14, 15]. *Sirt1* is the first homologous gene of this family identified in mammals. Some recent studies have found that the pharmacological activation or upregulation of Sirt1 expression showed neuroprotective effects in several models of neurodegenerative diseases [15–18]. Notably, Sirt1 is widely expressed in the entire adult brain [19] and involved in the maintenance of brain integrity regulating activities such as oxidative stress and neuronal degeneration [20]. However, the underlying roles of Sirt1 in astrocyte activation after brain injury are yet ill-understood.

Our previous studies found that mitogen-activated protein kinase (MAPK) cascades were involved in the glial activation [13] and resveratrol protects against striatum neuronal apoptosis induced by a nigrostriatal pathway injury in mice via MAPK pathway [21]. Moreover, some studies showed that Sirt1 participates in learning and memory through MAPKs. Sirt1 inhibition reduced the Ras/ERK1/2 pathway associating with resistance to oxidative damage, suggesting that a correlation between Sirt1 and MAPK pathways to protect against the central nervous system (CNS) injury through yet unknown mechanisms [22–25].

Thus, we hypothesize that both the Sirt1 and MAPK pathways, such as ERK, JNK, and p38, were involved in regulating the astrocyte activation, and some networks through yet unknown mechanisms promote the recovery of neural function via attenuation of the astrocyte activation. To test this hypothesis, we applied a nigrostriatal pathway injury in the mouse brain to mimic the traumatic brain injury in vivo and IL-1β stimulation model to induce astrocyte activation in vitro. Based on these in vitro and in vivo models, we analyzed the expression of Sirt1 and p-ERK, p-JNK, and p-p38 after stimulation or injury and monitored GFAP expression and astrocytes hypertrophy, as well as the interactions between Sirt1 and MAPK (ERK, JNK, p38MAPK) pathways after manipulation of Sirt1 and p-ERK, p-JNK, and p-p38 levels pharmacologically and genetically.

Methods

Reagents

Human recombinant IL-1β (1×10^9 IU/mg protein) was purchased from R & D Systems (Jiangsu, China). The cytokine was prepared as the previous study [4]. Medium, fetal bovine serum and penicillin-streptomycin solution were from Gibco-BRL/Thermo Fisher (Co., Ltd., USA); resveratrol (3,4,5′-trihydroxy-trans-stilbene) and dimethyl sulfoxide (DMSO) were provided by Sigma-Aldrich Inc. (St. Louis, MO, USA). U0126, SP600125, and SB203580 from Selleck. cn (Shanghai, China) were dissolved in 0.1% DMSO, which was used as a solvent control. Primary antibodies including Sirt1 and mitogen-activated protein kinases (MAPKs) proteins such as p-ERK, JNK, and p38 MAPK were obtained from CST (Shanghai, China), t-ERK/JNK/p38 MAPK from Proteintech (Wuhan, China), GFAP from Millipore (MA, USA), and GAPDH from Abcam (Shanghai, China). The secondary antibody for Western blot was HRP-conjugated anti-rabbit lgG from Zhongshan Company (Shanghai, China). Please contact the author for more detailed data requests.

Primary culture of mouse cortical astrocytes

Primary astrocytes were prepared from 1-day-old neonatal Kunming mice as described previously with some modifications [26]. Briefly, brain cortical tissues were dissociated in DMEM supplemented with 10% fetal bovine serum, 100 U/ml penicillin, and 100 μg/ml streptomycin. Cells were incubated at 37 °C for 24 h in 95% air and 5% CO_2. The medium was changed after 5 days and every 3 days thereafter. The cell cultures were used 9 days after plating. For pure astrocyte culture, astrocytes were isolated from culture flasks of confluent glial cultures by shaking at 250 rpm for 24 h. Astrocytes in the supernatant were collected by centrifugation at

1000 rpm for 5 min. Purified astrocytes were seeded into 24-well plates at 1×10^5 cells/ml. The purity of astrocytes was greater than 95% as determined by immunostaining using the marker of astrocyte glial fibrillary acidic protein (GFAP). The astrocytes were stimulated with 1 ng/ml IL-1β for the tested time course [4]. Cultures were pretreated with 10 μM U0126 (blocks the ERK pathway), 10 μM SP600125 (blocks the JNK pathway), 10 μM SB203580 (blocks the p38MAPK pathway), or DMSO (as a vehicle) for 30 min in serum-free media before stimulated with IL-1β.

Animal preparation

All experimental procedures were conducted in conformity with institutional guidelines for the care and use of laboratory animals, and protocols were approved by the Institutional Animal Care and Use Committee (CMU IACUC) in China Medical University (Shenyang, China). Male KM mice (CL) 8-week-old (25–30 g) were purchased from the Animal Department, China Medical University (Shenyang, China), and kept under a constant environment (12/12-h light/dark cycle). They were allowed free access to water and food. All the animals were randomly assigned into the following group: (i) sham injury, (ii) brain injury+DMSO, and (iii) brain injury+resveratrol or MAPK (ERK/JNK/p38MAPK) inhibitors. The resveratrol/inhibitors or DMSO was injected intracerebroventricularly 30 min prior to brain injury, respectively, including 3 μg/μl resveratrol [27], 400 μM U0126 (ERK inhibitor), 100 μM SP600125 (JNK inhibitor), and SB203580 (p38 kinase inhibitor) following previous studies [25, 28–30].

Behavioral testing

All behavioral tests were performed blindly with respect to drug administration. The test was conducted prior to and at 1 and 21 days after injury. Animals were pretrained for 3 days for all the tests. Behavioral studies were repeated two times with three different trials to validate the behavioral data.

The modified neurological severity score (mNSS) is a composite test, including motor, sensory, and reflex tests [31]. A scale of the 0–18 score was graded on the neurological function wherein the normal score was 0 and a maximal deficit score was 18. One point was given for the inability to perform each test or for the absence of a reflex.

Beam walking test—the beam walking test assessed fine motor coordination and function by measuring the ability of the animals to traverse an elevated narrow beam as described previously [32]. The time for the mouse to cross the beam (not to exceed 60 s) was recorded. The measurements were recorded 1 day before the brain injury (as the baseline) and at each tested time point after brain injury for all the tests.

For all the tests, three measurements per trial were recorded 1 day before brain injury (baseline) and at each tested time point after brain injury.

The model of nigrostriatal pathway injury

The nigrostriatal pathway injury in mouse was used as the traumatic brain injury model. Briefly, the mice were fixed in a stereotaxic apparatus (TME Technology Co., Ltd., Chengdu, China) with the incisor bar set 3 mm below the intraaural line under 10% chloral hydrate (30 mg/kg body weight) anesthesia. The mice were sheared and sterilized at first. The middle skin was incised on the preshaved scalp, periosteum was cleared from the cranium, and a small oval hole was made with a dental drill wherein a 2.0-mm razor blade knife was inserted [33, 34]. A rectangular gap was drilled at 1.5 mm right back of the bregma, exposing the brain. A 2.0-mm width cutter was fixed in a linear type space frame, and the tip of the knife was inserted into the right side of the brain at 0.5 mm lateral to the midline, 1.5 mm posterior to the bregma, and at a depth of 6.0 mm from the surface of the brain. Then, the cutter was slowly pulled out with hemostatic suture. The skull was only exposed in the sham group. For all mice, constant temperature operating table was used in the whole process of brain injury and the room temperature was controlled approximately at 25 °C in an air-conditioned room after the brain injury.

Adenovirus construction

To evaluate the potential effect of Sirt1 on activation of astrocytes in vitro, the astrocytes were transfected with control or Sirt1 for 24 h and then stimulated with 1 ng/ml IL-1β. The Sirt1-recombined adenoviral expression vector and the control vector were constructed (Invitrogen, Carlsbad, CA, USA) and performed at a multiplicity of infection (MOI) of 20 [35, 36]. The lacZ vector (Invitrogen) was added to control groups.

Cells (1×10^6) grown to 60–80% confluence in 24 wells were transfected with adenoviral vectors using a Lipofectamine 2000 kit (Invitrogen, cat. 11668–019) according to the procedure provided by the manufacturer. The cells were observed under a fluorescence microscope and harvested 24 h after transfection.

Western blot

Fresh brain tissues from injured part, which the area up and down 1 mm from the center of the lesion site including the nigrostriatal pathway, were taken and placed in cool PBS. The cerebral localization states briefly a rectangular area (2 × 2 mm) is 0.5 mm the posterior, 2.0 mm lateral from the bregma, and 5.5–6.0 mm deep from the cortex [13]. Western blot analysis was performed as previously described [37]. Briefly, equal amounts of protein (35 mg protein in 20 ml for tissue samples) were separated by sodium dodecyl sulfate-polyacrylamide gel, transferred to PVDF membranes (Millipore, US), and blocked using 5% bovine serum albumin (BSA). The primary antibodies were rabbit polyclonal anti-Sirt1 (1:1000), p-ERK/JNK/p38MAPK (1:1000), t-ERK/JNK/p38MAPK (1:2000), and mouse monoclonal anti-GAPDH (1:5000). All the antibodies were diluted by 5% BSA. In the following day, a goat anti-rabbit or goat anti-mouse secondary antibody (1:5000) labeled by horseradish peroxidase was added and incubated for 90 min at 37 °C. Bio-Rad was used for ECL luminescence.

Immunohistochemistry

Immunohistochemical analyses were performed according to our previous study [13]. Briefly, primary antibodies of chick anti-GFAP were diluted to 1:500 in 20 mM phosphate-buffered salines (PBS) and incubated overnight. In the following day, the sections or the cells were washed by PBS and cy3 (Jackson ImmunoResearch Labs, Donkey anti-Chick, 1:100) was added and incubated for 1 h at 37 °C. After washing by PBS, the fluorescence quenching agent was used to cover the slices. Fluorescent microscope (HMS Nikon Imaging Center, ECLIPSE 80i, Japan) was used to observe and a CCD spot camera was employed to collect photos. The photos were saved as TIF and processed by Adobe Photoshop 7.0 (Adobe Photoshop CS2).

Quantification and statistics

In the quantitative statistics of Western blot, the detection of gray value in p-ERK/JNK/p-38 bands used computer-assisted imaging analysis system (Bio-Rad) by drawing a rectangle with the same size to detect gray value of p-ERK/JNK/p-38 proteins. Because the total ERK/JNK/p-38 level did not change after the nerve injury, the gray level ratio of p-ERK and t-ERK, p-JNK and t-JNK, p-p38 MAPK and p38 MAPK, and the ratios of Sirt1 and GFAP to GAPDH were used as the relative expression level of the target protein. All the experiments were repeated for at least three times. Data are presented as the mean and standard error of the mean (mean ± SEM). The comparison of different groups was analyzed by one-way ANOVA followed by the post hoc Bonferroni evaluation using GraphPad Prism5. Differences were termed statistically significant at $P < 0.05$.

Results

IL-1β-stimulated model and stab brain injury model could induce astrocyte activation

As shown in Fig. 1a, compared to the control astrocytes, the GFAP expression was significantly increased within 0.5 h of IL-1β stimulation, indicating IL-1β-induced astrocyte activation. Compared with the control, the GFAP-positive astrocytes begin to proliferate with phenotypic changes and cell hypertrophy and the characteristics of the latter depend on the increased expression of GFAP in 1- and 4-day groups after IL-1β stimulation (Fig. 1c). In vivo, the protein level of GFAP was significantly increased at 1 and 4 days after brain injury. Compared with the sham group, the astrocytes became thicker and cell hypertrophy was noticeable around the lesion site at 1 and 4 days after brain injury (Fig. 1d). These results indicated that brain injury could induce astrocyte activation around the lesion site.

IL-1β-stimulated model and stab brain injury model could reduce the expression of Sirt1 and induce the activation of MAPK pathways

The results showed that the treatment with IL-1β significantly reduced the expression of Sirt1 protein from 0.5 h to 4 days. Concurrently, the ERK, JNK, and p38MAPK pathways were activated from 0.5 h and continued until 4 days. In addition, we also found that the p-ERK, p-JNK, and p-p38 proteins were at a high level within 1 day (Fig. 2a).

Compared with the sham group, the expression of Sirt1 in the injured groups was significantly decreased from 0.5 h to 4 days after brain injury (Fig. 2; $P < 0.01$ for all the evaluated time points). ERK, JNK, and p38MAPK pathways were activated significantly from 0.5 h and lasted for 4 days after brain injury compared with sham groups ($P < 0.01$ for all the evaluated time points). These results revealed that Sirt1 and MAPK pathways including ERK, JNK, and p38MAPK were also involved in the mechanism of astrocyte activation induced by brain injury, which was consistent with the in vitro results.

Sirt1 overexpression by transfected Sirt1 or pharmacological agonist resveratrol decreased the astrocyte activation in vitro and in vivo

The results revealed that the primary astrocytes transfected with Sirt1 appeared to elevate the Sirt1 expression and decrease the GFAP expression significantly as compared to those transfected with control vector after 24 h (Fig. 3a). As shown in Fig. 3c. As compared to the transfection with control, the Sirt1-transfected astrocytes showed fewer signs of cell hypertrophy and were similar to the control group.

As shown in Fig. 3b, as compared to pretreating with DMSO, pretreatment with resveratrol significantly increased the expression of Sirt1 at 1 day and reduced the expression of GFAP at 4 day after brain injury. Immunofluorescence staining revealed that resveratrol could remarkably improve the signs of astrocyte hypertrophy around the lesion site (Fig. 3d). The results

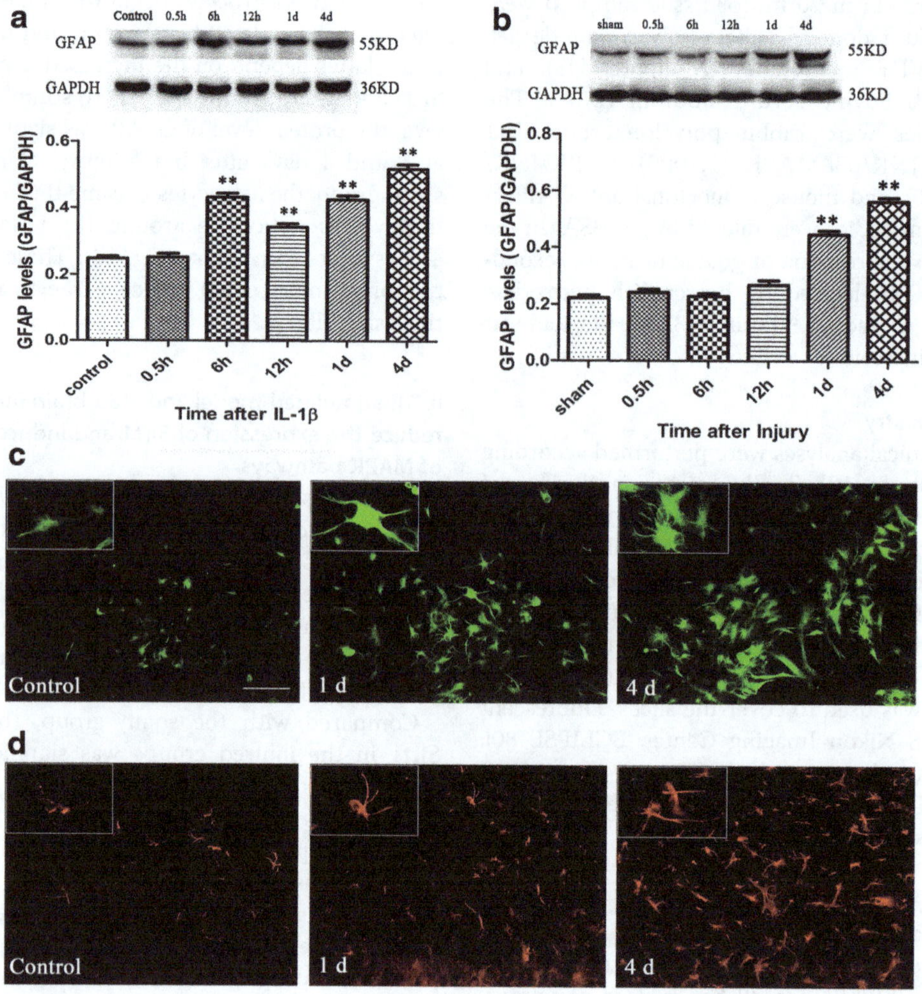

Fig. 1 Both the IL-1β stimulation and brain injury could induce the astrocyte activation. **a** Western blot showed that the GFAP expression after IL-1β stimulation, $^*P < 0.05$ and $^{**}P < 0.01$ vs. the control group, the control group: control without IL-1β stimulation. **b** The GFAP expression was showed after brain injury, $^*P < 0.05$ and $^{**}P < 0.01$ vs. the sham group. We also detected changes in astrocyte morphology by immunofluorescence staining in vitro; the GFAP-positive astrocytes were *green* (**c**) and in vivo and the GFAP-positive astrocytes were *red* (**d**) at 1 and 4 days, respectively. Scale bar = 50 μm

suggested that Sirt1 might function as a protective factor for astrocyte overactivation after brain injury in vivo.

Sirt1 overexpression upregulated ERK activation and downregulated JNK and p38MAPK activation induced by IL-1β-stimulation in vitro and brain injury in vivo

Compared with the transfection control, the results showed that transfected Sirt1 markedly upregulated the p-ERK expression and downregulated the p-JNK and p-p38MAPK expressions at 1 day after IL-1β stimulation in astrocytes (all $P < 0.05$; Fig. 4a). This suggested potential interactions between Sirt1 and MAPKs regulating the astrocyte activation induced by IL-1β stimulation.

The expressions of p-ERK, p-JNK, and p-p38 at 1 day after brain injury were shown in Fig. 4b. When the resveratrol-treated group significantly elevated the Sirt1 expression ($P < 0.01$; Fig. 3b), p-ERK expression was markedly increased and p-JNK/p-p38 MAPK expressions were reduced ($P < 0.05$ for p-ERK, $P < 0.01$ for p-JNK and p-p38MAPK; Fig. 4b), as compared to the treatment with DMSO in mice after brain injury. The results indicated that Sirt1 mediated the expression of ERK, JNK, and p-38MAPK pathways after mechanical brain injury in vivo.

The effects of inhibitors of MAPK pathways on ERK/JNK/p38 activation

As shown in Fig. 5a, when the ERK activation was inhibited by U0126, the JNK and p38 MAPK activation were not affected. Similarly, SP600125 or SB203580 could inhibit the JNK activation or p38MAPK activation, respectively, but did not affect the other two pathways.

The results showed that U0126 significantly inhibited the ERK activation but exerted no effect on the JNK or

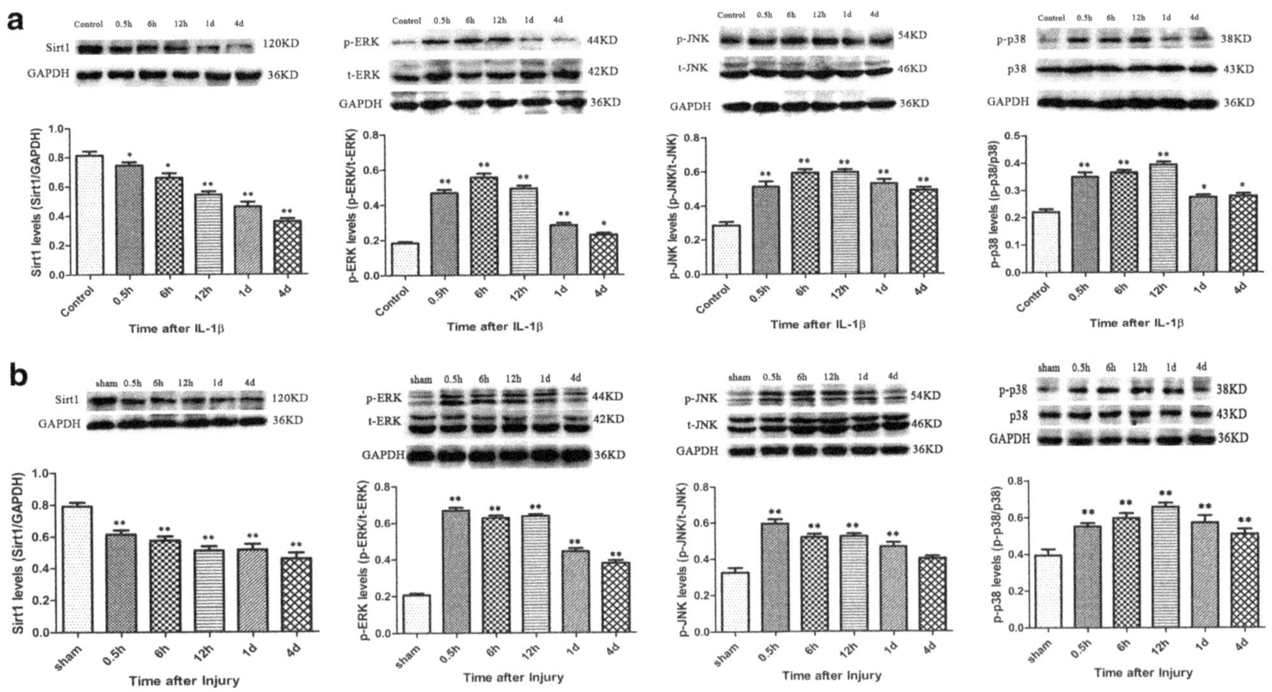

Fig. 2 The expression of Sirt1 and p-ERK/p-JNK/p-p38 after IL-1β stimulation and brain injury. The expression of Sirt1 is reduced and p-ERK, p-JNK, and p-p38 are elevated significantly for the time indicated in vitro (**a**) and in vivo (**b**). $n = 6$/group, *$P < 0.05$ and **$P < 0.01$ vs. the control or sham group

p38MAPK activation in comparison to the DMSO injection ($P < 0.05$ for ERK; $P > 0.05$ for JNK and p38MAPK; Fig. 5b). Similarly, P600125 significantly inhibited the JNK activation without affecting the ERK or p38MAPK activation as compared to the DMSO injection ($P < 0.05$ for JNK; $P > 0.05$ for ERK and p38MAPK; Fig. 5b). SB203580 significantly inhibited the p38MAPK activation but showed no effects on ERK or JNK activation as compared to DMSO injection ($P < 0.05$ for p38MAPK; $P > 0.05$ for ERK and JNK; Fig. 5b).

To further substantiate the in vitro finding, a stab wound brain injury was employed. When the ERK, JNK, or p38MAPK pathway was inhibited, the expression of Sirt1 was significantly elevated ($P < 0.05$ for all the inhibitors; Fig. 6b) and the GFAP level was attenuated as compared to DMSO ($P < 0.05$ for SB203580; $P < 0.01$ for U0126 and SP600125; Fig. 6b). We also detected a significant suppression of astrocyte hypertrophy and GFAP staining by immunofluorescence in vitro and in vivo (Fig. 6c, d).

Inhibiting ERK, JNK, or p38MAPK pathway activation elevated Sirt1 expression and attenuated astrocyte activation in vitro and in vivo

As shown in Fig. 6a, when the ERK, JNK, or p38MAPK pathway was inhibited at 1 day after IL-1β stimulation, the protein level of Sirt1 was significantly elevated in the primary astrocytes treated with the inhibitor as compared with the treatment with DMSO ($P < 0.05$ for U0126 and SB203580; $P < 0.01$ for SP600125). Moreover, Western blot demonstrated that the inhibition of ERK, JNK, or p38MAPK pathway significantly suppressed the GFAP protein level at 4 day after IL-1β stimulation in primary astrocytes ($P < 0.01$ for all; Fig. 6a). However, the DMSO control did not show any effect on GFAP protein level as compared to the primary astrocytes stimulated with IL-1β ($P > 0.05$, data not shown).

Elevating Sirt1 expression and inhibiting ERK, JNK, or p38MAPK pathway activation improved the neurobehavioral function after brain injury

As shown in Fig. 7a, the mean mNSS was significantly reduced in the resveratrol group (from 1 to 21 days all $P < 0.05$), U0126 group (from 4 to 21 days, $P < 0.05$), SP600125 group (from 7 to 21 days, $P < 0.05$), and SB203580 group (from 7 to 21 days, $P < 0.05$) as compared to the DMSO group. Moreover, the beam walk performances also showed significantly reduced latency to cross the beam from 4 to 21 days after injury (from 4 to 21 days, $P < 0.05$ for the resveratrol group; from 7 to 21 days, $P < 0.05$ for the U0126 group; from 7 to 21 days, $P < 0.05$ for the SP600125 group; from 7 to 21 days, $P < 0.05$ for the SB203580 group; Fig. 7b) as compared to the DMSO group.

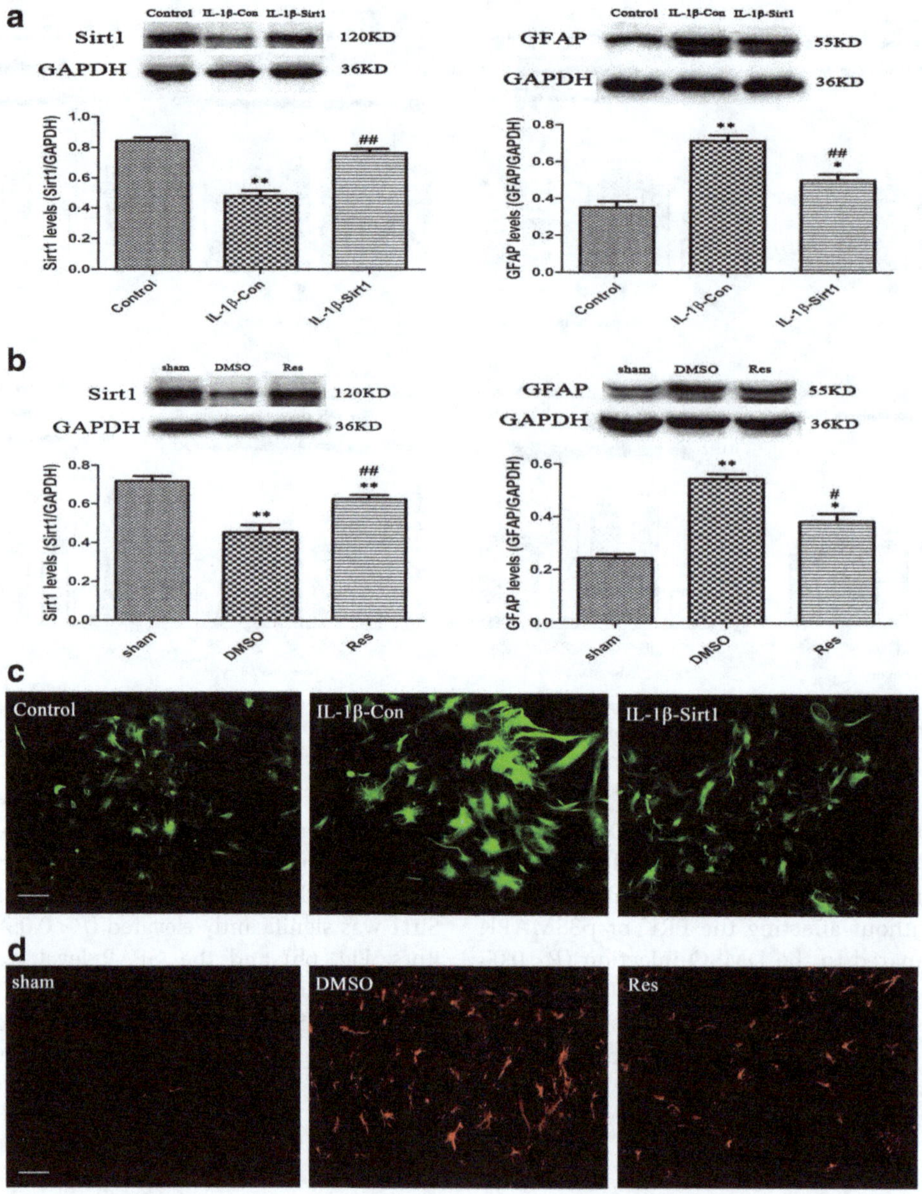

Fig. 3 Overexpression of Sirt1 attenuates astrocyte activation in vitro and in vivo. Overexpression of Sirt1 significantly reduced GFAP expression compared with transfection control in vitro (**a**), $n = 6$/group, $^{**}P < 0.01$ vs. the control group; $^{\#\#}P < 0.01$ vs. IL-1β-con; and in vivo (**b**), $^{*}P < 0.05$ and $^{**}P < 0.01$ vs. the sham group; $^{\#}P < 0.05$ and $^{\#\#}P < 0.01$ vs. the DMSO group. Immunofluorescence staining revealed that overexpression of Sirt1 improved the signs of astrocyte hypertrophy by immunodetection of GFAP in vitro (**c**, *green*) and in vivo (**d**, *red*)

Discussion

Astrocyte activation is presumed to depress neuronal regeneration after CNS injury due to the glial scar, a formation of a physical barrier, and overproduction of multiple proinflammatory cytokines, including IL-1β, IL-6, and TNFα, which further aggravate the glial activation and injure the remaining neurons through positive feedback [4, 31, 38, 39]. The recombinant IL-1β used in the present study was shown to be biologically active as previously demonstrated by its ability to induce astrocyte activation in an in vitro astrocyte activation model [4, 40–42]. Therefore, we speculate that our IL-1β stimulation model is suitable and credible for the detection of the astrocyte activation in vitro. Upregulation of GFAP and hypertrophy of astrocyte cellular processes play a major and prominent role in astrocyte activation and the formation of glial scar [6, 12]. In the present study, the IL-1β stimulation triggered an elevated level of GFAP and induced the astrocyte hypertrophy; this phenomenon was confirmed by the lesion site in a traumatic brain injury. The rational design of therapeutic interventions for CNS injury could be contingent critically

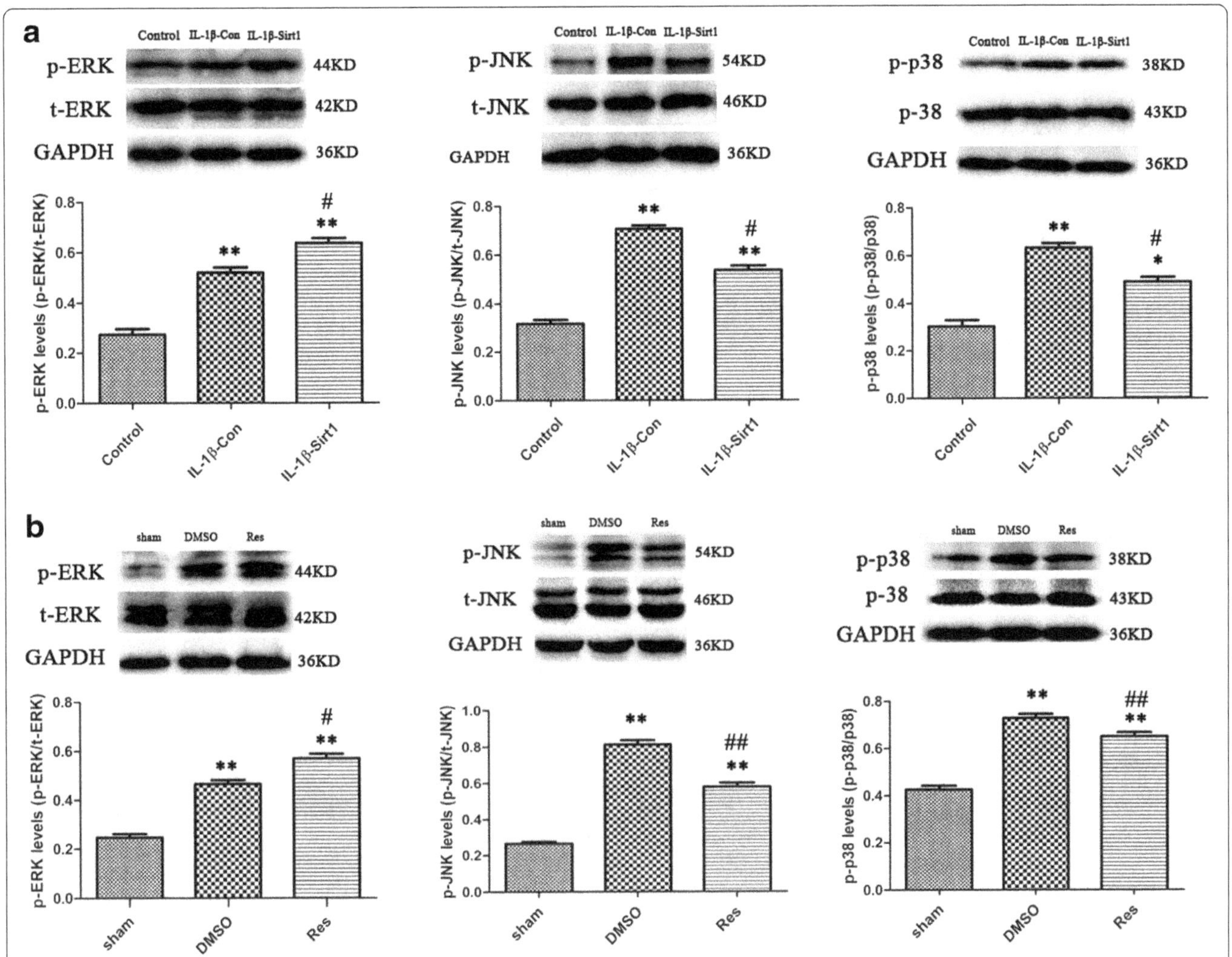

Fig. 4 The effects of Sirt1 overexpression on regulation of p-ERK/p-JNK/p-p38 in vitro and in vivo. **a** Overexpression of Sirt1 upregulates p-ERK and downregulates p-JNK and p-p38 compared to transfection control in vitro. $n = 6$/group, $^{**}P < 0.01$ vs. the control group; $^{\#}P < 0.05$ vs. IL-1β-con. **b** Elevated Sirt1 expression increased ERK activation and decreased JNK and p-38 activation in vivo. $n = 6$/group, $^{**}P < 0.01$ vs. the sham group; $^{\#}P < 0.05$ and $^{\#\#}P < 0.01$ vs. the DMSO group

upon a comprehensive understanding of the process of astrocyte activation, thereby necessitating an exploration of the mechanism of GFAP upregulation and astrocyte cellular hypertrophy after brain injury.

In recent years, Sirt1 has emerged as a strategy for the treatment of multiple neurodegenerative disorders [25, 43–46]. Although highly expressed in the brain, Sirt1 is also known to localize in the neurons and glial cells among various cell types [47–50]. In addition, investigators found that the expression of Sirt1 varies in different tissues or cell types' response to injury; some supported that the injury could induce Sirt1 activation and upregulate its expression [17, 25, 51], and others showed that Sirt1 expression was downregulated after the injury [52]. In the present study, we reported that the expression of Sirt1 was downregulated after brain injury in vivo; a similar result was obtained in primary astrocytes after stimulation with IL-1β in vitro. Moreover, the administration of resveratrol, a pharmacological Sirt1 agonist, attenuated astrocyte activation by decreasing the GFAP expression and improving the cell morphology in vivo. The overexpression of Sirt1 in primary astrocytes transfected with lentiviral vector Sirt1 in vitro also generated a similar result. The evidence suggests that Sirt1 expression was involved in the setting of astrocyte activation after injury in vivo or stimulation in vitro, which strongly supports the mechanism of the neuroprotective effect of Sirt1.

Previous study showed that overactivated astrocyte requires energy from mitochondrial biogenesis and the overenhanced mitochondrial respiration in astrocytes limits the substrate supply from astrocytes to neurons [53]. Recently, it was suggested that neurons can release and transfer damaged mitochondria to astrocytes for

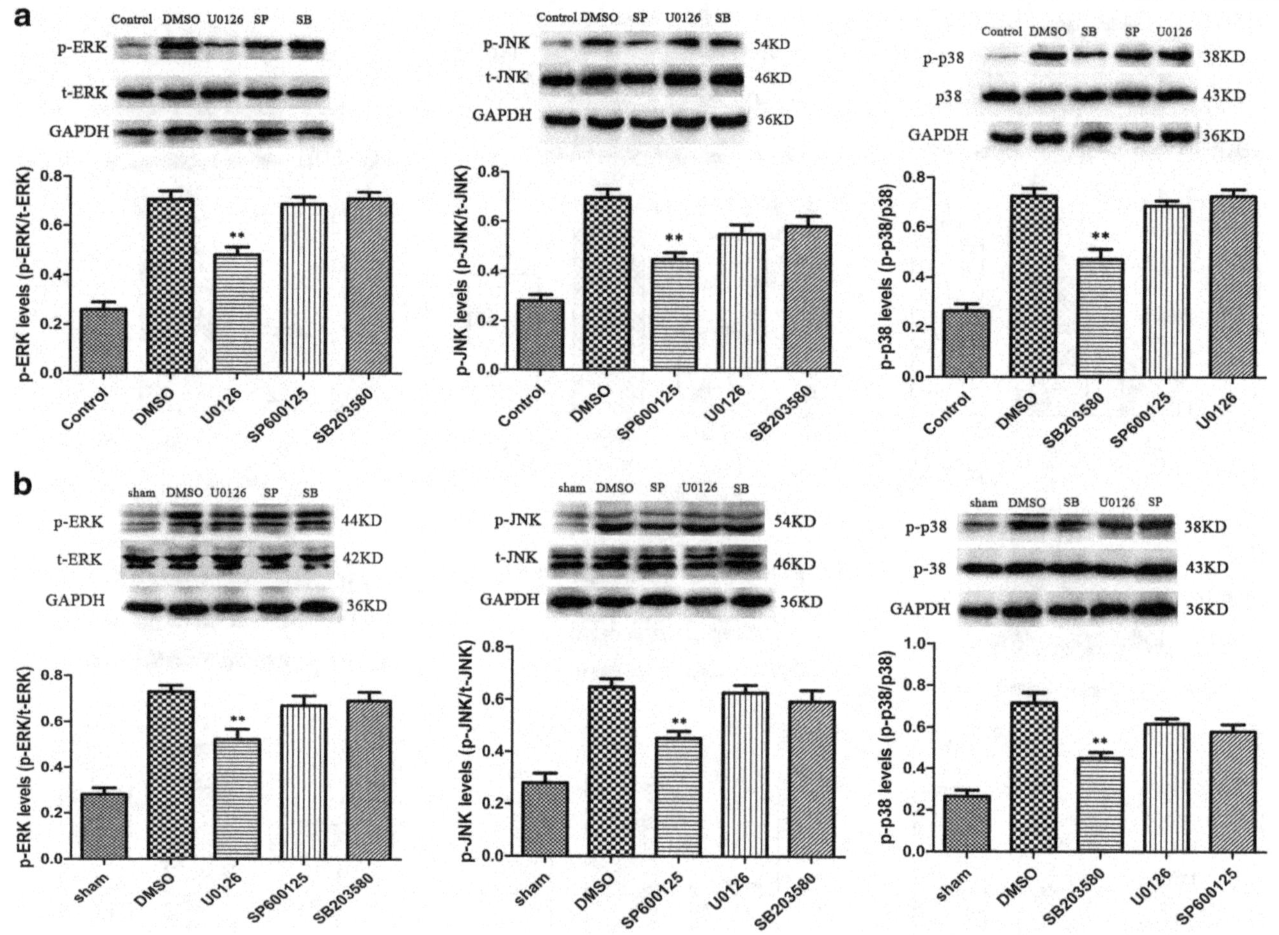

Fig. 5 The effects of inhibitors U0126, SP600125, and SB203580 on ERK, JNK, and p38 activation. **a** U0126, SP600125, and SB203580 (10 μM) significantly inhibited ERK, JNK, and p38MAPK activation respectively in vitro. $n = 6$/group, $^{**}P < 0.01$ vs. the DMSO group. **b** U0126 (200 μM), SP600125, and SB203580 (100 μM) significantly inhibited ERK, JNK, and p38MAPK activation respectively around the lesion site in vivo. $n = 6$/group, $^{**}P < 0.01$ vs. the DMSO group

disposal and recycling [54]. Mitochondrial function may be essential for these neuroglial protective mechanisms because damage of astrocytic mitochondria makes neurons vulnerable to cell death [55]. It may be surmised that increased mitochondrial function could support the functionality of astrocytes. As one of the major targeting organelles of Sirt1 (through PGC1α), mitochondrial function would be a highly possible candidate connection in neuroprotection of Sirt1. Resveratrol, one of the Sirt1 agonists, improves mitochondrial function and protects against metabolic disease by activating Sirt1 and PGC-1α [56]. In this study, we found that increased Sirt1 expression could attenuate the astrocyte activation and improve the neurobehavioral function after brain injury, the mechanism of which may be related to effects of Sirt1 on mitochondrial function in astrocytes. Further experiments are needed to verify this hypothesis.

After brain injury, MAPK family, including ERK, JNK, and p38MAPK, are highly expressed and inhibiting either of the cascades could alter the outcome of the brain injury [13, 57–61]. Though the ERK, JNK, and p38MAPK activation are proven to participate in a variety of injuries in vitro and in vivo, the roles of these three cascade activation in astrocyte stimulation in vivo and in vitro are yet controversial, which leads to the difficulties in exploring their effects on the mechanism of brain injury. Initially, our previous study has shown disparate roles of ERK stimulation in glial activation after brain injury in vivo [13]; however, some studies demonstrated that ERK activation also contributed to neuroprotection [62, 63]. Gao et al. (2013) identified that the inhibition of JNK, but not ERK and p38, suppressed GFAP upregulation in an astrocyte-scratched injury model in vitro, implying that JNK was involved in regulating astrocyte activation under physiological conditions. Several studies demonstrate that p38MAPK also mediates the expression of GFAP and various astrocyte-regulated molecules in vivo and in vitro [64–67]. In this study, we applied the inhibitors of

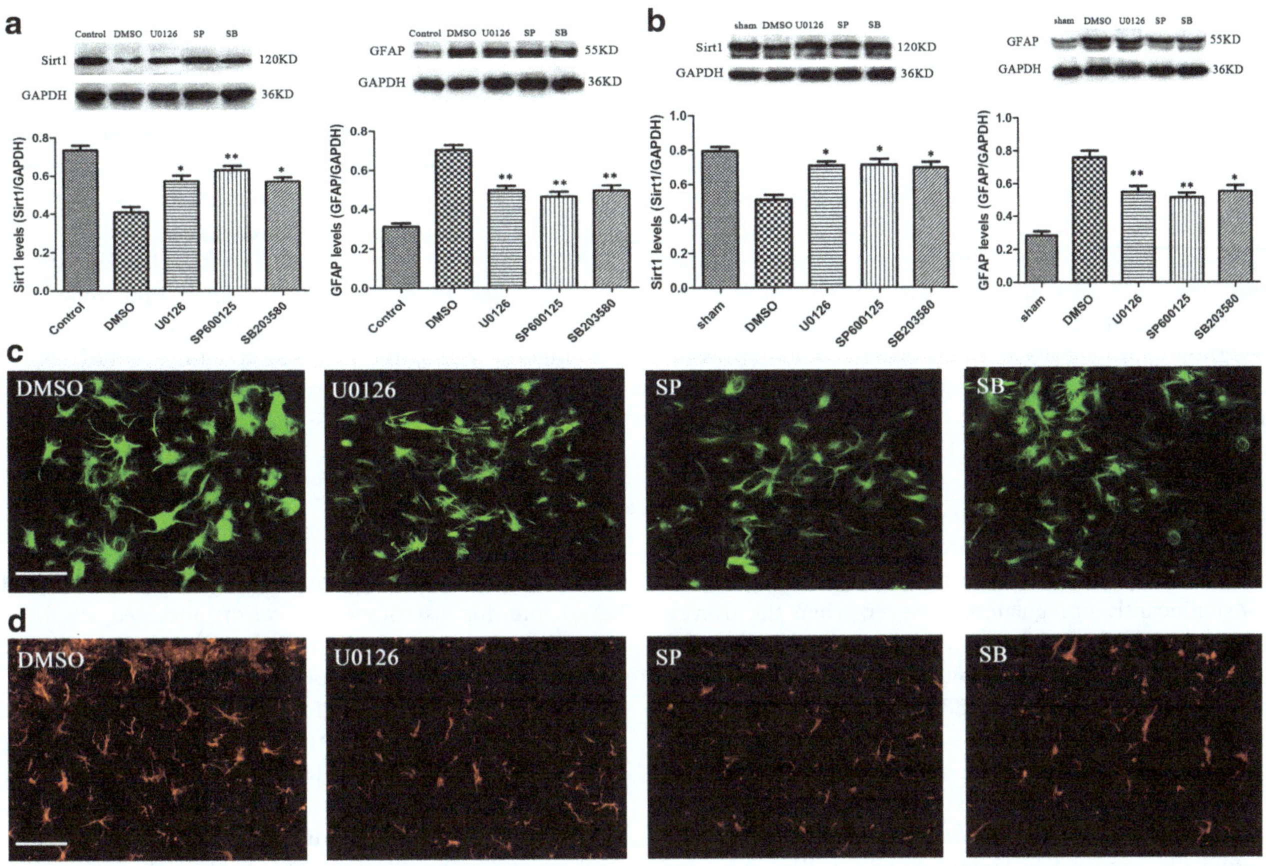

Fig. 6 Inhibiting MAPK pathway activation increases Sirt1 expression and alleviates astrocyte activation. **a** Levels of Sirt1 and GFAP protein in primary astrocytes after IL-1β stimulation in vitro. **b** Inhibiting MAPK pathway activation significantly increases Sirt1 expression but alleviates GFAP expression in vivo. $n = 6$/group, *$P < 0.05$ and **$P < 0.01$ vs. the DMSO group. Immunofluorescent image of GFAP in vitro and in vivo was showed in (**c**) and (**d**). Scale bar = 50 μm

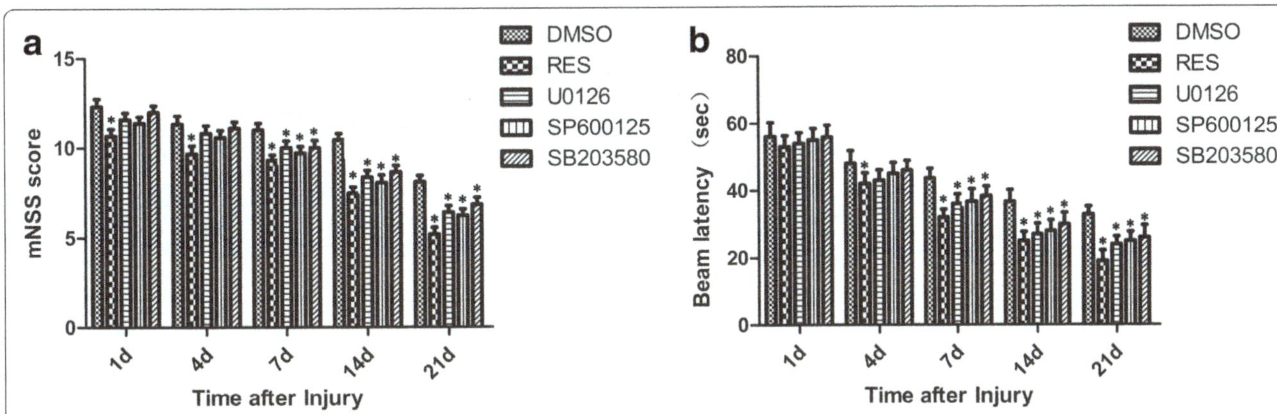

Fig. 7 The neuroprotection in mice pretreated with resveratrol to elevate Sirt1 expression or inhibitors to inhibit MAPK pathway activation. **a** The mNSS significantly reduced in mice with resveratrol and inhibitor groups. **b** Beam latency showed that resveratrol and inhibitor groups significantly decreased the time of mice to cross the beam compared to the DMSO group after brain injury. Values are showed as mean ± SEM. $n = 6$/group, *$P < 0.05$ vs. the DMSO group

ERK, JNK, and p38 to inhibit the expression of p-ERK, p-JNK, or p-p38, which could, in turn, suppress the GFAP upregulation and improve the cell hypertrophy.

Moreover, Zhao et al. (2012) showed that Sirt1 down-regulation induced by the pharmacological inhibitor salermide or RNA interference could attenuate the activation of ERK after brain injury. In addition, the inhibition of ERK activation could also decrease the Sirt1 expression, suggesting that there may be some interactions between Sirt1 and MAPK cascade activation.

In the present study, inhibition of ERK or JNK or p38 phosphorylation significantly upregulated the expression of Sirt1 and decreased the expression of GFAP in cultured cortical astrocytes and mice brain. The improved neurobehavioral function in ERK inhibitor, JNK inhibitor, or p38 inhibitor group indicated that these neuroprotective effects might be associated with alleviating the astrocyte activation. Interestingly, when the MAPK cascade activation was inhibited, the Sirt1 expression was significantly upregulated; however, when the overexpression of Sirt1 by pharmacological agonist (resveratrol) or Sirt1 interference was inhibited, the ERK activation was increased and the JNK and p38 activation were inhibited. These results further ravel some interactions between Sirt1 and MAPK activation after brain injury, although the precise mechanism remains to be further elucidated.

Herein, we have summarized the plausible dynamic relationship between Sirt1 and MAPK (ERK, JNK, and p38MAPK) pathways using a brain injury model in Fig. 8. The brain injury and IL-1β stimulation reduced Sirt1 and activated MAPK pathway leading to the astrocyte activation. The overexpression of Sirt1 by agonist or transfection-attenuated astrocyte activation regulated the MAPK pathway activation. The inhibition of MAPK pathway activation improved the astrocyte activation and elevated Sirt1 expression. Sirt1 interacted with MAPK activation via a synergic relationship to regulate astrocyte activation induced by brain injury in vivo or IL-1β stimulation in vitro, showing that both Sirt1 and MAPK pathways are potentially attractive therapeutic targets in the therapy of neurodegeneration induced by astrocyte activation. Thus, a new pharmacological product or endogenous method which could significantly elevate Sirt1 expression or activity might be a novel and efficient strategy for neuroprotection after brain injury.

Conclusions

In summary, this study found that Sirt1 is an important topic for astrocyte activation induced by IL-1β stimulation in vitro and traumatic brain injury in vivo; inhibition of ERK, JNK, or p38MAPK activation suppressed GFAP upregulation and improved the cell hypertrophy to attenuate the astrocyte activation; Sirt1 interacted with ERK pathway activation via a synergic way, but an antergic way with JNK and p38MAPK pathway activation to mediate the expression of GFAP and astrocyte morphology that is the astrocyte activation. Investigation of the regulation and levels of these and other signaling molecules may be a novel and effective strategy for neuroprotection after brain injury.

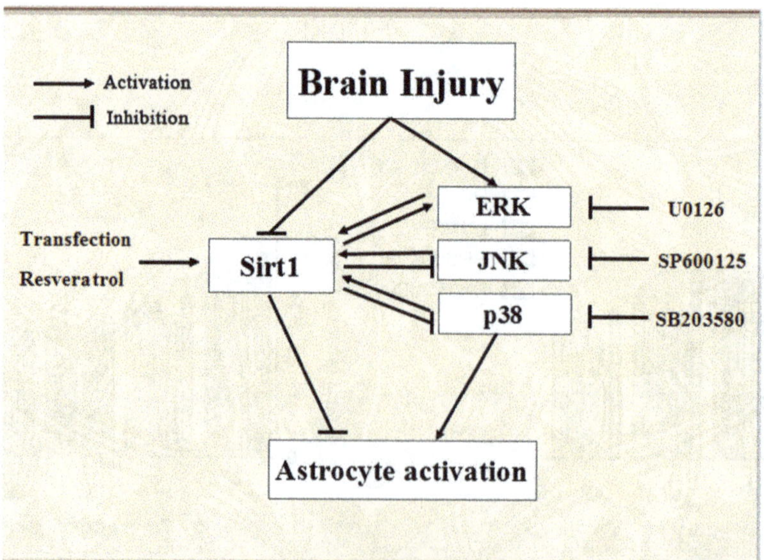

Fig. 8 The possible interactions between Sirt1 and ERK, JNK, or p38MAPK pathway in traumatic brain injury. The brain injury reduced endogenous Sirt1 level and activated ERK, JNK, and p38MAPK pathways. Overexpressed Sirt1 attenuated astrocyte activation and decreased ERK, JNK, and p38MAPK activation. Inhibition of ERK, JNK, or p38MAPK activation increased Sirt1 expression and attenuated astrocyte activation

Abbreviations

CNS: Central nervous system; GFAP: Glial fibrillary acidic protein; IL-1β: Interleukin-1β; MAPK: Mitogen-activated protein kinase; p-ERK: Phosphorylated extracellular regulated protein kinases; p-JNK: Phosphorylated c-Jun N-terminal kinase; p-p38: Phosphorylated p38 activation; Sirt1: Silent mating type information

Acknowledgements

This research was supported by the Hong-Peng Li's National Natural Science Foundation of China.

Funding

This research was supported by the National Natural Science Foundation of China (NSFC) (belongs to Hong-Peng Li), Grant No: NSFC-81171248.

Authors' contributions

DL, HK, H-HZ, XZ, and H-PL conceived and designed the experiments. DL, NL, LL H-HZ, XZ, and LZ performed the experiments. LT, NL, and HK analyzed the data. DL and H-PL wrote and revised the manuscript. All authors read and approved the final manuscript.

Competing interests

The authors declare that they have no competing interests.

Consent for publication

Not applicable.

Author details

[1]Department of Human Anatomy, College of Basic Medical Sciences, China Medical University, Shenyang, China. [2]Department of Health and Dietetics, Faculty of Health and Medical Science, Teikyo Heisei University, Tokyo 170-8445, Japan.

References

1. Graham DI, McIntosh TK, Maxwell WL, Nicoll JA. Recent advances in neurotrauma. J Neuropathol Exp Neurol. 2000;59:641–51.
2. Burda JE, Sofroniew MV. Reactive gliosis and the multicellular response to CNS damage and disease. Neuron. 2014;81:229–48.
3. Pekny M, Pekna M. Astrocyte reactivity and reactive astrogliosis: costs and benefits. Physiol Rev. 2014;94:1077–98.
4. Sticozzi C, Belmonte G, Meini A, Carbotti P, Grasso G, Palmi M. IL-1beta induces GFAP expression in vitro and in vivo and protects neurons from traumatic injury-associated apoptosis in rat brain striatum via NFkappaB/Ca(2)(+)-calmodulin/ERK mitogen-activated protein kinase signaling pathway. Neuroscience. 2013;252:367–83.
5. Eng LF, Ghirnikar RS. GFAP and astrogliosis. Brain Pathol. 1994;4:229–37.
6. Eng LF, Ghirnikar RS, Lee YL. Glial fibrillary acidic protein: GFAP-thirty-one years (1969–2000). Neurochem Res. 2000;25:1439–51.
7. Maragakis NJ, Rothstein JD. Mechanisms of disease: astrocytes in neurodegenerative disease. Nat Clin Pract Neurol. 2006;2:679–89.
8. Seifert G, Schilling K, Steinhauser C. Astrocyte dysfunction in neurological disorders: a molecular perspective. Nat Rev Neurosci. 2006;7:194–206.
9. Sofroniew MV, Vinters HV. Astrocytes: biology and pathology. Acta Neuropathol. 2010;119:7–35.
10. Pekny M, Pekna M. Astrocyte intermediate filaments in CNS pathologies and regeneration. J Pathol. 2004;204:428–37.
11. Ghirnikar RS, Yu AC, Eng LF. Astrogliosis in culture: III. Effect of recombinant retrovirus expressing antisense glial fibrillary acidic protein RNA. J Neurosci Res. 1994;38:376–85.
12. Yu AC, Lee YL, Eng LF. Astrogliosis in culture: I. The model and the effect of antisense oligonucleotides on glial fibrillary acidic protein synthesis. J Neurosci Res. 1993;34:295–303.
13. Li D, Tong L, Kawano H, Liu N, Yan HJ, Zhao L, Li HP. Regulation and role of ERK phosphorylation in glial cells following a nigrostriatal pathway injury. Brain Res. 2016;1648;90–100.
14. Donmez G. The neurobiology of sirtuins and their role in neurodegeneration. Trends Pharmacol Sci. 2012;33:494–501.
15. Houtkooper RH, Pirinen E, Auwerx J. Sirtuins as regulators of metabolism and healthspan. Nat Rev Mol Cell Biol. 2012;13:225–38.
16. Guo W, Qian L, Zhang J, Zhang W, Morrison A, Hayes P, Wilson S, Chen T, Zhao J. Sirt1 overexpression in neurons promotes neurite outgrowth and cell survival through inhibition of the mTOR signaling. J Neurosci Res. 2011; 89:1723–36.
17. Zhang F, Wang S, Gan L, Vosler PS, Gao Y, Zigmond MJ, Chen J. Protective effects and mechanisms of sirtuins in the nervous system. Prog Neurobiol. 2011;95:373–95.
18. Donmez G, Arun A, Chung CY, McLean PJ, Lindquist S, Guarente L. SIRT1 protects against alpha-synuclein aggregation by activating molecular chaperones. J Neurosci. 2012;32:124–32.
19. Sakamoto J, Miura T, Shimamoto K, Horio Y. Predominant expression of Sir2alpha, an NAD-dependent histone deacetylase, in the embryonic mouse heart and brain. FEBS Lett. 2004;556:281–6.
20. Chang HM, Wu UI, Lan CT. Melatonin preserves longevity protein (sirtuin 1) expression in the hippocampus of total sleep-deprived rats. J Pineal Res. 2009;47:211–20.
21. Li D, Liu N, Zhao L, Tong L, Kawano H, Yan HJ, Li HP. Protective effect of resveratrol against nigrostriatal pathway injury in striatum via JNK pathway. Brain Res. 2017;1654:1–8.
22. Becatti M, Taddei N, Cecchi C, Nassi N, Nassi PA, Fiorillo C. SIRT1 modulates MAPK pathways in ischemic-reperfused cardiomyocytes. Cell Mol Life Sci. 2012;69:2245–60.
23. Lemieux ME, Yang X, Jardine K, He X, Jacobsen KX, Staines WA, Harper ME, McBurney MW. The Sirt1 deacetylase modulates the insulin-like growth factor signaling pathway in mammals. Mech Ageing Dev. 2005;126:1097–105.
24. Li Y, Xu W, McBurney MW, Longo VD. SirT1 inhibition reduces IGF-I/IRS-2/Ras/ERK1/2 signaling and protects neurons. Cell Metab. 2008;8:38–48.
25. Zhao Y, Luo P, Guo Q, Li S, Zhang L, Zhao M, Xu H, Yang Y, Poon W, Fei Z. Interactions between SIRT1 and MAPK/ERK regulate neuronal apoptosis induced by traumatic brain injury in vitro and in vivo. Exp Neurol. 2012;237: 489–98.
26. Kong LY, McMillian MK, Maronpot R, Hong JS. Protein tyrosine kinase inhibitors suppress the production of nitric oxide in mixed glia, microglia-enriched or astrocyte-enriched cultures. Brain Res. 1996;729:102–9.
27. Falchi M, Bertelli A, Galazzo R, Vigano P, Dib B. Central antalgic activity of resveratrol. Arch Ital Biol. 2010;148:389–96.
28. Guan QH, Pei DS, Liu XM, Wang XT, Xu TL, Zhang GY. Neuroprotection against ischemic brain injury by SP600125 via suppressing the extrinsic and intrinsic pathways of apoptosis. Brain Res. 2006;1092:36–46.
29. Lennmyr F, Ericsson A, Gerwins P, Ahlstrom H, Terent A. Increased brain injury and vascular leakage after pretreatment with p38-inhibitor SB203580 in transient ischemia. Acta Neurol Scand. 2003;108:339–45.
30. Luo CL, Li QQ, Chen XP, Zhang XM, Li LL, Li BX, Zhao ZQ, Tao LY. Lipoxin A4 attenuates brain damage and downregulates the production of pro-inflammatory cytokines and phosphorylated mitogen-activated protein kinases in a mouse model of traumatic brain injury. Brain Res. 2013;1502:1–10.
31. Chen CC, Hung TH, Lee CY, Wang LF, Wu CH, Ke CH, Chen SF. Berberine protects against neuronal damage via suppression of glia-mediated inflammation in traumatic brain injury. PLoS One. 2014;9:e115694.
32. Chen CC, Hung TH, Wang YH, Lin CW, Wang PY, Lee CY, Chen SF. Wogonin improves histological and functional outcomes, and reduces activation of TLR4/NF-kappaB signaling after experimental traumatic brain injury. PLoS One. 2012;7:e30294.
33. Kawano H, Li HP, Sango K, Kawamura K, Raisman G. Inhibition of collagen synthesis overrides the age-related failure of regeneration of nigrostriatal dopaminergic axons. J Neurosci Res. 2005;80:191–202.
34. Yoshioka N, Hisanaga S, Kawano H. Suppression of fibrotic scar formation promotes axonal regeneration without disturbing blood-brain barrier repair

and withdrawal of leukocytes after traumatic brain injury. J Comp Neurol. 2010;518:3867–81.
35. Lee JH, Song MY, Song EK, Kim EK, Moon WS, Han MK, Park JW, Kwon KB, Park BH. Overexpression of SIRT1 protects pancreatic beta-cells against cytokine toxicity by suppressing the nuclear factor-kappaB signaling pathway. Diabetes. 2009;58:344–51.
36. Shen T, Yang C, Ding L, Zhu Y, Ruan Y, Cheng H, Qin W, Huang X, Zhang H, Man Y, et al. Tbx20 functions as an important regulator of estrogen-mediated cardiomyocyte protection during oxidative stress. Int J Cardiol. 2013;168:3704–14.
37. Chang CF, Chen SF, Lee TS, Lee HF, Chen SF, Shyue SK. Caveolin-1 deletion reduces early brain injury after experimental intracerebral hemorrhage. Am J Pathol. 2011;178:1749–61.
38. Pekny M, Nilsson M. Astrocyte activation and reactive gliosis. Glia. 2005;50: 427–34.
39. Sofroniew MV. Molecular dissection of reactive astrogliosis and glial scar formation. Trends Neurosci. 2009;32:638–47.
40. Pousset F, Cremona S, Dantzer R, Kelley K, Parnet P. Interleukin-4 and interleukin-10 regulate IL1-beta induced mouse primary astrocyte activation: a comparative study. Glia. 1999;26:12–21.
41. Pousset F, Cremona S, Dantzer R, Kelley KW, Parnet P. IL-10 and IL-4 regulate type-I and type-II IL-1 receptors expression on IL-1 beta-activated mouse primary astrocytes. J Neurochem. 2001;79:726–36.
42. Wu CY, Hsieh HL, Sun CC, Tseng CP, Yang CM. IL-1 beta induces proMMP-9 expression via c-Src-dependent PDGFR/PI3K/Akt/p300 cascade in rat brain astrocytes. J Neurochem. 2008;105:1499–512.
43. Martin A, Tegla CA, Cudrici CD, Kruszewski AM, Azimzadeh P, Boodhoo D, Mekala AP, Rus V, Rus H. Role of SIRT1 in autoimmune demyelination and neurodegeneration. Immunol Res. 2015;61:187–97.
44. Paraiso AF, Mendes KL, Santos SH. Brain activation of SIRT1: role in neuropathology. Mol Neurobiol. 2013;48:681–9.
45. Qu Y, Zhang J, Wu S, Li B, Liu S, Cheng J. SIRT1 promotes proliferation and inhibits apoptosis of human malignant glioma cell lines. Neurosci Lett. 2012; 525:168–72.
46. Tang BL, Chua CE. SIRT1 and neuronal diseases. Mol Aspects Med. 2008;29: 187–200.
47. Hisahara S, Chiba S, Matsumoto H, Tanno M, Yagi H, Shimohama S, Sato M, Horio Y. Histone deacetylase SIRT1 modulates neuronal differentiation by its nuclear translocation. Proc Natl Acad Sci U S A. 2008;105:15599–604.
48. Ramadori G, Lee CE, Bookout AL, Lee S, Williams KW, Anderson J, Elmquist JK, Coppari R. Brain SIRT1: anatomical distribution and regulation by energy availability. J Neurosci. 2008;28:9989–96.
49. Chen J, Zhou Y, Mueller-Steiner S, Chen LF, Kwon H, Yi S, Mucke L, Gan L. SIRT1 protects against microglia-dependent amyloid-beta toxicity through inhibiting NF-kappaB signaling. J Biol Chem. 2005;280:40364–74.
50. Cheng Y, Takeuchi H, Sonobe Y, Jin S, Wang Y, Horiuchi H, Parajuli B, Kawanokuchi J, Mizuno T, Suzumura A. Sirtuin 1 attenuates oxidative stress via upregulation of superoxide dismutase 2 and catalase in astrocytes. J Neuroimmunol. 2014;269:38–43.
51. Zhou XM, Zhang X, Zhang XS, Zhuang Z, Li W, Sun Q, Li T, Wang CX, Zhu L, Shi JX, Zhou ML. SIRT1 inhibition by sirtinol aggravates brain edema after experimental subarachnoid hemorrhage. J Neurosci Res. 2014;92:714–22.
52. Cheng Y, Di S, Fan C, Cai L, Gao C, Jiang P, Hu W, Ma Z, Jiang S, Dong Y, et al. SIRT1 activation by pterostilbene attenuates the skeletal muscle oxidative stress injury and mitochondrial dysfunction induced by ischemia reperfusion injury. Apoptosis. 2016;21:905–16.
53. Jiang T, Cadenas E. Astrocytic metabolic and inflammatory changes as a function of age. Aging Cell. 2014;13:1059–67.
54. Davis CH, Kim KY, Bushong EA, Mills EA, Boassa D, Shih T, Kinebuchi M, Phan S, Zhou Y, Bihlmeyer NA, et al. Transcellular degradation of axonal mitochondria. Proc Natl Acad Sci U S A. 2014;111:9633–8.
55. Voloboueva LA, Suh SW, Swanson RA, Giffard RG. Inhibition of mitochondrial function in astrocytes: implications for neuroprotection. J Neurochem. 2007; 102:1383–94.
56. Lagouge M, Argmann C, Gerhart-Hines Z, Meziane H, Lerin C, Daussin F, Messadeq N, Milne J, Lambert P, Elliott P, et al. Resveratrol improves mitochondrial function and protects against metabolic disease by activating SIRT1 and PGC-1alpha. Cell. 2006;127:1109–22.
57. Armstead WM, Kiessling JW, Riley J, Cines DB, Higazi AA. tPA contributes to impaired NMDA cerebrovasodilation after traumatic brain injury through activation of JNK MAPK. Neurol Res. 2011;33:726–33.
58. Armstead WM, Riley J, Cines DB, Higazi AA. Combination therapy with glucagon and a novel plasminogen activator inhibitor-1-derived peptide enhances protection against impaired cerebrovasodilation during hypotension after traumatic brain injury through inhibition of ERK and JNK MAPK. Neurol Res. 2012;34:530–7.
59. Wang LW, Tu YF, Huang CC, Ho CJ. JNK signaling is the shared pathway linking neuroinflammation, blood-brain barrier disruption, and oligodendroglial apoptosis in the white matter injury of the immature brain. J Neuroinflammation. 2012;9:175.
60. Wang Z-Q, Wu D-C, Huang F-P, Yang G-Y. Inhibition of MEK/ERK 1/2 pathway reduces pro-inflammatory cytokine interleukin-1 expression in focal cerebral ischemia. Brain Res. 2004;996:55–66.
61. Wei L, Zhang Y, Yang C, Wang Q, Zhuang Z, Sun Z. Neuroprotective effects of ebselen in traumatic brain injury model: involvement of nitric oxide and p38 mitogen-activated protein kinase signalling pathway. Clin Exp Pharmacol Physiol. 2014;41:134–8.
62. Chen T, Liu W, Chao X, Qu Y, Zhang L, Luo P, Xie K, Huo J, Fei Z. Neuroprotective effect of osthole against oxygen and glucose deprivation in rat cortical neurons: involvement of mitogen-activated protein kinase pathway. Neuroscience. 2011;183:203–11.
63. Guerra B, Diaz M, Alonso R, Marin R. Plasma membrane oestrogen receptor mediates neuroprotection against beta-amyloid toxicity through activation of Raf-1/MEK/ERK cascade in septal-derived cholinergic SN56 cells. J Neurochem. 2004;91:99–109.
64. Bellaver B, Souza DG, Bobermin LD, Souza DO, Goncalves CA, Quincozes-Santos A. Resveratrol protects hippocampal astrocytes against LPS-induced neurotoxicity through HO-1, p38 and ERK pathways. Neurochem Res. 2015; 40:1600–8.
65. Huang W, Lv B, Zeng H, Shi D, Liu Y, Chen F, Li F, Liu X, Zhu R, Yu L, Jiang X. Paracrine factors secreted by MSCs promote astrocyte survival associated with GFAP downregulation after ischemic stroke via p38 MAPK and JNK. J Cell Physiol. 2015;230:2461–75.
66. Nemoto W, Ogata Y, Nakagawasai O, Yaoita F, Tadano T, Tan-No K. Involvement of p38 MAPK activation mediated through AT1 receptors on spinal astrocytes and neurons in angiotensin II- and III-induced nociceptive behavior in mice. Neuropharmacology. 2015;99:221–31.
67. Zhu W, Li J, Liu Y, Xie K, Wang L, Fang J. Mesencephalic astrocyte-derived neurotrophic factor attenuates inflammatory responses in lipopolysaccharide-induced neural stem cells by regulating NF-kappaB and phosphorylation of p38-MAPKs pathways. Immunopharmacol Immunotoxicol. 2016;38:205–13.

15

TSG-6 attenuates inflammation-induced brain injury via modulation of microglial polarization in SAH rats through the SOCS3/STAT3 pathway

Ran Li, Wenchao Liu, Jian Yin, Yunchang Chen, Shenquan Guo, Haiyan Fan, Xifeng Li, Xin Zhang, Xuying He and Chuanzhi Duan*

Abstract

Background: An acute and drastic inflammatory response characterized by the production of inflammatory mediators is followed by stroke, including SAH. Overactivation of microglia parallels an excessive inflammatory response and worsened brain damage. Previous studies indicate that TSG-6 has potent immunomodulatory and anti-inflammatory properties. This study aimed to evaluate the effects of TSG-6 in modulating immune reaction and microglial phenotype shift after experimental SAH.

Methods: The SAH model was established by endovascular puncture method for Sprague–Dawley rats (weighing 280–320 g). Recombinant human protein and specific siRNAs for TSG-6 were exploited in vivo. Brain injury was assessed by neurologic scores, brain water content, and Fluoro-Jade C (FJC) staining. Microglia phenotypic status was evaluated and determined by Western immunoblotting, quantitative real-time polymerase chain reaction (qPCR) analyses, flow cytometry, and immunofluorescence labeling.

Results: SAH induced significant inflammation, and M1-dominated microglia polarization increased expression of TSG-6 and neurological dysfunction in rats. rh-TSG-6 significantly ameliorated brain injury, decreased proinflammatory mediators, and skewed microglia towards a more anti-inflammatory property 24-h after SAH. While knockdown of TSG-6 further induced detrimental effects of microglia accompanied with more neurological deficits, the anti-inflammation effects of rh-TSG-6 were associated with microglia phenotypic shift by regulating the level of SOCS3/STAT3 axis.

Conclusions: TSG-6 exerted neuroprotection against SAH-induced EBI in rats, mediated in part by skewing the balance of microglial response towards a protective phenotype, thereby preventing excessive tissue damage and improving functional outcomes. Our findings revealed the role of TSG-6 in modulating microglial response partially involved in the SOCS3/STAT3 pathway and TSG-6 may be a promising therapeutic target for the treatment of brain injury following SAH.

Keywords: Subarachnoid hemorrhage, Early brain injury, Microglial polarization, TSG-6, Anti-inflammation

* Correspondence: doctor_duanzj@163.com
Department of Neurosurgery, Zhujiang Hospital, The National Key Clinical Specialty, The Neurosurgery Institute of Guangdong Province, Guangdong Provincial Key Laboratory on Brain Function Repair and Regeneration, Southern Medical University, Guangzhou 510282, China

Background

Subarachnoid hemorrhage (SAH) constitutes 5 to 10% of all strokes worldwide [1]. Healthy people can harbor intracranial aneurysms noted in occasional examination or emerging with several symptoms, otherwise detected with SAH onset [2, 3]. Once intracranial aneurysm ruptures, SAH is usually catastrophic because there exists no effective therapy applied in concomitant brain injury [4]. Currently, early brain injury (EBI) and delayed cerebral ischemia (DCI) represent the main effects of SAH at two stages, and neuroprotection and anti-vasospasm are the most studied targets in numerous research [5, 6]. Though many putative agents demonstrate exciting therapeutic effects, little has been translated into clinical application, and many have failed clinical trials [7]. Only nimodipine has been widely used in clinical application and has proven effective in the treatment of SAH [8].

SAH can induce several external stress events, including rapid ascension of intracranial pressure, sharp reduction in cerebral perfusion pressure, brain edema, and heme burden from red blood cell lysis, all of which converged to result in cellular pathophysiological changes [9]. Several studies have indicated that inflammation is invariably associated with brain damage after SAH [10–12]. As shown in clinical data, a sign of early inflammation in aSAH patients is correlated with poor neurological outcome on admission [13]. Microglia may sense even small imbalances of environmental homeostasis and are rapidly activated in a mode of dynamic morphology and polarization [14]. Afterwards, activated microglia appear to be the predominant source for a plethora of inflammatory mediators in the central nervous system (CNS) [15]. The progression of a dysfunctional and highly reactive microglial activation results in releasing high levels of pro-inflammatory and cytotoxic mediators that contribute to neuronal dysfunction and cell death [16]. The secreted cytokines together with environmental toxins and endogenous proteins, combined with neuronal death, further provoke unregulated activation of microglia resulting in the production of toxic factors that can propagate inflammation-induced neuronal death [17]. Therefore, alternative strategies based on a clearer comprehension of microglia-mediated inflammation are pressingly warranted. Accordingly, microglia, the prominent responder during neuroinflammmtion, has been identified as the target in the present study.

Microglia polarization in different phenotypes exerting distinct responses is a central feature of disease progression involved inflammation [18]. Activated microglia are assumed to polarize into two extreme states: classical (M1, proinflammatory) and alternative (M2, anti-inflammatory) activation. Microglia dynamically transfer between M1 and M2 phenotypes after activation. Meanwhile, each phenotype can be identified by typical biomarkers. M1 phenotypic cells are characterized by the expression of CD86, CD68, iNOS, etc. Likewise, M2 phenotypic cells are associated with the expression of CD163, CD206, arginase-1(Arg-1), etc. In addition, M1 microglia are associated with a proinflammatory cellular state that has elevated expression of inflammatory cytokines, including IL-1β, TNF-α, and IL-6, which enhance brain damage. In contrast, M2 microglia release anti-inflammatory mediators, including IL-4, IL-10, and TGF-β, leading to beneficial neuroprotection [19, 20]. Though this M1/M2 paradigm is an oversimplified schema that simply divides the activated microglia populations into M1 and M2 phenotypes, it remains the most commonly used model to understand the role of microglia.

The phenomena of polarization of microglia has been carefully confirmed in several CNS diseases model. Fine-tuned microglia M1/M2 polarization has obtained positive therapeutic efficacy in experimental spinal cord injury (SCI), intracerebral hemorrhage (ICH), and ischemic brain injury models by suppressing the deleterious effects of inflammation, while boosting neuroprotective potential [21–23]. Largely, cues in the microenvironment and intertwined intracellular signals may determine how they polarize into M1 phenotype to exacerbate tissue injury or M2 phenotype to promote tissue recovery [24].

Recently, TSG-6 has emerged as a protective regulator against inflammation in cornea injury, peritonitis, autoimmune diabetes, asthma, and other inflammation-associated diseases. TSG-6 is a multifunctional glycoprotein composed of a hyaluronan-binding link domain and a CUB module in a contiguous fashion [25]. Normally, TSG-6 is upregulated in several pathological contexts especially related to inflammation. Collectively, the therapeutic effects of TSG-6 can be explained by participating in HA crosslinking and/or catalyzing the transfer of IαI heavy chains to HA [26]. It is, therefore, likely that TSG-6 acts as an endogenous inhibitor comprising part of a negative feedback loop in inflammation progression. Different from peripheral tissue, microglia play a major immune-response function instead of macrophages in the brain. However, the role of TSG-6 within CNS remains unclear. Our laboratory recently discovered that TSG-6 may preserve blood-brain barrier (BBB) by attenuating nitrative stress in an ICH model and improve outcomes in animal models of TBI by reducing the activation of microglia/macrophages [27, 28]. These results indicate that TSG-6 can play protective roles in CNS. However, whether TSG-6 impacts microglia polarization remains to be reported.

Herein, we aimed to address the possibility of TSG-6 in the regulation of microglia-mediated inflammation and the effects of TSG-6 on microglial polarization after

SAH injury, as well as its potential mechanism in a rat endovascular puncture model of SAH.

Methods

Animals

Sprague–Dawley male rats (280-320 g) were obtained from the Animal Experiment Center of Southern Medical University. All experimental procedures and animal care were approved by the Southern Medical University Ethics Committee and were in accordance with the guidelines of the National Institute of Health. All rats resided in a light and temperature-controlled environment with ad libitum access to food and water and adapted to the environment 1 week before the experiments.

Experimental design and animal groups

Time course and cell distribution

In this experiment, 84 male rats were divided into six groups at random (sham and, SAH 6, 12, 24, 48, 72 h after SAH). The mRNA and protein expression level and time course of TSG-6 were measured by qPCR and Western blot. Expression distribution was detected by FISH-ISH and double immunostaining to determine TSG-6 expression in different cell types of the brain in the sham group and 24 h after the SAH group. In additional study, qPCR and western blot were also employed to detect whether there was a statistical difference in TSG-6 gene and protein levels among the sham groups at 6 h, 12 h, 24 h, 48 h, and 72 h.

Outcomes of treatment

To assess the role of TSG-6 on early brain injury after SAH, 102 rats were randomly divided into the sham group, SAH group, SAH + vehicle group, SAH + rh-TSG-6 (1 μg), SAH + rh-TSG-6 (5 μg), SAH + scrambled siRNA group, and SAH + TSG-6 siRNA group. All the rats were sacrificed 24 h after SAH according to the results of the first experiment. siRNA transfection efficiencies of each sample were verified using western blot analysis. Neurological scores, brain water content, and fluoro-Jade C (FJC) analysis were conducted.

Correlation between TSG-6 and microglia polarization

To examine the effect of TSG-6 on microglia polarization, 60 rats were randomly assigned into the following groups: sham, SAH, SAH + vehicle, SAH + rh-TSG-6 (5 μg), SAH + scrambled siRNA group, and SAH + TSG-6 siRNA groups. Animals were sacrificed for brain tissue 24 h after SAH onsets. The samples were collected for qPCR, Flow cytometric analysis, ELISA, and immunofluorescence analysis. To clarify, we used samples partly from the first two for immunofluorescence (IF), qPCR, and WB experiments instead of having a separate cohort of SAH rats.

Therapeutic mechanism of action

To explore the potential mechanism of TSG-6 on modulating microglia polarization, 36 rats were randomly assigned into the following groups: sham, SAH, SAH + vehicle, SAH + rh-TSG-6 (5 μg), SAH + scrambled siRNA, and SAH + TSG-6 siRNA groups. Immunofluorescence and western blotting was performed 24 h after SAH induction.

Experimental SAH model

The SAH model was performed by endovascular puncturing for the induction of SAH as previously described [29]. Briefly, rats were deeply anesthetized by 1% pentobarbital sodium (40 mg/ kg, i.p.). A sharpened 4–0 nylon suture was inserted rostrally into the left internal carotid artery and perforated the bifurcation of the anterior and middle cerebral arteries until resistance was felt. Next, the suture was immediately withdrawn to allow blood reperfusion in the internal carotid artery, induced to SAH. Sham animals underwent the same procedures without vessel perforation.

SAH grade

After euthanasia and removal of the brain, the basal brain was photographed immediately and divided into six segments as previously described [30]. Based on the amount of blood clotting, each area was blindly assigned a score from 0 to 3. All area scores were summed as the total SAH grade (maximum SAH grade = 18). Experimental rats with mild SAH whose SAH grades ≤7 were excluded from the study.

Neurological score

The neurological scores were evaluated 24 h after SAH using the previously described modified Garcia scoring system [30]. Briefly, the evaluation included six tests scored from 0 to 3 or 1 to 3 and included the following: spontaneous activity, symmetry in the movement of four limbs, forelimbs outstretching, climbing ability, body proprioception, and the response to vibrissae stimulation. Possible scores ranged from 3 to 18. All the tests were evaluated by an observer who was blind to the treatment conditions. Higher scores represented better neurological function.

Brain water content analysis

Brains were removed at 24 h after SAH and were divided into four parts: left hemisphere, right hemisphere, cerebellum, and brainstem. Left and right hemispheres were weighed immediately to obtain the wet weight and were then oven dried at 105 °C for 24 h to obtain the dry weight. The percentage of water content was calculated as follows: [(wet weight − dry weight)/wet weight] × 100%.

Intracerebroventricular injection administration

In vivo transfection was performed as described previously [31]. TSG-6 siRNA (Santa Cruz Biotechnology, USA) and control scramble SiRNA (Santa Cruz Biotechnology, USA) transfection was performed with in vivo siRNA transfection reagent (Engreen Biosystem, Beijing, China) according to manufacturer protocols. TSG-6-siRNA was dissolved in RNase-free H_2O at concentrations of 1 μg/1 μl; an equivalent concentration of scrambled-sequence siRNA was transfected into the negative control. Next, 5 μL TSG-6 siRNA or control siRNA was diluted with 5 μL in vivo transfection reagent. Finally, the mixture was injected intracerebroventricularly using a 10 μl Hamilton microsyringe (Microliter No. 701; Hamilton Company, Switzerland) under the guidance of a stereotaxic instrument (Stoelting Company, USA) under anesthesia. The SAH model was established 48 h later. rh-TSG-6 was dissolved in sterile PBS to a final concentration of 1 μg/10 μL or 5 μg/10 μL. Then, 1 μg or 5 μg rh-TSG-6 was infused into the cerebroventricle using a Hamilton syringe with the guidance of a stereotaxic instrument 1.5 h after SAH induction. The dosage of rh-TSG-6 was determined based on a previous study. The vehicle group were administered the same volume of sterile PBS or RNase-free H_2O.

Quantitative real-time polymerase chain reaction

Quantitative real-time polymerase chain reaction (qPCR) was performed and analyzed as previously described [27]. Total RNA from brain tissues with blood clots was extracted using TRIzol (Invitrogen, USA). Total RNA was reverse-transcribed to cDNA using the PrimeScript™ RT reagent Kit with gDNA Eraser (Takara, China). Rt-PCR reactions were performed on the Illumina-Eco Real-Time PCR Detection System (Gene Company Limited, USA) using the SYBR Premix Ex TaqII kit (Takara, China). The running procedure was 30 s at 95 °C, 40 cycles of 5 s at 95 °C, and 30 s at 60 °C, following a melt curve. Gene expression was quantified with standard samples and normalized with β-actin. Data were expressed as normalized messenger RNA (mRNA) expression (fold mRNA increase). The real-time PCR primer sequences are listed in Table 1.

Western blotting

The cerebral cortex tissues with blood clots were collected at corresponding time-points after SAH. Western blot (WB) was performed as described previously [27]. The following primary antibodies were used for WB: mouse anti-TSG-6 (Santa Cruz Biotechnology; 1:800), rabbit anti-STAT3 (Cell Signaling Technology; 1:2000), rabbit anti-phosphorylated STAT3 at Tyr705 (Cell Signaling Technology; 1:1000), rabbit anti-SOCS3 (Abcam; 1:1000), mouse anti-CD163 (AbD Serotec; 1:500), rabbit anti-CD86 (ProteinTech; 1:600), rabbit anti-IL-6 (PeproTech; 1:800), rabbit anti-IL-10 (ProteinTech; 1:600), and rabbit anti-β-actin (Cell Signaling Technology; 1:1000). The blot bands were quantitated by ImageJ software (National Institutes of Health, USA). Quantitative data were expressed as the target protein OD/β-actin OD ratio.

Table 1 Real-time PCR primers used in this study

Primer name	Primer sequence	
TSG-6	Forward	CGTCTTGCAACCTACAAGCAGCTA
	Reverse	ACAGTTGGGCCCAGGTTTCA
CD86	Forward	GATTGCAGGTCCCAGTTCACTTC
	Reverse	CCACTGTCCTGCTTGGACTCAC
CD68	Forward	GGATTCAAACAGGACCGACAT
	Reverse	GGACACATTGTATTCCACTGCC
iNOS	Forward	TCCTCAGGCTTGGGTCTTGTTAG
	Reverse	TTCAGGTCACCTTGGTAGGATTTG
Arg-1	Forward	GCTGTGGTAGCAGAGACCCAGA
	Reverse	CATCCACCCAAATGACGCATAG
CD163	Forward	CTTTGGAATGGGCAAGAACAGAA
	Reverse	TGAGTGACAGCAGAGACGCTGA
CD206	Forward	TGGAGTGGCAGGTGGTTTATG
	Reverse	GGTTCAGGAGTTGTTGTGGGC
IL-1β	Forward	AATGCCTCGTGCTGTCTGA
	Reverse	GGATTTTGTCGTTGCTTGTCTC
IL-6	Forward	ATTGTATGAACAGCGATGATGCAC
	Reverse	CCAGGTAGAAACGGAACTCCAGA
TNF-α	Forward	TTCCAATGGGCTTTCGGAAC
	Reverse	AGACATCTTCAGCAGCCTTGTGAG
IL-4	Forward	TGCACCGAGATGTTTGTACCAGA
	Reverse	TTGCGAAGCACCCTGGAAG
IL-10	Forward	CAGACCCACATGCTCCGAGA
	Reverse	CAAGGCTTGGCAACCCAAGTA
TGF-β	Forward	CATTGCTGTCCCGTGCAGA
	Reverse	AGGTAACGCCAGGAATTGTTGCTA
β-actin	Forward	GGAGATTACTGCCCTGGCTCCTA
	Reverse	GACTCATCGTACTCCTGCTTGCTG

Fluorescent in situ hybridization (FISH)

Paraffin-embedded brain slices were sectioned at 4 μm. Fluorescence in situ hybridization was performed using custom TSG-6-specific FISH Probes (Bersinbio, Inc., Guangzhou, China). Following manufacturer instructions, brain slices were hybridized with a TSG-6 mRNA FISH Probe and labeled with Alexa Fluor Cy3 (Life Technologies, Inc., USA). Immunohistochemistry was then performed using rabbit anti-Iba-1(Abcam; 1:500), rabbit anti-NEUN (Abcam; 1:400), and rabbit anti-GFAP (Abcam; 1:400). Alexa Fluor 488-conjugated IgG (1:200, Invitrogen; 1:200) was applied as a secondary antibody. Photos were taken with confocal microscopes (LSM800, Carl Zeiss, Germany) following manufacturer instructions.

Immunofluorescence assay

Immunofluorescence staining was performed as previously described but with some modifications [27]. Briefly, brain sections were fixed in 4% paraformaldehyde for about 24 h. Coronal paraffin-embedded 4 μm thickness slices were conducted to Antigen retrieval and underwent blocking by 5% BSA for 1 h. After blocking, slices were incubated overnight at 4 °C with the following primary antibodies: mouse anti-NeuN (1:100, Millipore), rabbit anti-NeuN (1:400, Abcam), mouse anti-GFAP (1:300, R&D), rabbit anti-GFAP (1:400, Abcam), goat anti-Iba1 (1:300, Abcam), mouse polyclonal anti-TSG-6 (1:100, Santa Cruz Biotechnology), rabbit anti-CD163 (1:300, Abcam), rabbit anti-CD86(1:200, R&D), rabbit anti-pSTAT3 (1:400, Cell Signaling Technology), and rabbit anti-SOCS3 (1:500, Abcam). After washing with PBS, slices were then incubated with appropriate secondary antibodies for 1 h at room temperature. Following washing three times with PBS, the slices were re-stained by DAPI for 12 min before mounting. Then, images were obtained with a Leica DMi8 fluorescence microscope (Leica, Germany).

Fluoro-Jade C (FJC) staining

FJC staining was used to investigate neurodegeneration. Sections were subjected to FJC staining in accordance with the manufacturer instructions. Briefly, the sections were immersed in a solution of 1% sodium hydroxide in 80% alcohol for 5 min, 70% alcohol for 2 min, distilled water for 2 min, and followed by 0.06% potassium permanganate for 10 min with gently shaking. The sections were immersed in a solution of 0.0002% FJC (Millipore Corporation, USA) in 0.1% acetic acid for 30 min. The sections were then rinsed three times in distilled water and allowed to dry at 50 °C for 15 min before covering with DPX medium (Sigma, USA). FJC-positive cell counting was performed as previously described but with modifications. Six sections located inside in the injured region were analyzed and FJC-positive cells were counted in each image. Data were presented by the average number of FJC-positive neurons in the fields as cells/mm^2.

Microglia isolation

Microglia of left cerebral cortex tissues with blood clots were isolated using a Percoll density gradient as described previously [32]. Briefly, brain samples obtained from each group after perfusion with 200 ml sterile saline were dissociated with 800 U DNase I (sigma, USA) and 7 ml Cell Dissociation Reagent (StemPro™ Accutase™, Gibco, USA) at 37 °C for 30 min in an incubator. After filtration with 70-μm cell strainers (BD Falcon, USA) to generate a single cell suspension, immune cells were separated by centrifugation using 40% Percoll in PBS at 1700 rpm for 30 min.

Flow cytometry analysis

For flow cytometry analysis of microglial polarization status in the injured brain, the isolated microglia were stained with fluorescently labeled antibodies: CD11b-FITC (BD Biosciences), CD45-PE-Cy5 (BD Biosciences), CD163-APC (AbD Serotec), and CD86-PE (BD Biosciences) at 4 °C for 30 min. Flow cytometry was performed on a FACS VERSE apparatus (BD Bioscience) and obtained data were analyzed by Flow Jo software 7.6.1(Tree Star, USA).

Inflammatory cytokine measurements

Total protein concentrations were measured using a BCA Protein Assay Kit (Genecopoeia, USA). Frozen brain samples were mechanically homogenized and centrifuged at 12,000 rpm for 15 min at 4 °C. The levels of interleukin-6 (IL-6), interleukin-10 (IL-10), tumor necrosis factor alpha (TNF-α), and interleukin-1β(IL-1β) were measured using specific ELISA kits (eBIOSCIENCE, USA) according to manufacturer instructions. The concentration of the cytokines was determined by color intensity measured by spectrometry in a micro ELISA reader (Varioskan Lux, Thermo Scientific). The results are expressed as picogram per milligram for tissue samples.

Statistical analysis

All statistical analyses were performed using GraphPad Prism 6 (GraphPad software). Data are represented as a mean ± SD. Differences between two groups were analyzed with Student's t test (two-tailed), and data were analyzed by one-way analysis of variance (ANOVA) with post hoc Tukey test or Dunnett's test applied to assess multiple comparisons. Non-parametric data were analyzed using the Kruskal–Wallis H analysis followed by a Mann-Whitney U test. Statistical significance was set at a P value of < 0.05.

Results

No significant differences on TSG-6 mRNA expression and protein abundance were found in different time-points in sham

We found that there was no statistical difference of TSG-6 detected variables among sham groups at each time (Additional file 1A, B). Therefore, animals in sham group at 24 h after sham operation were chosen for further experiments.

Both mRNA and protein level of TSG-6 were upregulated after SAH injury

We first confirmed that brain TSG-6 increased in our SAH model. PCR and Western blot were performed to detect the time course of both mRNA and protein level of TSG-6 after SAH. The temporal profile of TSG-6 mRNA expression is shown in Fig. 1c. TSG-6 mRNA levels elevated immediately at 6 h after SAH ($p = 0.0127$) reached its peak value at 12 h, which almost six times that of the sham group. Afterwards, mRNA levels of TSG-6 gradually declined but were still significantly increased at 24 h, 48 h, and 72 h ($P = 0.0022$, $P = 0.0001$, $P = 0.0016$, respectively).

As shown in Fig. 1a, b, Western blotting revealed that the level of TSG-6 protein in the left temporal cortex increased over time. The level of TSG-6 protein abundance was weak in the sham group, while it increased significantly at 12 h ($P = 0.0015$), peaked at 24 h ($P = 0.0008$), and remained ascended at 72 h ($P = 0.0011$) post-SAH.

The endogenous TSG-6 was mainly expressed in microglia after SAH injury

We used FISH-ISH and double-labeling immunofluorescence to identify the cell distribution of TSG-6 at the peak activation of TSG-6 (at 12 h according to the PCR and 24 h according to the WB). FISH-ISH analysis showed that TSG-6 mRNA was expressed in microglia (Fig. 2a) at 12 h after SAH. Double staining confirmed that a low TSG-6 protein abundance in the microglia was observed in the sham group. Compared with the sham group, SAH augmented the relative TSG-6 protein abundance predominantly in microglia (Fig. 2c), but not neurons (Fig. 2d) or astrocytes (Fig. 2e). The co-expression of TSG-6 and Iba-1 was obviously more after SAH (Fig. 2f).

rh-TSG-6 alleviates SAH-induced brain injury (reduced brain water content and improved neurobehavioral outcomes) at 24 h after SAH

At 24 h after SAH, brain edema and neurobehavioral activity were examined in all groups. Two dosages of rh-TSG-6 (1 μg/10 μL and 5 μg/10 μL) were administrated intracerebroventricularly at 1.5 h after SAH. At 24 h, SAH insults induced poorer brain water content and neurological impairment compared to the sham group. No significant differences between SAH and SAH + vehicle groups in brain edema and neurological scores were observed. Both the two dosages of rh-TSG-6 dramatically ameliorated brain edema (Fig. 3a, b). However, only administration of high dosage rh-TSG-6 significantly improved neurobehavioral deficits (Fig. 3c) at 24 h post-ictus ($P = 0.0022$) vs. SAH + vehicle, $n = 6$. These results indicated that a high dosage is effective for reducing EBI; thus, a high dosage was selected for further studies.

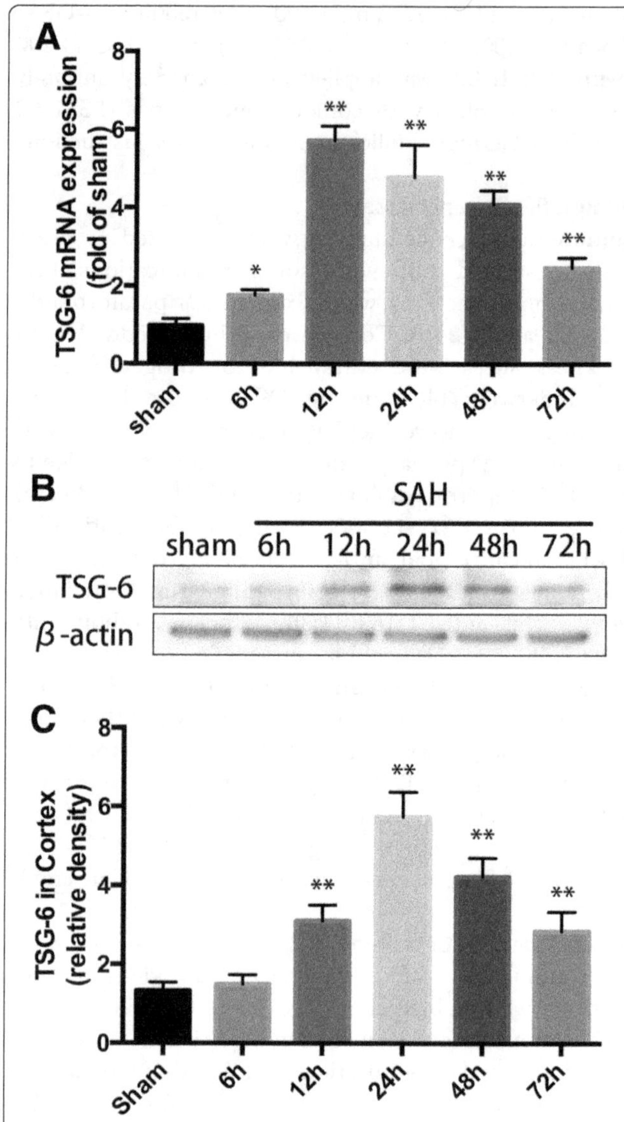

Fig. 1 Endogenous expression of TSG-6 in brain tissue after subarachnoid hemorrhage (SAH). **a** Quantification of TSG-6 mRNA level in rat temporal cortex. **b** Western blot analysis showed the level of TSG-6 protein abundance at 6, 12, 24, 48, and 72 h after SAH. **c** Quantification of the TSG-6 protein level as shown in **b**. All values are presented as means ± SD, $n = 6$ in each time point per group. *$p < 0.05$, **$p < 0.01$ versus sham group

rh-TSG-6 treatment attenuated SAH-induced brain cell injury

Neural loss is a key event in EBI after SAH. As shown in Fig. 4a, the procedure of SAH induced a large amount of neurodegeneration as revealed by FJC staining. Furthermore, there was no significant difference between the SAH and SAH + vehicle groups. When compared with the vehicle group at 24 h after SAH, the number of FJC^+

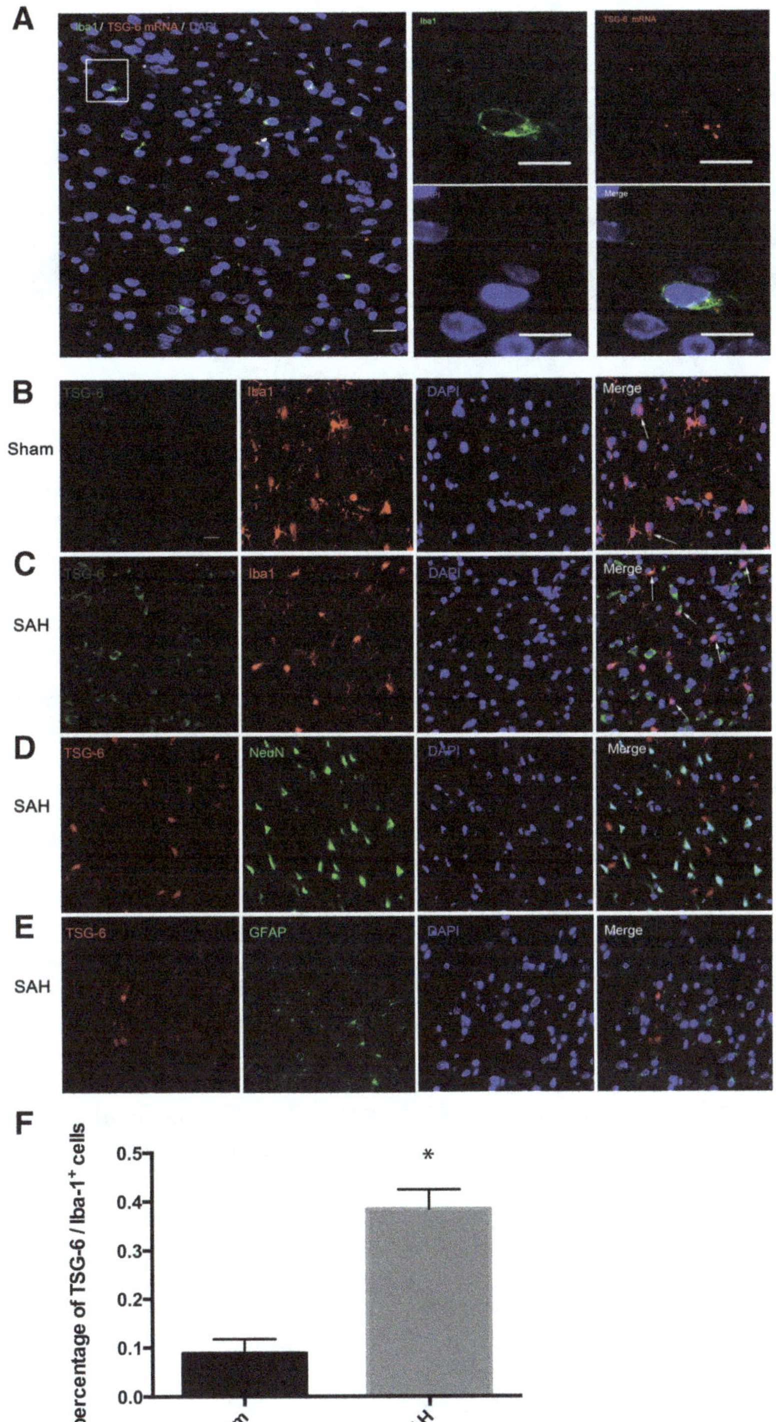

Fig. 2 Spatial distributions of endogenous TSG-6 after SAH. **a** After injury, TSG-6 mRNA expression was clearly seen in microglia (Iba1$^+$ cells). **b** Representative immunofluorescence staining slices of TSG-6 with calcium-binding adaptor molecule 1 (Iba1) in sham animals. **c** More Iba1-positive cells were observed after SAH when compared with sham group. Negative colocalization of TSG-6 with neurons (NeuN) (**d**) and astrocytes(GFAP) (**e**) at 24 h following SAH. Arrows point to TSG-6-positive microglia. $n = 6$ in each group. $^*p < 0.05$ versus sham group. Scale bars = 20 μm. Bars in higher magnification panels are 10 μm

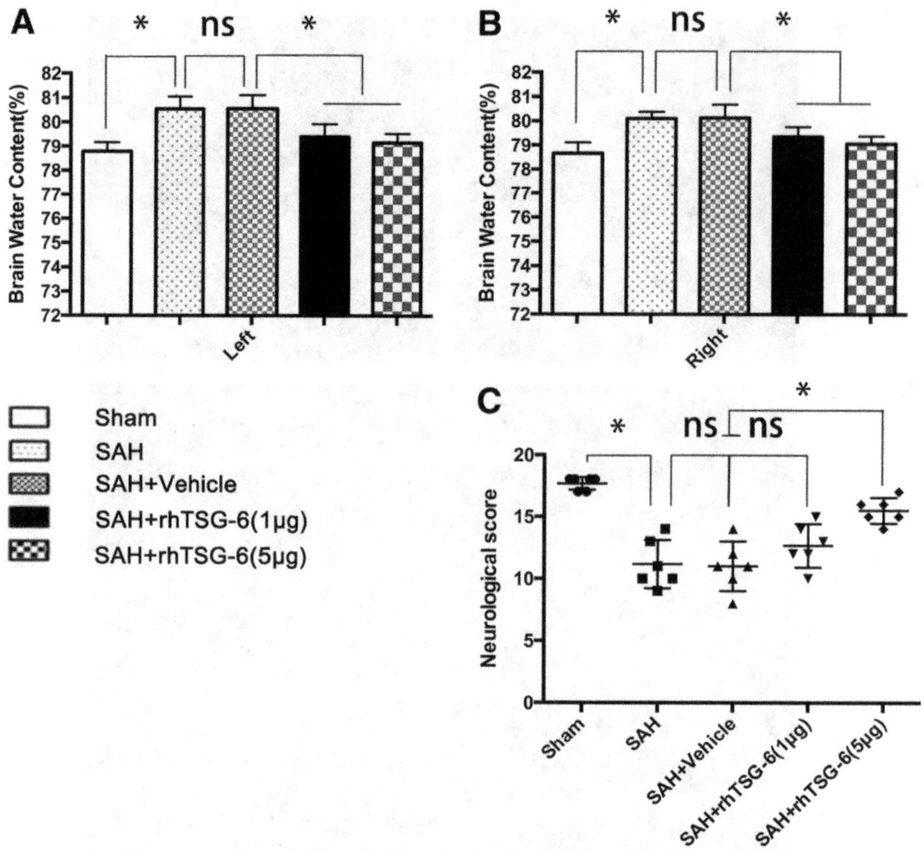

Fig. 3 Effects of rh-TSG-6 treatment on brain edema (**a**, **b**) and neurobehavioral deficits (**c**) at 24 h after SAH. Brain water content using a wet/dry weight method was measured at 24 h after SAH. Neurological scores were recorded at 24 h after SAH. High dosage of rh-TSG-6 effectively reduced brain edema (**a**, **b**) and improved neurological functions (**c**) at 24 h following SAH. Values are expressed as the mean ± SD, $n = 6$ in each group. *$P < 0.05$

cells was significantly decreased in the injured cortical region in rh-TSG-6-treated SAH rats ($P = 0.0022$) (Fig. 4a, b). Furthermore, the rh-TSG-6 group had a lower number of Fluoro-Jade C-stained neurons than the SAH-vehicle group at 72 h after SAH ($P = 0.0002$, Additional file 2A).

Knockdown of endogenous TSG-6 aggravated neural death and neurologic deficits after SAH

To further explore the role of TSG-6 in the pathogenesis of EBI, knockdown of endogenous TSG-6 was performed. TSG-6 siRNA was injected into the cerebroventricle at 48 h before SAH induction. Interfering efficiency of TSG-6 siRNA was verified using qPCR and WB experiments. Neurologic score evaluation was also performed 24 h after SAH. As shown in Fig. 5a–c, scramble siRNA had no effect on endogenous TSG-6 mRNA and protein expression compared to the SAH group, but knockdown of endogenous TSG-6 with siRNA decreased the mRNA and protein level of TSG-6 in the brain ($p = 0.0001$ and $p = 0.0004$, respectively; $n = 6$; $n = 6$). Furthermore, knockdown of endogenous TSG-6 significantly aggravated neurologic deficits 24 h after SAH (Fig. 5d).

SAH-induced activation of microglia and microglial M1 phenotype polarization was dominated during the SAH early phase

Activation of microglia is a hallmark of neuroinflammation. In this study, we investigated the characteristics of microglial activation in the early stages following SAH induction. We first detect whether microglia were markedly activated after SAH. Microscopic examination of whole brain sections stained for Iba1 confirmed that SAH-induced microglia were dramatically activated for whole brain sections compared to the sham group (Additional file 3). Next, we detected mRNA levels of markers of M1/M2 microglial cells and M1/M2-associated cytokines at corresponding times post-SAH. The data showed M1-associated markers CD68, CD86, and iNOS increased immediately and peaked at 24 h (iNOS) and 48 h (CD68, CD86) and remained at high levels for 72 h. M2-associated markers increased slowly and peaked at 48 h (CD206) and 72 h (Arg-1, CD206) and

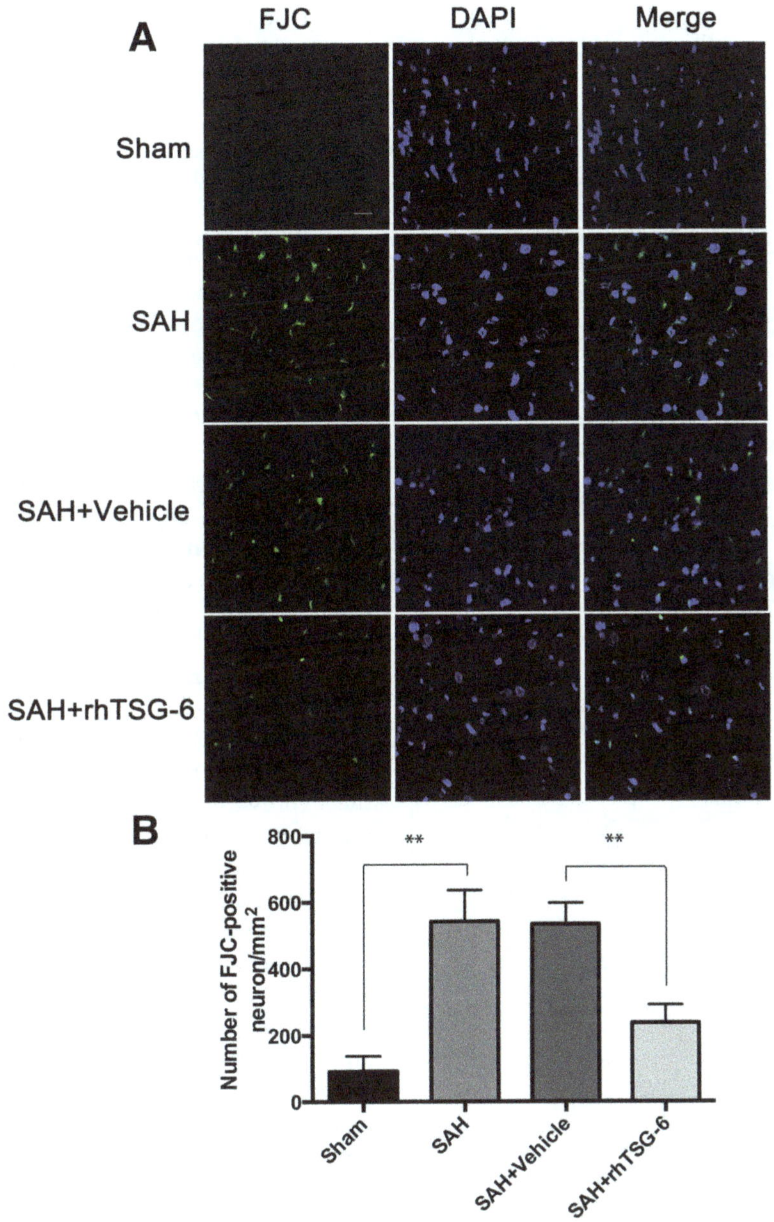

Fig. 4 Effects of rh-TSG-6 on neuronal degenerating at 24 h after subarachnoid hemorrhage (SAH). **a** Representative microphotographs of Fluoro-Jade C staining (FJC)-positive neurons in the Sham, SAH, Vehicle and rh-TSG-6 groups at 24 h following operation. **b** Quantitative analysis of FJC-positive cells was performed at the ipsilateral cortex. $n = 6$ in each group. Data are expressed as mean ± SD. $^{**}P < 0.01$. Scale bar = 20 μm

maintained a slight growth within 72 h after SAH (Fig. 6a).

Consistent with the M1/M2 marker qPCR results, mRNA expression levels of both pro-inflammatory and anti-inflammatory cytokines showed similar trends. Generally, the pro-inflammatory cytokine expression levels had a striking burst and peaked at 6 h (IL-1β) or 24 h (TNF-α, IL-6) post-SAH. In contrast, expression of anti-inflammatory cytokines was not augmented significantly until 6 h (TGF-β) or 24 h (IL-4, IL-10) and maintained a relatively gentle increase (Fig. 6b).

These results demonstrated that SAH induced a remarkable increase in both M1- and M2-type mRNA expression in the injured brains of rats compared with the sham groups. Moreover, SAH-induced activated microglia were mainly polarized to the M1 phenotype.

TSG-6 treatment provides neuroprotection in the brain under SAH conditions by modulating microglial phenotype and decreasing its pro-inflammation activity

Polarization of microglia was involved in the pathological progression of neurotoxic insults and strokes. To

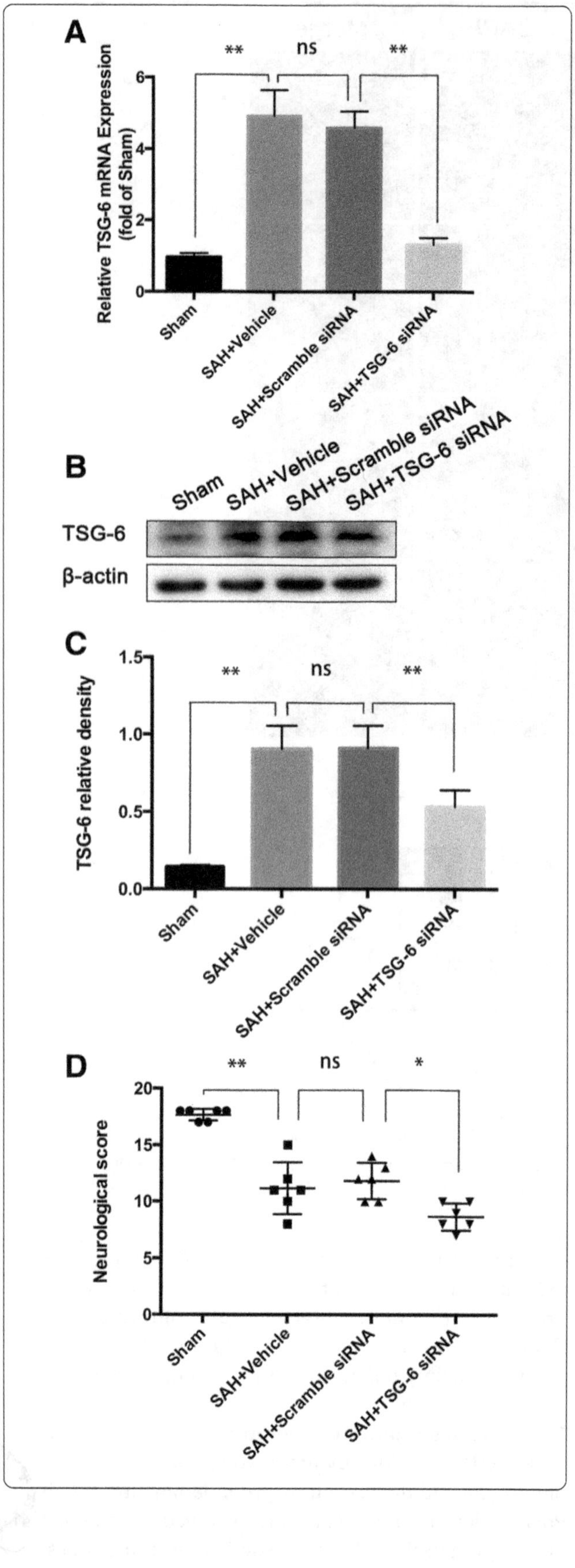

Fig. 5 Effects of TSG-6 siRNA pre-treatment in SAH rats. The expression of TSG-6 at mRNA (**a**) and protein (**b**) level at 24 h after intracerebroventricular injection of TSG-6 siRNA. **c** Neurologic score evaluation was also performed at 24 h after SAH. Knockdown of endogenous TSG-6 significantly worsened neurologic deficits at 24 h after SAH. ($n = 6$ rats/group). Values are reported as means ± SD. $^*p < 0.05$; $^{**}p < 0.01$

assess whether TSG-6 has a biological role in microglial polarization, the ipsilateral temporal lobe cortex was subjected to flow cytometry for the ratio of M1- and M2-type microglia measurement. Using flow cytometric analysis [33], we distinguished between activated microglia ($CD11b^+$ $CD45^{low}$) and infiltrating macrophages ($CD11b^+$ $CD45^{high}$) and detected changes in classical activation marker CD86 and alternative activation marker CD163 expression in specific cell populations. The gating strategy is shown in Fig. 7a. As shown in Fig. 7b, compared with the sham groups, the SAH and vehicle-treated group showed a higher percentage of $CD11b^+$ $CD45^{low}$ microglia labeled with markers for M1 (CD86) and M2 (CD163) phenotypes. In rats treated with rh-TSG-6 after SAH induction, the expression of CD163 was increased on $CD11b^+$ $CD45^{low}$ microglia than those in the vehicle treated group, while the expression of M1 marker (CD86) exhibited a remarkable attenuation. In accordance with declined M1 polarization elevating M2 phenotype after rh-TSG-6 treatment, there was a remarkable attenuation of TNF-α expression level and upregulated IL-10 expression level measured by ELISA in the rh-TSG-6 treatment group. As expected, no significant changes of either M1 or M2 ratio were noticed between the SAH and vehicle-treated groups.

Overall, these results demonstrated that rh-TSG-6 treatment partially retained SAH-driven M1 polarization and skewed the balance of M1/M2 ratio to a beneficial phenotype, thereby conferring its neuroprotective properties.

Deficiency of endogenous TSG-6 leads to an exaggerated pro-inflammatory microglial phenotype

To further determine the role of TSG-6 in modulatory effects of triggering phenotypic conversion of microglia, mice were subjected to TSG-6 siRNA treatment 48 h before SAH induction. The results of double immunofluorescent staining and western blot showed that the M1-associated marker CD86 (Fig. 8a, b, e) and M2-associated marker CD163 (Fig. 8c, d, f) were both significantly upregulated 24 h after SAH compared to the sham group. When TSG-6 was suppressed, the induction of SAH potentiated the protein expression of CD86, while the expression of M2 marker CD163 in Iba1 was lower than the scramble siRNA-treated group.

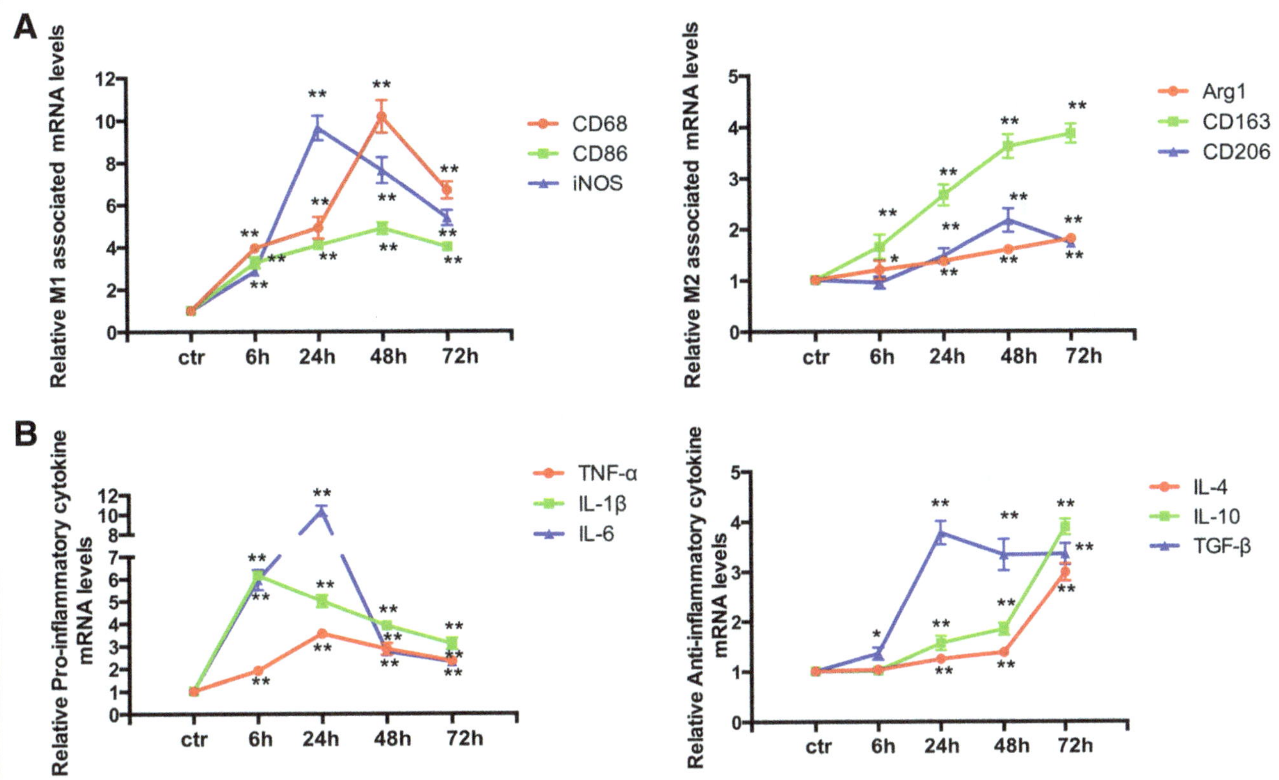

Fig. 6 Microglial phenotypic characteristics after SAH induction. **a** M1/M2 Markers of activated microglia increased over time after SAH. **b** Time course changes of mRNA expressions at 6 h, 24 h, 48 h, and 72 h for proinflammatory cytokines (TNF-α, IL-1β, IL-6) and anti-inflammatory cytokines (IL-4, IL-10, TGF-β) after SAH. Samples for PCR experiment sorted from left temporal brain lysates. Quantifications are expressed as the fold change compared to the sham group. $n = 5$ in each group. $^{*}P < 0.05$ and $^{**}P < 0.01$ vs. sham group. Ctr represents sham group

Considering the above results, we concluded that a loss of TSG-6 triggers microglial phenotypic changes with a bias towards pro-inflammatory activity, namely amplifying M1 polarization of activated microglia.

Effects of TSG-6 were involved in impeding the procedure of phosphorylation and the cellular location of Stat3

STAT3 is an important transcription factor associated with microglial polarization status. Overactivation of p-STAT3 can contribute to the upregulation of proinflammatory cytokines under some kinds of stroke. Since the activity of pSTAT3 was observed mainly in microglia/macrophages, but not in either neurons or astrocytes, therefore, immunofluorescence determined the expression of p-STAT3 in microglia in the rat cortex following SAH at 24 h. As shown in Fig. 9, fluorescence intensity of p-STAT3 was barely detected in the sham group. Obviously, rats which underwent SAH exhibited significantly increased p-STAT3 levels compared with sham-operated rats. Next, intervention with rh-TSG-6 diminished the level of phosphorylation of STAT3 in the SAH group. Correspondently, phosphorylation level of p-STAT3 was more enhanced in TSG-6 siRNA-pretreated rats. In addition, a reduction in nuclear translocation of STAT3 following rh-TSG-6 treatment and p-STAT3 immunoreactivity were more elevated following silencing treatment. Therefore, these results suggested that TSG-6 may be associated with the phosphorylation of STAT3.

The effects of TSG-6 on modulating microglial phenotype was involved in SOCS3/STAT3 pathway

Among the candidate signal pathways, the STAT3 signaling pathway can play a pivotal role in neuroinflammation and the activation of microglia within CNS. To further explore the underlying mechanism of TSG-6 in regulating microglia activation, factors in the STAT3 pathway pivotal to microglia polarization were tested. Results of Western blot (Fig. 10a) showed that after SAH, inflammatory responses occurred. Significant activation of STAT3 was observed accompanied with elevated expression of IL-6 rather than IL-10 and a raised SOCS3 levels in comparison with the sham group. However, the induction of SAH or TSG-6 was not observed to change the protein level of STAT3. Additionally, post-SAH TSG-6 upregulation was associated with an increase in IL-10 and SOCS3 levels and a decrease in

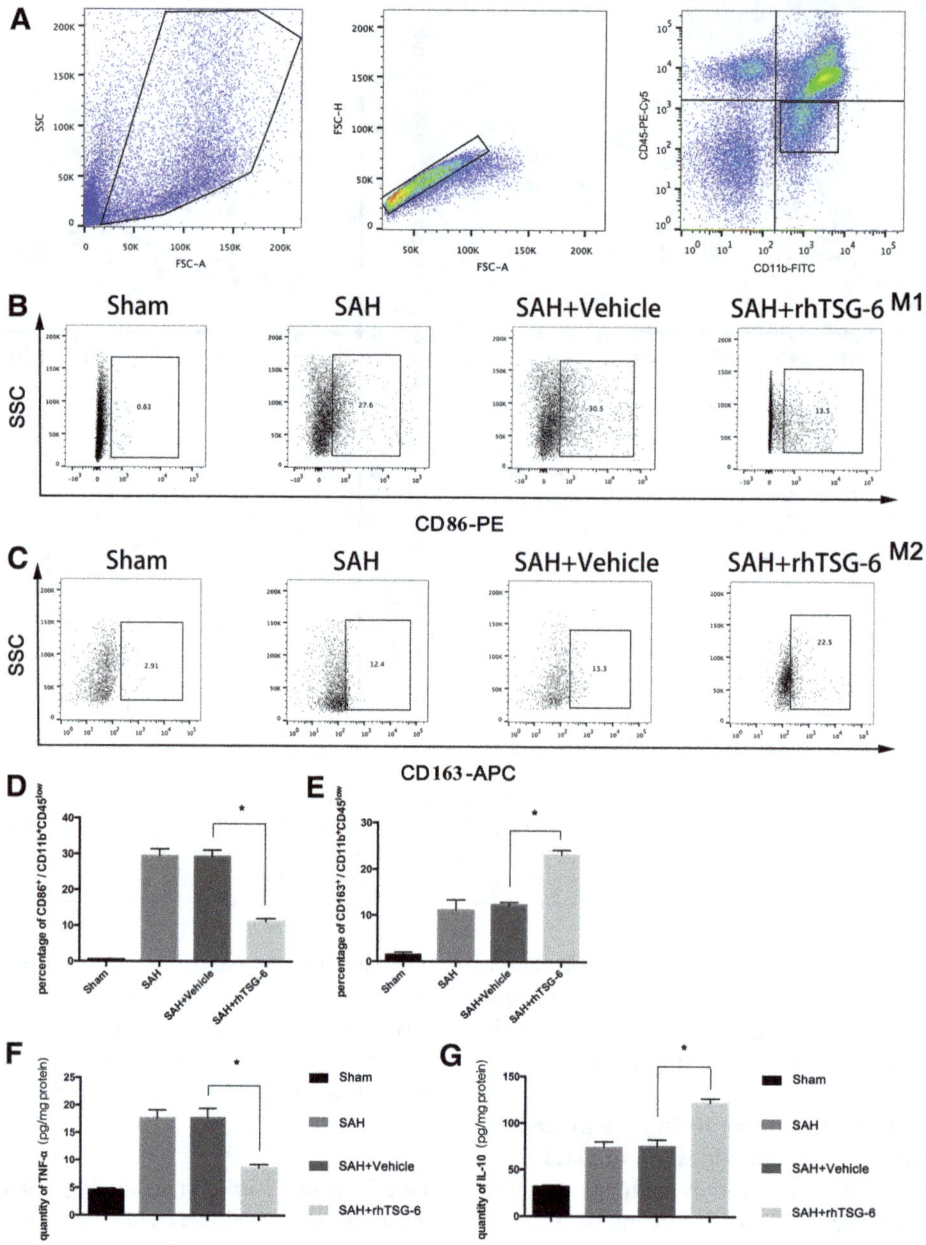

Fig. 7 Effects of rh-TSG-6 on SAH-induced microglia polarization. **a** Representative FACS plots showing gating strategy we use in flow cytometry analysis. Cells populations in the right dot plots defined as CD11b$^+$ CD45^{low} (microglia) were gated for further analysis. Representative dot plots showing the ratio of CD86-positive subsets (**b**) and CD163-positive subsets (**c**) in CD11b$^+$ CD45^{low} populations in the sham group, SAH group, SAH + vehicle group and SAH + rh-TSG-6 group. Bar graphs show quantitative analysis of CD86-positive subsets of CD11b$^+$ CD45^{low} populations (M1 microglia) (**d**) and CD163-positive subsets of CD11b$^+$ CD45^{low} populations (M2 microglia) (**e**) in different groups. Inflammatory mediators expressed in the brain cortex after SAH were detected with ELISA. Tissue TNF-α and IL-10 concentrations were analyzed from samples and standards in duplicates and expressed as pictograms per milliliter. rh-TSG-6 administration obviously reduced the level of TNF-α (**f**) and increased the level of IL-10 (**g**) in the brain tissue. Samples for FACS and ELISA experiments sorted from tissue lysates of left temporal lobe of the brain. The values (means ± SD) are representative of three independent experiments. *$p < 0.05$. $n = 6$/group. SSC = side scatter channel, FSC-A = forward scatter channel area, FITC = fluorescein isothiocyanate, PE = phycoerythrin, and APC = allophycocyanin

IL-6 and phospho-STAT3 levels in brain tissues 24 h after SAH. IL-6-mediated activation of STAT3 was inhibited in injured brain tissues of SAH rats treated with rh-TSG-6.

Finally, we knocked down endogenous TSG-6 to test the association between TSG-6 and the SOCS3/STAT3 axis (Fig. 10b). Conversely, deficiency of TSG-6 in SAH rats showed more increased pSTAT3 compared to

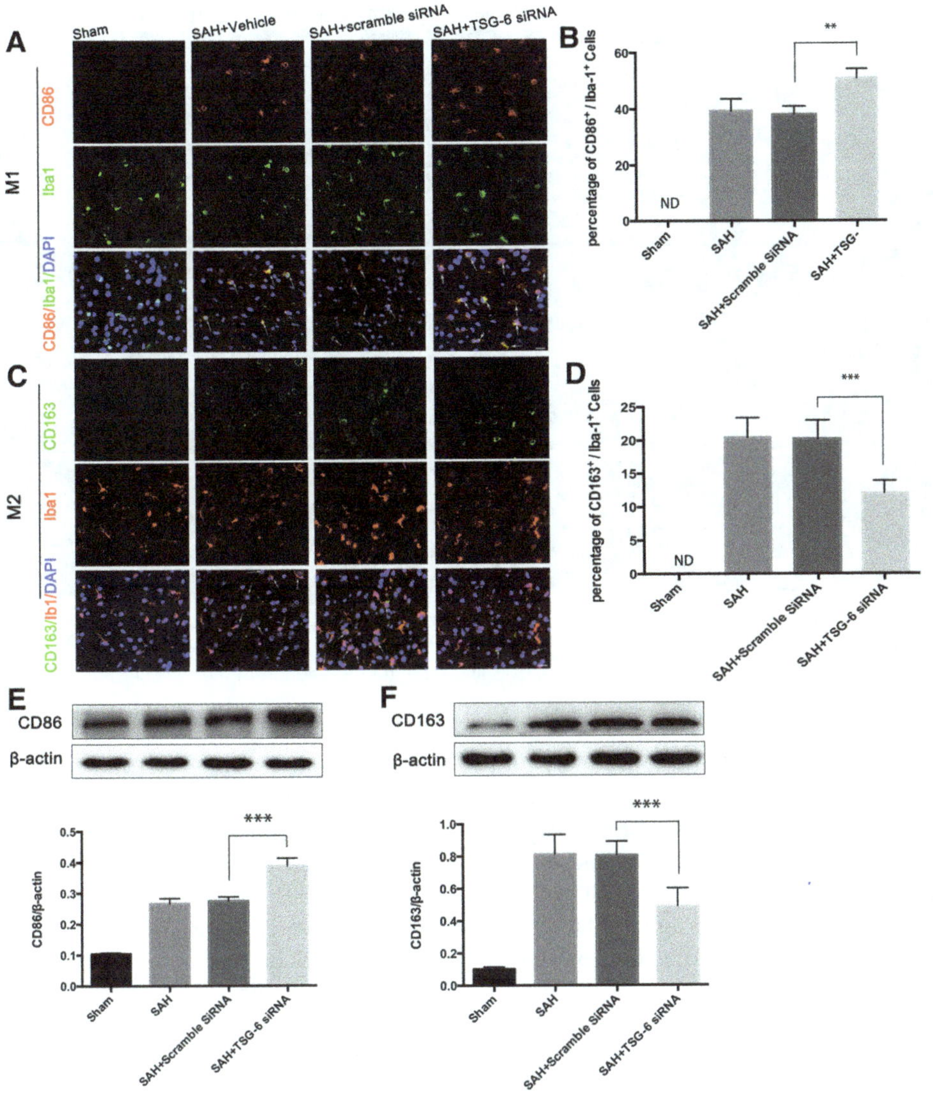

Fig. 8 Deficiency of endogenous TSG-6 leads to an exaggerated proinflammatory microglial phenotype. Immunofluorescence labeling and quantification analysis (**a**–**d**) and western blot (**e**, **f**) and showing that inhibition of TSG-6 further enhanced the increased levels of CD86 and the enhanced CD163 levels was decreased 24 h after SAH compared with the scramble siRNA group. The samples for western blot are tissue lysates obtained from the left temporal lobe of the brain. White arrows indicate typical cells. Values of the relative densitometric analysis are expressed as mean ± SD, Scale bar = 20 μm, $n = 6$ in each group. $^{**}P < 0.01$; $^{***}P < 0.001$

scramble siRNA treated rats. As expected, the two inflammatory cytokines indicated opposite trends (amplifying IL-6 expression and declining IL-10 expression) contributed by TSG-6 silencing treatment. Expression of SOCS3 showed a weaker response to SAH insult. Therefore, these results verified TSG-6 functions in altering microglial phenotypes by modulating SOCS3/STAT3 axis expression in inducible SAH rat model.

Discussion

In this study, we revealed a neuroprotective effect with emphasis on targeting the immunomodulatory functions afforded by TSG-6 in a rat model of SAH. Our data demonstrated that TSG-6 was upregulated in the brain cortex in a time-dependent manner after SAH. To further determine the role of TSG-6 following SAH, we continued our research in experimental rats. Exogenous TSG-6 greatly attenuated neurological deficits and brain water under inducible subarachnoid hemorrhage in vivo. After silencing endogenous TSG-6, early brain injury was further exacerbated. These results indicated that the neuroprotective effect of TSG-6 is associated with phenotypic modulation of the microglia shift. Signaling protein expression-associated STAT3 in brain tissue after SAH were investigated. The finding showed that levels of TSG-6 were involved in STAT3

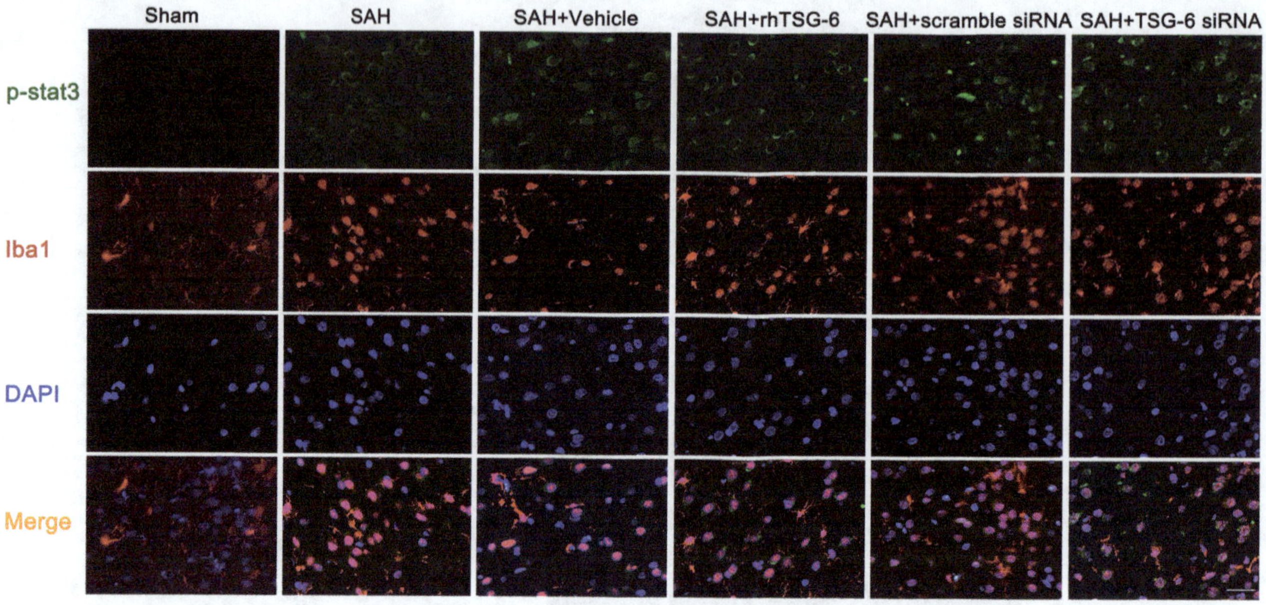

Fig. 9 The effects of rh-TSG-6 on phosphorylation of Stat3 and cellular location of p-STAT3. The phosphorylation of STAT3 was assessed by immunofluorescent double-labeling. Immunoreactivity for p-STAT3 is attenuated at 24 h in the SAH + rh-TSG-6 group, as compared with the SAH + vehicle group. TSG-6 deficiency increased the expression of p-STAT3 and more translocation from the cytosol to the nucleus occurs was observed. Scale bar = 20 μm

phosphorylation, which was an important factor for controlling microglial inflammatory subtypes. Accordingly, these results suggested that TSG-6 may play an endogenous brain protection role after SAH and an enhanced expression or supplementation of TSG-6 may induce a selective modulation of microglia polarization to anti-inflammatory phenotypes via the SOCS3/STAT3 pathways (Fig. 10).

TNF-stimulated gene-6 (TSG6) is a pleiotropic immunomodulatory protein activated rapidly in response to stimuli and functions at an early phase of inflammatory procedure. The protective effects of TSG-6 have been well studied in the brain, most of which focused on the anti-inflammatory aspect, especially its role in inhibiting activation of microglia/macrophages [27, 28, 34]. Given that the suppression of microglia/macrophages may also compromise the normal physiological defense mechanism of CNS and induce inevitable side effects [35, 36], the mechanism by which TSG-6 confers neuroprotection requires further investigation. In this study, the protein of TSG-6 was almost located in Iba1$^+$ microglia. However, this result was different from Coulson-Thomas et al.'s work, in which they found TSG-6 was only located in astrocytes in a SCI rat model [37]. As indicated in Fig. 2c, TSG-6 staining is positively co-expressed in not only microglia but also other cell types as well. According to the literature, blood-derived immunocytes, such as neutrophils and DC cells, can express TSG-6 under inflammation stimulation [26]. Therefore, under the circumstance that BBB is no longer intact after SAH insult, TSG-6 could originate from infiltrating peripheral immunocyte. Indeed, we cannot exclude the possibility that TSG-6 expressed by other cells also plays a role, but the proportion of infiltrating peripheral immune cells is relatively small compared to resident microglia, especially in the early stages [38, 39]. Thus, we assumed that data detected in the current study mainly reflects the biological function of microglial TSG-6. Correspondingly, by intervening in the concentration of TSG-6 (exogenous supplementary or knockdown), our results indicated that the level of microglial TSG-6 was closely associated with the severity of brain injury after SAH, which was in lines with several other studies that the level of TSG-6 can reflect the disease progression and act as a novel prognostic factor [40].

Some may argue that simply dividing microglia into the supposed dichotomy between M1 and M2 phenotypes is oversimplified [41]; however, this classification may provide a bridge for understanding the function of microglia in several brain diseases [24]. When irritated proinflammatory-status microglia dominates the inflammatory microenvironment, inflammation-induced developmental brain injury can be observed in some CNS diseases [42, 43]. Consistent with the findings of previous study [44], our study showed that, after induction of SAH, augmented microglia were identified by the panorama of brain slices and more strikingly elevated proinflammatory genes compared to anti-inflammatory genes within 72 h after SAH was revealed by PCR. rh-TSG-6 treatment significantly suppressed the prevailing M1

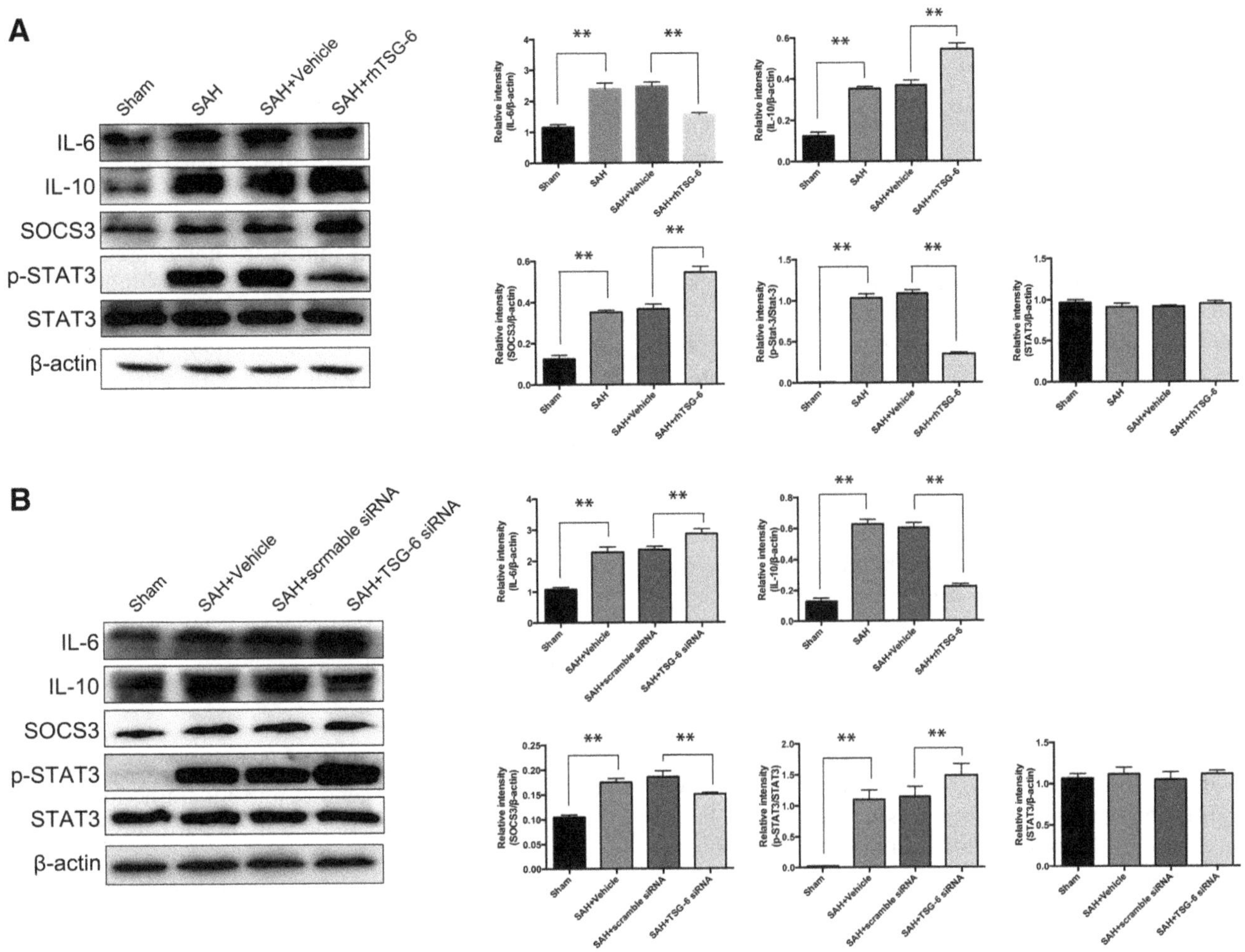

Fig. 10 Effects of rh-TSG-6 and TSG-6 siRNA treatments on SOCS3/STAT3 axis. **a** Effect of exogenous TSG-6 on STAT3 pathway expression was evaluated by western blot and the relative IL-6, IL-10, SOCS3, p-STAT3, and STAT3 densities were quantificationally evaluated. **b** The representative western blot analysis of STAT3 axis in SAH rats accepted intracerebroventricular injection of siRNA as indicated and quantification of the level of IL-6, IL-10, SOCS3, p-STAT3 and STAT3 after deficiency of TSG-6. Data are expressed as the mean ± SD from six rats. $^{**}P < 0.01$

phenotypes and observed a trend towards M2 phenotypes (Fig. 4). Resident microglia are major cells involved in inflammatory processes in the brain and are first to respond to the disturbed brain environment [38, 45]. Yet the time for microglia-mediated inflammation response to manifest occurred over hours to days, thereby creating an opportunity for clinical therapeutic intervention [46]. Accordingly, early limitation of microglia skewing towards proinflammatory phenotypes can help to preserve brain tissue. As expected, a lower abundance of endogenous TSG-6 protein led to the provocation of M1 phenotypic microglia after SAH and to be concomitant with the marked proinflammatory environment are degenerated neurons and upcoming unfavorable outcomes, while after administration of rh-TSG-6, the modified inflammatory milieu at the early stage of EBI through M1/M2 switching was accompanied by an improved outcome. A timely shift to beneficial M2 microglia can resolve neuroinflammation and create a microenvironment friendly to CNS repair [21]. However, long-term blockage of inflammation via suppressing M1 activation may not induce overall beneficial effects because deficiency of M1 phenotypic microglia will hinder clearing cell debris so as to prolong the inflammatory process. It is clear that cessation of inflammation progression before mounting to its peak is effective in alleviating brain injury. Accordingly, in the present study, we observed the effect of acute rh-TSG-6 treatment on early outcomes (24 h) in SAH rats. Modulation of the M1/M2 balance by TSG-6 is protective against neuronal injury 24 h after SAH. This effect also has a beneficial impact on neuronal survival at 72 h after SAH as indicated by our FJC data. Collectively, these results indicated a causal relationship between TSG-6 and the M1/M2 microglia switch.

Controlled neuroinflammation and immune cell infiltration within injured CNS were supposed to serve protective and beneficial functions [47]. However, to what extent and to what time inflammatory processes are deleterious and/or beneficial to brain recovery remain controversial. Therefore, a more precision modulation of microglial inflammation response remains to be explored. To date, there exists much uncertainty over which intracellular signaling pathways are involved in the mediation of the microglial shift in SAH. It is reported that STAT family members play various roles in microglial and macrophage polarization [48]. Our study discovered that microglial STAT3 was highly activated in the hemorrhagic hemisphere after experimental SAH. However, disparate functional outcomes from activated STAT3 were observed in different cerebral pathological conditions. Furthermore, whether microglial STAT3 activation during a pathologic condition results in inflammation or neuroprotection remains relatively controversial [49, 50]. Recent studies have shown that upstream kinase can regulate STAT3 and the subsequent downstream genes regulated by STAT3 [51]. Specifically, it has been demonstrated that both the proinflammatory mediator IL-6 and the anti- inflammatory cytokine IL-10 share the same STAT3 pathway [52]. Depending on different stimuli, IL-10-mediated STAT3 responses can lead to an anti-inflammatory phenotype associated with a higher expression of M2 neuroprotective markers [53]. However, under some sublethal strikes, a loss of normal feedback modulation on STAT3 from SOCS3 can result in overactivation of STAT3, thereby favoring IL-6 driven STAT3 [54, 55]. In good agreement with the previous studies [56], our results demonstrated that overactivation of STAT3 in microglia is detrimental, and a reduced phosphorylation of STAT3 may provide anti-inflammatory effects.

Regarding the possible mechanisms underlined in TSG-6-conferred neuroprotection, we discovered that treatment with rh-TSG-6 following SAH effectively decreased the expression of p-STAT3 accompanied by the increased of expression of SOCS3 as well as IL-10 and a decreased IL-6 expression related to the vehicle-treatment group, both of which correlated with a dominated anti-inflammatory microenvironment. In vivo TSG-6 knockdown further aggravated STAT3 activation and reversed the effects of IL-6, IL-10, and SOCS3 expression. As a result, a pronounced polarization to M1 phenotype microglia was linked with worsened brain injury, which is consistent with several previous works [23, 57]. Taken together, we speculated that TSG-6 appeared to play a unique role in M1/M2 polarization by modulating IL-6/STAT3 or/and IL-10/STAT3 activity through SOCS3 activation.

Recently, a study from Mittal et al. supported our finding whereby TSG-6 inhibited aberrant activation of STAT3 and primed the innate immunity response from a state of generating proinflammatory cytokines to a distinct anti-inflammatory status [58]. Although we have demonstrated that TSG-6 confers its neuroprotection partly depending on the SOCS3/STAT3 axis, the detailed mechanisms underlined require further investigation. Additionally, this study mainly focused on the role of TSG-6 in the early stage of SAH injury. The potential long-term roles of TSG-6 on M1/M2 phenotypic balance and responses to brain injury are not addressed herein and should be investigated in the future studies. Admittedly, injury-recovery is a continuously variable process. All immunotherapies may not achieve optimal clinical transformation if they do not compliment changes during the overall process. Likewise, whether the effect of TSG-6 beyond the EBI at a later time satisfies the demands of the CNS microenvironment will impact the recovery processes and the final neurological state. However, due to limitations inherit in the puncture SAH model, it is difficult to explore this research topic. A more perfect SAH model which is suitable for long-term research on SAH pathophysiological conditions is required.

Conclusions

In summary, we identified the protective effects of TSG-6, a novel endogenous anti-inflammation protein, after SAH insults by inhibiting inflammation through the SOCS3/STAT3 pathway. It was discovered that exogenous administration of rh-TSG-6 can provide neuroprotective effects related to modulating microglial polarization phenotypes. Our finding suggested that TSG-6 is a promising candidate for alleviating the degree of EBI following SAH, which may expand application in targeting microglial overactivation-mediated inflammation in cerebrovascular diseases.

Additional files

Additional file 1: Analysis of levels of TSG-6 gene and protein in different time-points in the sham (6 h, 12 h, 24 h, 48 h, 72 h). No significant differences of TSG-6 gene (A) and protein (B) were found among different groups. All values are presented as means ± SD, $n = 4$ in each time point per group.

Additional file 2: Effects of rh-TSG-6 on neuronal degenerating at 72 h after subarachnoid hemorrhage (SAH). Representative microphotographs and quantitative analysis of Fluoro-Jade C staining (FJC)-positive neurons in the sham, SAH, vehicle and rh-TSG-6 groups at 72 h following operation. $n = 6$ in each group. Data are expressed as mean ± SD. $^{***}P < 0.001$. Scale bar = 20 μm.

Additional file 3: Microglial phenotypic characteristics after SAH induction. Photomicrograph of microglia(red) and DAPI(blue) double immunostaining in a coronal section of the whole brain in sham and SAH groups. $n = 5$ in each group. Scale bar = 2000 μm.

Abbreviations

APC: Allophycocyanin; CNS: Central nervous system; EBI: Early brain injury; FITC: Fluorescein isothiocyanate; FJC: Fluoro-Jade C; GFAP: Glial fibrillary acidic protein; Iba1: Ionized calcium-binding adapter molecule 1; ICH: Intracerebral hemorrhage; NeuN: Neuronal nuclear protein; PE: Phycoerythrin; qRT-PCR: Quantitative real-time polymerase chain reaction; SAH: Subarachnoid hemorrhage; SCI: Spinal cord injury; SD: Sprague–Dawley; siRNA: Small interfering RNA; SOCS3: Suppressor of cytokine signaling 3; STAT3: Signal transducer and activator of transcription 3; TSG-6: TNF-α stimulated gene/protein 6

Funding
This study was supported by the National Natural Science Foundation of China (No. 81271315), the Science and Technology Project Foundation of Guangdong Province (Grant number 2016A020215098), and the Key Project of Clinical Research of Southern Medical University (Grant number LC2016ZD024).

Authors' contributions
CZD and RL conceived and designed the experiments. RL performed the experiments, drafted the manuscript, and analyzed the data. RL and WCL performed the animal model establishment. JY, YCC, SQG, HYF, XFL, XZ, and XYH provided the experimental technical support and assisted in completing the study at different stages. CZD reviewed and performed the edition of the paper. All authors checked and approved the final manuscript.

Consent for publication
Not applicable.

Competing interests
The authors declare that they have no competing interests.

References

1. Macdonald RL, Schweizer TA. Spontaneous subarachnoid haemorrhage. Lancet. 2017;389:655–66.
2. Brown RD, Broderick JP. Unruptured intracranial aneurysms: epidemiology, natural history, management options, and familial screening. The Lancet Neurology. 2014;13:393–404.
3. Korja M, Kaprio J. Controversies in epidemiology of intracranial aneurysms and SAH. Nat Rev Neurol. 2016;12:50–5.
4. de Oliveira Manoel AL, Goffi A, Marotta TR, Schweizer TA, Abrahamson S, Macdonald RL. The critical care management of poor-grade subarachnoid haemorrhage. Crit Care. 2016;20:21.
5. Macdonald RL. Delayed neurological deterioration after subarachnoid haemorrhage. Nat Rev Neurol. 2014;10:44–58.
6. Chen S, Feng H, Sherchan P, Klebe D, Zhao G, Sun X, Zhang J, Tang J, Zhang JH. Controversies and evolving new mechanisms in subarachnoid hemorrhage. Prog Neurobiol. 2014;115:64–91.
7. Young AM, Karri SK, Helmy A, Budohoski KP, Kirollos RW, Bulters DO, Kirkpatrick PJ, Ogilvy CS, Trivedi RA. Pharmacologic Management of Subarachnoid Hemorrhage. World Neurosurg. 2015;84:28–35.
8. Keyrouz SG, Diringer MN. Clinical review: prevention and therapy of vasospasm in subarachnoid hemorrhage. Crit Care. 2007;11:220.
9. van Lieshout JH, Dibué-Adjei M, Cornelius JF, Slotty PJ, Schneider T, Restin T, Boogaarts HD, Steiger HJ, Petridis AK, Kamp MA. An introduction to the pathophysiology of aneurysmal subarachnoid hemorrhage. Neurosurg Rev. 2017. https://doi.org/10.1007/s10143-017-0827-y.
10. Pradilla G, Chaichana KL, Hoang S, Huang J, Tamargo RJ. Inflammation and cerebral vasospasm after subarachnoid hemorrhage. Neurosurg Clin N Am. 2010;21:365–79.
11. Chen S, Ma Q, Krafft PR, Hu Q, Rolland W 2nd, Sherchan P, Zhang J, Tang J, Zhang JH. P2X7R/cryopyrin inflammasome axis inhibition reduces neuroinflammation after SAH. Neurobiol Dis. 2013;58:296–307.
12. He Y, Xu L, Li B, Guo ZN, Hu Q, Guo Z, Tang J, Chen Y, Zhang Y, Tang J, Zhang JH. Macrophage-inducible C-type lectin/spleen tyrosine kinase signaling pathway contributes to neuroinflammation after subarachnoid hemorrhage in rats. Stroke. 2015;46:2277–86.
13. Zheng VZ, Wong GKC. Neuroinflammation responses after subarachnoid hemorrhage: a review. J Clin Neurosci. 2017;42:7–11.
14. Ma Y, Wang J, Wang Y, Yang GY. The biphasic function of microglia in ischemic stroke. Prog Neurobiol. 2017;157:247–72.
15. Aguzzi A, Barres BA, Bennett ML. Microglia: scapegoat, saboteur, or something else? Science. 2013;339:156–61.
16. Brown GC, Vilalta A. How microglia kill neurons. Brain Res. 2015;1628: 288–97.
17. Iadecola C, Anrather J. The immunology of stroke: from mechanisms to translation. Nat Med. 2011;17:796–808.
18. Franco R, Fernandez-Suarez D. Alternatively activated microglia and macrophages in the central nervous system. Prog Neurobiol. 2015;131:65–86.
19. Bouhlel MA, Derudas B, Rigamonti E, Dievart R, Brozek J, Haulon S, Zawadzki C, Jude B, Torpier G, Marx N, et al. PPARgamma activation primes human monocytes into alternative M2 macrophages with anti-inflammatory properties. Cell Metab. 2007;6:137–43.
20. Tentillier N, Etzerodt A, Olesen MN, Rizalar FS, Jacobsen J, Bender D, Moestrup SK, Romero-Ramos M. Anti-inflammatory modulation of microglia via CD163-targeted glucocorticoids protects dopaminergic neurons in the 6-OHDA Parkinson's disease model. J Neurosci. 2016;36:9375–90.
21. Francos-Quijorna I, Amo-Aparicio J, Martinez-Muriana A, Lopez-Vales R. IL-4 drives microglia and macrophages toward a phenotype conducive for tissue repair and functional recovery after spinal cord injury. Glia. 2016; 64:2079–92.
22. Shi H, Zheng K, Su Z, Su H, Zhong M, He X, Zhou C, Chen H, Xiong Q, Zhang Y. Sinomenine enhances microglia M2 polarization and attenuates inflammatory injury in intracerebral hemorrhage. J Neuroimmunol. 2016;299:28–34.
23. Yang Y, Liu H, Zhang H, Ye Q, Wang J, Yang B, Mao L, Zhu W, Leak RK, Xiao B, et al. ST2/IL-33-dependent microglial response limits acute ischemic brain injury. J Neurosci. 2017;37:4692–704.
24. Xu H, Wang Z, Li J, Wu H, Peng Y, Fan L, Chen J, Gu C, Yan F, Wang L, Chen G. The polarization states of microglia in TBI: a new paradigm for pharmacological intervention. Neural Plast. 2017;2017:5405104.
25. Milner CM, Day AJ. TSG-6: a multifunctional protein associated with inflammation. J Cell Sci. 2003;116:1863–73.
26. Day AJ, Milner CM. TSG-6: a multifunctional protein with anti-inflammatory and tissue-protective properties. Matrix Biol. 2018. https://doi.org/10.1016/j.matbio.2018.01.011.
27. Chen M, Li X, Zhang X, He X, Lai L, Liu Y, Zhu G, Li W, Li H, Fang Q, et al. The inhibitory effect of mesenchymal stem cell on blood-brain barrier disruption following intracerebral hemorrhage in rats: contribution of TSG-6. J Neuroinflammation. 2015;12:61.
28. Zhang R, Liu Y, Yan K, Chen L, Chen XR, Li P, Chen FF, Jiang XD. Anti-inflammatory and immunomodulatory mechanisms of mesenchymal stem cell transplantation in experimental traumatic brain injury. J Neuroinflammation. 2013;10:106.
29. Schwartz AY, Masago A, Sehba FA, Bederson JB. Experimental models of subarachnoid hemorrhage in the rat: a refinement of the endovascular filament model. J Neurosci Methods. 2000;96:161–7.
30. Sugawara T, Ayer R, Jadhav V, Zhang JH. A new grading system evaluating bleeding scale in filament perforation subarachnoid hemorrhage rat model. J Neurosci Methods. 2008;167:327–34.
31. Zeng J, Chen Y, Ding R, Feng L, Fu Z, Yang S, Deng X, Xie Z, Zheng S. Isoliquiritigenin alleviates early brain injury after experimental intracerebral hemorrhage via suppressing ROS- and/or NF-kappaB-mediated NLRP3 inflammasome activation by promoting Nrf2 antioxidant pathway. J Neuroinflammation. 2017;14:119.
32. Frank MG, Wieseler-Frank JL, Watkins LR, Maier SF. Rapid isolation of highly enriched and quiescent microglia from adult rat hippocampus: immunophenotypic and functional characteristics. J Neurosci Methods. 2006;151:121–30.
33. Chang CF, Wan J, Li Q, Renfroe SC, Heller NM, Wang J. Alternative activation-skewed microglia/macrophages promote hematoma resolution in experimental intracerebral hemorrhage. Neurobiol Dis. 2017;103:54–69.
34. Watanabe J, Shetty AK, Hattiangady B, Kim DK, Foraker JE, Nishida H, Prockop DJ. Administration of TSG-6 improves memory after traumatic brain injury in mice. Neurobiol Dis. 2013;59:86–99.

35. Faustino JV, Wang X, Johnson CE, Klibanov A, Derugin N, Wendland MF, Vexler ZS. Microglial cells contribute to endogenous brain defenses after acute neonatal focal stroke. J Neurosci. 2011;31:12992–3001.
36. Fernandez-Lopez D, Faustino J, Klibanov AL, Derugin N, Blanchard E, Simon F, Leib SL, Vexler ZS. Microglial cells prevent hemorrhage in neonatal focal arterial stroke. J Neurosci. 2016;36:2881–93.
37. Coulson-Thomas VJ, Lauer ME, Soleman S, Zhao C, Hascall VC, Day AJ, Fawcett JW. Tumor necrosis factor-stimulated Gene-6 (TSG-6) is constitutively expressed in adult central nervous system (CNS) and associated with astrocyte-mediated glial scar formation following spinal cord injury. J Biol Chem. 2016; 291:19939–52.
38. Li T, Pang S, Yu Y, Wu X, Guo J, Zhang S. Proliferation of parenchymal microglia is the main source of microgliosis after ischaemic stroke. Brain. 2013;136:3578–88.
39. Pan J, Jin JL, Ge HM, Yin KL, Chen X, Han LJ, Chen Y, Qian L, Li XX, Xu Y. Malibatol A regulates microglia M1/M2 polarization in experimental stroke in a PPARgamma-dependent manner. J Neuroinflammation. 2015;12:51.
40. Wisniewski HG, Colon E, Liublinska V, Karia RJ, Stabler TV, Attur M, Abramson SB, Band PA, Kraus VB. TSG-6 activity as a novel biomarker of progression in knee osteoarthritis. Osteoarthr Cartil. 2014;22:235–41.
41. Ransohoff RM. A polarizing question: do M1 and M2 microglia exist? Nat Neurosci. 2016;19:987–91.
42. He Y, Ma X, Li D, Hao J. Thiamet G mediates neuroprotection in experimental stroke by modulating microglia/macrophage polarization and inhibiting NF-kappaB p65 signaling. J Cereb Blood Flow Metab. 2017;37:2938–51.
43. Jang E, Lee S, Kim JH, Kim JH, Seo JW, Lee WH, Mori K, Nakao K, Suk K. Secreted protein lipocalin-2 promotes microglial M1 polarization. FASEB J. 2013;27:1176–90.
44. Xie Y, Guo H, Wang L, Xu L, Zhang X, Yu L, Liu Q, Li Y, Zhao N, Zhao N, et al. Human albumin attenuates excessive innate immunity via inhibition of microglial Mincle/Syk signaling in subarachnoid hemorrhage. Brain Behav Immun. 2017;60:346–60.
45. Schilling M, Besselmann M, Leonhard C, Mueller M, Ringelstein EB, Kiefer R. Microglial activation precedes and predominates over macrophage infiltration in transient focal cerebral ischemia: a study in green fluorescent protein transgenic bone marrow chimeric mice. Exp Neurol. 2003;183:25–33.
46. d'Avila JC, Lam TI, Bingham D, Shi J, Won SJ, Kauppinen TM, Massa S, Liu J, Swanson RA. Microglial activation induced by brain trauma is suppressed by post-injury treatment with a PARP inhibitor. J Neuroinflammation. 2012;9:31.
47. Lucke-Wold BP, Logsdon AF, Manoranjan B, Turner RC, McConnell E, Vates GE, Huber JD, Rosen CL, Simard JM. Aneurysmal subarachnoid hemorrhage and neuroinflammation: a comprehensive review. Int J Mol Sci. 2016;17:497.
48. Liang Z, Wu G, Fan C, Xu J, Jiang S, Yan X, Di S, Ma Z, Hu W, Yang Y. The emerging role of signal transducer and activator of transcription 3 in cerebral ischemic and hemorrhagic stroke. Prog Neurobiol. 2016;137:1–16.
49. Satriotomo I, Bowen KK, Vemuganti R. JAK2 and STAT3 activation contributes to neuronal damage following transient focal cerebral ischemia. J Neurochem. 2006;98:1353–68.
50. Sehara Y, Sawicka K, Hwang JY, Latuszek-Barrantes A, Etgen AM, Zukin RS. Survivin is a transcriptional target of STAT3 critical to estradiol neuroprotection in global ischemia. J Neurosci. 2013;33:12364–74.
51. Oliva AA Jr, Kang Y, Sanchez-Molano J, Furones C, Atkins CM. STAT3 signaling after traumatic brain injury. J Neurochem. 2012;120:710–20.
52. Nakamura R, Sene A, Santeford A, Gdoura A, Kubota S, Zapata N, Apte RS. IL10-driven STAT3 signalling in senescent macrophages promotes pathological eye angiogenesis. Nat Commun. 2015;6:7847.
53. O'Shea JJ, Murray PJ. Cytokine signaling modules in inflammatory responses. Immunity. 2008;28:477–87.
54. Croker BA, Krebs DL, Zhang JG, Wormald S, Willson TA, Stanley EG, Robb L, Greenhalgh CJ, Forster I, Clausen BE, et al. SOCS3 negatively regulates IL-6 signaling in vivo. Nat Immunol. 2003;4:540–5.
55. Qin H, Yeh WI, De Sarno P, Holdbrooks AT, Liu Y, Muldowney MT, Reynolds SL, Yanagisawa LL, Fox TH 3rd, Park K, et al. Signal transducer and activator of transcription-3/suppressor of cytokine signaling-3 (STAT3/SOCS3) axis in myeloid cells regulates neuroinflammation. Proc Natl Acad Sci U S A. 2012; 109:5004–9.
56. Chen S, Dong Z, Cheng M, Zhao Y, Wang M, Sai N, Wang X, Liu H, Huang G, Zhang X. Homocysteine exaggerates microglia activation and neuroinflammation through microglia localized STAT3 overactivation following ischemic stroke. J Neuroinflammation. 2017;14:187.
57. Zhai Q, Li F, Chen X, Jia J, Sun S, Zhou D, Ma L, Jiang T, Bai F, Xiong L, Wang Q. Triggering receptor expressed on myeloid cells 2, a novel regulator of immunocyte phenotypes, confers neuroprotection by relieving neuroinflammation. Anesthesiology. 2017;127:98–110.
58. Mittal M, Tiruppathi C, Nepal S, Zhao YY, Grzych D, Soni D, Prockop DJ, Malik AB. TNFalpha-stimulated gene-6 (TSG6) activates macrophage phenotype transition to prevent inflammatory lung injury. Proc Natl Acad Sci U S A. 2016;113:E8151–e8158.

16

Natural IgM antibodies that bind neoepitopes exposed as a result of spinal cord injury, drive secondary injury by activating complement

Aarti Narang[1], Fei Qiao[1], Carl Atkinson[1], Hong Zhu[1], Xiaofeng Yang[1], Liudmila Kulik[2], V. Michael Holers[2] and Stephen Tomlinson[1,3*]

Abstract

Background: Natural IgM antibodies (Abs) function as innate immune sensors of injury via recognition of neoepitopes expressed on damaged cells, although how this recognition systems function following spinal cord injury (SCI) exposes various neoepitopes and their precise nature remains largely unknown. Here, we investigated the role of two natural IgM monoclonal Abs (mAbs), B4 and C2, that recognize post-ischemic neoepitopes following ischemia and reperfusion in other tissues.

Methods: Identification of post-SCI expressed neoepitopes was examined using previously characterized monoclonal Abs (B4 and C2 mAbs). The role of post-SCI neoepitopes and their recognition by natural IgM Abs in propagating secondary injury was examined in Ab-deficient Rag1−/− or wild type C57BL/6 mice using Ab reconstitution experiments and neoepitope-targeted therapeutic studies, respectively.

Results: Administration of B4 or C2 mAb following murine SCI increased lesion size and worsened functional outcome in otherwise protected Ab-deficient Rag1−/− mice. Injury correlated with colocalized deposition of IgM and C3d in injured spinal cords from both mAb reconstituted Rag1−/− mice and untreated wild-type mice. Depletion of peritoneal B1 B cells, a source of natural Abs, reduced circulating levels of IgM with B4 (annexin-IV) and C2 (subset of phospholipids) reactivity, reduced IgM and complement deposition in the spinal cord, and protected against SCI. We therefore investigated whether the B4 neoepitope represents a therapeutic target for complement inhibition. B4-Crry, a fusion protein consisting of a single-chain Ab derived from B4 mAb, linked to the complement inhibitor Crry, significantly protected against SCI. B4-Crry exhibited a dual function in that it inhibited both the binding of pathogenic IgM and blocked complement activation in the spinal cord.

Conclusions: This study identifies important neoepitopes expressed within the spinal cord after injury. These neoepitopes are recognized by clonally specific natural IgM Abs that activate complement and drive pathology. We demonstrate that these neoepitopes represent novel targets for the therapeutic delivery of a complement inhibitor, and possibly other payload, to the injured spinal cord.

Keywords: Complement, Spinal cord injury, Natural antibodies, IgM, Neoepitope, Therapy

* Correspondence: tomlinss@musc.edu
[1]Department of Microbiology and Immunology, Medical University of South Carolina, 173 Ashley Ave, CRI 213, Charleston, SC 29425, USA
[3]Ralph H Johnson VA Medical Center, Charleston, SC, USA
Full list of author information is available at the end of the article

Background

Traumatic spinal cord injury (SCI) results in severe debilitation, often with complete paralysis and loss of sensory function below the injury site. Following a primary mechanical insult, a secondary wave of cell death ensues, that is accompanied by ischemia, vascular damage, glutamate excitotoxicity, ionic dysregulation, and inflammation. The area of secondary injury emanating from the site of trauma represents a therapeutic target.

There is strong evidence that complement plays an important role in secondary SCI, and both the classical [1] and alternative [1, 2] pathways of complement activation have been implicated in propagating injury (reviewed in [3]). The alternative pathway functions as an amplification loop for the classical and lectin pathway of activation, although the role of the lectin pathway has not been investigated in SCI. Also, complement fragment levels have been found to be elevated in sera of spinal cord injury patients [4]. In an experimental model, it has been shown that complement activation and the propagation of SCI can be caused by pathogenic autoantibodies that arise following SCI-mediated activation of B cells [5, 6]. However, the role of naturally occurring pre-existing self-reactive antibodies (nAbs) produced by innate B1 B cells, and how complement is activated acutely after SCI, has not been investigated. Since SCI shares some pathophysiological characteristics with ischemia reperfusion injury (IRI), and since IRI is driven by natural IgM Ab-mediated activation of complement in some organs [7–10], we investigated a role for natural IgM Abs in propagating SCI.

Tissue ischemia exposes neoepitopes known as damage-associated molecular patterns (DAMPs) on the cell surface, and these neoepitopes are recognized by circulating natural IgM Abs that subsequently activate complement [11]. Some of these post-ischemic neoepitopes have been identified in the context of IRI and include non-muscle myosin [8], annexin IV [9], and various phospholipids [10, 12]. However, the nature of the neoepitopes exposed as a result of trauma on the injured spinal cord has not been investigated. Natural IgM Abs differ from adaptive immune Abs in that they are germline encoded, arise without exogenous antigen stimulation, and are produced by the B1 subset of B cells. B1 cells differ from conventional B2 cells by their phenotype, self-renewing capacity, and production of natural Abs. Although most natural IgM Abs are polyreactive, the subsets that initiate IRI are unique in that they recognize a specific set of epitopes or patterns and, importantly, are specific for neoepitopes on stressed or injured cells. Here, we investigate a pathogenic role for natural IgM Abs in promoting spinal cord injury, but it is important to note that natural Abs also have important physiological roles, such as protection from pathogens and the removal of cellular and molecular waste [13, 14]. Indeed, a monoclonal IgM Ab corresponding to a natural Ab specificity is currently undergoing clinical evaluation as a potential therapeutic for multiple sclerosis [15, 16].

We previously isolated two natural IgM mAbs from unmanipulated mice, B4 mAb that recognizes annexin IV and C2 mAb that recognizes a subset of phospholipids, and demonstrated that these mAbs specifically bind to the intestine [9], brain [10], and heart [17] tissue following ischemia and reperfusion. In this study, we make use of these mAbs to investigate neoepitope expression post-SCI.

Methods

IgM mAbs and annexin IV purification

Hybridomas expressing B4 and C2 IgM mAbs were isolated after fusion of splenocytes from unmanipulated C57BL/6 mice with SP2/0-AG14 myeloma cells, with screening of hybridomas for specificity to apoptotic cells [9]. B4 mAb has been shown to recognize annexin IV [9] and C2 mAb to recognize a subset of phospholipids [10]. F632 and D5 IgM mAbs recognize 4-hydroxy-3-nitrophenylacetyl [17] and cytokeratin-19 [9], respectively, and were used as control mAbs. The D5 mAb was isolated from the same panel of hybridomas from which B4 and C2 mAbs were isolated, and does not bind to apoptotic cells. The IgM mAbs were purified from culture supernatant by affinity chromatography using an agarose bead column conjugated with goat anti-mouse IgM (Sigma-Aldrich, St Louis, MO) as described [17]. Recombinant annexin IV, the B4 ligand, was expressed in 293 F cells and purified from culture supernatant as described [9].

Injury model and treatments

Mice used in this study were female C57BL/6 mice and Rag1−/− mice on a C57BL/6 background, weighing between 18 and 22 g and between 6 and 8 weeks old, and obtained from Harlan Labs (Indianapolis, IN). Before the procedure, mice were anesthetized with ketamine/xylazine anesthesia (80 mg/kg/10 mg/kg, i.p.) and subjected to laminectomy T9-T12. Contusion injury was performed at T10 using an Infinite Horizon impactor (Precision Systems and Instrumentation, LLC, Lexington, Kentucky) at 80 Kdynes [18]. Sham control mice underwent laminectomy without contusion injury. Mice were kept on a temperature-controlled heating pad until the animals regained their mobility, after which they were placed back in a recovery cage on Alpha dri bedding. Mice were monitored, and bladders were voided twice daily until the bladder function was restored. For IgM mAb reconstitution experiments, Rag1−/− mice were randomized into different mAb treatment groups and a control group. Rag1−/− mice were injected i.v. with 100 μg C2, B4 or control mAbs 30 min after surgery. For therapeutic studies, animals were randomized into vehicle and B4Crry treatment groups and a single dose of 0.2 mg of protein was administered i.v. 30 min after injury. All procedures were approved by the Institutional Animal Care and Use Committee (IACUC) at the Medical University of South Carolina.

B1 B cell depletion

Peritoneal B1 cell depletion was achieved by a modification of the method described by Peterson et al. [19]. Briefly, starting at 4 weeks of age, mice were administered progressively increasing amounts of distilled water, injected i.p. once per week over a 6-week period (2 injections each of 0.2, 0.5, and 1 ml). One group of mice received PBS injections as control. One day after the final injection, mice were used for procedures. For analysis of B1 B cell depletion, peritoneal cells were obtained by injecting 5 ml of ice cold PBS into the peritoneal cavity, gently massaging the cavity, and collecting lavage fluid containing peritoneal cells using a 22-gauge needle. Single-cell suspensions of these cells were incubated with CD16/32 for 5 min at 4 °C to block Fc receptor binding [19] and were then analyzed by flow cytometry using flourochrome-conjugated Abs: anti-mouse CD19 APC and CD45R (B220) FITC (eBioscience, San Diego, CA). Gate was placed on live (7-Aminoactinomycin D viable stain) peritoneal cells, and $CD19^+$ IgM^{hi} $B220^{lo}$ populations were quantified.

Natural IgM levels in mouse serum

Blood was collected immediately following harvest of peritoneal cells, and serum prepared. Levels of anti-annexin IV and anti-phosphatidylcholine IgM Abs in mouse serum were quantified by ELISA using purified recombinant annexin IV (see above) and PC-BSA (Sigma) as capture reagents as previously described [10]. An ELISA kit was used to measure bound IgM in mouse serum according to the manufacturer's instructions (Bethyl Laboratories, Montgomery, TX).

Behavioral tests

Open-field assessment of locomotor function was done using the BMS scoring system with a scale of 0–9. The BMS scale is based on operational definitions of hind limb movement. Briefly, individual mice were simultaneously observed by two blinded investigators for a 4-min testing period, during which hind limb movements, trunk/tail stability, and forelimb-hind limb coordination were assessed and then graded according to published methods [20]. All mice subjected to contusion injury exhibited a BMS score of 0 immediately after injury. The grip walk test (also referred to as the foot fault task), modified from the grid walk/ladder rung walking task [21], assesses deficits in descending motor control and is a test of motor coordination [22]. The apparatus consists of a grid floor with the grid raised above the surface. Mice were placed at one end of the grid and monitored from the side as they walked across the grid. The number of hind limb grips instead of placement errors as the animal traverses the grid was scored. Each time the paw gripped the bar was counted and compared between different treatment groups. All analyses were performed by investigators blinded to the treatment groups.

Tissue histology

Spinal cord tissue obtained from mice at 72 h, 7 days, or 21 days after injury was fixed in 10% formalin and embedded in paraffin. Seven-micrometer transverse sections were cut using a microtome and stained with standard hematoxylin and eosin stains for stereological analysis. Photographic documentation was made using Axio Vision Software (Carl Zeiss) at the resolution of 1024 × 1024 pixels. The hemorrhaged area and lesional tissue area was outlined using the measure tool from axiovision (refer to Additional file 1: Figure S2), and the extent of hemorrhage and lesion expressed as percentage of the total area per section. This analysis was done using 100-μm step sections across the length of 1 mm starting at 100 μm from the epicenter on each side [22].

Immunohistochemistry and immunoflourescence

Spinal cord tissue was embedded in OCT on dry ice and frozen sections were fixed in acetone for 6 min, air dried, and then equilibrated in PBS. For paraffin sections, tissue was fixed in 10% formalin and processed by standard techniques. Deposition of the complement activation product, C3d, was detected using a goat anti-mouse C3d Ab (1:30, R&D Systems, Minneapolis, MN) with rabbit anti-goat IgG AlexaFluor-555 conjugate as secondary Ab (1:100, Invitrogen, Carlsbad, CA). IgM binding was detected using a goat anti-mouse IgM FITC conjugate (1:100, EMD Millipore, Billerica, Massachusetts). The images were taken using Olympus Fv10i Confocal microscope, images were processed using Adobe Photoshop CS6 software (Adobe System Inc., San Jose, CA, USA), and manipulations were limited to brightness/contrast functions.

ImageJ and Fiji plugin (NIH) were used for analysis of images for fluorescence intensity. The intensity was measured and averaged from 100-μm step sections across a length of 1 mm, centered at the epicenter and starting at 100 μm from the epicenter on each side.

Statistical analysis

Statistical differences between parametric data were assessed using one-way analysis of variance (ANOVA) test with Bonferroni's multi-group comparison, and non-parametric data were compared with the Kruskal-Wallis test with Dunn's comparison (Prism 5.0,

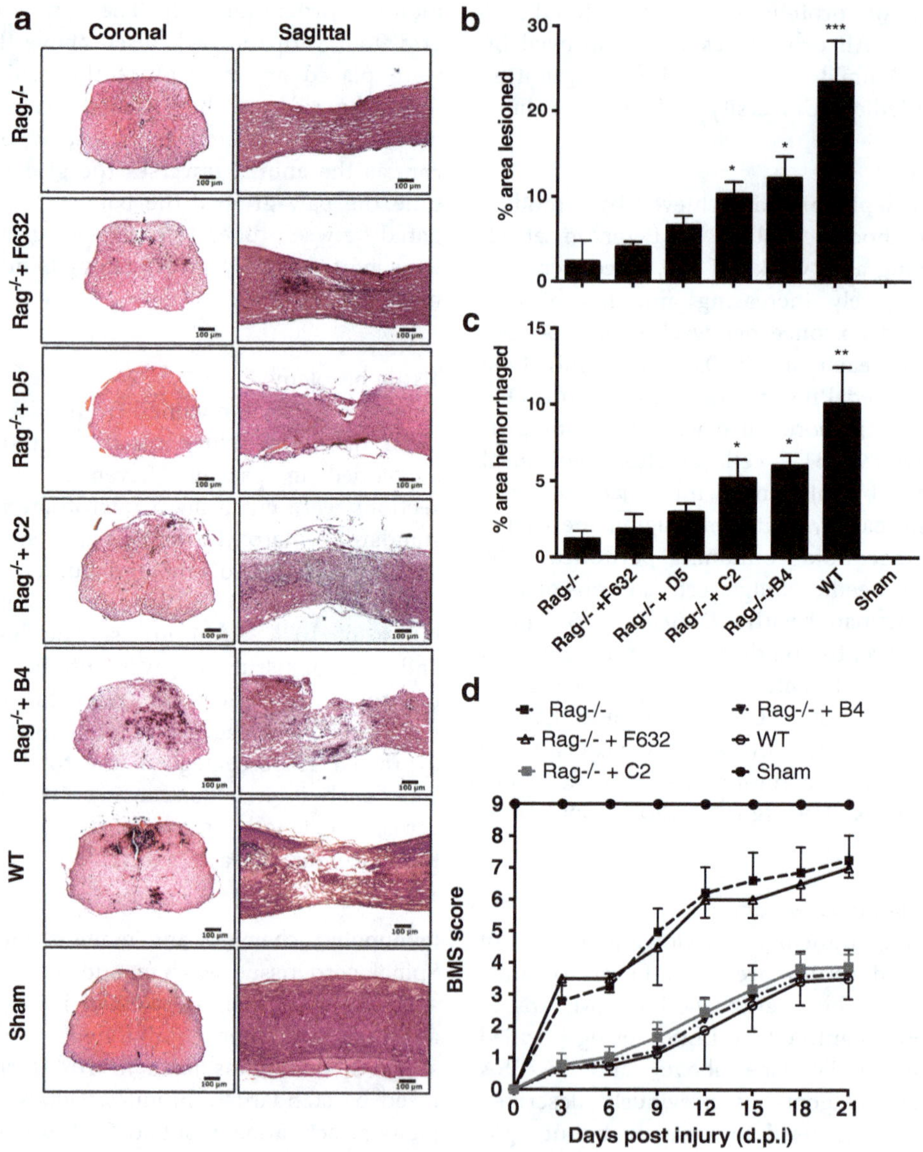

Fig. 1 Specific IgM mAbs restore injury in otherwise protected Rag1−/− mice. **a** Representative H&E stained coronal and sagittal sections of WT mice, Rag1−/− mice, and Rag1−/− mice reconstituted with indicated mAb. As quantified in subsequent panels, histopathology revealed Rag1−/− mice were protected from injury, B4 and C2 mAbs restored injury in Rag1−/− mice, and control F632 and D5 mAbs had no significant effect on injury in Rag1−/− mice. **b** Lesion size determined from step sections obtained across 1-mm distance from the epicenter and expressed as percentage of total area of each section analyzed. Mean ± SE, ***$p < 0.001$, **$p < 0.01$, *$p < 0.05$ represent comparisons to Rag1−/−, $n = 6$ per group. **c** Hemorrhaged area determined from step sections obtained across 1-mm distance from the epicenter and expressed as percentage of total area of each section analyzed, Mean ± SE, ** $p < 0.01$, *$p < 0.05$ represent comparisons to Rag1−/−, $n = 6$ per group. **d** Open field 10-point BMS score to assess functional recovery over a 21-day period after SCI. A score of 9 represents no impairment of locomotor activity. Groups consisted of WTC57/bl6 and Rag1−/− mice, and Rag1−/− mice reconstituted with indicated IgM mAb. Mean ± SE, *$p < 0.05$, $n = 6–8$. Starting at day 3, significant differences were seen between Rag1−/− mice and Rag1−/− mice treated with control mAb vs. WT mice and Rag1−/− mice reconstituted with B4 and C2 mAbs

GraphPad). Differences between data were considered statistically significant when $p < 0.05$.

Results

Specific IgM mAbs restore SCI in otherwise protected Rag1−/− mice

Recognition of ischemic tissue by natural self-reactive IgM promotes injury in various organs subsequent to reperfusion. To better understand the pathophysiology of inflammatory secondary damage following SCI, we investigated whether a similar IgM recognition system is involved in promoting secondary injury to the spinal cord after trauma. Antibody deficient Rag1−/− mice were protected from SCI, but injury outcomes worsened when Rag1−/− mice were injected with either B4 or C2 IgM mAb within 30 min of injury. We found

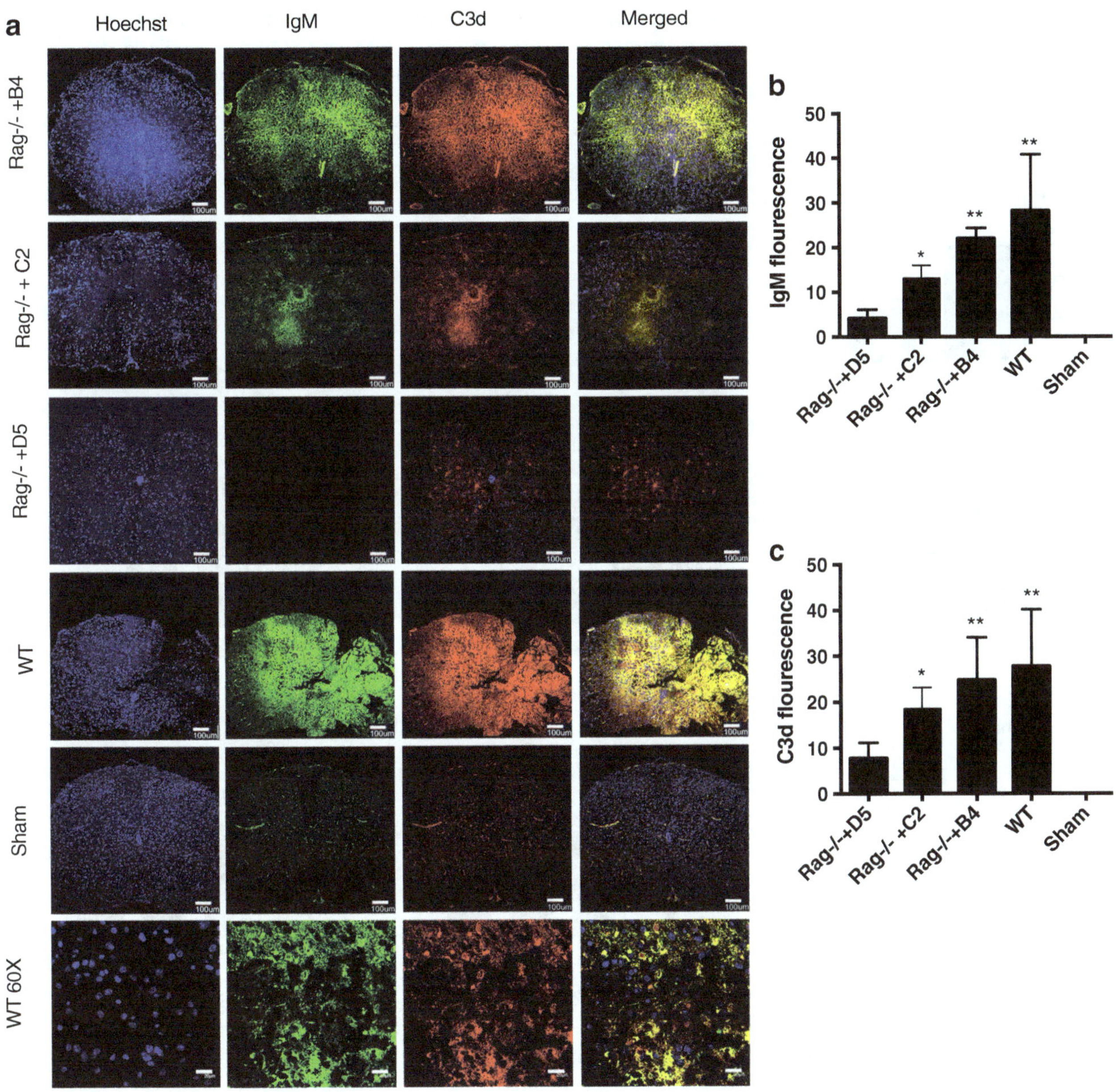

Fig. 2 IgM binding and C3 deposition in injured spinal cords of wt and B4 mAb reconstituted Rag1−/− mice. Coronal step sections were obtained up to 0.5 mm each side from epicenter of contusion injury, 72 h after SCI. **a** Analysis of IgM and C3d deposition in spinal cords isolated from wt mice or Rag1−/− mice reconstituted with either B4 mAb or D5 mAb (control). Composite image (merged) indicates co-localization. Bottom panel shows high mag images of injured WT spinal cord. **b**, **c** Quantification of IgM binding and C3d deposition was done by measuring intensity from step sections across the length of 1 mm, centered at the epicenter and starting at 100 μm from the epicenter on each side. Mean ± SE, $^{*}p < 0.05$, $^{**}p < 0.01$, $n = 6$ per group. Scale bar = 100 μm

significantly reduced lesion size and hemorrhaging at 3 days post-injury in Rag−/− mice after injury (Fig. 1a–c). Injection of specific natural Abs caused greater extent of injury in otherwise protected Rag−/− mice. Reconstitution of Rag1−/− mice with control F632 mAb or D5 mAb (Fig. 1a–c) did not alter outcome measures, demonstrating that the enhanced injury phenotype is neoepitope specific. We utilized one of these two specificities as controls for further studies. Compared to wild-type (wt) mice, Rag1−/− mice had significantly improved locomotor activity over a 21-day period post-injury (Fig. 1d). BMS measures in Rag1−/− mice were significantly worse upon reconstitution with B4 or C2 mAb, while injection of F632 mAb did not cause any significant changes.

Analysis of IgM binding and C3 deposition following SCI

Complement has been shown to play a key role in modulating the progression of SCI, and we investigated the specificity of B4 mAb binding to the injured spinal cord together with analysis of complement activation. Spinal cord sections obtained from wt mice at the lesion site 3 days post injury demonstrated co-localization of IgM and the complement activation fragment C3d (Fig. 2). Co-localization of IgM and C3d was similarly demonstrated in Rag1−/− mice reconstituted with B4 mAb, but not in

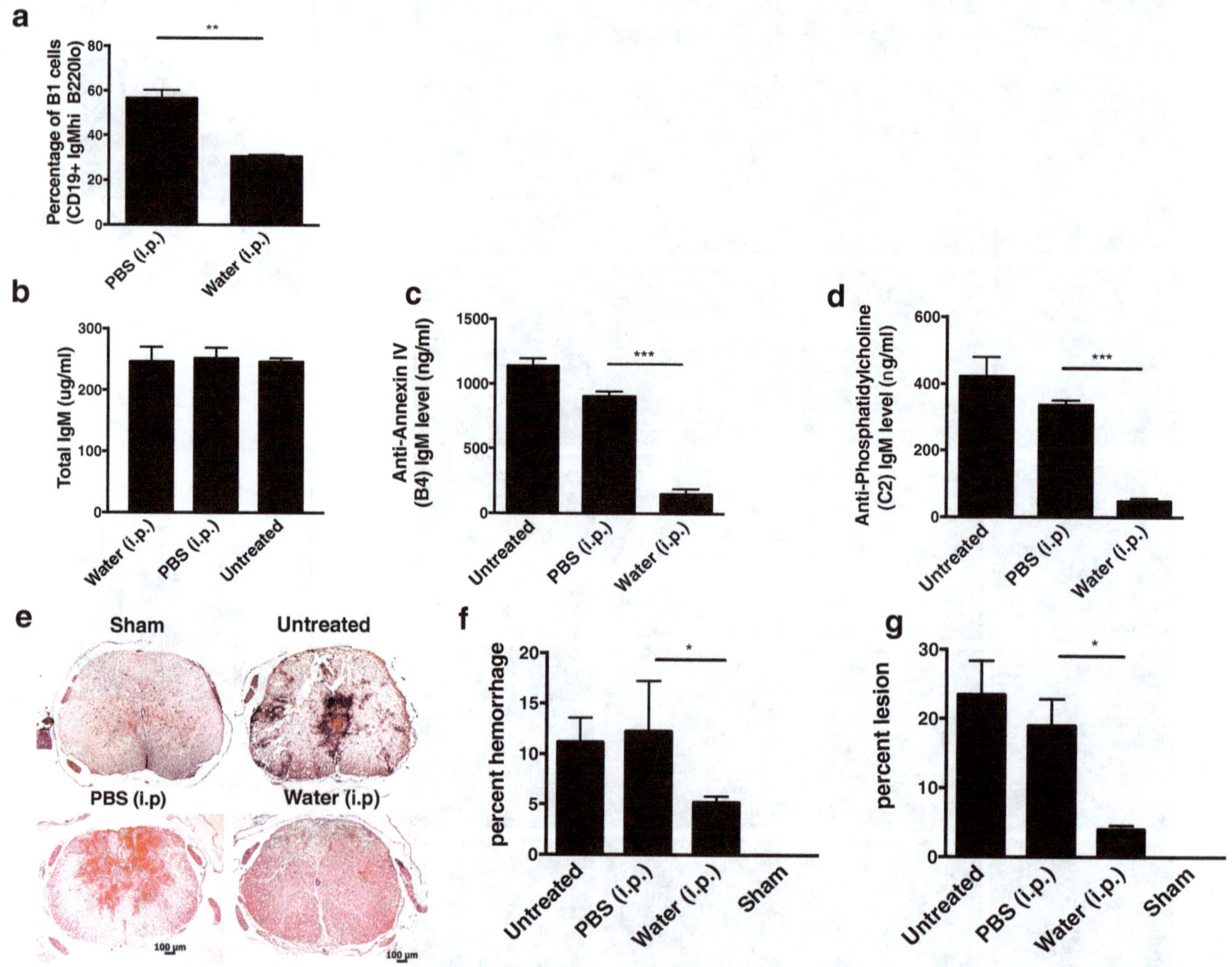

Fig. 3 B1 B cell depletion reduces circulating levels of neoepitope-specific natural IgM Abs and protects against SCI. **a** Quantification of B1a B cell depletion by flow cytometry analysis of peritoneal cells following a 6-week hypotonic shock procedure, demonstrating depletion of peritoneal B1 B cells ($B220^{lo}CD5^{+}$). Mean ± SE, *$p < 0.05$, $n = 3$, and data is representative of three separate experiments. **b–d** Analysis of serum levels of total IgM, specific natural IgM antibodies with B4 mAb reactivity (annexin-IV) and C2 reactivity (phosphatidylcholine), determined by ELISA. Serum from mice treated with peritoneal injections of either PBS or water, as well as serum from WT mice, was analyzed. Mean ± SE, *$p < 0.01$, $p < 0.001$ respectively, $n = 3$–5. **e** Following B1 cell depletion or a control procedure, WT mice were subjected to SCI, and spinal cords isolated 72 h later for analysis. **f**, **g** Hemorrhaged area and lesion size and from step sections obtained across 1-mm distance, 0.5 mm from each side of the epicenter, and expressed as percentage of total area of each section analyzed. *$p < 0.05$, **$p < 0.01$, ***$p < 0.001$, $n = 6$ animals per group

Rag1−/− mice reconstituted with control D5 mAb, correlating with the injury profiles shown above. Together with previous data showing an important role for complement in SCI, these results indicate specific IgM-mediated activation of complement is propagating injury.

Peritoneal B1 B cell depletion reduces levels of circulating pathogenic natural IgM antibodies and provides protection in the acute phase of injury

Natural IgM Abs are produced by innate like B1 B cells that are capable of self-renewal and are present in high numbers in the peritoneum. To confirm that the pathogenic effect in this model is mediated by natural Abs, we investigated the effect of peritoneal B1 B cell depletion on SCI in wt mice. B1 B cells were depleted using a hypotonic shock method involving intraperitoneal injection of water, and depletion was confirmed by flow cytometric analysis that demonstrated water treatment resulted in a significant reduction in $CD19^{+}$ $B220^{lo}$ peritoneal cells (Fig. 3a) (see also additional file Figure S2). As previously shown [19], peritoneal B cell depletion did not result in a reduction of total circulating IgM (Fig. 3b). However, peritoneal B1 B cell depletion did result in a significant decrease in circulating Abs of B4 and C2 specificities, further indicating the natural Ab status of anti-annexin IV and anti-phospholipid IgM mAbs (Fig. 3c, d). Analysis of spinal cord sections 3 days post injury revealed significantly less hemorrhaging in spinal cords from B1 B cell-depleted mice compared to controls, and this correlated with significantly less IgM and C3d deposition (Figs. 3f, g, Fig. 4). Taken together, the data demonstrate that SCI is propagated in large part by peritoneal-derived B cell natural IgM and its recognition of annexin IV and phospholipid neoepitopes in the injured spinal cord that subsequently activate complement. Further, the recognition of tissue and enhanced injury is neoepitope specific.

Targeting complement inhibition to IgM recognition sites in the injured spinal cord

On the basis of the above data and previous data showing both efficacy and safety benefits of site targeted

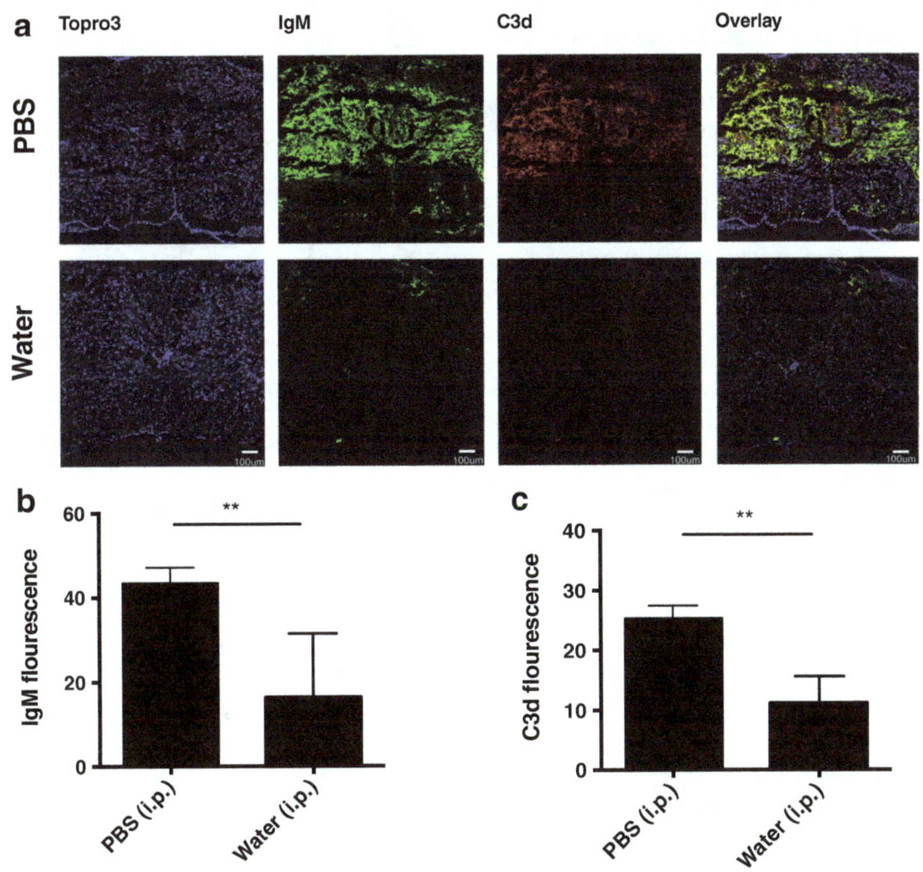

Fig. 4 B1 B cell depletion reduced IgM deposition and complement activation in the injured spinal cord. **a** Immunofluorescence images of IgM and C3d deposition in cords isolated from control and B1 B cell depleted mice. Coronal step sections (100 um) were obtained across 1 mm from epicenter of contusion injury, and intensity measured and averaged. Composite image (merged) indicates co-localization. Representative images, $n = 6$. **b**, **c** Quantification of IgM binding and C3d deposition, respectively. Mean ± SE, $^{**}p < 0.01$, $n = 6$

complement inhibition [17, 23], we investigated whether the B4 neoepitope is a therapeutic target for complement inhibition post-SCI. We recently described the construction and functional characterization of B4-Crry, a fusion protein consisting of a scFv derived from B4 mAb linked to the mouse complement inhibitor Crry [17]. Administration of B4-Crry to WT mice 30 min after SCI significantly improved locomotor activity compared to vehicle-treated mice, and locomotor functional activity was restored by day 21 in B4-Crry-treated mice (Fig. 5a). B4-Crry treatment also significantly improved performance on a grip walk test, indicating improved restoration of sensorimotor function (Fig. 5b). The percentage lesion area per section was averaged over step sections obtained across 1 mm around the epicenter. We found significant reduction in lesion size and hemorrhaged area with B4-Crry treatment (Fig. 6).

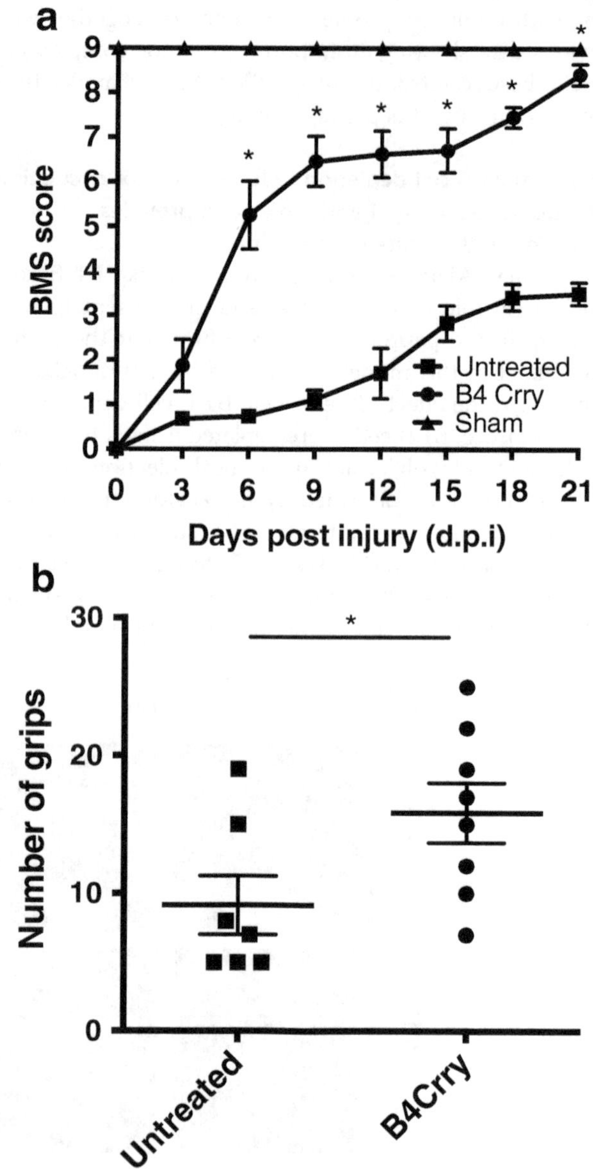

Fig. 5 Neoepitope-targeted complement inhibition with B4-Crry improves functional outcome after SCI. **a** Assessment of locomotor activity over a 21-day period post-SCI using the 10-point BMS scale. A score of 9 represents no impairment of locomotor activity. Groups consisted of untreated injured WT C57bl/6 mice and B4-Crry-treated mice. Mean ± SE, *$p < 0.001$, $n = 6–8$. **b** Grip Walk test performed at 21 days post-SCI. Groups as above. Mean ± SE, *$p < 0.05$, $n = 6–8$

Effect of B4-Crry on IgM deposition and complement activation in the injured spinal cord

Immunoflourescence microscopy of spinal cord sections demonstrated that B4-Crry reduced IgM binding and abolished C3d deposition at the injury epicenter (Fig. 7a), as well as rostrocaudally as indicated by analysis of longitudinal sections (Fig. 7b). Quantification of both IgM and C3d fluorescence signal suggested that the animals treated with B4Crry had significant decrease in both these signals 3 days post injury (Fig. 7c). These data indicate a dual functionality of B4-Crry in providing protection from SCI, since it not only blocks complement activation, but also inhibits the binding of endogenous pathogenic self-reactive IgM in the context of a full natural Ab repertoire.

Discussion

Natural Abs are present from birth and are germline encoded without a requirement for exogenous antigen exposure, and it is increasingly recognized that subsets of natural Abs have varying and distinct roles. Natural IgM Abs can have homeostatic roles, for example by recognizing DAMPs expressed on stressed or dying cells and facilitating their clearance, and they can serve protective roles by a variety of cellular mechanisms [13]. However, they can also have pathogenic roles as has been shown in models of ischemia and reperfusion injury where pathogenic levels of IgM bind to ischemic tissue and activate complement [11].

It has been shown previously that following murine SCI, B cells become activated and produce pathogenic autoantibodies that propagate secondary injury in the spinal cord and impair recovery. Precisely, how traumatic injury to the spinal cord results in B cell dysfunction and autoantibody production is not clear, but pathology is caused, at least in part, via complement activation and Fc receptor ligation [6]. However, while there is accumulating evidence that B cell activation and autoantibody production play an important role in propagating SCI (reviewed in [24]), the mechanisms by which secondary spinal injury is initiated and therein the functional significance of self-reactive natural IgM Abs (as opposed to autoreactive Abs resulting from a pathogenic adaptive immune response) in this process have

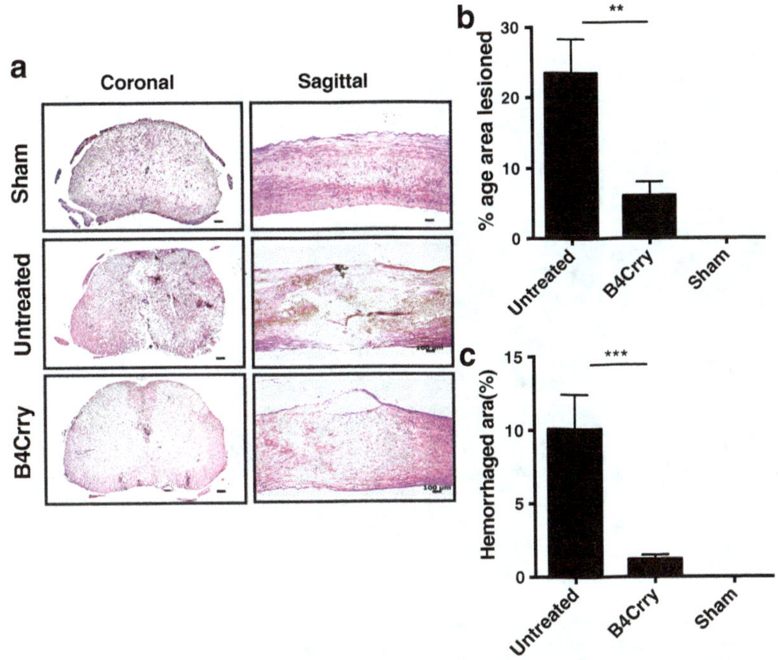

Fig. 6 Histopathology of spinal cords from B4-Crry treated showed reduced spread of lesion 72 h after SCI. **a** H&E stained coronal and sagittal sections from epicenter of contusion injury after B4-Crry or PBS treatment. Representative images, $n = 6$. **b**, **c** Quantification of lesion and hemorrhage. Lesion size and hemorrhaged area were determined from step sections obtained across 1-mm distance from the epicenter and expressed as percentage of total area of each section analyzed. Mean ± SE, $^{**}p < 0.01$, $^{***}p < 0.001$, $n = 6$.

not been investigated. Here, we show a role for a specific subset of natural IgM Abs in activating complement and propagating secondary injury after trauma to the spinal cord and show that SCI mimics the pathological paradigm of IgM-mediated IRI in other tissues. Thus, in addition to a role for an adaptive autoantibody response in contributing to post-SCI pathology, we demonstrate a role for pre-formed self-reactive IgM Abs in an innate immune response to SCI.

Identification of the human counterpart of murine B1 B cells has been controversial, partly because CD5 is an activation marker on human B cells. However, studies have identified $CD20^+CD27^+CD43^+$ B cells as the human B1 cell equivalent [25, 26]. Although B1 cells had been thought to be located predominantly in the peritoneal and pleural cavities of mice, recent evidence indicates that the bone marrow and spleen may be an important source [27]. Nevertheless, the current study indicates that peritoneal B1 cell-derived natural IgM plays an important role in propagating SCI, since peritoneal depletion of B1 B cells both significantly reduced levels of circulating pathogenic IgM of B4 and C2 specificity and significantly improved recovery. Both our data and previous studies have shown that these B1 depletion procedures do not alter total IgM levels [28]. Together, these data suggest a role for distinct subsets of naturally occurring IgM Abs and raise the possibility of different Ab repertoires originating from different B1 cell locations.

The B4 and C2 IgM mAbs that we utilize in this study have been previously described: B4 recognizes a post-translational modification of annexin IV [9] and C2 recognizes a subset of phospholipids [10].The natural Ab status of these mAbs is indicated by the fact that they were derived from unmanipulated mice, they are universally present in C57BL/6 mice, and the circulatory levels of IgM Abs of B4 and C2 specificity are reduced following peritoneal B1 cell depletion. Also, natural IgM Ab recognition of neoepitopes is the accepted paradigm for complement activation following ischemia and reperfusion of other tissues. We show here that the B4 and C2 antigens represent DAMPs expressed in the injured spinal cord. Injury was contingent upon specific recognition of the injured spinal cord, since unlike B4 and C2 mAbs, control IgM mAbs, including one that was isolated from the same panel containing the B4 and C2 mAbs, neither bound within the injured spinal cord nor reconstituted injury in otherwise protected Ab-deficient Rag1−/− mice. In an earlier report, Rag2−/− mice were shown to have improved recovery following spinal cord contusion compared to wt mice, with improved locomotor function and increased axonal regrowth [29]. Improved recovery in Rag2−/− mice was associated with decreased

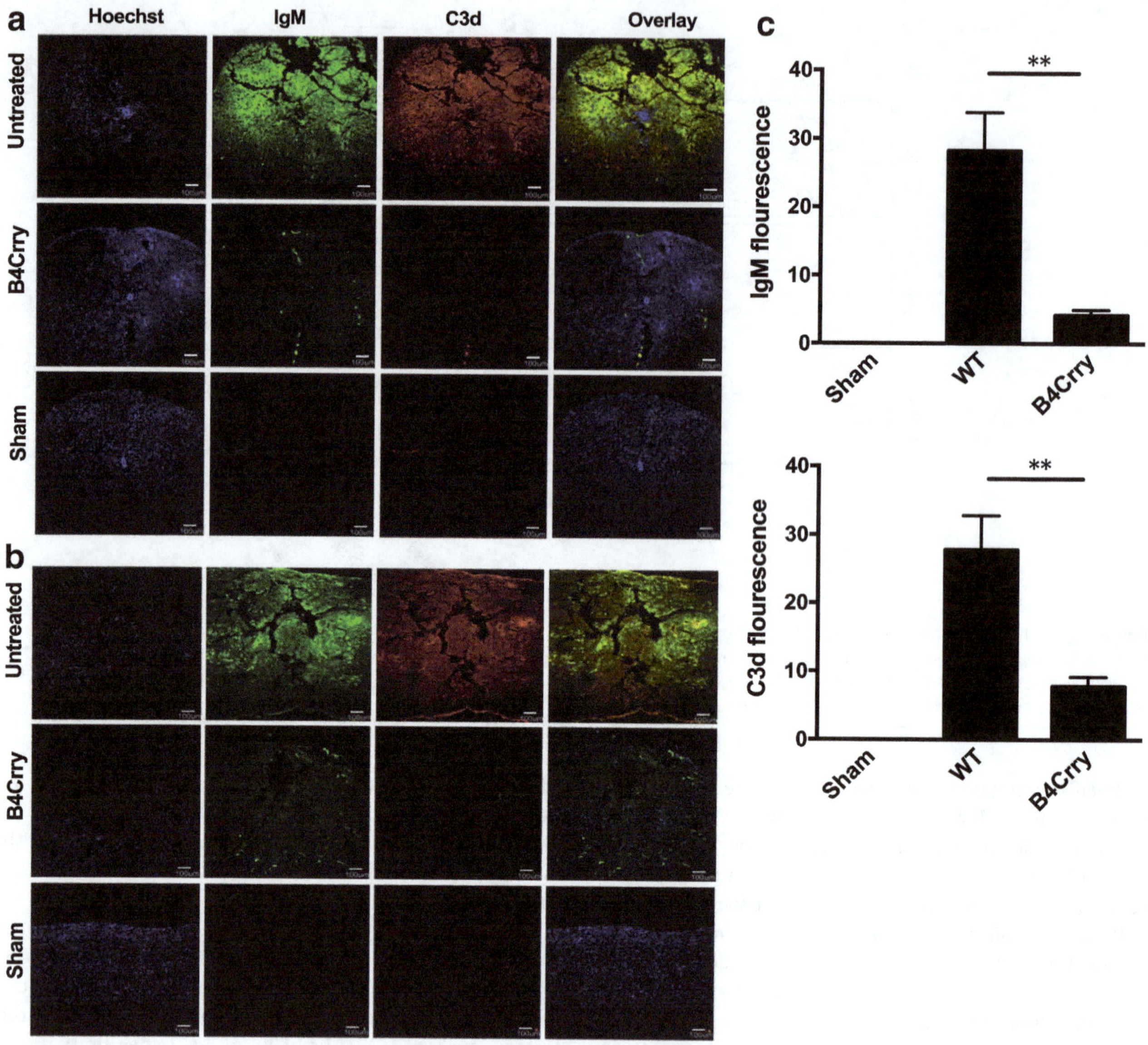

Fig. 7 B4-Crry treatment reduces both IgM binding and C3d deposition after SCI. Analysis of of IgM and C3d deposition in vehicle treated, B4-Crry treated, and in sham operated animals at 72 h after SCI. Composite image (merged) indicates co-localization. **a** Representative coronal sections from epicenter of contusion injury. **b** Representative sagittal sections showing rostrocaudal deposition. **c** Quantification of C3d and IgM fluorescence. Quantification of IgM binding and C3d deposition was done by measuring intensity from step sections across the length of 1 mm, centered at the epicenter and starting at 100 μm from the epicenter on each side

microglia/macrophage infiltration, which the authors attributed to the absence of T cell-derived cytokines. Certainly, this could be a contributing mechanism of injury, besides the critical role for natural Abs in activating complement and initiating injury.

It is interesting that specific natural IgM Abs are also implicated in CNS repair mechanisms, beyond their role in identifying injured and dying cells for removal, and some IgM mAbs have shown potential for therapeutic application following CNS injury (reviewed in [16]). These protective Abs appear to function by providing intracellular signals that promote neuron or glial cell survival. The mechanistic relationship between pathogenic and protective natural Abs is not clear. There may be quantitative and/or qualitative, as well as temporally acting or context-dependent differences between Abs that are involved in injury vs. repair. It is also noteworthy that complement activation products can have both neurodegenerative and neuroregenerative effects following CNS injury [30, 31]. While complement-mediated protective mechanisms likely become more important in the subacute phase after CNS injury [32], this balance between complement-mediated injury and repair is an area in need of further investigation.

Based on the identification of neoepitopes exposed in the injured spinal cord and the pathogenic and complement-activating properties of mAbs recognizing these neoepitopes, we investigated a site-targeted therapeutic strategy for the local delivery of a complement inhibitor. Site-targeted complement inhibition obviates the need for systemic inhibition, increases bioavailability, and markedly increases efficacy (over 10-fold) [23]. We have also shown previously that unlike systemic inhibitors, therapeutic doses of site-targeted complement inhibitors do not adversely affect important physiological functions such as host defense [17, 23]. This latter point is an important consideration for the treatment of SCI patients, since CNS injury is immunosupressive and there is a high incidence of morbidity and mortality caused by infection in neurotrauma and SCI patients.

In our therapeutic paradigm, we used our recently described fusion protein consisting of a single chain (scFv) derived from the B4 hybridoma linked to Crry, a murine orthologue of human sCR1 [17]. In our previous report, we also demonstrated that B4-Crry does not increase susceptibility to infection [23, 33]. Here, the protective effect of B4-Crry correlated not only with significantly reduced complement activation, but also reduced IgM deposition at the injury site. This indicates that in addition to complement inhibition, B4-Crry is inhibiting the binding of IgM Abs to the injured spinal cord in the context of a full natural Ab repertoire. This could be due to B4 scFv competing for IgM binding sites, but also due to decreased complement-mediated injury with a reduction in the associated exposure of neoepitopes. While it can be expected that there is much redundancy in IgM and neoepitope specificities, we have nonetheless shown that B4 scFv alone can significantly reduce IgM binding in the post-ischemic heart [17]. A possible explanation for this effect of a single scFv specificity on overall IgM binding is that there is a requirement for recognition of exposed neoepitopes in a chronological sequence, such that disrupting any one of these interactions ameliorates complement activation. Another possibility is that recognition of these neoepitopes on multiple cell types is critical for complement dependent injury, and blocking even one of these specificities is consequential for the overall complement mediated injury response.

Conclusions

This study identifies important neoepitopes expressed within the spinal cord after injury, that are recognized by clonally specific natural IgM Abs that activate complement and drive secondary injury. Peritoneal B1 cells are a source of a subset of pathogenic self-reactive Abs that contribute to pathology by activating complement. Post-SCI expressed neoepitopes represent novel targets for the targeted delivery of therapeutics to the injured spinal cord, and we show that targeted delivery of a complement inhibitor significantly improves recovery following trauma to the spinal cord. With regard to the potential translation of this therapeutic strategy to the clinic, it has been shown that the B4 annexin IV neoepitope is also expressed on stressed and injured human cells [10]. Therefore, this antibody based targeting strategy presents a new therapeutic payload delivery option in an injury site specific manner.

Additional file

Additional file 1: Figure S1. (A) Spinal cord tissue analyses were done across the length of 1 mm centered at the epicenter (B). Examples of hemorrhaged (red) and lesioned (gray) area are outlined. The outlined area for each section measured using a Nikon eclipse E600 with axiovision outline tool and was expressed as a percentage of total area of each section measured. **Figure S2.** (A) After B1 cell depletion procedure, the peritoneal fluid was analyzed by flow cytometry to confirm a decrease in $CD19^{+}IgM^{hi}B220^{lo}$ populations. Initial gate was placed on live cells and viability determined by 7-AAD (7-Aminoactinomycin D) staining followed by gating on CD19+ and IgMhi cells. The $B220^{lo}$ subpopulation from the gated population was used for comparison among different groups (B). The mice that received PBS injections as control were used for these analyses. $n = 6$.

Abbreviations

Ab: Antibody; IRI: Ischemia reperfusion injury; mAb: Monoclonal antibody; scFv: Single-chain antibody; SCI: Spinal cord injury

Acknowledgements

We gratefully acknowledge Dr. Bei Liu, Medical University of South Carolina, for her assistance with flow cytometry analysis.

Funding

This work was supported by grants from the Department of Veterans Affairs (Merit Award 1I01RX001141 and 1BX001218), the National Institutes of Health (DK102912 and CA158179), and the South Carolina Spinal Cord Injury Research Fund.

Authors' contributions

AN performed experiments, analyzed data, and drafted the manuscript. FQ and XY performed experiments and analyzed data, CA analyzed data, HZ performed experiments, and LK and VMH provided reagents and edited the manuscript. ST conceived and planned the study, analyzed data, and drafted the manuscript. All authors read and approved the final manuscript.

Competing interests

Tomlinson, Atkinson, Kulik and Holers have a patent pending for targeted delivery of complement inhibitors to post-ischemic neoepitopes. The authors Aarti Narang,Fei Qiao,Hong Zhu and Xiao Feng Yang do not have any competing interests.

Consent for publication

Not applicable.

Author details

[1]Department of Microbiology and Immunology, Medical University of South Carolina, 173 Ashley Ave, CRI 213, Charleston, SC 29425, USA. [2]Departments of Medicine and Immunology, University of Colorado School of Medicine, Denver, CO, USA. [3]Ralph H Johnson VA Medical Center, Charleston, SC, USA.

References

1. Anderson AJ, Robert S, Huang W, Young W, Cotman CW. Activation of complement pathways after contusion-induced spinal cord injury. J Neurotrauma. 2004;21:1831–46.
2. Qiao F, Atkinson C, Kindy MS, Shunmugavel A, Morgan BP, Song H, Tomlinson S. The alternative and terminal pathways of complement mediate post-traumatic spinal cord inflammation and injury. Am J Pathol. 2010;177:3061–70.
3. Peterson SL, Anderson AJ. Complement and spinal cord injury: traditional and non-traditional aspects of complement cascade function in the injured spinal cord microenvironment. Exp Neurol. 2014;258:35–47.
4. Rebhun J, Madorsky JG, Glovsky MM. Proteins of the complement system and acute phase reactants in sera of patients with spinal cord injury. Ann Allergy. 1991;66:335–8.
5. Ankeny DP, Lucin KM, Sanders VM, McGaughy VM, Popovich PG. Spinal cord injury triggers systemic autoimmunity: evidence for chronic B lymphocyte activation and lupus-like autoantibody synthesis. J Neurochem. 2006;99:1073–87.
6. Ankeny DP, Guan Z, Popovich PG. B cells produce pathogenic antibodies and impair recovery after spinal cord injury in mice. J Clin Invest. 2009;119:2990–9.
7. Chan RK, Ibrahim SI, Verna N, Carroll M, Moore Jr FD, Hechtman HB. Ischaemia-reperfusion is an event triggered by immune complexes and complement. Br J Surg. 2003;90:1470–8.
8. Zhang M, Austen Jr WG, Chiu I, Alicot EM, Hung R, Ma M, Verna N, Xu M, Hechtman HB, Moore Jr FD, Carroll MC. Identification of a specific self-reactive IgM antibody that initiates intestinal ischemia/reperfusion injury. Proc Natl Acad Sci U S A. 2004;101:3886–91.
9. Kulik L, Fleming SD, Moratz C, Reuter JW, Novikov A, Chen K, Andrews KA, Markaryan A, Quigg RJ, Silverman GJ, et al. Pathogenic natural antibodies recognizing annexin IV are required to develop intestinal ischemia-reperfusion injury. J Immunol. 2009;182:5363–73.
10. Elvington A, Atkinson C, Kulik L, Zhu H, Yu J, Kindy MS, Holers VM, Tomlinson S. Pathogenic natural antibodies propagate cerebral injury following ischemic stroke in mice. J Immunol. 2012;188:1460–8.
11. Fleming SD. Naturally occurring autoantibodies mediate ischemia/reperfusion-induced tissue injury. Adv Exp Med Biol. 2012;750:174–85.
12. Fleming SD, Egan RP, Chai C, Girardi G, Holers VM, Salmon J, Monestier M, Tsokos GC. Anti-phospholipid antibodies restore mesenteric ischemia/reperfusion-induced injury in complement receptor 2/complement receptor 1-deficient mice. J Immunol. 2004;173:7055–61.
13. Gronwall C, Silverman GJ. Natural IgM: beneficial autoantibodies for the control of inflammatory and autoimmune disease. J Clin Immunol. 2014;34 Suppl 1:S12–21.
14. Panda S, Ding JL. Natural antibodies bridge innate and adaptive immunity. J Immunol. 2015;194:13–20.
15. Leslie M. Cleanup crew. Science. 2005;347:1058–9. 1061.
16. Wootla B, Watzlawik JO, Warrington AE, Wittenberg NJ, Denic A, Xu X, Jordan LR, Papke LM, Zoecklein LJ, Pierce ML, et al. Naturally occurring monoclonal antibodies and their therapeutic potential for neurologic diseases. JAMA Neurol. 2015;72:1346–53.
17. Atkinson C, Qiao F, Yang X, Zhu P, Reaves N, Kulik L, Goddard M, Holers VM, Tomlinson S. Targeting pathogenic postischemic self-recognition by natural IgM to protect against posttransplantation cardiac reperfusion injury. Circulation. 2015;131:1171–80.
18. Lee JH, Streijger F, Tigchelaar S, Maloon M, Liu J, Tetzlaff W, Kwon BK. A contusive model of unilateral cervical spinal cord injury using the infinite horizon impactor. J Vis Exp. 2012;65:3313.
19. Peterson LK, Tsunoda I, Fujinami RS. Role of CD5+ B-1 cells in EAE pathogenesis. Autoimmunity. 2008;41:353–62.
20. Pajoohesh-Ganji A, Byrnes KR, Fatemi G, Faden AI. A combined scoring method to assess behavioral recovery after mouse spinal cord injury. Neurosci Res. 2010;67:117–125.
21. Metz GA, Whishaw IQ. The ladder rung walking task: a scoring system and its practical application. J Vis Exp. 2009;28:1204.
22. Yu CG, Geddes JW. Sustained calpain inhibition improves locomotor function and tissue sparing following contusive spinal cord injury. Neurochem Res. 2007;32:2046–53.
23. Atkinson C, Song H, Lu B, Qiao F, Burns TA, Holers VM, Tsokos GC, Tomlinson S. Targeted complement inhibition by C3d recognition ameliorates tissue injury without apparent increase in susceptibility to infection. J Clin Invest. 2005;115:2444–53.
24. Zhang Y, Popovich P. Roles of autoantibodies in central nervous system injury. Discov Med. 2011;11:395–402.
25. Griffin DO, Holodick NE, Rothstein TL. Human B1 cells in umbilical cord and adult peripheral blood express the novel phenotype CD20+ CD27+ CD43+ CD70. J Exp Med. 2011;208:67–80.
26. Covens K, Verbinnen B, Geukens N, Meyts I, Schuit F, Van Lommel L, Jacquemin M, Bossuyt X. Characterization of proposed human B-1 cells reveals pre-plasmablast phenotype. Blood. 2013;121:5176–83.
27. Savage HP, Baumgarth N. Characteristics of natural antibody-secreting cells. Ann N Y Acad Sci. 2015;1362:132–42.
28. Renner B, Strassheim D, Amura CR, Kulik L, Ljubanovic D, Glogowska MJ, Takahashi K, Carroll MC, Holers VM, Thurman JM. B Cell Subsets Contribute to Renal Injury and Renal Protection after Ischemia/Reperfusion. J Immunol. 2010;185(7):4393–400.
29. Wu B, Matic D, Djogo N, Szpotowicz E, Schachner M, Jakovcevski I. Improved regeneration after spinal cord injury in mice lacking functional T- and B-lymphocytes. Exp Neurol. 2012;237:274–85.
30. Yanamadala V, Friedlander RM. Complement in neuroprotection and neurodegeneration. Trends Mol Med. 2010;16:69–76.
31. Alexander JJ, Anderson AJ, Barnum SR, Stevens B, Tenner AJ. The complement cascade: Yin-Yang in neuroinflammation—neuro-protection and -degeneration. J Neurochem. 2008;107:1169–87.
32. Alawieh A, Elvington A, Tomlinson S. Complement in the homeostatic and ischemic brain. Front Immunol. 2015;6:417.
33. Yanamadala V, Friedlander RM: Complement in neuroprotection and neurodegeneration. Trends in molecular medicine. 2010;16:69–76.

Permissions

All chapters in this book were first published in JNI, by BioMed Central; hereby published with permission under the Creative Commons Attribution License or equivalent. Every chapter published in this book has been scrutinized by our experts. Their significance has been extensively debated. The topics covered herein carry significant findings which will fuel the growth of the discipline. They may even be implemented as practical applications or may be referred to as a beginning point for another development.

The contributors of this book come from diverse backgrounds, making this book a truly international effort. This book will bring forth new frontiers with its revolutionizing research information and detailed analysis of the nascent developments around the world.

We would like to thank all the contributing authors for lending their expertise to make the book truly unique. They have played a crucial role in the development of this book. Without their invaluable contributions this book wouldn't have been possible. They have made vital efforts to compile up to date information on the varied aspects of this subject to make this book a valuable addition to the collection of many professionals and students.

This book was conceptualized with the vision of imparting up-to-date information and advanced data in this field. To ensure the same, a matchless editorial board was set up. Every individual on the board went through rigorous rounds of assessment to prove their worth. After which they invested a large part of their time researching and compiling the most relevant data for our readers.

The editorial board has been involved in producing this book since its inception. They have spent rigorous hours researching and exploring the diverse topics which have resulted in the successful publishing of this book. They have passed on their knowledge of decades through this book. To expedite this challenging task, the publisher supported the team at every step. A small team of assistant editors was also appointed to further simplify the editing procedure and attain best results for the readers.

Apart from the editorial board, the designing team has also invested a significant amount of their time in understanding the subject and creating the most relevant covers. They scrutinized every image to scout for the most suitable representation of the subject and create an appropriate cover for the book.

The publishing team has been an ardent support to the editorial, designing and production team. Their endless efforts to recruit the best for this project, has resulted in the accomplishment of this book. They are a veteran in the field of academics and their pool of knowledge is as vast as their experience in printing. Their expertise and guidance has proved useful at every step. Their uncompromising quality standards have made this book an exceptional effort. Their encouragement from time to time has been an inspiration for everyone.

The publisher and the editorial board hope that this book will prove to be a valuable piece of knowledge for researchers, students, practitioners and scholars across the globe.

List of Contributors

Alex P. Di Battista, Shawn G. Rhind, Syed Hassan and Maria Y. Shiu
Defence Research & Development Canada, Toronto Research Centre, Toronto, ON, Canada

Andrew J. Baker
Institute of Medical Science, University of Toronto, Toronto, ON, Canada
Department of Surgery, St. Michael's Hospital, University of Toronto, Toronto, ON, Canada

Michael G. Hutchison
Faculty of Kinesiology & Physical Education, University of Toronto, Toronto, ON, Canada

Jane Topolovec-Vranic
Keenan Research Centre, Li Ka Shing Knowledge Institute, St. Michael's Hopsital, Toronto, ON, Canada

Kenji Inaba
Division of Trauma & Critical Care, University of Southern California, Los Angeles, CA, USA
LA County+ USC Medical Center, Los Angeles, CA, USA

Sandro B. Rizoli
Department of Critical Care, St. Michael's Hospital, University of Toronto, Toronto, ON, Canada
Department of Anesthesia, St. Michael's Hospital, University of Toronto, Toronto, ON, Canada
Department of Surgery, St. Michael's Hospital, University of Toronto, Toronto, ON, Canada

Antonio Capone Neto
Institute for Healthcare Improvement (IHI) Fellow, Cambridge, MA, USA

Xiaosong He, Xiaohong Lin and Dahong Long
Key Laboratory of Neuroscience, the Second Affiliated Hospital Guangzhou Medical University, Guangzhou, China
Department of Anatomy, School of Basic Medical Science, Guangzhou Medical University, Guangzhou, China

Yanqun Liu
Department of Neurology, Changhai Hospital, Naval Military Medical University, Shanghai, China

Falei Yuan
Hailisheng Biomarine Research Institute, Zhoushan, China

Zhijun Zhang and Yongting Wang
Neuroscience and Neuroengineering Research Center, Med-X Research Institute and School of Biomedical Engineering, Shanghai Jiao Tong University, Shanghai, China

Guo-Yuan Yang
Department of Neurology, Ruijin Hospital, School of Medicine, Shanghai Jiao Tong University, Shanghai, China
Med-X Research Institute and School of Biomedical Engineering, 1954 Hua-shan Road, Shanghai 200030, China

Aiguo Xuan
Department of Anatomy, Guangzhou Medical college, Guangzhou 511546, China

Dulguun Batbold and Satoshi Yamaguchi
Department of Oral and Maxillofacial Surgery, Graduate School of Medical and Dental Sciences, Tokyo Medical and Dental University, 1-5-45 Yushima, Bunkyo-ku, Tokyo 113-8549, Japan

Masamichi Shinoda, Kuniya Honda and Koichi Iwata
Department of Physiology, School of Dentistry, Nihon University, 1-8-13 Kandasurugadai, Chiyoda-ku, Tokyo 101-8310, Japan

Akihiko Furukawa and Ryuta Akasaka
Department of Clinical Medicine, School of Dentistry, Nihon University, 1-8-13 Kandasurugadai, Chiyoda-ku, Tokyo 101-8310, Japan

Momoko Koizumi
Department of Dentistry, Jikei University School of Medicine, 3-25-8 Nishi-Shimbashi, Minato-ku, Tokyo 105-8461, Japan

Nicole M. Smith, Charlotte Bailey and K. Swaminathan Iyer
School of Molecular Sciences, The University of Western Australia, Stirling Hwy, Perth, Western Australia 6009, Australia

Marcus K. Giacci, Alexander Gough and Sarah A. Dunlop
Experimental and Regenerative Neurosciences, School of Biological Sciences, The University of Western Australia, Stirling Hwy, Perth, Western Australia 6009, Australia

Terence McGonigle, Anna M. B. Black, Thomas O. Clarke and Carole A. Bartlett
Curtin Health Innovation Research Institute, Curtin University, Verdun St, Nedlands, Western Australia, Australia

Melinda Fitzgerald
Perron Institute for Neurological and Translational Science, Sarich Neuroscience Research Institute, Verdun St, Nedlands, Western Australia 6009, Australia

Denis Grandgirard, Michelle Buri, Michael Perny and Stephen L. Leib
Neuroinfection Laboratory, Institute for Infectious Diseases, University of Bern, Friedbühlstrasse 51, 3001 Bern, Switzerland

Lukas Muri
Graduate School for Cellular and Biomedical Sciences (GCB), University of Bern, Freiestrasse 1, 3012 Bern, Switzerland

Fan Liu, Zhiyao Wang, Chunyan Li, Yikuan Xie and Chao Ma
Department of Human Anatomy, Histology and Embryology, Institute of Basic Medical Sciences, Chinese Academy of Medical Sciences, School of Basic Medicine, Peking Union Medical College, Beijing 100005, China

Yue Qiu, Min Wei, Le Shen and Yuguang Huang
Department of Anesthesiology, Peking Union Medical College Hospital, Chinese Academy of Medical Sciences, Peking Union Medical College, Beijing 100730, China

Yue Zhou, Zhenjie Zhu, Yuming Hu and Aisong Guo
Department of Rehabilitation Medicine, Affiliated Hospital of Nantong University, Nantong 226001, People's Republic of China

Yingjie Wang, Xuejie Zhang, Wenjuan Wang, Nan Du, Tiancheng Song and Yongjun Wang
Key Laboratory of Neuroregeneration of Jiangsu and Ministry of Education, Co-innovation Center of Neuroregeneration, Nantong University, Nantong 226001, People's Republic of China

Wei Guo
School of Basic Medical Sciences, Nanjing Medical University, Nanjing, People's Republic of China

Kaini Yang and Zongyu Guan
Medical College, Nantong University, Nantong 226001, People's Republic of China

Anna Badner, Justin Hacker, James Hong, Mirriam Mikhail and Reaz Vawda
Division of Genetics and Development, Krembil Research Institute, University Health Network, 60 Leonard Ave, Toronto, Ontario M5T 2S8, Canada
Institute of Medical Science, University of Toronto, 1 King's College Circle, Toronto, Ontario M5S 1A8, Canada

Michael G. Fehlings
Division of Neurosurgery, Toronto Western Hospital, 399 Bathurst St. Suite 4WW-449, Toronto, Ontario M5T 2S8, Canada

Jing Chang, Yue Huang, Meihau Cai and Mazhong Zhang
Department of Anesthesiology and Pediatric Clinical Pharmacology Laboratory, Shanghai Children's Medical Center, Shanghai Jiao Tong University School of Medicine, 1678 Dongfang Road, 200127 Shanghai, China

Xingrui Gong
Department of Anesthesiology, Shiyan Taihe Hospital (Affiliated Hospital of Hubei University of Medicine), Shiyan, Hubei, China

Michael G. Edwards
Bioinfo Solutions LLC, Parker, CO, USA

Yongmei Chen
Department of Laboratory, Shiyan Taihe Hospital (Affiliated Hospital of Hubei University of Medicine), Shiyan, Hubei, China

Joy E. Tomlinson, Emilija Žygelytė, Jennifer K. Grenier and Jonathan Cheetham
Cornell University College of Veterinary Medicine, Ithaca, NY, USA

Yuanyuan Ma, Liping Wang and Zhen Jiang
Department of Neurology, Ruijin Hospital, School of Medicine, Shanghai Jiao Tong University, Shanghai 200025, China

Yaning Li, Lu Jiang, Yongting Wang and Zhijun Zhang
Neuroscience and Neuroengineering Research Center, Med-X Research Institute and School of Biomedical Engineering, Shanghai Jiao Tong University, 1954 Hua Shan Road, Shanghai 200030, China

Fu-yi Liu, Jing Cai, Chun Wang, Wu Ruan, Guo-ping Guan, Hai-zhou Pan, Jian-ru Li, Cong Qian, Jing-sen Chen, Lin Wang and Gao Chen
Department of Neurosurgery, The Second Affiliated Hospital of Zhejiang University School of Medicine, Hangzhou, China

Jane A. Lindborg, Jon P. Niemi, Madeline A. Howarth, Kevin W. Liu, Christian Z. Moore, Deepti Mahajan and Richard E. Zigmond
Department of Neurosciences, School of Medicine, Case Western Reserve University, Cleveland, OH, USA

Madeline A. Howarth
Science and Engineering Program, Hathaway Brown School, Shaker Heights, OH, USA

Richard E. Zigmond
Department Neurosciences, School of Medicine, 10900 Euclid Avenue, Robbins E701, Cleveland, OH 44106-4975, USA

Dan Li, Nan Liu, Hai-Hua Zhao, Xu Zhang, Lu Liu, Liang Zhao and Hong-Peng Li
Department of Human Anatomy, College of Basic Medical Sciences, China Medical University, Shenyang, China

Hitoshi Kawano
Department of Health and Dietetics, Faculty of Health and Medical Science, Teikyo Heisei University, Tokyo 170-8445, Japan

Ran Li, Wenchao Liu, Jian Yin, Yunchang Chen, Shenquan Guo, Haiyan Fan, Xifeng Li, Xin Zhang, Xuying He and Chuanzhi Duan
Department of Neurosurgery, Zhujiang Hospital, The National Key Clinical Specialty, The Neurosurgery Institute of Guangdong Province, Guangdong Provincial Key Laboratory on Brain Function Repair and Regeneration, Southern Medical University, Guangzhou 510282, China

Aarti Narang, Fei Qiao, Carl Atkinson, Hong Zhu and Xiaofeng Yang
Department of Microbiology and Immunology, Medical University of South Carolina, 173 Ashley Ave, CRI 213, Charleston, SC 29425, USA

Liudmila Kulik and V. Michael Holers
Departments of Medicine and Immunology, University of Colorado School of Medicine, Denver, CO, USA

Stephen Tomlinson
Ralph H Johnson VA Medical Center, Charleston, SC, USA

Index

www.ingramcontent.com/pod-product-compliance
Lightning Source LLC
LaVergne TN
LVHW080656210926
848485LV00003B/384